Green and Richmond

PEDIATRIC DIAGNOSIS

Fourth Edition

Interpretation of Symptoms and Signs in Different Age Periods

MORRIS GREEN, M.D.

Perry W. Lesh Professor and Chairman, Department of
Pediatrics, Indiana University School of Medicine;
Physician-in-Chief, James Whitcomb Riley Hospital for Children,
Indianapolis, Indiana

1986   W. B. SAUNDERS COMPANY
Philadelphia, London, Toronto, Mexico City, Rio de Janeiro, Sydney, Tokyo, Hong Kong

W. B. Saunders Company: West Washington Square
                         Philadelphia, PA   19105

Library of Congress Cataloging in Publication Data

Green, Morris.

Pediatric diagnosis.

At head of title: Green and Richmond.

Includes bibliographies and index.

1. Children—Diseases—Diagnosis.   I. Richmond, Julius B.,
   (Julius Benjamin), 1916–   II. Title. [DNLM:
   1. Diagnosis—in infancy & childhood. WS 141 G797p]

RJ50.G7 1986   618.92′0075   85–11916

ISBN 0–7216–1829–4

Listed here is the latest translated edition of this book together with the
language of the translation and the publisher.

Spanish—*Third Edition*—Editorial Alhambra, S.A., Madrid, Spain

Acquisition Editor: Dana Dreibelbis
Production Manager: Frank Polizzano
Compositor: W. B. Saunders Company
Printer: W. B. Saunders Company Press

Pediatric Diagnosis   ISBN 0-7216-1829-4

Last digit is the print number: 9   8   7   6   5   4   3   2   1

In loving memory of
RHEE RICHMOND
warm, generous, and courageous friend

PREFACE

This fourth edition has been prepared to reflect recent advances in pediatric diagnosis. Written to meet a need in pediatric education and practice not fully addressed by encyclopedic textbooks of pediatrics, synopses, handbooks or the various monographs on specific diseases, organ systems and age periods, this book is based on the observation that children are brought to the doctor because of symptoms and signs or for health supervision. The clinician must be prepared to deal effectively with whatever symptom or sign that a child may present. The information and the approach utilized in this book are in the service of that expectation. I am pleased that the kind of problem-oriented approach introduced in the previous editions continues to be helpful in serving as a guide to pediatric physical examination and diagnosis for medical students, pediatric residents, pediatricians, family practitioners, pediatric nurses and allied health professionals who care for children. Health supervision is included in *Ambulatory Pediatrics*, with Robert J. Haggerty as co-editor.

Chapters added in this edition include pelvic pain, giftedness, and psychosocial symptoms such as school refusal, out-of-control toddler behavior, personality change, phobias, masturbation, lying, stealing, fire-setting, conduct disorder and psychotic behavior. The chapter on the pediatric history has been revised to include an extensive discussion of the principles of interviewing. Physical findings and symptoms in adolescents and youth are more thoroughly included in this edition. Numerous other revisions, additions and elaborations in the text enlarge its coverage and reflect new pediatric knowledge and practice.

I am indebted to all those who have contributed to my knowledge of pediatric diagnosis and who shared with me their observations and suggestions. Dr. Julius B. Richmond has, as always, been most generous with his encouragement, support and thoughtful advice. Mr. Dana Dreibelbis, Medical Editor of the W. B. Saunders Company, with whom I have worked in the preparation of this fourth edition, has been a valued advisor. Mrs. Glenna Clark, who cheerfully assisted greatly in the organization of this material and typed the manuscript through multiple drafts, deserves special commendation. I appreciate deeply her dedication and skill.

MORRIS GREEN

CONTENTS

Part One   THE PHYSICAL EXAMINATION

Part Two SIGNS AND SYMPTOMS

Part One

THE PHYSICAL EXAMINATION

1 / APPROACH TO THE PHYSICAL EXAMINATION

Besides supplying information about the status of physical findings, a comprehensive and skillful physical examination considerably reassures the patient and his family. Parents are favorably impressed by the physician who does a complete physical appraisal; less satisfied with the physician whose examination is hurried and incomplete. Once the parents are confident that the examination has been thorough, they are generally able to accept the findings. In addition, the adolescent, child and even the infant can sense the physician's expertise and tend to respond cooperatively and confidently. To fulfill this role the physician must be highly competent and self-confident. Only intensive training and practice can help the physician develop these necessary skills. A physician cannot have too much experience.

The assessment begins the moment the physician sees the child and the parents. The experienced clinician immediately begins to gather information that will make his time with the patient productive. His initial impressions help direct the subsequent interview and physical examination. They are not intended to encourage impetuous diagnoses. Instead, the experienced physician's ability to quickly assess the overall clinical picture allows him to rapidly and accurately formulate provisional diagnoses and therapeutic possibilities, and to arrive at a prognostic outlook, any or all of which may be modified or discarded upon completion of a more detailed examination, history-taking, and laboratory tests and through continuing observation. Assessment of the patient's physical and psychologic status contributes importantly to the physician's overall impression. This assessment is largely based on inspection of the patient's facies, physical development, activity, and affect and observance of the patient's, as well as his parents', behavior.

Characteristic facies or facial appearance has been described for patients with numerous disorders. A number of excellent atlases that illustrate and describe a wide variety of facies are available (see references on page 6). Coarse facies occur in the Coffin-Siris syndrome, generalized gangliosidosis, hyperimmunoglobulin recurrent infection (Job's) syndrome, hypothyroidism, Leroy I-cell syndrome, mucopolysaccharidoses, multiple neuroma syndrome, multiple sulfatase deficiency, sialic acid storage disease with sialuria, Sotos' syndrome and Williams syndrome. Expressionless or mask-like facies occur with depression, Möbius' syndrome, infantile botulism, Wilson's disease, myotonic dystrophy, facioscapulohumeral muscular dystrophy and Prader-Willi syndrome. Triangular facies is seen with the Russell-Silver's, Mulibrey nanism and Turner's syndromes.

The patient's position and activity during the assessment may be informative. Thus the child with epiglottitis is observed to be sitting up and leaning forward, not lying down; the child with peritonitis lies quietly and does not thrash about; the child with meningitis may lie on his side with the thighs flexed on the abdomen or in a position of opisthotonos; the patient with postencephalitic sequelae may demonstrate perseveration and hyperactivity. Certain clinical states that may be apparent on general assessment warrant special emphasis. These include biomedical conditions such as dehydration, malnutrition, acidosis, sepsis, respiratory failure and shock and those of a psychologic nature such as depression, anxiety or inappropriate behavior.

Throughout the assessment, a number of descriptive terms may evoke definite mental images to the experienced clinician. These include: vigorous, alert, cooperative, robust, weak, dull, exhausted, listless, lethargic, acutely ill, chronically ill, seriously ill, apprehensive, fearful, worried, complacent, writhing, comatose, delirious, malnourished, cachectic, moribund, confused, uncooperative, irritable, fretful, sad, prostrate, restless, anxious and toxic. One of the most difficult judgments for the student or young physician to make is the severity of a patient's illness. This comes with experience (e.g., the baby who is seriously ill usually cannot be made to smile).

The seasoned clinician learns to telescope these observations on the basis of experience. Because he's adept and flexible in the procedures and findings of physical diagno-

3

sis, he is able to continue the interview while examining the patient, to observe meaningfully the behavior of both parents and child, and to determine something about the interpersonal relations between parents and child and their interaction with himself.

The physician can gain his patients' cooperation by learning and anticipating the reactions and responses characteristic of various age groups and through insight into each patient's emotional development. The physician who is confident, enjoys children and is patient with them will find physical examination productive and pleasant. The physician who is hurried, annoyed, disinterested or impersonal may find his experiences frustrating and unrewarding.

To help assure a positive experience for everyone involved, the physician should maintain a friendly, warm, seemingly unhurried and informal attitude throughout the assessment. Before beginning the direct examination, the physician should spend a few moments talking to the parents or becoming acquainted with the child, perhaps by admiring her bracelet or shoes or allowing the child to hold or play with a ball or other small toy. These gestures often prove time-saving in the long-run. The physician should address children by their names. If the child is reticent, appears frightened or is irritable, the physician should take a more impersonal attitude and conduct the examination as rapidly as possible. Sometimes whispering "secrets" into a young child's ear and encouraging him to whisper back or saying, "You know, I like you," may place the child at ease. The physician's adaptability to the individual situation will determine to a considerable extent his ability to establish a good patient relationship. Children usually respond positively to persons whom they sense like them.

The physical examination can also be an important psychotherapeutic tool. Because it facilitates questions about bodily concerns, the interview can continue in such a way as to reassure adolescents about their normalcy and to teach them about their bodies. The physician should encourage dialogue with a statement such as: "As we go through the examination, this is a convenient time to bring up questions that you may have about your body and its changes— things that you sometimes wonder about." Rather than wait until the physical examination is complete, the adolescent should receive appropriate reassurance as the examination proceeds. For example: "Your heart is fine. Your blood pressure is normal.

Your breasts are normal, etc." Abnormalities, if detected, e.g., scoliosis, should be presented matter-of-factly along with an explanation of what can be done to correct them.

Patients should be completely undressed for each examination. Room temperature should, of course, be comfortable. Adolescents and some younger children wish to be treated with the same attention to privacy as adults, if not more so. Appropriate gowns should be provided for the child and adolescent. When a pelvic examination is indicated, careful attention should be given to draping the adolescent girl. A nurse or the mother should be present during the examination. Sometimes a young child will object to being undressed in the physician's presence; hence, the patient should be given time to undress before the physician enters the room. If the child objects to removing all his clothes at once, the physician might remove the child's clothing gradually, a piece at a time, as the examination proceeds and the child's anxiety lessens.

The physical examination should be conditioned by the patient's age. The physician specifically looks for physical findings that characterize the child's particular age group. The order of the examination also varies according to the patient's age. With older children, the physician may begin with the head, then proceed to the chest, and so on. In infants and younger children, however, the order of the examination is adapted to the individual situation. An infant's routine developmental examination should be woven into the physical examination. Questions about developmental achievements may be most naturally asked at this time.

Since children tend to tire readily and are less cooperative when tired, the physical examination should not require much time. In making requests during the examination, it is sometimes best to make positive statements such as, "Open your mouth, Johnny," rather than "Will you open your mouth for me?" The latter may be an open invitation to negativism.

In general, infants are not apprehensive until seven or eight months of age. The baby who as early as the fourth month seems to recognize that the physician is a stranger and to manifest resistance when approached is rare. Actually, most infants eight months and under enjoy the examination period and smile or babble in response to the physician. After this period, however, infants often show apprehension, poor cooperation and, occasionally, even terror. At this age, if the child appears timid or about to cry, the physician should begin the examination with the parent holding the child. If necessary, the physician should complete the examination in this manner, or with the child lying across the parent's lap. Often the physician can examine the child's ears most easily if the child sits on his parent's lap. The parent holds the child's head against her shoulder with one hand, keeping the other available to restrain his free arm, if necessary.

If the child appears friendly and not frightened, the parent or nurse may place him on the examining table and the physician can begin the examination. Most children feel more secure if they sit or stand during the examination, rather than lie supine. So the physician should complete as much of the examination as possible with the patient in these positions. Infants who have just learned to sit up may especially object to being placed supine. Such resistance may be avoided if the parent or the nurse, rather than the physician, lays the infant down. If two children in a family are to be examined, the one less likely to cry should be examined first. The physician should avoid looking directly at the infant or young child who is about to cry. In these instances the physician is wise to begin the examination by auscultating the back of the child's chest while the child looks the other way.

Negativism and resistance to examination in young children are normal maturational events. Although such situations may be infrequent, they inevitably occur, no matter how the physician approaches the examination. The physician may quiet a highly active child by talking to him slowly and quietly and rubbing his back.

If the child struggles when the physician begins to remove his clothes or to examine him, and a complete examination is not imperative at the time, it may be wise to continue the examination at a later date when the child is more willing to cooperate. With anxious children, a number of brief "social" visits may be necessary before much progress occurs. At these times the child should be greeted in a gentle, friendly manner and given a balloon or tongue depressor. In unusual instances, of course, the physician may wish to determine why the child demonstrates such excessive anxiety and unusual resistance. As the parents observe that the physician proceeds with understanding and kindness, even though the child is uncooperative and irritable, they may undertake to mention their child-rearing difficulties. This is especially true with the parents of a patient who is retarded or has congenital anomalies. The fact that the doctor holds and talks to the baby seems to convey that he accepts the baby. And his actions serve as powerful, positive nonverbal communication.

The physician should always wash and warm his hands before the examination, then wash them again when the examination is complete. Parents watch for this practice, and young children are sometimes intrigued by the soap dispenser. The stethoscope bell or diaphragm should also be warm and clean. It is sometimes well to allow children to become familiar with the diagnostic instruments before they are used. They may carefully scrutinize the stethoscope or try to listen with it.

Before using the otoscope, the physician may ask the child to try to blow out the light, as the physician flips the switch on and off at the appropriate time. Younger children sometimes enjoy this. Before darkening the room for the ophthalmoscopic examination, the physician should tell the child that the light will be turned out for a moment.

A pacifier may promote cooperation in small infants during the eye examination and may quiet a crying baby during the abdominal examination. Infants and young children who grab for the stethoscope or otoscope when the physician is using them, can be distracted by giving them a tongue depressor for each hand.

He can also distract the child, especially during the abdominal examination by talking quietly with him about his pets, school, home or siblings. Some children cooperate well until the examination of the ears, nose and mouth; hence, these often are best left until last. The physician can allay apprehension by acting as though this portion of the examination were a game. At best, however, examinations of the ears, nose and throat are not pleasant. So the physician should perform them quickly and with minimal discomfort. Before examining the throat, he may ask to see the patient's teeth. He can then introduce a tongue depressor, and after examining the patient's teeth say, "Let's look way back there. This will just take a second, then we'll be all through."

It is important to inform the child in an understandable way what he should expect before performing any painful or unfamiliar procedure, such as a throat swab, blood pressure determination, lumbar puncture, venipuncture or intradermal test. The physician should also answer the child's questions truthfully. If the procedure will be painful, the child should be told that it will hurt somewhat. Likening a procedure such as an intradermal injection to some familiar sensation, such as a mosquito bite, may be helpful. When necessary, the physician should apply manual restraint effectively and with dispatch and complete the procedure promptly, evoking as little anxiety as possible. He should tell the child that the restraint is just to hold still until the procedure is completed, after which he will be released. Children often repeatedly ask, "All done?" as the physical examination or procedure nears completion. The physician may say "Almost" or have the child count slowly with him until he is finished, at which time he can announce "All done!" If a child cries because of anxiety or in response to pain, he should, of course, not be made to feel inadequate or that he must be the Stoic implied by the statement, "Big boys don't cry."

GENERAL REFERENCES

Bergsma, D.: Birth Defects Compendium. 2nd ed. New York, Alan R. Liss, Inc., 1979.
Gellis, S., and Feingold, M.: Atlas of Mental Retardation Syndromes—Visual Diagnosis of Facies and Physical Findings. Washington, D.C., U.S. Government Printing Office, 1968.
Goodman, R. M., and Gorlin, R. J.: Atlas of the Face in Genetic Disorders. St. Louis, C. V. Mosby Co., 1977.
Gorlin, R. J., Pindborg, J. J., and Cohen, M. M., Jr.: Syndromes of the Head and Neck. 2nd ed. New York, McGraw-Hill Book Co., 1976.
Hatzilevich, B.: Mental Retardation: An Atlas of Diseases with Associated Physical Abnormalities. New York, The Macmillan Co., 1972.
McKusick, V. A.: Heritable Disorders of Connective Tissue. 4th ed. St. Louis, C. V. Mosby Co., 1972.
Smith, D. W.: Recognizable Patterns of Human Malformation. Philadelphia, W. B. Saunders Co., 1976.
Warkany, J.: Congenital Malformations. 2nd ed. Chicago, Year Book Medical Publishers, Inc., 1971.

2 / THE HEAD

HEAD CONTROL

A young infant's head control is an early indication of motor development. When he is raised to a sitting position during the first month of life, the infant's head lags and remains overextended. In the sitting position, the head falls forward, with perhaps an occasional erect bob. In the supine position the infant lies with his head to one side, occasionally raising the side of his face. In the prone position, most newborn infants can transiently raise their heads slightly so that their chin just clears the surface. The head, however, cannot be maintained in the midline.

The *asymmetric tonic neck reflex (TNR)* describes the infant's posture. With TNR the infant's head is turned to one side, the ipsilateral arm is extended and the contralateral arm is flexed. The TNR appears between two weeks and two months of age and disappears normally between four and six months of age.

By the end of the second month, the infant can maintain his head in the midline for a short time in the prone position and intermittently raise it 2 or 3 inches. Toward the end of the third month, the infant, when held in a sitting position, begins to hold his head erect, though wobbly and unsteadily. By four months of age, he steadily holds his head forward in the sitting position; however, if his head is rotated much, control may disappear. During the fifth month, the head position is not disturbed by sudden rotation.

Failure to achieve head control by four months, persistence of the tonic neck attitude after six months or presence of an obligatory TNR are indications of neuromotor retardation and may be the earliest clinical manifestation of cerebral palsy, other neurologic deficit or mental retardation. Loss of head control may occur in infantile botulism.

CIRCUMFERENCE (Figs. 2–1 and 2–2)

During infancy, the head should be routinely measured at its maximum occipitofrontal circumference. In the term infant, head circumference is usually about 2 cm

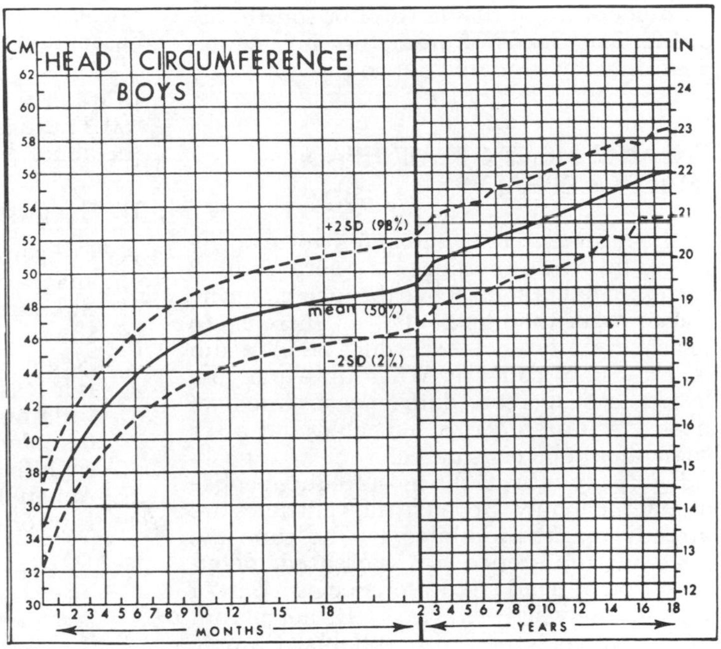

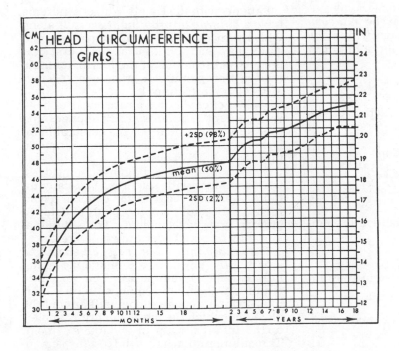

FIGURE 2–1. Composite graph for males from birth through 18 years. (From Nellhaus, G.: Head circumference from birth to 18 years: Practical composite international and interracial graphs. Pediatrics 41:106, 1968.)

FIGURE 2–2. Composite graph for females from birth through 18 years. (From Nellhaus, G.: Head circumference from birth to eighteen years: Practical composite international and interracial graphs. Pediatrics 41:106, 1968.)

greater than that of the chest. In the premature infant the difference is even greater. If scalp edema or cranial molding is present, measurement of head circumference may be inaccurate until the third or fourth day of life. The heads of premature infants appear disproportionately large.

ENLARGEMENT OF THE HEAD (MACROCEPHALY)

The term *macrocephaly* refers to an occipitofrontal circumference of more than 3 standard deviations above the mean. During the first six months of life, an increase in head circumference exceeding 2 cm/month is a cause of concern. When an expanding lesion is suspected, daily measurement of head circumference is indicated and a CT scan should be considered.

Hydrocephalus is the most frequent cause of macrocephaly. Because the ventricles are already markedly dilated by the time the head circumference has increased, determination of head circumference as a part of well-infant visits will, in itself, not permit early diagnosis of hydrocephalus. Chronic cerebrospinal fluid shunt insufficiency, for example, may cause head circumference to enlarge only slightly beyond the normal rate. For this reason careful attention needs to be routinely given to the fontanels, sutures, skin texture, eye movement, symptoms and to the use of ultrasonography.

Hydrocephalus, which may be *noncommunicating* owing to blockage within the ventricular system or at the foramina, may be caused by the following:

I. CONGENITAL ANOMALIES

A. Atresia, stenosis or obstruction of the aqueduct of Sylvius or foramina of Luschka and Magendie
B. Arnold-Chiari malformation
C. Platybasia
D. Achondroplasia
E. Dandy-Walker syndrome

II. TRAUMA, owing to organization of hemorrhage

III. POSTHEMORRHAGIC HYDROCEPHALUS largely in the preterm but also in the full-term infant

IV. NEOPLASMS, such as tumors and cysts

V. INFLAMMATORY

A. Brain abscess

B. Complication of meningitis
C. Late-onset Group B neonatal streptococcal infection

Communicating hydrocephalus may be associated with

I. INCREASED PRODUCTION OF CEREBROSPINAL FLUID, e.g., hypertrophy or papilloma of the choroid plexus

II. DECREASED ABSORPTION

A. Congenital failure of subarachnoid space formation
B. Subdural and subarachnoid hemorrhage
C. Neoplasms, such as gliomatosis, posterior fossa tumors
D. Inflammatory: bacterial, including tuberculosis; toxoplasmosis; congenital syphilis
E. Achondroplasia
F. Intracranial arteriovenous fistula

Chaplin, E. R., Goldstein, G. W., Myerberg, D. Z., Hunt, J. V., and Tooley, W. H.: Posthemorrhagic hydrocephalus in the preterm infant. Pediatrics 65:901, 1980.
Hill, A., and Volpe, J. J.: Normal pressure hydrocephalus in the newborn. Pediatrics 68:623, 1981.
Raimondi, A. J.: A critical analysis of the clinical diagnosis, management and prognosis of the hydrocephalic child. Adv. Pediatr. 18:265, 1971.

Patients with the Dandy-Walker syndrome have a *bulging or prominent occiput* along with hydrocephalus. A suboccipital dermal sinus may lead to an intracranial cyst that produces obstruction of the fourth ventricle and hydrocephalus. A prominent occiput also occurs in trisomy 18.

Hydranencephaly is a rare cause of head enlargement in infants. The meninges and the skull are normal, but the cerebral hemispheres are not developed. Transillumination of the head is positive.

Porencephaly is a diagnostic consideration in infants with seizures, especially infantile spasms, focal motor deficits, asymmetry of the skull, macrocephaly or delay in growth and development. Transillumination may be noted over the cystic area.

Transillumination of the skull should be a part of the physical examination of young infants under 1 year of age. The procedure requires a flashlight equipped with a narrow, opaque, sponge rubber cuff around the glass end which the physician firmly applies to the infant's scalp in a darkened room. Transillumination is an important screening procedure in infants with macrocephaly, and those suspected of having a subdural effusion, subdural hematoma, hydrocephalus, hydranencephaly, porencephaly or increased intracranial pressure. Translucency that extends beyond 2 to 2.5 cm in the frontal area or over 1 cm in the occipital region may be abnormal. Subdural effusions may cause increased transillumination in the fronto-parietal area. Suboccipital transillumination may suggest dilatation of the fourth ventricle as in the Dandy-Walker malformation. Transillumination is impaired by the presence of a caput succedaneum, cephalohematoma, scalp edema, infiltration of scalp vein infusions, thick black hair and the examiner's lack of dark adaptation. Transillumination in hydrocephalus and porencephaly will not occur if the cortex is thicker than 1 cm.

Sjogren, I., and Engsner, G.: Transillumination of the skull in infants and children. Acta Paediatr. Scand. 61:426, 1972.
Swick, H. M., Cunningham, M. D., and Shield, L. K.: Transillumination of the skull in premature infants. Pediatrics 58:658, 1976.

Subdural hematoma may cause head enlargement with or without hydrocephalus. A posterior fossa subdural hematoma, which rarely occurs in newborns, causes lethargy, irritability, tense anterior fontanel, head enlargement, respiratory difficulty, and bloody cerebrospinal fluid.

Serfontein, G. L., Rom, S., and Stein, S.: Posterior fossa subdural hemorrhage in the newborn. Pediatrics 65:40, 1980.

Subdural effusions may complicate bacterial meningitis.

Cerebral arachnoid cysts in young infants produce signs that may suggest a subdural hematoma or hydrocephalus (e.g., excessive size or growth of the head, tense fontanels, suture width, localized bulging of the skull and transilluminability.)

A rapid increase in head circumference may be the first clinical manifestation of an *intracranial tumor* in infants and young children.

Thickening of the skull may be noted in osteopetrosis, osteogenesis imperfecta, orodigitofacial dysostosis, craniometaphyseal dysplasia, epiphyseal dysplasia, pyknodysostosis, leontiasis ossea and progressive diaphyseal dysplasia.

Megalocephaly or macrocephaly may reflect brain growth at the upper limits of normal or a benign familial pattern with one parent and often a sibling also found to have a large head. A large head is also a physical finding in cerebral gigantism, fragile X syndrome, achondroplasia, the mucopolysaccharidoses, generalized gangliosidosis, neurofibromatosis, Klippel-Trenaunay-Weber syndrome, cutis marmorata telangiectatica congenita, and the Weaver syndrome. Macrocephaly occurs along with lipomas and hemangiomas in the Bannayan syndrome. Macrocephaly, osteopathia striata and cranial sclerosis constitute an autosomal dominant malformation syndrome.

Higginbottom, M. C., and Schultz, P.: The Bannayan syndrome: An autosomal dominant disorder consisting of macrocephaly, lipomas, hemangiomas and risk for intracranial tumors. Pediatrics 69:632, 1982.
Robinow, M., and Unger, F.: Syndrome of osteopathia striata, macrocephaly, and cranial sclerosis. Am. J. Dis. Child. 138:821, 1984.

Caravan's disease (spongy degeneration of the central nervous system) is an autosomal recessive disorder in Ashkenazi Jews. The disease is characterized by megalocephaly in early infancy, developmental slowing and regression, hypotonia and an opisthotonic response to auditory, visual and tactile stimuli. *Alexander's disease* is also characterized by head enlargement owing to obstruction of the aqueduct of Sylvius, mental retardation, spasticity and seizures.

Day, R. E., and Schutt, W. H.: Normal children with large heads—benign familial megalencephaly. Arch. Dis. Child. 54:512, 1979.
DeMyer, W.: Megalencephaly in children. Neurology 22:634, 1972.
Lorber, J., and Priestley, B. L.: Children with large heads: A practical approach to diagnosis in 557 children, with special reference to 109 children with megalencephaly. Dev. Med. Child Neurol. 23:494, 1981.

The *Russell dwarf* has a pseudohydrocephalus, that is, a normal-sized head with a dwarfed face and body.

Mulibrey nanism is characterized by pseudohydrocephalus, triangular facies, failure to thrive, prominent veins on the forehead and neck, muscular hypotonia, hepatomegaly, yellow dots on the fundi and constrictive pericarditis.

MICROCEPHALY

Microcephaly is characterized by a head circumference of more than three standard deviations below the mean for age, sex, height and weight.

Cerebral dysgenesis or hypoplasia is often accompanied by microcephaly, since failure of brain growth provides a diminished stimulus for skull enlargement. At birth the brain has normally achieved about 25 per cent of its adult volume; at 1 year of age, about 75 per cent. *Primary* or *familial microcephaly,* an autosomal recessive or dominant disorder, is characterized by a low crown, receding forehead, occiput flattening and, perhaps, skin wrinkling. Sex-linked microcephaly may be associated with spastic diplegia. *Secondary microcephaly* occurs as a result of trauma, radiation, or central nervous system disorders and infections. Microcephaly also occurs with the following syndromes: incontinentia pigmenti, cat-cry, Cockayne's, Smith-Lemli-Opitz, Wolf-Hirschhorn, Rothmund-Thomson, fetal alcohol, fetal hydantoin and trisomy 13. The Miller-Dieker syndrome (lissencephaly) is characterized by bitemporal grooving of a high, narrow forehead, microcephaly, ptosis, micrognathia, and striking hypotonia.

Jones, K. L., Gilbert, E. F., Kaveggia, E. G., and Opitz, J. M.: The Miller-Dieker syndrome. Pediatrics 66:277, 1980.

Congenital viral infections (e.g., cytomegalovirus, rubella and toxoplasmosis) may cause microcephaly, which may be present at birth or evident toward the end of the child's first year of life. Microcephaly also occurs in fetal drug syndromes.

Haslam, R. H., and Smith, D. W.: Autosomal dominant microcephaly. J. Pediatr. 95:701, 1979.
Smith, D. W.: Fetal drug syndromes: Effects of ethanol and hydantoins. Pediatr. Rev. 1:165, 1979.

Premature synostosis of the sutures or *craniosynostosis* may cause microcephaly or asymmetry of the head.

Infants with *Down's syndrome* usually have a small, brachycephalic head.

Avery, G. B., Meneses, L., and Lodge, A.: The clinical significance of "measurement microcephaly." Am. J. Dis. Child. 123:214, 1972.
Martin, H. P.: Microcephaly and mental retardation. Am. J. Dis. Child. 119:128, 1970.

SKULL DEFECTS

Craniotabes refers to thin, parchment-like, soft, mushy areas which can be indented like a ping-pong ball. These areas are most commonly present along suture lines and in the parietal bones at the vertex. Craniotabes may be physiologic up to three months of age. Rickets, hydrocephalus, syphilis, osteogenesis imperfecta or hypervitaminosis A may also be accompanied by craniotabes. A soft skull occurs in premature infants with hypophosphatasia.

Lacunar skull is characterized by thin areas in the skull owing to defective formation of the diploe and inner tables. These lesions resemble craniotabes on palpation. *Craniofenestria,* a defect caused by a localized absence of membranous bone in the skull, is accompanied, at times, by herniation of cranial contents. Lacunar skull and craniofenestria usually occur in the parietal bones. Spina bifida is often an accompanying defect.

Enlarged *parietal foramina,* in which bilateral, sharply demarcated, and irregular depressions are found in the posterior portion of the parietal bones along the sagittal sutures, may be large enough to admit the tip of a finger.

Small, localized, rounded *depressions* sometimes seen in the frontal and parietal bones at birth are presumably secondary to abnormal intrauterine pressure associated with unusual fetal posture. These defects disappear during the neonatal period.

Meningoceles or *encephaloceles* are rounded, compressible, usually midline tumors. They may also present through a suture line or bony defect elsewhere. *Meckel syndrome,* an autosomal recessive disorder, consists of an occipital encephalocele, polydactyly and polycystic kidneys among other anomalies.

Delayed cranial ossification, large fontanels, widely-open suture lines and frontal, parietal and occipital bossing may occur with *cleidocranial dysostosis.* Cranial findings may not be accompanied by abnormality of the clavicles.

ASYMMETRY OF THE HEAD OR FACE

Molding of the skull with some overlapping of the bones during birth commonly causes temporary asymmetry. Normal head shape is largely regained by the end of the first week. Molding is not present in infants born by caesarean section or breech extraction.

Facial asymmetry may result from abnormal intrauterine pressure. A rounded depression may be present under the angle of the jaw on the involved side. Occasionally, this concavity may occur further anteriorly or extend posteriorly to the ear. When the lips are separated, the alveolar processes on the involved side are noted to touch, while those on the contralateral side do not. Usually the asymmetry is minimal and gradually disappears. Infants with breech or face presentations may demonstrate transient facial asymmetry owing to mandible displacement.

Plagiocephaly or a rhomboid head shape may also occur in newborns owing to intrauterine constraint (position of comfort) or may develop over months in infants with congenital torticollis.

Cranial changes associated with *familial metaphysial dysplasia* include diffuse symmetrical hyperostosis of the skull and mandible, hypertelorism and cranial nerve palsies.

Bumps on the head may be noted with *myositis ossificans progressiva.*

Fibrous dysplasia of the facial bones is characterized by a firm, painless bone swelling with considerable asymmetry and deformity of facial structures. The bones most commonly involved include the maxilla, zygoma, mandible and calvarium. The orbits and teeth may be displaced.

Infants who lie predominantly in one position may develop *flattening of the occiput.* During the latter half of the first year such flattening suggests that the infant is not held often or that he is retarded. A high association exists between head flattening and brain maldevelopment. Infants who are very hypotonic may also develop asymmetry of the head if permitted to always lie in the same position. Infants with hydrocephalus are also prone to occipital flattening.

An asymmetrical skull enlargement may suggest a cystic lesion on the enlarged side or an atrophic or malformed cerebral hemisphere on the smaller side. But an etiologic diagnosis cannot be established by inspection. Such asymmetry may be especially evident when looking down from above at the top of the infant's head.

Facial asymmetry may also occur in children with premature synostosis of the cranial sutures.

Hemifacial atrophy (Romber's syndrome) is characterized by progressive atrophy of the skin and underlying tissues. It quickly affects the temporal and buccinator muscles, then extends to involve one entire side of the face. Skin pigmentation, seizures and trigeminal neuralgia may also occur.

FONTANELS

Because overriding of the sutures may be present immediately after the newborn's delivery, the anterior fontanel may appear barely open. A few days later, after normal separation of the sutures, the anterior fontanel has an average diameter of about 2.5 cm and in some infants the diameter may be as much as 4 to 5 cm. The anterior fontanel may normally enlarge somewhat in the first months of life. The posterior fontanel may remain palpable for four to eight weeks.

Variability in the shape, size and time of closure of the anterior fontanel ranges widely. Closure usually occurs between 4 and 26 months of age. Ninety per cent close between the ages of 7 and 19 months; 2.7 per cent by 6 months; 13.5 per cent by 9 months; and 41.6 per cent by the end of the first year. If head growth is proceeding normally and no suture ridging has occurred, early closure of the fontanel should cause no concern. In premature and other infants with delayed ossification of the membranous bones, the anterior fontanel may be large, and the sagittal suture may extend almost to the base of the nose. The slight depression which may be present for a time after the anterior fontanel closes is not to be confused with a sunken or open fontanel.

Delayed closure or a large open anterior fontanel is seen in rickets, hydrocephalus, syphilis, congenital hypothyroidism, osteogenesis imperfecta, Down's syndrome, cleidocranial dysostosis, mucopolysaccharidoses, achondroplasia, Alpert's syndrome, hypophosphatasia, pyknodysostosis, Hallermann-Streiff syndrome, malnutrition, progeria, congenital rubella, Russell-Silver's syndrome, trisomy 13, trisomy 18 and the syndromes of cutis laxa, ligamentous laxity and delayed development.

Popich, G. A., and Smith, D. W.: Fontanels: Range of normal size. J. Pediatr. 80:749, 1972.

An unusually *small fontanel* may occur in infants with slow brain growth and with craniosynostosis.

Though a slight depression of the fontanel is often present in normal infants, a *sunken fontanel* is an important sign of dehydration in infants who have experienced a 10 per cent body weight loss.

On palpation, the anterior fontanel is slightly depressed relative to the frontal and parietal bones. With crying the fontanel bulges, but remains pulsatile. Such normal fullness should be differentiated from true bulging, a sign of great clinical importance. Pulsation of the anterior fontanel occurs in normal infants held upright. In the hydrocephalic infant the anterior fontanel is usually not visibly pulsatile and almost always bulges.

In the neonatal period, bulging of the anterior fontanel may be associated with intraventricular hemorrhage.

Mitchell, W., and O'Tuama, L.: Cerebral intraventricular hemorrhages in infants: A widening age spectrum. Pediatrics 65:35, 1980.

A bulging fontanel in an infant should always suggest meningitis and may be the only early physical indication of that disorder. This finding also occurs with a subdural hematoma, including bleeding secondary to whiplash, shaking abuse, intracranial tumors, other space-occupying lesions and obstruction of a cerebrospinal fluid shunt. Bulging is also noted with maple syrup urine disease, vitamin A poisoning, vitamin D–dependent rickets, hypophosphatasia and pseudohypophosphatasia. A bulging fontanel and jaundice in a young infant suggests the possibility of galactosemia. Transient, unexplained, benign bulging of the fontanel may also occur in some normal infants and rarely with roseola infantum.

Huttenlocher, P. R., Hillman, R. E., and Hsia, Y. E.: Pseudotumor cerebri in galactosemia. J. Pediatr. 76:902, 1970.

SUTURES

Sutures are fibrous septa between the cranial membranous bones. After spontaneous correction of the overlap of these bones, which may occur in the newborn infant, the sutures may be as much as one fourth inch in width. Although suture lines are normally not palpable after the fifth or sixth month, final closure does not occur until early adult life. The metopic suture is an exception in that it fuses in the early neonatal period.

During infancy, cranial bones grow predominantly at their borders. Interference with such growth, as occurs with premature suture synostosis, seriously hampers normal enlargement of the cranial vault. If the sutures close during the first two years of life, brain compression and blindness follow unless decompression is accomplished early. Craniostenosis may occur in some infants with the severe form of idiopathic hypercalcemia, phenylketonuria, hypophosphatasia, rickets and thyrotoxicosis.

Johnsonbaugh, R. E., Bryan, R. N., Hierlwimmer, U. R., and Georges, L. P.: Premature craniosynostosis: A common complication of juvenile thyrotoxicosis. J. Pediatr. 93:188, 1978.

Premature synostosis of the sutures or craniosynostosis may lead to cranial distortions. A palpable ridge along a suture line occurs in premature metopic closures, most sagittal closures and some unilateral or bilateral coronal closures. A ridge may also be present along the sagittal and metopic sutures in normal infants. The metopic suture is prominent in infants with the fetal hydantoin syndrome.

Cranial growth in the anterior-posterior plane is compromised with craniosynostosis of the coronal suture. But growth continues along the sagittal and, sometimes, the lambdoidal sutures. The result is widening of the head, shortening of the anteroposterior diameter and, at times, a smaller than normal circumference. Other congenital anomalies, especially choanal atresia, are often present. With synostosis of the coronal, lambdoidal and sagittal sutures, growth occurs only in the region of the anterior fontanel, resulting in a rounded pointing of the skull (oxycephaly, acrocephaly or tower skull). Unilateral synostosis of the coronal suture produces cranial asymmetry (plagiocephaly). With craniosynostosis of the sagittal suture, continued growth at the coronal and lambdoidal sutures leads to an elongated, narrow head (dolichocephaly) which may be ridged (scaphocephaly) and may simulate an inverted boat. (A dolichocephalic head also occurs with cerebral gigantism.) Premature or prenatal closure of the metopic suture between the frontal bones produces a prominent mid-keel forehead (trigonocephaly). While such closure usually occurs alone, it may be associated with arhinencephaly. The anterior fontanel may be open even with premature closure of the metopic, sagittal or coronal sutures.

Cranial dysostosis, or *Crouzon's disease,* is characterized by oxycephaly, exophthalmos, exotropia, optic atrophy, a beak-shaped nose and protrusion of the mandible. The Saethre-Chotzen syndrome is comprised of brachycephaly or acrocephaly, broad forehead, ptosis of eyelids, beaked nose, brachydactyly and cutaneous syndactyly.

Friedman, J. M., Hanson, J. W., Graham, C. B., and Smith, D. W.: Saethre-Chotzen syndrome: A broad and variable pattern of skeletal malformations. J. Pediatr. 91:929, 1977.

Carpenter's syndrome is characterized by acrocephaly, brachysyndactyly of the fingers, polydactyly and syndactyly of the toes and mental retardation.

Pfeiffer's syndrome is characterized by premature closure of various sutures, usually the coronal; downward slanting palpebral fissures; short nose; short fingers with hypoplasia or absence of the middle phalanges; and thumbs that are broad and radially deviated.

Alpert's syndrome is characterized by flattening of the occiput and prominence of the forehead owing to premature closure of the coronal sutures. Hypertelorism and ocular proptosis may also be noted. Marked syndactyly results in a "mitten" hand or "sock" foot.

Stewart, R. E.: Craniofacial malformations. Clinical and genetic considerations. Pediatr. Clin. North Am. 25:485, 1978.

Separation or widening of the sutures. Because the sutures are not fused in infants and children, enlargement of the head owing to hydrocephalus or space-occupying lesions may readily occur. Abnormal separation of the sutures can sometimes be detected by palpation. In infants with hydrocephalus, the splitting of the sutures occurs in the following sequence: first, the superior portion of the coronal sutures; then the sagittal suture from the anterior to the posterior fontanel; and, finally, the lambdoidal sutures. With such spontaneous decompression, other signs of increased intracranial pressure either disappear or are delayed. Separation of the sutures is frequent in patients with subtentorial tumors. In *cleidocranial* dysostosis, the sutures are wide and contain numerous wormian bones.

OTHER CRANIAL FINDINGS

Cranial *bossing,* characterized by rounded prominences in the center of the parietal and frontal bones, may occur in infants as an early manifestation of rickets. Bossing may also occur with congenital syphilis, cleidocranial dysostosis, pyknodysostosis, fetal face syndrome, generalized gangliosidosis Type I, Lowe's syndrome, hypohidrotic ectodermal dysplasia, thalassemia and 10p depletion syndrome.

A *prominent forehead* is seen in patients with chondrodystrophy, mucopolysaccharidoses, craniofacial dysostosis, Laron's dwarfism, congenital ectodermal dysplasia and the following syndromes: Goldenhar, Ehlers-Danlos, Williams, nevoid basal cell carcinoma, frontodigital, Pfeiffer's, Sotos, Alagille and Larsen's.

Osteomas may rarely arise in the membranous skull. Small cartilaginous exostoses may appear at the base of the skull. Ectopic cartilage may also cause a parietal protuberance between the mastoid process and the occiput.

Nodding of the head once or twice a second, either up and down or side to side, along with nystagmus, occurs with *spasmus nutans.* Nodding may be greater in the sitting than the supine position. In older children transient periods of head nodding or drooping may be a manifestation of petit mal epilepsy. Head nodding may also occur in infants with ocular albinism. Poor head control, nodding and cog-wheel nystagmus occurs in *Pelizaeus-Merzbacher disease.* Head banging, head nodding and other periodic movements may occur in emotionally deprived and retarded infants and in some normal children.

Head bobbing in infants that is synchronous with breathing may be a sign of respiratory distress and an indication of the infant's use of the accessory muscles of inspiration. The infant's head, supported by his mother's forearm, bobs forward with each inspiration. *The bobble-head doll syndrome,* characterized by an unusual to-and-fro tremor of the head and trunk occurs in patients with hydrocephalus secondary to a lesion in the third ventricle region. The rhythmic oscillation occurs from side-to-side or up-and-down and is similar to the continuous bobbing seen in dolls with weighted heads set on a coiled spring. The head bobbling does not occur during sleep and can be stopped voluntarily.

Russman, B. S., Tucker, S. H., and Schut, L.: Slow tremor and macrocephaly: Expanded version of the bobble-head doll syndrome. J. Pediatr. 87:63, 1975.

Tilting of the head to one side may be an early sign of herniation of cerebellar tonsils secondary to increased intracranial pressure. Head tilt, neck stiffness and headaches may be caused by basilar impression of the skull.

Head banging or *head rolling* may be associated with environmental stresses, deprivation, mental retardation and autism. It may occasionally occur in normal children.

Auscultation over the orbits and skull is indicated when an intracranial aneurysm is suspected. An *intracranial bruit* occurs in 10 to 15 per cent of normal children, especially in the temporal area. Such bruits are rare, however, in infants under four months of age. Infants and young children with purulent meningitis have cranial bruits that may persist for one to four days after initial treatment. Recurrence of a bruit on the third to sixth day in a child with meningitis suggests a subdural effusion. Other conditions associated with bruits include fever, increased intracranial pressure, anemia, thyrotoxicosis and loud cardiac murmurs.

Cohen, M., and Levin, S. E.: Significance of intracranial bruits in neonates, infants, and young children. Arch. Dis. Child. 53:592, 1978.

Macewen's sign, a "cracked-pot" sound on percussion of the skull, may be present with hydrocephalus, increased intracranial pressure or suture spreading. It is also simulated in many normal infants.

Osteomyelitis of the frontal bone is characterized by local pain, increasing edema, especially of the upper eyelid on the involved side, and systemic toxicity.

HEAD INJURIES

Head injuries are also discussed on page 335.

The internal table of the infant's skull is largely absent at birth except frontally in the region of the sinuses. The remainder of the inner table develops during the child's first two years. Because of this, *skull fractures* in infants are usually linear, not comminuted, and do not produce depressions of the inner table, as in older children. Linear fractures in the infant or young child may be caused by physical abuse. Depressed skull fractures ("ping-pong ball") in infants involve only the external table.

During cranial growth, osseous remolding occurs with bony resorption in the center of the frontal, parietal and occipital bones. The dural attachments in these areas are relatively weak, and potential spaces exist for an *extradural hematoma*. If the ruptured vessel responsible for an extradural hematoma is not large, and if the child's skull can expand to some extent, a latent period may occur before symptoms or signs of increased intracranial pressure appear. The child's neurologic status may then rapidly deteriorate. Epidural hematomas, which may be caused by a fall from a high chair, are frequently associated with mildly depressed skull fractures; on the other hand, no fracture may be detected. Local swelling of the scalp is the most common finding, followed by hemiparesis and stupor. Persistent restlessness, irritability or pallor in a young child after a closed head injury are causes for concern.

Cephalohematoma is caused by a subperiosteal collection of blood over one or more of the flat bones of the skull secondary to separation of the periosteum from the underlying bone. Since the periosteum is bound down at the edges of these bones, the swelling, unlike that of caput succedaneum, is limited by the edges of the affected bone and, therefore, does not cross suture lines. At birth, a developing hematoma obscured by an overlying caput succedaneum may not be apparent until the second day with maximal size usually reached by the third day. Cephalohematomas are usually unilateral, but may be bilateral. The parietal bone is most commonly affected, but the occipital bone may also be involved. The swelling usually disappears by the third or sixth week. Because the elevated periosteum may rapidly produce new bone around the edge of the hematoma and, occasionally, over the clot, eggshell crepitation over the area may be noted after a few weeks. A peripheral ridge or parietal bossing may persist for months. An underlying skull fracture may be present, especially with bilateral cephalohematomas in newborn infants. Skull roentgenograms should be obtained four to six weeks and three to four months after a skull fracture in children under the age of three. If the fracture line has widened, a leptomeningeal cyst ("growing skull fracture") is a diagnostic possibility.

Rothman, L., Rose, J. S., Laster, D. W., and Tenner, M.: The spectrum of growing skull fracture in children. Pediatrics 57:26, 1976.

SCALP

Scalp hair is discussed on pages 15 to 17.

A *scalp abscess* at the site of electrode application may occur secondary to intrapartum, internal, fetal heart rate monitoring.

Caput succedaneum is a diffuse, soft, boggy swelling of the scalp which usually disappears by the end of the first day or two. Ecchymoses and petechial hemorrhages may be present over the involved area.

In infants with *hydrocephalus*, the skin of the scalp is thin and shiny.

Seborrheic dermatitis or cradle cap in infants may cause adherent scales and crusts that are large, moist, greasy, and dirty yellow. In older children, fine scales are present either diffusely or at the scalp borders and behind the ears. Psoriasis, which may begin in the scalp, requires differentiation from seborrhea.

Distention of the scalp veins may occur secondary to hydrocephalus or other causes of increased intracranial pressure in infants, dural venous thrombosis and neonatal copper deficiency.

The occipital area may be bald in infants who lie chiefly on their backs and in patients who are confined to bed for long periods of time. Localized loss of hair is also noted in young children with persistent head banging.

A localized, coin-sized (0.5 to 6 cm), congenital *absence of scalp* covered by a thin epithelial membrane or a serosanguineous exudate may occur at the vertex, especially in the midline. The defect heals with an atrophic, scarred area of alopecia. Pressure necrosis of the scalp over the parietal prominences may also occur in newborn infants. Scalp defects are present in the the following syndromes: trisomy 13, Wolf-Hirschhorn, focal dermal hypoplasia and incontinentia pigmenti.

Subcutaneous nodules may occur over the scalp, especially in the occipital area, with rheumatic fever or rheumatoid arthritis. The lesions of chickenpox, lymphosarcoma, eosinophilic granuloma and xanthomatosis may also be present in the scalp. A painful swelling may be associated with eosinophilic granuloma. Monilial infection of the scalp may cause keratinous horns.

Dermoid tumors of the scalp may occur over the bridge of the nose, along the midline of the head or in the occipital areas.

Absence of skin pigmentation over the forehead and of a triangular area of hair in the midfrontal portion of the scalp may be accompanied by white skin spotting. A *white forelock* may be noted in Waardenburg's syndrome.

Nevus sebaceus is a flat or slightly-raised, waxy, yellow-orange or orange-brown scalp plaque with a granular surface devoid of hair. It may be present on the scalp or face at birth or appear in the first year of life. Lesions greater than 6 cm in diameter may be accompanied by mental retardation and seizures. A *subgaleal hematoma*, at times extensive, may be caused by hair pulling associated with child abuse or by minor head trauma, including combing.

SCALP HAIR

The *hair of premature infants* is fine, wooly and bunched, while that of term infants is silky, single stranded, flat, and often long and dark. Hair present at birth is usually lost by four to six weeks of age and then gradually regrows.

In *congenital ectodermal dysplasia* hair may be absent, scant or light brown with a shiny and smooth scalp. Infants with hypothyroidism may have dry, thin, lusterless, brittle and coarse hair that extends low on the forehead. In chronic idiopathic hypoparathyroidism, the hair of the scalp, eyebrows and eyelashes may be thin, patchy and coarse.

Progeria is characterized by fine hair which later may be entirely lost. Abnormally fine, silky, sparse hair and short-limbed dwarfism occur in the *cartilage-hair hypo-plasia syndrome*. The hair breaks off easily, and baldness may occur. Hair pigmentation does not occur in children with albinism. Thinning or loss of hair, especially in the frontoparietal area, may occur in congenital syphilis. Vitamin A poisoning may also cause sparse hair. Brittle hair may occur in patients with anorexia nervosa.

Fragility, beading and longitudinal splintering of the hair shaft ("paint-brush" hair) occurs with *trichorrhexis nodosa,* the most common hair shaft anomaly. Unusual dryness of the hair caused by too frequent shampooing and the trauma of excessive combing and brushing are contributory etiologic factors. Proximal trichorrhexis nodosa, which occurs only in black children, causes the hair to be extremely fragile and to grow not more than a few centimeters in length. Trichorrhexis nodosa also occurs in Menke's disease and in argininosuccinicaciduria, along with seizures, ataxia and mental retardation. *Monilethrix,* usually a familial disorder, is characterized by beaded, sparse, short, wiry stubble along with horny follicular papules (keratosis pilaris) over the upper back and shoulders. *Pili torti* or *twisted hairs* also causes sparse, short, shiny, brittle, brown scalp hair which shimmers in reflected light. Alopecia is evident by two or three years of age, especially over the occiput. On microscopic examination, the hairs are seen to be twisted through 180 degrees at irregular intervals along the long axis. Other ectodermal defects and sensorineural hearing loss may be present. *Bamboo hair* is associated with ichthyosiform skin changes and an atopic diathesis. *Pili annulati* is characterized by light and dark bands when observed in reflected light.

Kinky hair disease, which occurs in boys as the clinical expression of a sex-linked recessive trait, is characterized by stubby, sparse, white, kinky hair and seizures, especially myoclonic jerks. Hypothermia, susceptibility to infection, failure to thrive, drowsiness and lethargy may be presenting symptoms. The hair may appear normal in the affected newborn infant.

Danks, D. M., Campbell, P. E., Stevens, B. J., Mayne, V., and Cartwright, E.: Menkes's kinky hair syndrome. An inherited defect in copper absorption with widespread effects. Pediatrics 50:188, 1972.

Unruly scalp hair which tends to stand up persistently over the top of the head, occurs in about 2 per cent of normal infants, but more commonly with microcephaly.

Smith, D. W., and Greely, M. J.: Unruly scalp hair in infancy: Its nature and relevance to problems of brain morphogenesis. Pediatrics 61:783, 1978.

Hypopigmented or white hair occurs in sialic acid storage disease with sialuria.

Premature graying of the hair appears in patients with ataxia-telangiectasia.

Uveomeningoencephalitic syndrome is characterized by progressive whitening of the hair and eyelashes (poliosis) and alopecia, uveitis, meningeal symptoms, vitiligo and hearing impairment or tinnitus.

Pili annulati ("spangled" hair), characterized by alternating dark and light bands, also shimmers in reflected light.

Protein-calorie malnutrition or *kwashiorkor* may be associated with sparse, straight, thin, easily pluckable, lackluster, gray or red-streaked, depigmented or flag-sign hair.

The scalp hair in patients with *homocystinuria* is fine, fair, friable and easily removed by brushing. Alopecia also occurs in dyskeratosis congenita.

In *hypohidrotic ectodermal dysplasia* the scalp hair is fine, stiff, short and blond.

Hypotrichosis involving the scalp (bald spots), eyelashes and eyebrows occurs in the *Hallermann-Streiff* syndrome.

Hair loss may be categorized as either *anagen effluvium,* affecting hair in its anagen or active growth phase; or *telogen effluvium*, with the hair in the telogen or resting stage. The former is characterized by obvious hair loss beginning 7 to 14 days after cancer chemotherapy, epilating cranial radiation or thallium ingestion; the latter is characterized by an onset of 2 to 4 months after etiologies such as hyperpyrexia; severe infection, e.g., Kawasaki disease; toxic shock syndrome; major psychologic stress; crash diets; anorexia nervosa; and drugs, including valproic acid. Hair loss may also occur as a result of zinc deficiency, systemic lupus erythematosus, arsenic poisoning, dermatomyositis, sarcoidosis and hyperthyroidism. A subset of patients with vitamin D–dependent rickets, type II, have alopecia totalis.

Rosen, J. F., Fleischman, A. R., Finberg, L., Hamstra, B. S., and DeLuca, H. F.: Rickets with alopecia: An inborn error of vitamin D metabolism. J. Pediatr. 94:729, 1979.

Congenital alopecia may be complete, patchy or characterized by diffuse hypotrichosis.

Loss of hair occasionally occurs in *hypothyroid infants* after the initiation of thyroid therapy.

Trichotillomania, in which the child pulls out and, perhaps, swallows his hair, may lead to partial alopecia. Areas most commonly involved include those within ready reach of the dominant hand, such as the eyebrows, eyelashes and parts of the scalp, especially the crown and occipital areas. Twirling causes the hairs to break off close to the scalp so that the hair follicles appear as black dots. Occasionally, the involved areas appear circular. When multiple areas are involved, trichotillomania may be confused with alopecia areata, except that hair loss is incomplete, remaining hairs vary in length, and the margins of involved areas are poorly demarcated.

Muller, S. A., and Winkelmann, R. K.: Trichotillomania. Arch. Dermatol. 105:535, 1972.

Alopecia areata is characterized by a sudden loss of hair, perhaps overnight, leaving round, well-demarcated patches (1 to 5 cm) of smooth white scalp. "Exclamation point" hairs, colorless and thin at their roots, may occur at the border. With peripheral extension of involved areas, the entire scalp may become bald (alopecia arcata totalis). Alopecia areata universalis is characterized by total loss of body hair. Pitting and ridging of the nails may also occur.

Traction alopecia, owing to trauma and traction on the hair from pony tails, braids, night rollers, curlers, barrettes or combing, may cause non-inflammatory hair loss along the hair margins or part lines. Alopecia and subgaleal hematoma secondary to hair pulling may be a manifestation of child abuse.

Alopecia with loss of hair from the scalp, eyebrows and eyelashes occurs one to two weeks after ingestion of thallium. Ataxia or tremors may precede or accompany the hair loss.

Alopecia of the scalp, eyebrows and eyelashes occurs in *acrodermatitis enteropathica* along with vesicular and pustular dermatitis around the mucocutaneous orifices and on the extremities.

Tinea capitis, or ringworm of the scalp, is most frequently caused by *Trichophyton tonsurans* of the involved hairs. The hairs are broken off flush with the scalp and appear as black dots under magnification. Hair loss that is either diffuse, irregularly patchy or minimal, with diffuse or patchy scaling that simulates seborrheic dermatitis, may be noted. Fluorescence with the Wood's light does not occur. In the presence of alopecia, a negative Wood's lamp examination and a negative KOH scalp scraping preparation, a KOH mount and fungus culture should be obtained on one of the plucked, involved hairs. Ringworm caused by *Microsporum canis* or *M. audouini* is characterized by bald, discrete, slightly inflamed, round, scaling patches, ½ to 2 inches in diameter, which fluoresce under a Wood's light. Several patches are usually present. Hairs are gray and lusterless and break off close to the scalp. Involved areas may become erythematous, edematous, crusted and pruritic. Purulent folliculitis and kerion formation may cause localized or weeping masses.

Rasmussen, J. E.: Hair loss in children. Pediatr. Rev. 3:85, 1981.

Stroud, J. D.: Hair loss in children. Pediatr. Clin. North Am. 30:641, 1983.

In patients with *pediculosis,* large numbers of ova or "nits," each the size of a small grain of sand, attach firmly to the hair near the scalp. Lice may also be observed moving about. Suboccipital and postauricular adenopathy may develop. The presenting complaint is pruritus of the scalp.

Hair casts, which may be mistaken for the nits of pediculosis in the absence of microscopic confirmation, are shiny, white, firm cylinders, 2 to 7 mm in length, which encircle and can be moved along the scalp hairs.

In patients with an abnormally short neck, owing to the Klippel-Feil syndrome or other anomaly, scalp hair appears to extend far down on the neck posteriorly.

A tongue-shaped growth of scalp hair may extend onto the cheek in patients with mandibulofacial dysostosis.

Orentreich, N.: Disorders of the hair and scalp. Pediatr. Clin. North Am. 18:953, 1971.

Price, V. H.: Disorders of the hair in children. Pediatr. Clin. North Am. 25:305, 1978.

3 / THE EYES

The newborn infant should be examined for the *red reflex.* Using the "0" ophthalmoscopic lens from a distance of about 10 inches, the physician focuses the light upon the infant's pupil. In white infants, the pupillary area is seen as a bright orange-red circle, while in black infants the reflex may be yellow-orange. The presence of a normal red reflex indicates that the lens is clear. If the reflex is not clearly seen, the pupils should be dilated and the eyes reexamined. Newborn infants usually resist separation of their eyelids. Examination for a red reflex may, therefore, be delayed until the infant spontaneously opens his eyes. If the infant's head is placed lower than the trunk, the eyes may spontaneously open.

The possible occurrence of retinopathy of prematurity makes routine ophthalmologic examination mandatory in premature infants.

DEVELOPMENT OF VISION

The premature infant's eyes are closed most of the time. Occasionally the infant may transiently and partially or completely open one or both eyes. The newborn infant responds to the flashing of a bright light by frowning, blinking and with other withdrawal reactions. The eyes may move about, but do not fixate at this time. Larger premature infants are able to follow a dangling ring through an arc of 45 degrees.

The newborn term infant is able to differentiate between light and darkness. Pupillary contraction, blinking of the eyelids and contraction of the orbicularis muscle occur in response to the flashing of a bright light. A pupillary light reflex indicates that the peripheral visual apparatus is probably functional, and, unless cortical blindness is present, that the infant has some vision. Thrusting the examiner's hand toward the baby's eyes to elicit blinking is an unreliable test of vision.

A *fixation* reflex in which a baby instinctively looks at a light is present shortly after birth. A red ball or the examiner's face held 8 to 12 inches from the infant's eyes serves as a useful visual stimulus for newborn infants, especially if the baby is alert and the room not too brightly lighted. During the early weeks of life, the eyes move about, seemingly with no particular fixation or perception. Occasional pauses do occur, however, during which the infant stares at a wall, a window or other source of light. He may transiently open one or both eyes but spends most of his time sleeping. In response to a visual stimulus the infant may demonstrate monocular fixation and generalized diminution of bodily activity, as if giving almost total attention to the stimulus. Monocular fixation for near objects continues until about 16 weeks of age. The nonfixating eye may be kept closed, partially open or moving about. At one month of age, the infant can follow an object 60 degrees on each side of the midline. Absence of visual fixation and following by 3 to 4 months of age is an indication for ophthalmologic consultation.

Not until the fifth or sixth week does an infant become capable of binocular fixation and prolonged visual contact with an adult. For the next three or four months the power of fusion is so weak that frequent deviations from parallelism occur. By the fifth or sixth month a moderate degree of binocular fixation has developed. Convergence ability begins during the second month in a jerky and poorly coordinated fashion. Similar incoordination of eye movements occurs when the infant follows moving objects.

During the third and fourth months, the infant performs convergence and ocular following movements comparatively well. This increased coordination and visual acuity are a result of both progression in neuromuscular control of the ocular muscles and the more complete development of the macula during the third month. At three or four months of age the infant can perceive a small pellet. With attainment of improved head control at this time the infant is able to follow his mother as she moves about the room. Babies of this age also enjoy looking at their hands. At 12 weeks of age the infant can follow a dangling ring through an arc of 180 degrees. Some color perception may also develop by about four months. Between five and six months true coordination of eyes and hands begins to appear.

The eyeballs of most infants are relatively shorter in their anteroposterior diameter than is the case later; thus, most infants have hyperopia, possibly of several diopters. Hyperopia in older children is usually caused by an abnormally short longitudinal axis of the eye. The eye may attempt to compensate for this refractive error through accommodation. Overactivity of the internal rectus muscle may, however, occur with the development of a convergent strabismus. The normal lengthening of the anteroposterior diameter of the eye that occurs with growth accounts for the appearance or increase of myopia in some children. An infant's eyes are relatively large compared to other facial features. But as the infant's head grows, the eyes appear less prominent.

VISUAL ACUITY

Visual acuity in the newborn is estimated to be 20/400 utilizing the optokinetic nystagmus and forced choice preferential techniques; and 20/100 to 20/200 by visually evoked potential. At four months of age, visual acuity ranges from 20/200 to 20/80, depending upon the technique used. At 1 year it is between 20/40 and 20/60; at 2 years about 20/20. Since macular development is not complete until 6 or 7 years of age, a visual acuity of 20/30 or 20/40 as determined by the Snellen test charts may be considered normal at age 4 or 5. On the Snellen test charts 20/20 vision is not usually demonstrated until age five or six.

Vision impairment is usually caused by a refractive error, most frequently myopia. In evaluating young infants' vision, the examiner checks the pupillary light reaction and the infant's ability to blink in response to a bright light, fixate monocularly or binocularly and follow a bright object or light.

Infants with possible decreased vision may be evaluated with the optokinetic drum or tape, forced choice preferential looking or visually evoked potential.

Under the age of two to four years the determination of a child's visual acuity may be difficult without refraction, unless the examiner determines the child's ability to recognize standard objects. Such objects include various-sized white marbles placed at standard distances in the examining room. At a distance of 18 to 20 feet, recognition of a marble 1½ inches in diameter indicates a visual acuity of 20/200; of a ¾ inch marble, an acuity of 20/80. Recognition of a dime at a distance of five feet is consistent with at least 20/50 vision.

If the child has not learned to recognize the letters of the regular Snellen chart, the modified or illiterate Snellen chart should be used. On this latter chart the letter "E" is printed with bars up or down and to the right or left. The child is instructed to duplicate with his fingers the direction in which the bars of the "E" point. By age three or four, children can usually be successfully tested with the illiterate Snellen "E" chart. Such assessment is an essential part of the general physical examination in order to detect myopia and amblyopia at an age when treatment may still be effective.

The use of the Snellen test charts alone, however, has limitations. Though myopia and amblyopia may be detected, hyperopia and strabismus, latent or manifest, may be overlooked. The first part of the Massachusetts screening test for visual testing in children uses a Snellen type chart. The 20/20 line was originally recommended. However, the test may be more helpful for children aged 6 to 8 if ophthalmologic referral is based on the child's inability to read correctly four of the six symbols on the 20/30 line. The following levels of visual acuity may be used as an indication for ophthalmologic referral: 20/50 or less in a 3 year old; 20/40 or less in 4 and 5 year olds; one or more line difference in visual acuity between the two eyes; and 20/30 for children in the fourth grade and above. The second portion of the test screens for hyperopia. With a plus 1.50 lens placed before each eye, the ability to read the 20/20 or the 20/30 line with each eye is regarded as an indication for referral. Since some degree of hyperopia is normal in children, The National Society for the Prevention of Blindness recommends that a plus 2.25 sphere be used in children in the first three grades and a plus 1.75 for those in the fourth grade and above.

The Allen Picture Cards, the Sjögren Hand, the Landolt Ring charts and the Titmus screener are all reliable visual acuity tests. Screening of children 3 years of age or older for stereopsis can be performed with the TNO Random Dot E test. The Titmus stereo tester with Polaroid glasses may also be used for determination of stereopsis. The Titmus fly test for stereoacuity usually is not helpful before age 7.

In addition to referrals made on the basis of these screening tests, children with headache and ocular pain should have an ophthalmologic examination with refraction unless the complaints are attributable to causes other than eyestrain.

Greenwald, M. J.: Visual development in infancy and childhood. Pediatr. Clin. North Am. 30:977, 1983.

Nelson, L. B., Rubin, S. E., Wagner, R. S., and Breto, M. E.: Developmental aspects in the assessment of visual function in young children. Pediatrics 73:375, 1984.

Color vision may also be checked by a variety of charts. The incidence of benign red/green color blindness is 0.5 per cent in girls and 8 per cent in boys.

IMPAIRED, DISTORTED OR ATYPICAL VISION. AMAUROSIS.

Developmental retardation and aberration in infants may be caused by defective vision.

Motor development, especially activities such as rolling over and sitting, which require orientation in space, may be delayed in infants who are blind or severely myopic. Babies with impaired vision may demonstrate nystagmoid eye movements and may rub their eyes excessively.

Children with *infantile autism* may appear to look through the examiner. Infants with *psychosocial failure to thrive* may also demonstrate gaze avoidance or fleeting eye contact. "Radar-like" visual activity is characteristic of infants with rumination. These patients are also exceedingly visually alert.

Blindness may be a sequela of cataracts, retrolental fibroplasia, optic atrophy, glaucoma, macular degeneration, retinoblastoma, chorioretinitis, trauma, meningitis, encephalitis, ocular infections, occipital encephalocele, hydranencephaly or porencephaly, and a variety of cerebral degenerative diseases, including adrenoleukodystrophy. The initial symptom in Spielmeyer-Vogt (Batten's) disease may be progressive loss of vision.

Hysterical amblyopia may occur in children. In these children, the visual fields are constricted and tubular.

Acute cortical blindness, characterized by vision loss, normal pupillary reflexes and absence of ophthalmologic disease, may be a complication of meningitis, head trauma, increased intracranial pressure, uremia, hypoxia, carbon monoxide poisoning, hydrocephalus, seizures, migraine syndrome and cardiac arrest. Recovery of vision occurs rapidly after head trauma but less rapidly with other disorders. Transient blindness may be a manifestation of a vaso-occlusive central nervous system episode in sickle cell anemia. The onset of acute cortical blindness is a sensitive sign of *cerebrospinal fluid shunt dysfunction.*

Barnet, A. B., Manson, J. I., and Wilner, E.: Acute cerebral blindness in children. Neurology 20:1147, 1970.

Nelson, I. B.: The visually handicapped child. Pediatr. Rev. 6:173, 1984.

Scheiner, A. P., and Moomaw, M.: Care of the visually handicapped child. Pediatr. Rev. 4:74, 1982.

Tepperberg, J., Nussbaum, E., and Feldman, F.: Cortical blindness following meningitis due to *Hemophilus influenzae* type B. J. Pediatr. 91:434, 1977.

Vision loss or a change in visual fields not accompanied by fundus changes suggests an *intracranial neoplasm.* Young children with brain tumors do not complain of diminished visual acuity until papilledema is advanced. Disk elevation may be present for many months without report of impaired vision. Vision loss occurs with papillitis and with retrobulbar neuritis.

High grade, progressive myopia may occur in infants. In the *Stickler syndrome* (hereditary arthro-ophthalmopathy), sudden, spontaneous retinal detachment may occur in the first decade of life.

Migraine may be accompanied by diverse visual symptoms, including scotomas, bright flashes, wavy vision, geometric designs, stars, visual field defects, blurred vision, micropsia, macropsia, zoom vision, inversion, alteration in motion perception and visual hallucinations.

Hachinski, V. C., Porchawka, J., and Steele, J. C.: Visual symptoms in the migraine syndrome. Neurology 23:570, 1973.

Blurred vision may be secondary to neuropathies caused by diphtheria or botulism, diabetes, increased intracranial pressure, pseudotumor cerebri, conversion disorder, hypertensive encephalopathy and *Candida* endophthalmitis.

Metamorphopsia or distorted visual perception of an object's size (micropsia, macropsia), shape or position (teleopsia in which an object looks more distant) occurs with complicated migraine, partial seizures, the use of hallucinogenic drugs and emotional disorder. Formed hallucinations of figures or scenes are usually attributable to temporal lobe lesions, while unformed hallucinations or light sensations are usually associated with occipital, anterior visual pathway or retinal lesions.

Cooperman, S. M.: "Alice in Wonderland" syndrome as a presenting symptom of infectious mononucleosis in children. Clin. Pediatr. 16:143, 1973.

Smith, D. L.: Micropsia. Clin. Pediatr. 19:297, 1982.

EYELIDS

Ptosis. Newborn infants often have one eye widely open while the other eyelid droops or is closed. This pseudoptosis disappears with further maturation. *Congenital ptosis* is usually unilateral and sporadic. In the *Marcus Gunn phenomenon* (jaw-winking reflex), which is associated with congenital ptosis, protrusion or movement of the jaw to one side causes elevation of the ptosed eyelid on the contralateral side. In infants, sucking may produce a similar response.

The triad of ptosis, blepharophimosis, and epicanthus inversus is inherited.

Myotonic dystrophy may cause congenital ptosis that precedes by many years other signs of that disorder.

A pseudoptosis may occur with paralysis of the superior rectus muscle along with hypotropia of the involved eye and drooping of the upper lid. An epicanthal fold may also be present.

Ptosis may also be caused by paralysis of the oculomotor nerve, encephalitis, thallitoxicosis, cervical neuroblastoma, infant botulism, myasthenia gravis (unilaterally or bilaterally), ocular myopathy, pineal tumors, Horner's syndrome, tuberculous meningitis and ocular rhabdomyosarcoma. Ptosis also occurs in the Fisher, Aarskog, Noonan, Möbius, Leigh, multiple pterygium, whistling face, fetal alcohol, Saethre-Chotzen, Smith-Lemli-Opitz and the Kearns-Sayre syndromes.

Oculosympathetic paralysis occurring during the course of acute otitis media in children is manifested by a slight droop of the upper eyelid. The lid can, however, be fully elevated.

Elevation or retraction of the upper lids in advanced hydrocephalus exposes the sclera above the cornea and produces an apparent exophthalmos or downward displacement of the eyes. Widening of the palpebral fissure owing to exophthalmos and retraction of the lids may cause a staring expression in children with *hyperthyroidism*; the *lid lag sign,* characterized by the upper eyelid lagging behind the eyeball when the patient looks downward, may also be present along with increased lacrimation, chemosis and conjunctival injection.

An *"eye-popping" appearance* created by a sudden transient widening of the palpebral fissures may be noted in some infants when the examining light is removed after testing pupillary reflexes or when the lights in a room are turned off. A simultaneous downward deviation of the eyes may be noted.

Perex, R. B.: The eye-popping reflex of infants. J. Pediatr. 81:87, 1972.

Lower *eyelid colobomas* or notches are present in the Treacher-Collins syndrome. A unilateral upper eyelid coloboma may be present in Goldenhar's syndrome.

Excessive *blinking* of the eyes may indicate eyestrain or tic.

Squinting or narrowing of the palpebral fissures is an indication for an ophthalmologic examination. Narrowing of the palpebral fissure also occurs secondary to puffy, edematous eyelids and with Duane's retraction syndrome.

Blepharospasm occurs in the Schwartz-Jampel syndrome; congenital glaucoma with marked photophobia and secondary to a corneal ulceration; conjunctivitis; or keratitis.

Palpebral fissure length may be measured by sighting over a ruler held across the eye's greatest horizontal axis from the medial to lateral canthus. The mean length at 40 weeks' gestation in white infants is 1.85 ± 0.13 cm; in black infants, 2.00 ± 0.22; and in Hispanic newborns, 1.95 ± 0.20. Short palpebral fissures are found in syndromes such as fetal alcohol, Williams whistling face and the 10p deletion, as well as with microphthalmia.

Fuchs, M., Iosub, S., Bingol, N., and Gromisch, D. S.: Palpebral fissure size revisited. J. Pediatr. 96:77, 1980.

Jones, K. L., Hanson, J. W., and Smith, D. W.: Palpebral fissure size in newborn infants. J. Pediatr. 92:787, 1978.

In *Duane's retraction syndrome*, sometimes confused with sixth nerve palsy, eye adduction is accompanied by narrowing of the palpebral fissure, eyeball retraction and superior or inferior deviation of the globe. A decrease or loss of abduction with widening of the palpebral fissure on lateral gaze also occurs. Esotropia is present in the primary position. In *Brown's* syndrome, the eye cannot be elevated in adduction.

Staring episodes may occur with petit mal epilepsy. A fixed stare may be a sign of phenothiazine toxicity. Staring episodes may also be reported in some emotionally disturbed children.

Slanting of the palpebral fissures from the lateral to the medial canthus occurs in children with Down's syndrome and occasionally in normal infants. Antimongoloid slanting occurs in Alport's, Pfeiffer's, cri du chat, Treacher-Collins, whistling face and the 10p depletion syndromes. A droop at the outer canthus can also be seen in patients with the Treacher-Collins syndrome. Almond shaped eyes with upslanting palpebral fissures are present in the Prader-Willi syndrome.

Hordeolum or *stye,* a localized staphylococcal infection that occurs at the edge of the eyelid, is a painful, red and tender swelling, usually surmounted by a yellow punctum.

Chalazion, or *meibomian cyst,* is a firm, discrete, nonpainful nodule on the bulbar aspect of the lid adjacent to the tarsal plate.

Swelling of the eyelid may be the first sign of an *orbital rhabdomyosarcoma.* Embryonal rhabdomyosarcoma occurs most often at the upper inner angle of the orbit.

A *hemangioma* may cause bluish enlargement of an eyelid.

Bleeding into the eyelids may occur in the Henoch-Schönlein syndrome.

Thickening and eversion of the eyelid margins and pedunculated nodules on the palpebral conjunctiva may occur in the *multiple mucosal neuroma syndrome.*

Thickening and distortion of the upper eyelid may occur with *neurofibromatosis,* especially when associated with a glioma of the optic nerve.

A *dermoid cyst* may present as a lump in the lateral part of the upper lid, most commonly under the left eyebrow.

Pollard, Z. F., Harley, R. D., and Calhoun, J.: Dermoid cysts in children. Pediatrics 57:379, 1976.

Marginal blepharitis is characterized by persistent erythema, scaling and crusting of the edges of the eyelids. *Staphylococcal blepharitis* produces tenacious scales which on removal leave small ulcerated lesions. Pustules may develop about the base of the eyelashes, and the meibomian glands may contain pus. Some of the eyelashes may be lost. In seborrheic dermatitis, the scales are greasy, waxy and easily removed.

A red and swollen eye may be caused by periorbital or preseptal cellulitis, orbital cellulitis and cavernous sinus thrombosis.

Orbital cellulitis may be caused by *Staphylococcus aureus, Streptococcus pyogenes, Escherichia coli, Streptococcus pneumoniae* and *Haemophilus influenzae, type B.* In addition to the sudden onset of redness and swelling of the lids, findings of orbital cellulitis may include conjunctival injection and edema, proptosis, tenderness, impaired visual acuity, pain and restricted eye movements. Computed tomography may be indicated. *Haemophilus influenzae* cellulitis often causes a blue-purple discoloration of the eyelids. A similar discoloration occurs in infections caused by *Streptococcus pneumoniae.* Adenoviruses and influenza viruses may also cause periorbital cellulitis.

Barkin, R. M., Todd, J. K., and Amer, J.: Periorbital cellulitis in children. Pediatrics 62:390, 1978.

Teele, D. W.: Management of the child with a red and swollen eye. J. Pediatr. Infect. Dis. 2:258, 1983.

Thirumoorthi, M. C., Asmar, B. I., and Danani, A. S.: Violaceous discoloration in pneumococcal cellulitis. Pediatrics 62:492, 1978.

An *atopic pleat* (Morgan's fold or Dennie's line), a bilateral wrinkle or fold of skin just below the lower eyelid, is present in some atopic individuals.

Children with *dermatomyositis* develop a lilac or heliotrope discoloration and scaling dermatitis of the eyelids which, along with periorbital edema, is virtually pathognomonic.

EYELASHES AND EYEBROWS

Eyelashes and eyebrows are usually absent in premature infants.

Long, curved eyelashes may be inherited. They are also frequent in chronically ill children and in the De Lange syndrome.

Pediculosis confined to the eyelashes may be detected only by careful examination. Frequent rubbing of the eyes or marginal blepharitis may be noted.

In patients with albinism the eyelashes are not pigmented. Poliosis or progressive whitening of the eyelashes is seen in the *uveomeningitis syndrome.*

Distichiasis or extra eyelashes may accompany familial lymphedema.

Eyelashes may be absent on the inner two thirds of the lower eyelid in patients with the Treacher-Collins syndrome. Patients with the Hallermann-Streiff and cartilage hair syndromes have hypotrichosis of the eyebrows and eyelashes.

Children with Hurler's syndrome have bushy eyebrows. In the De Lange and Waardenburg syndromes, the eyebrows meet in the midline.

The Coffin-Siris syndrome is characterized by hypertrichosis of the eyebrows and eyelashes and hypotrichosis of the scalp.

Carey, J. C., and Hall, B. D.: The Coffin-Siris syndrome: Five new cases including two siblings. Am. J. Dis. Child. 132:667, 1978.

SWELLING OF EYELIDS AND PERIORBITAL TISSUES

In the newborn, silver nitrate *chemical conjunctivitis* often produces eyelid edema. Prolonged crying may also cause mild edema. The eyelids in infants with hypothyroidism are characteristically puffy.

Acute ethmoid sinusitis may cause swelling of the periorbital region, especially medially. Initially, the swelling may be minimal and, therefore, easily overlooked.

Slight puffiness of the eyelids and dark circles about the eyes may be seen in children with frequent respiratory infections or nasal allergy ("allergic shiners").

Other causes of lid edema include pollen allergy and conjunctivitis. Swelling of the eyelids may be noted in infants with pertussis after paroxysms of coughing. Measles and infectious mononucleosis may be accompanied by puffiness of the lids. In dermatomyositis the eyelids may be edematous and have a heliotrope color. The upper lids may also be swollen in trichinosis. Nephritis and nephrosis are classically characterized by puffy eyelids. Other causes of periorbital edema include angioedema, osteomyelitis of the frontal bone, cavernous sinus thrombosis, the superior vena caval syndrome and orbital infarction owing to sickle cell vaso-occlusive crisis.

Blowout fracture of the orbital floor following trauma to the orbit by baseball-sized objects may cause periorbital swelling, ecchymosis and conjunctival hemorrhage. If the inferior rectus or inferior oblique muscles herniate through the orbital floor into the maxillary sinus as a result of the injury, eyeball mobility is reduced and enophthalmos ensues. The patient may complain of diplopia, especially on upward gaze.

Heller, R. M.: The clinical and radiological presentation of blowout fracture of the orbit in children. Pediatrics 46:796, 1970.

EPICANTHUS

A fold of skin extending down from the upper lid to cover the medial canthus of the eye may be noted in normal newborns. The fold usually disappears in one to three months.

In Down's syndrome the epicanthic fold is usually prominent and extends down at the inner canthus. As the child becomes older this fold may disappear.

Epicanthal folds occur in patients with congenital ptosis of the eyelids, glycogenosis Type II (Pompe's disease) and in the following syndromes: cerebrohepatorenal, De Lange, Smith-Lemli-Opitz, Ehlers-Danlos, leopard, Möbius, Noonan's, Turner, cri du chat, Williams, fetal alcohol and hydantoin.

A pronounced semicircular epicanthic fold extends from the forehead downward onto the cheek in infants with bilateral renal agenesis (Potter's syndrome). These infants also have wide-spaced eyes.

SPACING OF THE EYES

Ocular hypertelorism refers to abnormally wide spacing of the eyes and a broadened bridge of the nose owing to maldevelopment of the sphenoid bone. A number of physical findings, including epicanthal folds, flat nasal bridge or widely spaced eyebrows, may give a misleading impression of ocular hypertelorism. The interpupillary distance between the center of the eyes has diagnostic usefulness in evaluating craniofacial dysostoses and, with the exception of Waardenburg's syndrome, is the best indicator of ocular hypertelorism. Pryor has suggested the following formula: interpupillary distance is A − B/2 + B where A is the distance between the two outer angles of the palpebral fissures and B the distance between the two median angles. Determination of these distances is facilitated if measured while the patient looks upward. Because racial differences in cranial configuration exist, appropriate normative values should be used.

Juberg, R. C., Sholte, F. G., and Touchstone, W. J.: Normal values for intercanthal distances of 5- to 11-year-old American blacks. Pediatrics 55:431, 1975.

Ocular hypertelorism is also present in these syndromes: Aarskog's, Noonan's, Apert's, craniofacial dysostosis, cerebral gigantism, craniometaphyseal dysostosis, multiple lentigines, nevoid basal cell carcinoma, Rubinstein-Taybi, whistling face, orofaciodigital dysostosis, otopalatodigital, cri du chat, Ehlers-Danlos, fetal hydantoin, cerebrohepatorenal, chromosome 4p, Coffin-Lowry, Crouzon, DiGeorge, Larsen, Robinow, fetal face, Weaver, Williams and Turner.

An unusually wide distance between the inner canthi of the eyes (dystopia canthorum), a broad nasal root, lateral displacement of the inferior lacrimal points, confluence of the eyebrows, heterochromia of the irises, white forelock and congenital deafness constitute *Waardenburg's syndrome*. The inner canthi are laterally displaced in the Carpenter's, orofaciodigital and multiple nevoid basal cell carcinoma syndromes.

The orofaciodigital syndrome is characterized by lateral displacement of the inner canthi, hypoplasia of the alar cartilages and broad nasal root.

Orbital hypotelorism, a decrease in the distance between the orbits, is found in the arhinencephaly group of malformations. These median faciocerebral defects include *cyclopia*, in which a single orbit is present in the nasal region, usually with a superior proboscis; *ethmocephaly* with extreme hypotelorism, separate orbits and proboscis; *cebocephaly* in which a flat, rudimentary nose similar to that of the platyrrhine monkey is present; and *arhinencephaly* with

median or lateral cleft palate or with trigonocephaly.

LACRIMAL GLAND AND NASOLACRIMAL DUCT

Most term or almost-term babies secrete tears.

In perhaps one third to two thirds of term infants, complete patency of the nasolacrimal duct has not been established at the time of birth. The lower end of the nasolacrimal duct is usually separated from the inferior meatus by a thin membrane. Patency of the duct is usually present some weeks after birth, but if occluded, watering of the eye is noted with the tears running over onto the cheek. Persistence of obstruction past the sixth month is an indication for ophthalmologic consultation. Failure of drainage may predispose to dacryocystitis with swelling, tenderness and erythema that is medial and inferior to the inner canthus. A persistent conjunctivitis often develops in which the eyelids may stick together during sleep, and purulent material may be expressed from the duct opening.

Familial dysautonomia and acquired postganglionic cholinergic dysautonomia are characterized by an absence or near absence of tears.

Inamdar, S., Easton, L. B., and Lester, G.: Acquired postganglionic cholinergic dysautonomia: Case report and review of the literature. Pediatrics 70:976, 1982.

Epiphora, or excessive tearing, may occur with inflammatory disease, a corneal ulcer, foreign body plugging of the nasolacrimal duct, exophthalmos, or as an allergic reaction.

Sjögren's syndrome, characterized by dry eyes, dry mouth and parotitis, may occasionally occur in children with polyarticular, seropositive juvenile rheumatoid arthritis.

EXOPHTHALMOS, PROPTOSIS

Whereas minimal exophthalmos cannot be measured directly, progression or unilateral differences may be assessed by comparative readings.

Neuroblastomas, which frequently metastasize to the orbit, may cause periorbital ecchymosis and unilateral or bilateral exophthalmos. Orbital sarcoma, lymphoma, retinoblastoma, glioma of the optic nerve, and retro-orbital tumors and abscesses may also cause protrusion of the orbit.

Progressive, unilateral, nonpulsatile proptosis in association with diminishing visual acuity is usually the presenting finding in *intraorbital glioma*. Café-au-lait spots may also be noted. Neurofibromatosis may also cause overgrowth of the greater wing of the sphenoid bone and a bony defect in the posterior orbit followed by an orbital proptosis which is more prominent when the patient stands.

Other causes of exophthalmos, proptosis or prominent eyes include:
Congenital cystic eye
Hyperthyroidism

Uretsky, S. H., Kennerdell, J. S., and Gutai, J. P.: Graves' ophthalmopathy in childhood and adolescence. Arch. Ophthalmol. 98:1963, 1980.

Histiocytosis X; Hand-Schüller-Christian syndrome
Ocular rhabdomyosarcoma causes a rapidly progressive proptosis.
Cavernous hemangioma; lymphangioma
Cavernous sinus thrombosis
Arteriovenous fistula. Pulsation may be present.
Orbital and retro-orbital hemorrhage caused by trauma or a bleeding disorder
Orbital cellulitis
Crouzon's disease or other craniosynostosis
Giant cell reparative granuloma of nonspecific etiology
Osteomyelitis of the maxilla
Apert's syndrome
Fibrous dysplasia of the facial bones
Basal skull fracture
Anterior meningocele or encephalocele. Pulsation may be present.
Acrocephalosyndactyly
Leopard syndrome
Pycnodysostosis
Sickle cell disease with proptosis, eyelid edema and impairment of function of extraocular muscles.

Blank, J. P., and Gill, F. M.: Orbital infarction in sickle cell disease. Pediatrics 67:879, 1981.

Progressive unilateral proptosis may be an early sign of *cystic fibrosis*.
Mucormycosis may cause unilateral ophthalmoplegia, proptosis and extensive necrosis. A serosanguinous nasal discharge and necrotic nasal mucosa may occur. Leukemia and diabetes mellitus are predisposing diseases.
Congenital glaucoma is characterized by eyeball enlargement.

OTHER ORBITAL FINDINGS

Sunken, expressionless eyes may be noted in malnourished or severely dehydrated infants who have lost 10 per cent or more of their body weight.
Periorbital hemorrhage ("raccoon eyes") may occur with child abuse, neuroblastoma or basal skull fracture.
Microphthalmia may occur in patients with persistent tunica vasculosa lentis, retinal dysplasia or encephalo-ophthalmic dysplasia, retinopathy of prematurity, toxoplasmosis, trisomies 13 and 18 and the focal dermal hypoplasia, Hallermann-Streiff and Lenz's microphthalmia syndromes. In infancy, many cataracts are associated with microphthalmia.
Deeply set eyes, overhanging forehead, pointed chin and liver disease characterize arteriohepatic dysplasia.
Anophthalmos, or congenital absence of the eye, is a rare anomaly. The eye may be replaced by a large cyst, or an ocular cyst occurring below a congenitally small eye may cause lower eyelid protrusion.
A *meningocele* may rarely present as a cystic protrusion in the orbit's anteromedial aspect.
Prominent *supraorbital ridges* are noted in the congenital ectodermal dysplasia, Hurler's, Marfan's and frontometaphyseal dysplasia syndromes.
Wrinking of the skin about the eyes is noted in ectodermal dysplasia with atopic eczema and in older adolescents with pituitary dwarfism.
"Allergic shiners" are dark circles under the eyes in patients with nasal allergy.

CONJUNCTIVA

Subconjunctival hemorrhage, commonly seen in newborn infants as a bright red, complete or incomplete band around the iris, generally has no clinical significance and disappears rapidly. Similar hemorrhage may occur after trauma in toxic shock syndrome, in patients with pertussis after paroxysms of severe coughing, in hemorrhagic disorders, in Henoch-Schönlein purpura, and as a result of physical abuse by shaking.
Conjunctivitis. Small vessels around the periphery of the bulbar conjunctiva that radiate toward the cornea become reddened and engorged. The palpebral conjunctiva also demonstrate hyperemia and edema. Secretions may be watery, mucopurulent or purulent.

Hammerschlag, M. R.: Conjunctivitis in infancy and childhood. Pediatr. Rev. 5:285, 1984.

Ophthalmia neonatorum (conjunctivitis of the newborn) has a number of etiologies. Shortly after birth, about 90 per cent of infants demonstrate *chemical conjunctivitis* with edema of the eyelids as a reaction to silver nitrate instillation. This occurs on the first day, about the same time that gonorrheal infections become evident.

Chlamydial conjunctivitis, the most common type of infectious neonatal conjunctivitis, usually occurs late in the first week and during the second week. Only mild erythema of the bulbar conjunctiva or a copious mucopurulent discharge, edema of the eyelids and diffuse conjunctival injection may occur. Chlamydial conjunctivitis cannot be differentiated from bacterial infection on clinical findings alone. Chlamydial and gonorrheal ophthalmia may occur concomitantly.

Hammerschlag, M. R.: Chlamydial infections. Pediatr. Rev. 3:77, 1981.
Rowe, D. S., Aicardi, E. Z., Dawson, C. R., and Schachter, J.: Purulent ocular discharge in neonates: Significance of *Chlamydia trachomatis*. Pediatrics 63:628, 1979.

Redness, watering of the eyes and swelling of the caruncle occur in patients with measles. Conjunctivitis, frequently petechial, is often present in Rocky Mountain spotted fever. Conjunctivitis is infrequently caused by herpes simplex virus, varicella-zoster virus, Epstein-Barr virus and New Castle disease virus. Injection of the blood vessels of the bulbar conjunctiva without generalized suffusion or discharge may last for 3 to 5 weeks in Kawasaki syndrome. Bilateral conjunctivitis may occur with Reiter's disease. Leptospirosis may cause a conjunctivitis as well as iritis and iridocylitis.

Acute mucopurulent or catarrheal conjunctivitis, caused by *Staphylococcus aureus, Streptococcus pneumoniae*, Koch-Weeks bacillus, *Haemophilus influenzae, Neisseria meningitidis* and *Streptococcus viridans*, is characterized by a mucopurulent discharge, swelling and redness of the conjunctiva and sticking of the lids on awakening ("pink eye"). *Haemophilus influenzae* is the most common cause of acute conjunctivitis, followed by *Streptococcus pneumoniae*. Bacteriologic studies are indicated with purulent conjunctivitis. Gonorrheal conjunctivitis is a special hazard during the immediate newborn period.

Oculoglandular tularemia is characterized by conjunctivitis, usually unilateral, and by preauricular and cervical lymphadenopathy. *Cat-scratch disease* also causes preauricular adenopathy when the primary lesion is in the conjunctiva.

Carithers, H. A.: Oculoglandular disease of Parinaud. Am. J. Dis. Child. 132:1195, 1978.

Adenovirus is the etiologic agent in about 20 per cent of the instances of acute conjunctivitis in children. Pharyngoconjunctival fever, caused by adenovirus types 3, 7 and 14, is characterized by conjunctivitis, pharyngitis and preauricular lymphadenopathy.

Trachoma, caused by *Chlamydia trachomatis*, occurs in a limited population of Navaho Indians in the Southwest United States. Characteristically the onset is insidious, with few eye complaints. Physical findings include follicles on the upper tarsal conjunctiva and extension of limbal vessels.

Severe conjunctivitis occurs frequently with the *Stevens-Johnson syndrome.*

Vernal conjunctivitis has an allergic etiology, occurs most frequently during the spring and summer, and is characterized by intense pruritus, photophobia and lacrimation. The palpebral conjunctiva has a bluish-white, cobblestone appearance, and plaques may be noted on the bulbar conjunctiva. A stringy, mucoid secretion is present.

Epidemic keratoconjunctivitis, caused by adenovirus type 8, is initially characterized by prominent follicles on the conjunctiva, along with edema of the eyelids and ocular conjunctiva. Epiphora, pruritus, pain and photophobia are also present. A pseudomembrane may appear on the lids. Preauricular lymphadenopathy may be noted. Some days later, punctate corneal opacities appear, and vision is temporarily impaired. Resolution occurs slowly.

Acute hemorrhagic conjunctivitis is usually caused by enterovirus 70, coxsackievirus A 24 or an adenovirus. The conjunctival infection is characterized by rapid onset with swollen eyelids, bulbar conjunctival hemorrhages, tearing, and follicular conjunctival reaction.

Phlyctenular keratoconjunctivitis is characterized by pinhead-sized, yellowish or grayish-white, conical, papular lesions accompanied by injection of the surrounding conjunctival vessels. Ciliary injection may also be present. These lesions may occur on the cornea, the bulbar conjunctiva or at the limbus. Photophobia, blepharospasm and epiphora may be notable, and ulceration may occur.

Conjunctivitis may occur in preschool children following overexposure to sunlight.

OTHER CONJUNCTIVAL FINDINGS

Pallor of the conjunctiva is a good clinical sign of anemia. Marijuana causes conjunctival injection.

Vitamin A deficiency produces drying and injection of the bulbar conjunctiva. Yellowish patches *(Bitot's spots)* may occur on the bulbar conjunctiva.

The *ataxia-telangiectasia syndrome* is characterized by bulbar *conjunctival telangiectasis*, usually noted between two and eight years of age. Other findings include progressive cerebellar ataxia; nystagmus; oculomotor apraxia; choreoathetosis; cutaneous telangiectasia of the face, pinnae, eyelids and arms; and recurrent pulmonary infections.

Careful examination of the conjunctiva is indicated when subacute bacterial endocarditis is suspected, since petechiae in the conjunctiva may be an embolic phenomenon.

Pinguecula is a slightly elevated, yellowish, wedge-shaped benign lesion which extends from the outer canthus. Rare in infants and young children, this lesion is observed in Gaucher's disease.

Pterygium is a rare triangular membranous fold. The fold's apex involves the cornea, while its base is continuous with the conjunctiva. Exposure to wind, dust and sun is thought to be etiologic.

Epibulbar dermoids and/or *lipodermoids* are present in children with *Goldenhar syndrome* (oculoauriculovertebral dysplasia) along with auricular appendices, preauricular fistulas and vertebral anomalies. The dermoid is a yellow or white, flat or ellipsoidal lesion usually seen at the corneal margin in the lower outer quadrant. The lipodermoid is usually noted in the upper outer quadrant.

Feingold, M., and Baum, J.: Goldenhar's syndrome. Am. J. Dis. Child. 132:136, 1978.

SCLERA

The sclerae of infants and young children are usually bluish. Blue sclerae are also seen in patients with osteogenesis imperfecta, glaucoma and in the Russell-Silver's, Ehlers-Danlos, Hallermann-Streiff and Marfan's syndromes.

Melanin deposits in the form of nevi or freckles are frequently seen in the sclera. Ota's nevus may cause small patches or almost complete blue "spilt ink" staining of the affected eye. Hyperpigmentation of the orbit may also occur.

Fikar, C. R., and Lee, M. A.: Picture of the month: Ota's nevus. Am. J. Dis. Child. 134:1083, 1980.

Icterus may first be evident in the sclera. Pigmentation associated with carotenemia is manifest in the skin but not in the slcera.

CORNEA

The cornea in newborn infants has a diameter of 9 to 10 mm. Between 6 and 12 months of age, the cornea reaches the adult size of about 12 mm.

Congenital anomalies of the cornea include abnormalities of size and curvature. A cone-shaped cornea is a rare anomaly. Hereditary abnormal eye enlargement *(megalocornea or macrophthalmia)* occurs almost exclusively in boys. The diameter of the cornea and depth of the anterior chamber are increased. The pupil is contracted, the iris may be tremulous and the lens subluxated.

Primary or *congenital glaucoma* is usually present bilaterally at birth, but may begin insidiously in the first year of life. The diameter of the cornea increases to greater than 10.5 to 11 mm and may be cloudy. Depth of the anterior chamber also increases. Dilatation of the pupil occurs, and the sclerae appear thin and bluish-white. The cornea may appear clear, hazy or white. Photophobia, epiphora or excessive lacrimation and blepharospasm, usually the earliest symptoms, may be present for weeks before corneal hazing and enlargement are noted. *These findings should always arouse suspicion of congenital glaucoma.* In infants under one year of age, photophobia is the first sign of congenital glaucoma in 50 per cent of cases. Because the eye often appears red and irritated, glaucoma may intially be confused with conjunctivitis.

Some patients with unilateral glaucoma also have an ipsilateral capillary hemangioma (Sturge-Weber syndrome). Lowe's syndrome in males is characterized, in part, by glaucoma and cataracts along with mental retardation, hypotonia and aminoaciduria. Glaucoma also occurs in homocystinuria, retinoblastoma, congenital anirida, neurofibromatosis, tuberous sclerosis and congenital rubella. It may occur in the Stickler and the cerebrohepatorenal syndromes and as a complication of retinopathy of prematurity.

In the systemic mucopolysaccharidoses, corneal clouding occurs in these syndromes: Hurler's, Morquio's, Scheie's, Hurler-Scheie, Maroteaux-Lamy's and beta-glucuronidase deficiency (MPS VII). The lysosomal storage diseases associated with corneal clouding include GM$_1$ gangliosidosis and mannosidosis. Corneal clouding also occurs in the mucolipidoses. Corneal opacities or haziness, best visualized with the slit lamp, may occur in children with cystinosis owing to the deposition of cystine crystals in the cornea. In the newborn, birth trauma with contusion of the eye, rupture of Descemet's membrane and edema of the cornea may cause transient corneal clouding. Unilateral corneal opacity always raises the possibility of congenital glaucoma.

Interstitial keratitis owing to congenital syphilis may occur during the latter half of the first decade. Initially, involvement is usually unilateral. The cornea is cloudy, ground-glass and reddish-gray in appearance. Photophobia, blepharospasm and lacrimation may be intense. Injection of the ciliary vessels occurs around the limbus of the cornea. Uveitis may also develop.

Corneal ulceration caused by the herpes virus is characterized by a grayish or yellow infiltration of the cornea, conjunctival and ciliary injection, intense pain, photophobia, lacrimation and blepharospasm.

Corneal hypesthesia is present in children with familial dysautonomia. The corneal reflex is absent.

Corneal arcus is usually present by age 10 in children with familial hypercholesterolemia.

PUPILS

Pupillary contraction, blinking and eyelid closure occur in normal newborn infants in response to bright light; however, the pupil at rest is small and contracts or dilates more slowly than in older infants or children.

A *unilateral contracted pupil* indicates involvement of the cervical sympathetic chain. The pupil reacts to light and dilates with instillation of a cyloplegic drug. *Horner's syndrome* consists of constriction of the pupil, slight drooping of the upper lid, and enophthalmos. Vasodilatation and anhidrosis may occur on the involved side. A cervical neuroblastoma may cause Horner's syndrome.

Oculosympathetic paralysis, characterized by a slight ptosis of the upper eyelid and miosis of the ipsilateral pupil, may occur as a complication of acute otitis media. Unequal pupil size is more evident in dim than in bright light. The pupillary reaction to light is normal.

Peri- or intraventricular hemorrhage in the newborn, if catastrophic in character, causes nonreactive pupils and the absence of extraocular movements.

Because of the importance of the comparative size and activity of pupils in children who have sustained a head injury, mydriatics should not be used. Asymmetry of the pupils indicates unilateral brain damage. Dilatation of one pupil suggests ipsilateral, localized intracranial hemorrhage.

Mydriasis, loss of pupillary light reflexes and doll's eye phenomenon in the first 12 hours of life may be associated with *poisoning with mepivacaine or lidocaine* used in local anesthesia for episiotomy or for paracervical, pudendal or epidural maternal anesthesia.

Dilatation of the pupil may occur in *retinoblastoma,* along with a yellow to gray-green, "cat's eye" pupillary reflex, visual impairment and squinting.

Glaucoma is characterized by dilatation of the pupil.

Pupils respond poorly to light in patients with botulism.

The pupils are widely dilated as a result of atropine or Jimson weed poisoning; overdosage of tricyclic antidepressants; use of amphetamines, cocaine or some hallucinogens; and with narcotic withdrawal.

Adie's syndrome (tonic pupil), a rare childhood finding, occurs in some children with familial dysautonomia or after a neurotropic viral infection. The characteristic finding is unilateral pupillary dilatation, which slowly increases in the dark. Conversely, the pupil will contract in bright light, often after a delay of minutes, and then return to its original size when the light is removed. Pupillary contraction during accommodation-convergence for near vision occurs slowly, but may be marked. Absence of tendon reflexes, especially the ankle jerks, and segmental hypohydrosis may be associated phenomena.

The *Marcus Gunn* pupil occurs with neuritis or optic nerve tumor. With the child looking at a distant target, a flashlight is moved slowly and rhythmically from pupil to pupil. With direct stimulation of the normal eye, the pupils of both the direct and consensual eye contract; however, with stimulation of the visually impaired eye, both pupils dilate rather than constrict. Esotropia may also be present in the affected eye.

Enlarged pupils may occur during migraine episodes.

Pineal tumors may be accompanied by Argyll Robertson pupils. Dilatation and inequality of the pupils and impaired reaction to light may be noted in children with brain stem tumors.

Miosis in comatose patients may follow ingestion of narcotics, barbiturates, phenothiazines, ethanol, propoxyphene and phencyclidine.

Nonreactive miosis occurs with organophosphate insecticide poisoning. A dilated, poorly reactive pupil in an unresponsive child raises the possibility of herniation of the uncus of the *temporal lobe*. Bilateral, *dilated and fixed pupils* unresponsive to light indicate damage to cranial nerve III owing to transtentorial herniation, brain stem compression and death. Marked but transient anisocoria may occur during seizures.

A *"white pupil"* or *leukokoria* may be caused, in order of frequency, by cataracts, persistent hyperplastic primary vitreous, retinopathy of prematurity, retinal dysplasia, retinoblastoma and larval granulomatosis.

LENS

Cataracts are circumscribed, central opacities of the lens that cause a white pupillary reflex. Ophthalmoscopically, the cataract appears as an opaque density surrounded, if the cataract is not complete, by a red fundal reflex. The examiner should use a positive ophthalmoscope lens (+8 to +15) and stand a few inches away from the child. Microphthalmia may be present.

Congenital cataracts may be present at birth or appear in early infancy. Some are bilateral and complete; others bilateral, but incomplete; still others unilateral. With small central cataracts the infant may have some vision when the pupils are dilated, but not when they are constricted. Transient cataracts have been reported as an unusual finding in low birth weight infants.

Alden, E. R., Kalina, R. E., and Hodson, W. A.: Transient cataracts in low-birth-weight infants. J. Pediatr. 82:314, 1973.

Congenital rubella, toxoplasmosis, herpes simplex and cytomegalovirus infections may cause cataracts. Congenital cataracts may be inherited on an autosomal dominant basis. Fifty per cent of cataracts in infants are of sporadic, unknown etiology.

Systemic processes that may be accompanied by cataracts include galactosemia, galactokinase deficiency, hypoparathyroidism, aspartylglycosaminuria, Lowe's syndrome, osteopetrosis, diabetes, homocystinuria and mannosidosis.

Other disorders associated with cataracts include these syndromes: pachyonychia congenita, Hallermann-Streiff, Rothmund-Thomson, chondrodysplasia punctata (Conradi disease), incontinentia pigmenti, Cockayne, Marinesco-Sjögren's, Stickler, mandibulodysostosis, Marfan's, cerebrohepatorenal, Smith-Lemli-Opitz, trisomy 13, 18, 21 and Turner's.

High-dose, long-term systemic corticosteroid therapy may produce translucent posterior subcapsular cataracts. Uveitis and trauma to the orbit as in perforating wounds may also lead to cataract formation.

Congenital dislocation of the lens leading to myopia may occur in Marfan's syndrome and with homocystinuria. Patients with the *Marchesani syndrome* have a small spherical lens with associated myopia and glaucoma. The lens may also be dislocated. Other clinical features are short stature and stubby fingers.

Kohn, B.: The differential diagnosis of cataracts in infancy and childhood. Am. J. Dis. Child. 130:184, 1976.

RETROLENTAL MEMBRANES

Persistent tunica vasculosa lentis. During fetal life the hyaloid artery and its supporting connective tissue, which constitutes the tunica vasculosa lentis, passes through the vitreous and supplies blood vessels to the posterior surface of the lens. Uncommonly, part of this tissue persists in fullterm infants and produces a retrolental opacity which is most marked centrally and from which long ciliary processes extend peripherally. If part of the vitreous can be visualized, the persistent hyaloid artery may be seen. Involvement is usually unilateral, and some degree of microphthalmos may develop. Occasionally, a posterior cortical cataract results in complete opacity of the lens.

Persistent hyperplastic primary vitreous (PHPV) causes a white pupil in term infants owing to a retrolental fibrovascular mass. Involvement, usually unilateral, is present at birth. Bilateral PHPV may be associated with trisomy 13.

Persistent pupillary membrane appears in premature infants as a brown or gray filamentous strand which projects across the pupil from the anterior surface of the iris to the lens or across the lens to the opposite side of the pupil.

Retinal dysplasia (Reese) or *encephaloophthalmic dysplasia* (Krause) is characterized by a white pupil, retrolental membrane and, usually, by microphthalmia.

Retinopathy of prematurity is classified as to the location, the extent and the stage of retinopathy. Early changes in infants with retinopathy of prematurity can be seen only with indirect ophthalmoscopy.

The earliest evidence of retinopathy of prematurity usually appears between the second and fifth weeks of life; uncommonly in the first week. Peripheral retinal neovascularization is the earliest finding, followed by ingrowth into the vitreous. Dilatation of the retinal vessels, especially the veins, and tortuosity, especially of the arteries, then occur. Next, grayish-yellow elevations of the retina are evident at the extreme periphery. Fuzziness of the disk appears, and a grayish membrane owing to folds of detached retina can be noted in the retrolental space. A number of vitreous bands then develop. The mild proliferative stage of retinopathy of prematurity spontaneously regresses in some infants. The acute phase lasts through the third and fourth months and is followed by organization and cicatrization. Microphthalmos, enophthalmos and dark circles about the eyes are late manifestations.

An international classification of retinopathy of prematurity. Pediatrics 74:127, 1984.
McCormick, A. Q.: Retinopathy of prematurity. Cur. Probl. Pediatr. 7:3, 1977.

UVEAL TRACT

In *ciliary injection* the vessels radiate from the limbus toward the periphery and are not as brightly injected as in conjunctivitis.

The iris of newborn white infants is gray-blue, slate-colored or grayish-brown. In black and brown races the iris is brown or grayish-brown. The permanent color of the iris appears in about 50 per cent of infants by the age of six months and in the others by the end of the first year.

In children with *albinism* the iris is pink, pale blue or dull gray. The iris transilluminates well when the sclera is illuminated by a light in contact with the orbit. In *ocular albinism* only the eye lacks pigmentation. The choroidal vessels are easily seen through the low-pigmented fundus. Visual acuity is low, especially in bright light. Pendular horizontal nystagmus and photophobia are noted. Oculocutaneous albinism occurs in the Chédiak-Higashi syndrome.

"Salt and pepper" speckling of the iris (*Brushfield spots*) is noted in infants with Down's syndrome. However, the condition may occur in patients with other types of mental retardation, such as the cerebrohepatorenal syndrome, as well as in normal children.

In many patients with neurofibromatosis, pigmented or non-pigmented iris nodules (Lisch spots), visible to the naked eye or on slit lamp examination, occur bilaterally, especially after five years of age.

A child may normally have one blue and one brown iris. Some instances of *heterochromia*, however, are associated with a chronic, low-grade iridocyclitis and secondary cataract formation in the eye with the lighter-colored iris (heterochromic iridocyclitis of Fuchs). Heterochromia may be noted in Waardenburg's syndrome.

Heterochromia may be associated with a Horner's syndrome present at birth, with the ipsilateral eye remaining blue. In cervical or mediastinal neuroblastoma, the iris on the involved side may be lighter in color.

Jaffe, N., Cassady, J. R., Filler, R. M., Petersen, R., and Traggis, D.: Heterochromia and Horner syndrome associated with cervical and mediastinal neuroblastoma. J. Pediatr. 87:75, 1975.

Iridodonesis, a quivering movement of the iris, may be caused by dislocation of the lens in patients with Marfan's syndrome or homocystinuria.

Coloboma is a congenital notching or absence of part of the iris, lens, choroid or retina. A keyhole effect is produced in the iris. When the choroid and retina are affected, a depigmented area is noted on funduscopy. Colobomas occur in the focal dermal hypoplasia, trisomy 13 and Wolf-Hirschhorn syndromes.

The "cat eye" syndrome, in which a lower, vertical iridal and choroidal coloboma causes a slitlike pupil, is attributable to a translocation involving chromosome 22. A number of congenital anomalies are present, including preauricular pits, imperforate anus and congenital heart disease.

Freedom, R. M., and Gerald, P. S.: Congenital cardiac heart disease and the "cat eye" syndrome. Am. J. Dis. Child. 126:16, 1973.

Aniridia, or absence of the iris, is inherited as an autosomal dominant disorder. Nonfamilial aniridia may be associated with Wilms' tumor and neoplasms of the adrenal cortex and liver. Aniridia and hypoplastic iris also occur in Rieger's syndrome.

Haick, B. N., and Miller, D. R.: Simultaneous occurrence of congenital aniridia, hamartoma, and Wilms' tumor. J. Pediatr. 78:497, 1971.

The *Kayser-Fleischer ring,* a unilateral or bilateral, complete or incomplete, golden brown or grayish-green ring at the limbus of the cornea, may be seen in Wilson's disease, in some familial cholestatic syndromes, and in chronic active hepatitis with cirrhosis. The findings may be visible to the naked eye or with simple magnification. However, in some patients, slit-lamp ophthalmoscopy is required. The pigmentary deposits, which are most prominent at the 12 and 6 o'clock positions, are always present in the patient with neurologic findings. They may be absent, however, in those with hepatic disease.

The *"setting sun"* sign, in which the irises appear to sink beneath the lower eyelids when the infant is quickly lowered from a sitting to supine position, may occur in normal premature and some term infants. But it is also present in kernicterus, hydrocephalus, lesions of the brain stem and Laron's dwarfism.

Uveitis is termed *anterior* when the iris and ciliary body are involved; *posterior* when the choroid and retina are affected; and *panuveitis* when all components are included. This disorder may occur in systemic diseases such as sarcoidosis, rheumatoid arthritis, tuberculosis, syphilis, brucellosis, Crohn's disease or leptospirosis. Most instances, however, are idiopathic.

Iritis or *iridocyclitis* is characterized by a deep, perilimbal flush, and dulling and discoloration of the iris; a contracted, sluggishly reacting, irregular pupil; ciliary injection; photophobia; epiphora; impairment of vision; and ocular pain. The aqueous may be cloudy, and precipitates may appear on the posterior surface of the cornea. Exudates may be seen as opacities in the vitreous.

Iridocyclitis may occur as a complication of pauciarticular rheumatoid arthritis. Since early anterior uveitis may be asymptomatic, children with this form of rheumatoid arthritis should have slit-lamp examinations four times a year. The parents should be instructed to contact the physician promptly if photophobia, red eye, eye pain or decreased visual acuity occurs. Iridocyclitis may precede or follow joint symptoms.

The *uveomeningoencephalitic syndrome* (Vogt-Koyanagi-Harada) is characterized by uveitis, signs of meningeal irritation, other central or peripheral nervous system symptomatology, progressive whitening of hair and cyclashes (poliosis), vitiligo, alopecia, hearing impairment or tinnitus.

Behçet's syndrome is manifest by recurrent uveitis along with oral and genital ulcerations, meningoencephalitis, synovitis and cutaneous vasculitis.

Choroiditis and chorioretinitis produce chorioretinal atrophy characterized by irregular, white patches and clumps of black pigment. Toxoplasmosis, cytomegalic virus infection, syphilis and tuberculosis may be etiologic. When caused by a congenital infection, chorioretinitis may not be evident until weeks after birth. In some instances, the retinopathy is confined to the periphery, but macular involvement is more common. Toxoplasmosis may cause solitary, yellow-white or gray cotton-like patches. The Aicardi syndrome in girls consists of infantile spasms, mental retardation and chorioretinopathy characterized by discrete, yellow-white holes with sharp borders and little pigmentary change in the surrounding retina. Disseminated candidiasis in immunosuppressed patients may cause white "cotton-ball" areas of choreoretinitis. In endophthalmitis, which may occur as a complication of *Haemophilus influenzae*, type b bacteremia and meningitis, the anterior chamber is so cloudy that the fundus cannot be visualized.

O'Connor, G. R.: Manifestations and management of ocular toxoplasmosis. Bull. N.Y. Acad. Med. 50:192, 1974.

Willis, J., and Rosman, N. P.: The Aicardi syndrome versus congenital infection: Diagnostic considerations. J. Pediatr. 96:235, 1980.

Chorioretinal and vitreous degeneration occurs in the Stickler syndrome.

RETINA

Funduscopic examination is usually readily performed in the older child, and mydriatics permit adequate visualization in infants. In infants, sedation may be required, but a pacifier or moistened sugar nipple may facilitate the examination. An associate may hold the infant's head steady and retract one of the lids while the examiner retracts the other. Older children may be helped to hold their eyes reasonably fixed if the mother is asked to hold a colored object at an appropriate spot as a point of fixation. A brief respite is advisable if the examination is prolonged, since funduscopy may rapidly fatigue the child. Supporting the back of the child's head in the upright position or performing the examination with the child lying down may facilitate cooperation. To observe the peripheral fundus adequately in the newborn, 7 mm of dilatation is required. If a mydriatic is necessary, 2.5 per cent phenylephrine (Neo-Synephrine) or 1 per cent tropicamide (Mydriacyl) is a satisfactory agent.

Following some order in the examination of the retina is desirable. One may examine, in sequence, the disk, the vessels, the remainder of the fundus and the macular area. The macula appears as a dark, yellow-orange area lateral to and slightly below the optic disk. A bright light reflex is present around the fovea. The normal ratio of the caliber of the arterioles to that of the veins is 3:5.

Pulsation of the veins is present in most normal children. Disappearance of spontaneous venous pulsation is an early sign of papilledema. Venous pulsations in the retinal veins as they enter the optic nerve head indicate normal intracranial pressure. In infants the optic disks are pale, while in children they are light pink. The lateral portion of the disk is frequently pale, especially in children who are light-complexioned or anemic. This normal pallor is to be differentiated from that of optic atrophy. A partial or complete brown or black pigmented ring is commonly present around the border of the disk. The medial edge of the disk may normally appear somewhat fuzzy.

A funduscopic examination to rule out increased intracranial pressure should be routinely performed before lumbar puncture. Funduscopy is also important in children with impaired vision, convulsive disorders, retardation, microcephaly, headache, recurrent vomiting or other findings that suggest neurologic disease. In most instances differentiating between a normal and an abnormal fundus is not difficult; however, considerable normal variation exists, and, at times, such differentiation is difficult.

Retinal hemorrhage is seen commonly in the normal newborn infant as well as those with a hemorrhagic disorder. Preretinal and retinal hemorrhages occur in most children with a subdural hematoma. Hemorrhagic retinopathy accompanied by retinal exudates may be present in the shaken, abused child.

Tomasi, L. G., and Rosman, N. P.: Purtscher retinopathy in the battered child syndrome. Am. J. Dis. Child. 129:1335, 1975.

Retinal edema, hemorrhage and engorgement of the retinal veins may be caused by cavernous sinus thrombosis. Increased intracranial pressure, especially when sudden, may lead to subhyaloid (preretinal) hemorrhages. Retinal hemorrhages and exudates may occur in hypertension. Although fundus changes are uncommon in children with diabetes, capillary aneurysms and small round hemorrhages may appear. Retinal cytoid bodies resembling the cotton wool exudates seen in hypertensive disease and diabetic retinopathy may appear in lupus erythematosus and dermatomyositis.

Candida endophthalmitis in immunosuppressed children may produce blurred vision and "cotton-ball" areas of choreoretinitis.

Baum, J. D., and Bulpitt, C. J.: Retinal and conjunctival haemorrhage in the newborn. Arch. Dis. Child. 45:344, 1970.
Fruman, L. S., Sullivan, D. B., and Petty, R. E.: Retinopathy in juvenile dermatomyositis. J. Pediatr. 88:267, 1976.

The so-called *cherry red spot*, usually more of an orange-red colored area surrounded by a grayish-white areola, indicates involvement of the macula with GM_1 gangliosidosis, GM_2 gangliosidosis I (Tay-Sachs), GM_2 gangliosidosis II (Sandhoff's disease), infantile Gaucher's disease or Niemann-Pick disease. Macular cherry-red spots may also occur in patients with the cherry-red spot myoclonus syndrome (sialidosis, Type I), metachromatic leukodystrophy and mucolipidosis I. The macular area should be carefully examined in all infants in whom degenerative disease is suspected. In late infantile amaurotic idiocy, fine brown pigment replaces the macular light reflex. Macular changes may also occur in Alport's syndrome.

Menkes, J. H., Andrews, J. M., and Cancilla, P. A.: The cerebral retinal degenerations. J. Pediatr. 79:183, 1971.

Lipemia retinalis, characterized by a peculiar milky-white, pink, waxy appearance of the retinal vessels, rarely occurs in diabetic children and may be a finding in familial type I hyperlipoproteinemia.

Retinoblastoma usually appears during the first three to five years of life, generally as a unilateral, but often as a bilateral, gray or yellow-white, glistening vitreous mass. If the macula is involved, esotropia may be the first sign. Tortuous vessels and hemorrhage may be present on the surface of the neoplasm. Unless the tumor is small, a whitish appearance or a grayish-yellow reflex through the pupil or unilateral dilatation of the pupil may be noted. *Nematode endophthalmitis* caused by *Toxocara canis* may produce blindness, a white pupillary reflex and an intraocular tumor, findings that are suggestive of a retinoblastoma.

Rubella retinitis is characterized by unilateral or bilateral involvement of the posterior pole, especially the macula, with small, black, irregular masses or fine to gross pigmentary speckling.

Tuberous sclerosis causes a glistening, nodular, mulberry-like mass or oval, gray, flat areas in the retina. These lesions may be present in infancy. The retinal lesions of tuberculosis and neurofibromatosis may simulate those of tuberous sclerosis. *Retinal angiomatosis* (von Hippell's disease; the von Hippel-Lindau syndrome) is often associated with cerebellar as well as retinal involvement. One or more pairs of dilated and tortuous arterioles and veins may be followed from the disk into a peripherally placed, white tumor mass.

In glycogenosis Type I, multiple, bilateral, flat yellow lesions may be noted around the macula.

Retinitis pigmentosa is characterized by degeneration, atrophy and pigmentation of the retina. Night blindness results from progressive constriction of the visual fields. The Laurence-Moon-Biedl syndrome consists of retinitis pigmentosa, obesity, mental retardation, hypogenitalism and polydactyly. Retinitis pigmentosa also appears in Refsum's syndrome with polyneuritis and ataxia; Cockayne's syndrome with dwarfism and deafness; Usher syndrome with deafness; Kearns-Sayre syndrome with progressive external ophthalmoplegia and heart block; and Bassen-Kornzweig syndrome with acanthocytosis and abetalipoproteinemia.

Coat's disease (exudative retinitis) occurs in boys between the ages of eight months and eight years. Strabismus and a detached retina may be present.

Norrie's disease is a sex-linked recessive disorder consisting of retinal detachment, deafness and mental retardation.

Macular degeneration produces a reddish or pigmented atrophic area in the macula.

Eller, A. W., and Brown, G. C.: Retinal disorders of childhood. Pediatr. Clin. North Am. 30:1087, 1983.

PAPILLEDEMA

Papilledema is caused by increased intracranial pressure and edema of the nerve fibers as they cross the disk. The optic disk becomes blurred and elevated. Elevation of the disk is expressed by the number of diopters' difference in the ophthalmoscopic lenses used to see clearly a vessel or other area on the disk or elsewhere on the retina. The continuity of the vessels becomes interrupted at the edge of the disk. Engorgement of the retinal veins, loss of venous pulsation and hemorrhages on or around the disk occur as the process advances. Obliteration of the physiologic cup occurs and the blind spot increases. Secondary optic atrophy and impairment of visual acuity do not occur until papilledema has been present for a long time. With the onset of atrophy, swelling of the disk may recede.

Griffith, J. F., and Brasfield, J. C.: Increased intracranial pressure. Pediatr. Rev. 2:269, 1981.

Papilledema is most commonly secondary to such space-occupying lesions as tumor, tuberculoma, abscess or intracranial hematoma. Premature synostosis of the cranial sutures may be etiologic. Choking of the disk may also occur in patients with encephalitis, meningitis, Guillain-Barré syndrome, chronic vitamin A intoxication or lead poisoning, hypertensive encephalopathy, rarely with hypoparathyroidism, as well as in patients being treated with corticosteroids and in those with severe anemia or hypercapnia.

Bilateral papilledema may also be associated with *pseudotumor cerebri*, a syndrome in which the neurologic examination, electroencephalogram and computed tomography are normal.

Rothner, A., and Brujt, J.: Pseudotumor cerebri. Arch. Neurol. 30:110, 1974.

Papilledema is present in 90 per cent of children with *brain tumors*. Elevation of the disk is an almost constant finding with cerebellar neoplasms, but is much less frequent with a pontine glioma. Papilledema is usually bilateral. Unilateral differences are not of localizing value.

Papilledema, venous distention and tortuosity, retinal hemorrhages and cystic macular changes have been observed either separately or jointly in some patients with moderate to severe pulmonary disease owing to *cystic fibrosis* or cyanotic *congenital heart disease*.

Petersen, R. A., and Rosenthal, A.: Retinopathy and papilledema in cyanotic congenital heart disease. Pediatrics 49:243, 1972.

Optic disc edema may occur in *diabetes*.

Pavan, P. R., Aiello, L. M., Wafai, M. Z., Briones, J. C., Sebestyen, J. G., and Bradbury, M. J.: Optic disc edema in juvenile-onset diabetes. Arch. Ophthalmol. 98:2193, 1980.

Early differentiation of *true* and *pseudopapilledema* may be difficult. In pseudopapilledema, which occurs in about 5 per cent of the population, especially Caucasians, some blurring of the optic disk is present. Elevation of the disk, if it occurs, is central rather than peripheral as with true papilledema. The vessels demonstrate preretinal branching, the disk does not obscure the origin of the vessels, and venous pulsations are present. The blind spot is not enlarged. Since pseudopapilledema tends to be inherited, ophthalmologic examination of relatives may reveal others with similar blurring or anomaly of the disk.

Conditions that may be confused with papilledema include medullated nerve fibers, drusen or hyaloid bodies and papillitis. When *myelination of the optic nerve* continues beyond the usual termination at the optic disk, whitish-yellow, feather-edged areas may radiate from the disk into the retina. *Drusen* of the optic nerve, which are hyaline bodies in front of the lamina cribrosa that protrude through the disk, are the most common cause of pseudopapilledema.

OPTIC NEURITIS

Acute optic neuritis causes edema of the disk or papillitis. The ophthalmoscopic findings of optic neuritis and papilledema may be similar, and, at times, the two disorders cannot be differentiated. In optic neuritis, visual acuity is reduced early. A similar loss of vision does not occur until papilledema is advanced. Loss of vision in patients with acute optic neuritis may be largely central or complete. In the former, the retrobulbar pupillary reaction is present (e.g., pupillary contraction occurs in response to light), followed rapidly, with continued exposure to light, by dilatation. In the latter, the pupillary light reflex is absent. Visual acuity and visual fields should be obtained in patients who have edema of the disks. In optic neuritis, moderate elevation and haziness of the disk occur, and the vessels, especially the veins, are widened and engorged. The disk is also hyperemic and may be covered by exudate and hemorrhages. Edema of the disk in optic neuritis may increase initially; however, the swelling usually begins to disappear within two or three weeks, and pallor then becomes evident. In *retrobulbar neuritis*, which may occur as a side effect of the antituberculosis drug ethambutol, the disk may appear normal, but the patient has no vision in the affected eye. Secondary optic atrophy may occur.

Optic neuritis may occur as a complication of meningitis, chickenpox, measles, pertussis, mumps, influenza and, possibly, infectious mononucleosis. The condition has also been reported to follow diphtheria immunization and to be associated with lead poisoning. Multiple sclerosis in children may begin with optic neuritis.

Neuromyelitis optica, an uncommon condition in childhood, is characterized by gradual vision impairment that may progress to total blindness. Neurologic findings, which may precede or follow ocular symptoms, may simulate transverse myelitis. The patient's difficulty in walking and talking may also suggest multiple sclerosis. Cerebrospinal fluid examination reveals elevation of protein, cells and pressure. Usually, normal vision returns after some weeks. The neurologic symptoms may, however, recur.

OPTIC ATROPHY

With optic atrophy the disk is almost completely white, the margins well-demarcated and the vessels and lamina cribrosa normal. Impairment of visual acuity and visual field defects also occur. Pallor of the disk, in itself, is not a reliable criterion for the diagnosis of optic atrophy in young children since the disks are normally pale at that age, and other factors may cause the pallor. Distinction between primary and secondary optic atrophy may be impossible on ophthalmologic examination.

Optic atrophy may occur with tuberous sclerosis, Hurler's syndrome, toxoplasmosis, GM_1 gangliosidosis, Tay-Sachs disease, Schilder's disease, Krabbe's disease, Pelizaeus-Merzbacher's disease, premature synostosis of the cranial sutures, osteopetrosis, craniometaphyseal dysostosis (leontiasis ossea), craniopharyngioma, optic glioma, Friedreich's ataxia, Cockayne syndrome, Conradi's disease, intracranial hemorrhage, hydrocephalus, lead poisoning, thallium intoxication, optic neuritis or retrobulbar neutritis. Optic atrophy, high frequency hearing loss and diabetes insipidus may occur in association with juvenile diabetes mellitus.

Gunn, T., Borttolussi, R., Little, J. M., Anderman, F., Fraser, F. C., and Belmonte, M. D.: Juvenile diabetes mellitus, optic atrophy, sensory nerve deafness, and diabetes insipidus—a syndrome. J. Pediatr. 89:565, 1976.

Optic nerve hypoplasia is characterized by a pale or gray optic disk, one-third to one-half normal size, surrounded by a proximal, mottled, yellow halo encircled by a darkly pigmented ring. Presenting complaints are impaired vision, searching-eye movements and strabismus.

Margalith, D., Jan, J. E., McCormick, A. Q., Tze, W. J., and Lapointe, J.: Clinical spectrum of congenital optic nerve hypoplasia: Review of 51 patients. Dev. Med. Child. Neurol. 26:311, 1984.

Central loss of vision may be the first clinical manifestation of central nervous system degenerative disease.

STRABISMUS

Strabismus represents nonparallelism of the visual axes in the various fields of gaze. Ocular deviation is a common and physiologic occurrence in infants three to six months of age before coordinated ocular movements develop. Occasionally, the deviation is so definite or constant that a true squint can be diagnosed sooner and an ophthalmologic consultation obtained. Up to 18 months of age, transient unilateral deviation of an eye may normally occur for a few seconds. After this time, however, such deviation is not normal. The flat, relatively wide naso-orbital configuration of young infants may create the illusion of an internal strabismus. If constant or intermittent strabismus persists, an ophthalmologic consultation should be obtained.

Conditions which may predispose to strabismus include muscular defects, hyperopia, cerebral injury, differences in the refractive power of the two eyes, impairment of fusion ability and hereditary factors. An eye with impaired vision will tend to deviate inward in young children and outward in older children. Infants with cerebral palsy may demonstrate strabismus. Strabismus may occur suddenly with intracranial hemorrhage, abscess or tumor, encephalitis, the Guillain-Barré syndrome, tuberculous meningitis, diphtheria, measles, lead poisoning and myasthenia gravis. Transient strabismus may occur with hypoglycemia. The sudden appearance of strabismus suggests the possibility of an intracranial, intraocular or intraorbital tumor. Unilateral or bilateral esotropia, often observed in children with intracranial tumors, may cause diplopia. Usually the increase in intracranial pressure is well-established before it causes strabismus owing to pressure on the abducens nerve.

External ophthalmoplegia, ataxia and absent or decreased deep tendon reflexes may be noted in Fisher's syndrome. Ophthalmoplegia with diplopia may occur in botulism. Extraocular palsies also occur in Leigh's syndrome and in some older children with chronic cholestasis.

Ophthalmoplegic migraine consists of episodes of severe pain involving the eye, forehead or hemicranium followed by ipsilateral third nerve palsy with mydriasis, ptosis and possibly paresis of the cranial nerves IV and

VI. The ophthalmoplegia may persist for several days.

Raymond, L. A., Tew, J., and Fogelson, M. H.: Ophthalmoplegic migraine of early onset. J. Pediatr. 90:1035, 1977.

External ophthalmoplegia may be caused by echo 9 viral infection and by ocular myopathy or neuropathy. The Kearns-Sayre syndrome consists of external ophthalmoplegia, ptosis, retinitis pigmentosa, cerebellar signs and complete heart block. Impaired extraocular muscle function (orbital apex syndrome) may occur with orbital infarction in sickle cell disease.

Because of pressure on the corpora quadrigemina, patients who have a pineal tumor may be unable to elevate their eyes. This finding may also be present with tumors of the cerebellum, the fourth ventricle, the pons and the diencephalon or with diencephalic, midbrain or cerebellar herniation owing to increased intracranial pressure. Tumors of the pons may cause paralysis of conjugate movement of the eyes. Deviation of one eye upward and laterally and the other downward and medially (skew deviation) suggests the presence of a neoplasm in the posterior fossa. Paralysis of the ipsilateral third nerve may follow temporal lobe herniation. Rarely, a congenital aneurysm may cause ophthalmoplegia.

A phoria or tendency for strabismus may become converted to a tropia or manifest strabismus when a child is tired, emotionally disturbed or acutely ill.

Classification of Strabismus

Esotropia—convergent strabismus (eye turns medially)

Exotropia—divergent strabismus (eye turns laterally)

Hypertropia—upward deviation of the eye

Hypotropia—downward deviation of the eye

Esophoria—tendency to converge

Exophoria—tendency to diverge

Concomitant (nonparalytic) strabismus is characterized by a constant angle of deviation of the eyes in all fields. Concomitant strabismus may be congenital or precipitated by a febrile illness, head injury, fatigue or emotional upset. In *incomitant or paralytic strabismus,* the angle of deviation of the visual axes is not constant in all directions but increases in the direction of movement normally produced by the paretic muscle. The paralysis may be congenital or acquired. *Constant (monocular) strabismus* is constantly present in the nonfixing eye. In *alternating strabismus* the eyes alternate in fixing and squinting. Esotropia is usually an alternating type of strabismus. Children with monocular strabismus, even though the deviation is barely detectable, are at risk for amblyopia.

Since accommodation and convergence are closely associated movements, overactivity of the internal rectus muscle may lead to esotropia when the eye attempts to accommodate for a refractive error. Hyperopia is thus a common cause of convergent concomitant squint, which may become apparent during infancy or in early childhood. When first noted, the strabismus may be intermittent; later, it becomes constant and is either monocular or alternating in character. Impairment of fusion is an important factor in this development. Although myopia may be present in patients with convergent concomitant strabismus, this refractive error is usually associated with the less common divergent concomitant strabismus.

Screening Tests for the Detection of Strabismus. FRANK STRABISMUS (TROPIA). The child is asked to look at an otoscope light held about 13 to 15 inches in front of his eyes; meanwhile, the examiner, seated in front of the child, sights the position of the light reflex on the subject's pupil. The reflex should fall nearly in the center of each pupil. In children with strabismus, the reflex falls somewhere between the center of the pupil and the limbus. If lateral displacement of the reflex occurs, the patient has a convergent squint; with medial displacement, a divergent strabismus exists. To evaluate the presence of strabismus when fixing on distant objects, the child is asked to look at a toy or Snelling chart 20 feet away. The examiner then determines the position of the light reflex. When one eye appears to be deviant, the other may be covered with a card. If the uncovered eye has been convergent, it will then move temporally. If divergent, it will move nasally. If no movement occurs, strabismus is not present.

TENDENCY TO STRABISMUS (PHORIA). The child is asked to focus on a close and then a distant target straight ahead and then up and down with both eyes uncovered. One eye is then covered with a card. When the card is removed, the examiner observes any eye movement. When a phoria is present, the eye will move from the convergent or divergent position assumed when covered to its original fixing position. If a child objects to occlusion of one eye, amblyopia may be present in the other.

Reinecke, R. D.: Current concepts in opthalmology: Strabismus. N. Engl. J. Med. 300:1139, 1979.

The oculomotor nerve also supplies the levator palpebrae superioris, the ciliary muscle and the sphincter of the pupil. The dilator of the pupil is supplied by sympathetic fibers. In older patients, diphtheritic neuritis may produce dysfunction of the ciliary muscle with resultant inability to read or do other work that requires close accommodation. Patients receiving large doses of hydantoin may have difficulty with accommodation.

Head tilting or *ocular torticollis* may follow impaired function of the superior oblique. The head is tilted to the side opposite the involved muscle.

Infants with athetosis secondary to kernicterus are often unable to move their eyes upward and downward.

Bell's phenomenon is the automatic upward rotation of the eyes when the patient closes or, in the case of facial paralysis, attempts to close his eyes.

Third nerve palsies lead to ipsilateral ptosis, dilatation of the pupil and exotropia.

Ataxia-telangiectasia may be characterized by a pseudopalsy in which the child is unable to make rapid eye movements. The eyes tend to turn up on focusing.

VISUAL FIELDS

Examination of the visual fields is indicated when edema of the optic disks is present or an intracranial space-occupying lesion is suspected. The confrontation test may be used as a screening examination. A more exact delineation of the visual fields requires the use of a perimeter. In the confrontation test the patient, seated about three feet from the examiner and with his back to the light, is asked to cover one eye and to look with his uncovered eye toward the examiner's opposite eye. Using his finger or a small object, the examiner moves the test object from outside the patient's visual field toward his line of focus, keeping the object about 20 inches from the patient's eyes. This movement is performed in each of the principal meridians. Constriction of the visual fields may be noted in some patients with conversion disorder. Enlargement of the blind spot is an absolute criteria of papilledema. In children four to five years of age, finger counting may be used in which the child is requested to hold up the same number of fingers as the examiner. Quantitative perimetry may be used after five to seven years of age.

DIPLOPIA

Diplopia may occur in the Guillain-Barré syndrome, encephalitis, myasthenia gravis, pseudotumor cerebri, botulism, Fisher syndrome, Sydenham's chorea and central nervous system leukemia. An intracranial tumor is a diagnostic possibility when diplopia is precipitated by an acute paralytic strabismus. Transient diplopia may occur secondary to a stroke in a child with sickle cell anemia. A child in whom double vision has suddenly developed may rub his eyes or squint, as if photophobia were present, but he will not object to the ophthalmoscope light as he would with photophobia. Patching one eye relieves the child of the disturbing double vision. Diplopia may occur in patients receiving hydantoin or with a blowout fracture of the orbit. Vertebrobasilar occlusive vascular disease or basilar artery migraine are characterized by intermittent episodes of diplopia, vertigo, nausea, vomiting and mental confusion.

DeVivo, D. C., and Farrell, F. W.: Vertebrobasilar occlusive disease in children. Arch. Neurol. 26:278, 1972.

PHOTOPHOBIA

Photophobia may be noted in the following conditions:
Measles
Rocky Mountain spotted fever
Vernal conjunctivitis
Foreign body
Iridocyclitis owing to injury, bacterial infection or systemic illness
Corneal ulcer
Phlyctenular keratitis
Interstitial keratitis
Chronic idiopathic hypoparathyroidism
Xeroderma pigmentosa
Albinism
Cystinosis
Congenital glaucoma. *Photophobia may be the initial symptom.*
Migraine headaches
Acrodermatitis enteropathica
Exposure to bright light
Botulism
Toxic shock sydrome
Photophobia, partial albinism, atypical granules in the leukocytes and recurrent infections characterize the *Chédiak-Higashi syndrome.*

NYSTAGMUS

Nystagmus is a rhythmic, usually rapid movement of the eyes which may be horizontal, vertical, rotatory or mixed. The tremor may be about equal in rate in all directions (*pendular nystagmus*) or have a quicker movement or component in one direction than in the other (*jerk nystagmus*). The direction in which the fast component occurs is used to signify the direction of the nystagmus. The slight oscillating or nystagmoid movement (*end-point nystagmus*) with the fast component in the direction of gaze, which often occurs normally when children look out of the far corners of their eyes, is not true nystagmus.

The etiologic factors in nystagmus may broadly be regarded as neurologic, vestibular or ocular. In vestibular and neurologic disturbances, jerk nystagmus is usually present. Ocular defects are generally associated with the pendular type.

Ocular causes of nystagmus include cataracts, retrolental fibroplasia, astigmatism or other refractive errors, albinism, and weakness of the extraocular muscles. An unexplained congenital type of nystagmus may occur. Persistent vertical or horizontal nystagmus may be associated with intraventricular hemorrhage in preterm infants. In infancy, pendular nystagmus and wandering of the eyes in an aimless searching fashion suggest a visual defect. Ocular nystagmus may not be present, however, when total blindness has existed since birth or early infancy.

Vestibular causes of nystagmus, usually associated with labyrinthitis or other labyrinth disease, are discussed on page 345.

Neurologic disorders associated with nystagmus include encephalitis, tuberculous meningitis, Friedreich's ataxia and Werdnig-Hoffman disease. Nystagmus caused by an intracranial tumor suggests an infratentorial rather than supratentorial location. Nystagmus, usually on horizontal gaze, is present in most patients who have a posterior midline cerebellar tumor and is frequently found with tumors of the cerebellar hemispheres. This type of nystagmus is usually not spontaneous, as is common with vestibular disturbances, but develops when the patient focuses upon some point (*fixation nystagmus*). When the patient looks toward the side of the tumor, the nystagmus is slow and coarse. When the gaze is toward the opposite side, nystagmus is either not present or is quick and minimal. In patients with a brain stem tumor, nystagmus is often noted on horizontal and, occasionally, on upward gaze, Nystagmus may occur with cerebral palsy or organic brain damage. It may also be associated with systemic infections and drugs (e.g., large doses of hydantoin). Fixation nystagmus is seen in ataxiatelangiectasia. Cog-wheel rotatory nystagmus, delayed head control and head nodding are seen in Pelizaeus-Merzbacher disease. Nystagmus also occurs in the craniofacial dysostosis and cerebrohepatorenal syndromes.

Spasmus nutans, or nodding spasm, is an uncommon disorder that occurs chiefly during the latter half or two thirds of the first year in infants who have received relatively little environmental stimulation. The infant's history may also indicate inadequate environmental lighting. The principal symptom is periodic, slight, up-and-down or side-to-side nodding or rolling of the head that is most prominent when the infant is in the sitting position and tends to disappear when supine. These movements occur once or twice a second for either brief or prolonged periods. Unilateral or bilateral, intermittent, rapid nystagmus may appear some weeks before the nodding. Spasm nutans must be differentiated from similar symptomatology caused by tumors of the hypothalamic and chiasmal areas.

Antony, J. H., Ouvrier, R. A., and Wise, G.: Spasm nutans: A mistaken identity. Arch. Neurol. 37:373, 1980.

Opsoclonus ("dancing eyes"), characterized by rapid, chaotic, irregular jerking of the eyes in all planes, but mainly horizontal, may be associated with occult neural crest tumors, especially neuroblastoma. In the Kinsbourne syndrome in infants or young children, opsoclonus is accompanied by myoclonic ataxia and extreme irritability.

Moe, P. G., and Nellhaus, G.: Infantile polymyoclonia-opsoclonus syndrome and neural crest tumors. Neurology 20:756, 1970.

Roving eye movements, nystagmus and extreme hyperactivity may be caused by *scorpion envenomation.*

Rimsza, M. E., Zimmerman, D. R., and Bergeson, P. S.: Scorpion envenomation. Pediatrics 66:298, 1980.

The *doll's eye phenomenon* or oculocephalic reflex is present in the first 10 days of life and disappears shortly thereafter. With the infant in the supine position, the baby's eyes lag behind when the head is turned gradually from side to side. Loss of eye movement on the doll's head maneuver may be secondary to neonatal drug intoxication owing to a local maternal anesthetic agent or to intraventricular hemorrhage. The doll's eye maneuver may also be used in the evaluation of the older comatose child. Holding the patient's head first in a neutral position and with the eyelids held open, the examiner quickly rotates the head up and down and from side to side. In response to this maneuver, the eyes should move in a direction opposite to that of the head. Absence of doll's eye movements implies damage to the brain stem secondary to increased intracranial pressure and transtentorial herniation. Caution is advised if a possibility of a cervical fracture exists or if resistance is experienced to the head turning.

GENERAL REFERENCES

Coles, R. S.: Ocular manifestations of connective tissue disease. Hosp. Pract. 20:70, 1985.
Goldberg, M. E. (ed.): Genetic and Metabolic Eye Disease. Boston, Little, Brown and Co., 1974.
Harley, R. D.: Pediatric Opthalmology. Philadelphia, W. B. Saunders Co., 1975.
Helveston, E. M., and Ellis, F. D.: Pediatric Opthalmology Practice. St. Louis, C. V. Mosby Co., 1980.

4 / THE EARS

HEARING

Normally, the newborn infant reacts to loud, sharp and sudden noises either with a startle response or by crying. In the second month he may demonstrate transient cessation of activity in response to sound. A month or two later the sound of the mother's voice brings anticipation. The five- or six-month-old child with well-developed head control often turns his head toward the source of sound. Deaf infants, although visually aware and attentive, may demonstrate a generalized indifference to sound. The five- to six-month-old infant enjoys squealing and cooing. A monotonal quality, diminution or an absence of such sound experimentation suggests deafness.

When seeing infants during the first months of life, the physician should inquire about the infant's vocalizations and whether the parent believes that the infant can hear. In the older child, delayed speech development, difficulty in enunciating sibilants and a gradual loss of or a change in speech are indications for hearing appraisal. When hearing is lost, speech disappears within a matter of weeks. In the younger child, the disappearance is more rapid.

Deafness or hearing impairment in a young child may be difficult to diagnose. Deafness refers to hearing that is nonfunctional for ordinary purposes, even with a hearing aid. A *conductive* hearing loss is caused by a problem in the external or middle ear, while *sensorineural* or *nerve deafness* is attributable to a disorder medial to the stapes, e.g., in the inner ear, the auditory nerve or brain. A conductive hearing loss is seldom more severe than 60 decibels. A mixed hearing loss consists of combined conductive and sensorineural impairments.

An infant's ability to babble, perhaps to say "da-da," or apparently to notice the ringing of a telephone, the rumbling of a truck or similar noises does not assure adequate hearing for speech perception. His response to the slamming of a door may be tactile or proprioceptive rather than auditory. Young children with impaired hearing for the higher frequencies may appear to understand many words and even begin to speak. A child with a loss of 30 to 45 decibels will be able to understand conversational speech from 3 to 5 feet but will have difficulty if the sound is faint or the speaker's face not visible.

Some parents first suspect a problem when they walk, undetected, into a room while their infant is looking in another direction. The baby with hearing impairment appears startled when the parent finally comes into his line of vision. An infant with normal hearing and head control usually swings his head around almost instantly whenever someone enters the room.

Sometimes parents are concerned about a possible hearing loss because the child turns up the volume of the radio or television until the sound is very loud. Usually this is a normal activity and does not indicate the presence of a hearing loss; however, the possibility cannot always be immediately ruled out. A careful hearing assessment is important whenever one suspects hearing loss in an infant.

Matkin, N. D.: Early recognition and referral of hearing-impaired children. Pediatr. Rev. 6:151, 1984.

A child may be characterized as deaf if his hearing threshold across the speech frequencies is depressed 80 decibels in the better ear. Hearing impairment and deafness may be conductive or perceptive. Deafness may be genetic or acquired. Over 60 types of hereditary deafness exist, including autosomal recessive, autosomal dominant and sex-linked. Deafness may occur with diseases such as:

Alport's syndrome—hereditary nephritis and deafness
Congenital malformations of the ear
Hurler's syndrome; Hunter's syndrome
Keratopachydermia, digital constriction and deafness
Knuckle pads, leukonychia and hearing loss
Leopard syndrome
Osteogenesis imperfecta
Osteopetrosis
Pendred's syndrome of deafness and goiter
Recessive albinism
Retinitis pigmentosa (Usher syndrome)
Surdocardiac syndrome—characterized by deafness, electrocardiographic abnormalities (remarkably prolonged Q-T interval), syncopal attacks and sudden death
Treacher-Collins syndrome
Trisomies
Waardenburg's syndrome

Other children at risk of hearing loss include those affected by a maternal prenatal viral infection, such as rubella or cytomegalovirus; neonatal hyperbilirubinemia; cleft palate; micotia; atresia of external auditory canal; perinatal hypoxia; and those who weigh less than 1500 gm.

Acquired deafness may be caused by infections, such as measles, meningitis and mumps; ototoxic drugs (kanamycin, gentamicin); anoxia; and trauma. Deafness, usually severe and bilateral, or hearing impairment occurs as a complication of meningitis usually appearing on the first or second day in 3 to 30 per cent of patients. Hearing evaluation should be routinely accomplished on recovery from meningitis.

Dodge, P. R., et al.: Prospective evaluation of hearing impairment as a sequela of acute bacterial meningitis. N. Engl. J. Med. 311:869, 1984.
Kaplan, S. L., Catlin, F. I., Weaver, T., and Feigin, R. D.: Onset of hearing loss in children with bacterial meningitis. Pediatrics 73:575, 1984.

Serous otitis media is a common cause of a conductive hearing loss. Twenty-five per cent of children with cleft palates are estimated to have impaired hearing.

Infants and children with severe *mental retardation* may show little attentiveness or response to speech.

Unilateral sensorineural deafness may be associated in some children with deficits in auditory and psycholinguistic skills as well as educational difficulties.

Bess, F. H., and Tharpe, A. M.: Unilateral hearing impairment in children. Pediatrics 74:206, 1984.

Dysacusis is characterized by an ability to hear but not to discriminate sound. Discrimination impairment is an added handicap with neurosensory hearing losses.

Psychogenic deafness or *pseudohypacusis,* characterized by an indifference to speech, is a conversion disorder characterized by a discrepancy between the child's purported inability to hear ordinary conversation and his performance on repeated audiologic screening tests. The threshold response to pure tones and to voice is inconsistent. Because of their lack of speech response, psychotic children may be referred for a supposed hearing problem.

Veniar, F. A., and Salston, R. S.: An approach to the treatment of pseudohypacusis in children. Am. J. Dis. Child. 137:34, 1983.

HEARING TESTS

Evaluating the status of hearing in infants and young children is often difficult without careful observation over time and repeated hearing tests. Because of the complexity of the tests and the need for familiarity with their application, exact delineation of hearing loss in infants and children is usually a specialized procedure. Auditory brain stem response (auditory evoked potential) is a noninvasive technique that may provide a quantitative assessment of hearing status in infants and in children who are autistic, mentally retarded or unable to cooperate. This examination is also useful in the diagnosis of functional hearing loss.

The use of pure tones for testing may result in unreliable responses in infants and in many children under the age of three or four years. Tuning forks to test for air conduction or bone conduction in the young child are of no value. A watch is usually not a satisfactory screening tool because the ability to hear ticking, a high frequency sound, does not necessarily mean that speech perception is adequate.

Behavioral observation audiometry is used for hearing assessment in infants under 24 months of age. The *aural-palpebral reflex* refers to blinking of the eyes in response to an intense sound.

Turning of the head in response to a sound stimulus is another useful reflex (orientation or localization response) between the ages of five and nine months. A number of noise-producing devices, including dog and police whistles, a squeaky toy mouse, cup and spoon, cowbells, cymbals, tom-toms, tambourines and ratchets, may be sounded out of the child's sight as qualitative office tests of hearing in young children. Cessation of activity or reflex turning of the head and eyes indicates an ability to hear. Some quantitation can be obtained if the frequency and intensity of sound produced by these devices at various distances from the subject are known. Such assessment may be difficult unless the examiner has had extensive experience and the circumstances of the test are carefully controlled. Infants and young children normally respond to an auditory stimulus a few times, but they rapidly lose interest and then fail to do so.

The *conditioned reflex* or play audiometry is used as a hearing test in children above the age of 2½ years. A number of variations such as the peep show technique have been devised with the conditioned reflex as their basis. In some situations the child may be conditioned to react to various sounds with responses such as moving a block, pushing a button or picking up a ring and placing it on a stand when he hears the word "Go," which is stated at gradually decreasing intensities. Similarly, the child who understands some language may be seated at a table with a few familiar objects or a picture book and asked to "Show me the cow," and the like, the intensity of the request being varied each time. Use of the audiometer without conditioned reflex responses is generally not possible before the age of five years. Even then, pure tone testing does not always permit a complete evaluation of a child's ability to perceive speech.

Downs, M. P.: Auditory screening. Otolaryngol. Clin. North Am. 11:611, 1978.
Fria, T. J.: Assessment of hearing. Pediatr. Clin. North Am. 28:757, 1981.

Rinne's test compares loudness of sound from a vibrating 512-cycle tuning fork placed next to the external auditory canal and then held in contact with the mastoid process. A normal or positive Rinne is obtained when the child hears the sound twice as long by air as by bone conduction. A child with conductive hearing loss has difficulty hearing a 512-cycle tuning fork held near his ear but not when the handle is applied to the mastoid bone. With a sensorineural hearing loss, both air and bone sound conduction are reduced, more so through the latter. In addition to hearing loss, children with severe deafness have problems with speech discrimination.

The *Weber test* utilizes a vibrating 512-cycle tuning fork placed on the center of the forehead. In the presence of unilateral conductive loss, the sound will lateralize to the affected side. In unilateral sensorineural loss, the lateralization will be to the unimpaired ear.

Lesions of the vestibular branch of the auditory nerve may be detected by the use of the vestibular function tests described on page 115.

Bess, F. H.: Childhood Deafness. Causation, Assessment, and Management. New York, Grune and Stratton, 1978.

PINNAE

In the premature infant, the ears lie flat against the scalp with only slight incurving of the superior part of the pinnae occurring at about 33 to 34 weeks' gestation. Because the ear contains no cartilage in preterm infants, it remains folded when bent forward in early preterm babies. By 36 weeks of gestation, the pinna springs back after folding. Incurving has occurred over two thirds of the ear by 38 to 40 weeks' gestation.

Anomalies of the pinna, because they may be associated with deformities of the middle ear ossicles and a congenital hearing loss, are an indication for a hearing evaluation. Anatomic landmarks of the pinna are illustrated in Figure 4–1.

Jaffe, B. F.: Pinna anomalies associated with congenital conductive hearing loss. Pediatrics 57:332, 1976.

Preauricular papillomas or tubercles are caused by maldevelopment of the first branchial arch. Single or multiple in number, they occur on the cheek just anterior to the tragus and between the tragus and the corner of the mouth. Other anomalies of the external ear may be present, as in Goldenhar's syndrome.

Congenital aural fistulas or pits appear as unilateral or bilateral, pinpoint or slitlike openings from which a greasy, cheesy, white material can sometimes be expressed. The fistula is usually present immediately anterior and superior to the tragus or, more unusually, in the helix. Infection leads to inflammatory changes in the surrounding tissue.

A *darwinian tubercle* appears as a small nodule or thickening along the posterior segment of the helix near the tip of the auricle.

Abnormally protruding ears occur not infrequently. Patients with Marfan's syndrome may have prominent ears with pointing of the tips. Large, prominent ears are one of the phenotypic abnormalities in the *fragile X syndrome*.

Infants with *Down's syndrome* have small low-set ears measuring 3.4 cm or less in their greatest vertical axis. The superior helix of the ear may be turned downward more than normally, and this border may be straight instead of curved.

Soft blister-like lesions or swellings occur in the first few days or weeks in newborn infants with *diastrophic dwarfism*. Spontaneous resolution of the lesions occurs after three to four weeks, leaving cartilaginous

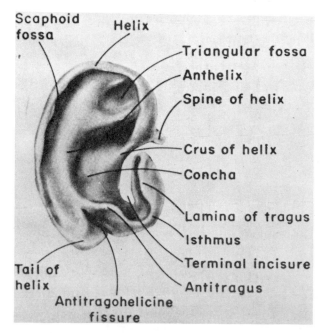

FIGURE 4–1. Anatomic landmarks of lateral aspect of right pinna. (From Jaffe, B. F.: Pinna anomalies associated with congenital conductive hearing loss. Pediatrics 57:332, 1976.)

thickening and deformity. The lesions may later calcify. Infants with *bilateral renal agenesis* may have low-set, large, and unusually floppy ears. Deformity of the pinna, microtia, atresia or stenosis of the external meatus and deafness may occur with the *Treacher-Collins* and *Goldenhar syndromes*. In the latter, the maxillary, temporal and malar bones are unilaterally hypoplastic. Blind fistulas and extra skin tags may occur between the tragus and the angle of the mouth. Preauricular pits and tags, imperforate anus, ocular colobomata, congenital heart defects and renal abnormalities (*cat eye syndrome*) is caused by a chromosome 22 translocation.

The ears may appear to be *low-set* in children with hydrocephalus and those with the following syndromes: Apert's, camptomelic; Carpenter's; cri du chat; DiGeorge's; fetal hydantoin; Hallermann-Streiff; leopard; Noonan's; Pierre Robin; Potter's; Smith-Lemli-Opitz; Treacher-Collins; trisomy 13, 18, and 21; Turner's; Williams; and Wolf-Hirschhorn.

Robinow, M., and Roche, A. F.: Low-set ears. Am. J. Dis. Child. 125:482, 1973.

Linear indentations of the ear lobes in the form of an inverted Y is a frequent finding in the *Beckwith-Wiedemann syndrome*. Notched ears may occur in the DiGeorge syndrome.

Tophi may occur in the ears of patients with the Lesch-Nyhan syndrome.

MASTOID

In infants with otitis media, the mastoid area should be examined for swelling and tenderness. With acute mastoiditis, the pinna is displaced forward, and the anteroposterior diameter of the meatus narrowed. Xanthomatosis is a rare cause of swelling in the mastoid region. Occasionally an enlarged lymph node is present over the mastoid area. Hemorrhage over the mastoid (Battle's sign) may occur with a basal skull fracture.

EXTERNAL AUDITORY CANAL

External otitis may be caused by bacterial or fungal infection. A history of water in the external auditory canal is usually obtained. Itching is the most common complaint, but exquisite pain may be present, especially if inflammatory edema occurs.

Tenderness may be elicited with movement or pressure on the tragus. A wet, slimy aural discharge may occur. Otitis externa is common in patients with the hyperimmune E recurrent infection (Job's) syndrome.

Marcy, S. M.: Infections of the external ear. Pediatr. Infect. Dis. 4:192, 1985.

A *foreign body* in the ear may cause a purulent or a serosanguineous discharge.

Cerumen, often in large amounts and sometimes impacted, may be softened with one or two instillations of hydrogen peroxide, warm sweet oil or light mineral oil. It may then be readily removed by washing gently with warm water providing no perforation has occurred and no polyethylene tubes are present. In the child above the age of five or six years, the cerumen may be cleansed out with a Waterpik or ear syringe once the procedure has been carefully explained and demonstrated to the child and he has been permitted to feel the stream of water against his palm. Cerumen may also be removed through an operating otoscope head with a Billeau earloop or spoon designed for the purpose. This procedure may be largely atraumatic in the older and cooperative child. However, because the skin covering the external auditory canal is highly vascular, the procedure may cause traumatic bleeding in infants and young children unless the patient is firmly restrained.

The *Ramsay Hunt syndrome* consists of herpes zoster of the auricle and external auditory canal with paralysis of the facial nerve which persists a few days to two weeks.

TYMPANIC MEMBRANE

The manner of holding the otoscope depends upon the examiner's preference. One method which permits flexibility of movement consists of grasping the upper end of the handle of the otoscope between the thumb and index finger so that the case rests on the metacarpophalangeal joint of the index finger perpendicular to the palm of the hand. Grasping the otoscope handle so that it is parallel to the palm does not permit the same range of motion. It is important that the illumination be bright.

In the examination of infants, it is critical that the head be held steady. The infant may be placed in the prone position with the head turned to each side and secured by the examiner's forearm while the examiner holds the otoscope in the other hand. A parent can hold an older infant against her chest, using one hand to hold the child's head tightly against her body while the examiner checks one ear, then turns the baby's head and checks the other.

In children, visualization of the tympanic membrane is facilitated if the auricle is pulled upward, outward and backward and if the speculum is directed anteriorly and superiorly. During infancy, the auricle should be pulled slightly downward. The speculum may have to be rotated slightly to permit visualization of the entire tympanic membrane. A sketch of the normal tympanic membrane with landmarks is presented in Figure 4–2. These are easily seen in the older child but may be less distinct in the infant. With a bulging drum, the malleus handle and short process are not evident, whereas with a retracted tympanic membrane, the short process is accentuated. The vertical and horizontal inclinations of the tympanic membrane observed in older children are greater in the early weeks of life, when the drum lies in an almost horizontal position with the postero-superior portion of the membrane nearest the examiner. Differentiating between the distal part of the external auditory canal and the proximal edge of the pars flaccida may be difficult.

On the first day of life, the tympanic membrane in the newborn is covered by vernix caseosa in the external canal. If the drum must be examined, this debris may be irrigated away with a small-tipped medicine dropper and light mineral oil. A 2- or 3-mm speculum should be used in the newborn.

Normally, the /eardrum is slightly concave, so absence of concavity or a bulge,

noted initially at the periphery, is consistent with increased air pressure, effusion or suppuration in the middle ear. Retraction of the drum may be attributable to negative air pressure or adhesions in the middle ear.

The ear drum is pearl gray or ground glass in color and not as translucent in infants as in older children. In young infants, the tympanic membrane may appear dull. The degree of luster or the presence or absence of a light reflex is not diagnostically helpful in determining the presence or absence of middle ear effusion or infection. Slight injection along the manubrium and the drum periphery may be noted in normal infants and children and slight generalized erythema may be induced by crying.

Otitis media occurs frequently in early life, especially between 4 and 12 months of age, but also may occur in the newborn. *Streptococcus pneumoniae* is the most frequent cause of acute otitis media. *Haemophilus influenzae,* usually nontypable, is frequently the etiologic agent in children under four years of age. Group A beta-hemolytic *Streptococcus* and *Staphylococcus aureus* are uncommonly involved. *Pseudomonas aeruginosa* and other gram-negative enteric bacilli may be associated with chronic or recurrent middle ear disease. Cultures of the nasopharynx or oropharynx are not helpful in determining the bacterial etiology in otitis media. Needle aspiration is recommended if (1) the child is critically ill; (2) chronic otitis media is present; (3) clinical response does not occur within 48 hours; or (4) the patient is immunodeficient. Otitis media is to be considered when children present with symptoms of ear pain, fever, irritability or screaming. Acute and persis-

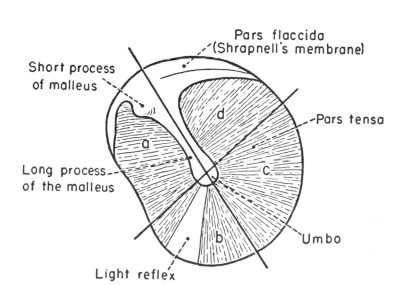

FIGURE 4–2. Diagram of left tympanic membrane. *a,* Anterior-superior quadrant; *b,* anterior-inferior quadrant; *c,* posterior-inferior quadrant; *d,* posterior-superior quadrant.

tent crying may be noted in infants with otitis media. Perforation of the drum and drainage may occasionally occur without pain. Some infants pull at the involved ear while others do not. Tugging at an ear or head shaking may be a habit rather than a sign of otitis media.

With suppurative otitis media, hyperemia or intense redness along the handle of the malleus, the periphery and pars flaccida of the drum occurs early. The color of the drum may be red, pale yellow or white. Later, it becomes diffusely opaque and may have an air-fluid level. With continuation of the process, bulging appears, usually first in the posterior-superior quadrant and then moving forward. Drum mobility is usually diminished.

The diagnosis of otitis media in the newborn is difficult since the symptoms of irritability, anorexia, vomiting, lethargy, cough, diarrhea or rhinorrhea are non-specific, and the tympanic membrane often normally looks dull, red and thickened. Since normally the short process of the malleus is almost always seen, its obliteration is diagnostic. Etiologic agents include *Escherichia coli, Staphylococcus aureus* and *Klebsiella pneumoniae.*

Gentle squeezing of the bulb of the pneumatic otoscope permits observation of the tympanic membrane's mobility in response to positive pressure; releasing of the bulb allows evaluation of the response to negative pressure. The ear drum normally moves inward with positive pressure and outward with negative pressure. To satisfactorily evaluate tympanic mobility, a close fit must be obtained in the external ear canal, and air must not leak around the lens frame or the attachment of the speculum. Rubber tubing slipped on the end of the ear speculum contributes to an air-tight seal between the external canal and the speculum. Fluid in the middle ear, scarring or adhesions impede drum mobility. A retracted drum usually does not move inward with positive pressure; but with negative pressure it moves somewhat outward.

In babies and young children, the diagnosis of otitis media is often difficult because of the presence of cerumen and because retraction or fullness and changes in color, translucency and mobility may be subtle. Tympanometry has been helpful in differentiating a normal middle ear from one with effusion in the evaluation of middle ear function in infants over 6 months of age in the office and in the clarification of uncertain otoscopic diagnoses. A flat curve may be demonstrated in children with middle ear effusion.

Paradise, J. L., Smith, G. G., and Bluestone, C. D.: Tympanometric detection of middle ear effusion in infants and young children. Pediatrics 58:198, 1976.

Scars, perforations or *retraction pockets* may also appear on the tympanic membrane.

Blebs or bullae (bullous myringitis) containing a serous or hemorrhagic fluid are occasionally noted on the tympanic membrane with acute otitis media owing to a bacterial or viral infection. At first glance, these may simulate a perforation. At other times, hemorrhagic flecks may be noted on the drum. Severe otalgia and hearing impairment may be associated symptoms.

Roberts, D. B.: The etiology of bullous myringitis and the role of mycoplasmas in ear disease: A review. Pediatrics 65:4, 1980.

Nonsuppurative otitis with effusion (serous otitis media) is a common cause of acute or chronic hearing loss. Although the older child may complain of a feeling of fullness or "water" in the ear, the disorder is usually asymptomatic. Hearing loss, often unsuspected, is usually detected on routine audiometric evaluation. The appearance of the tympanic membrane varies. Some retraction is usually present, but the drum may be normal or slightly bulging. A thickened, opaque tympanic membrane with obscured bony landmarks may be difficult to differentiate from a bulging drum. A fluid level or bubble may be present. The tympanic membrane, which may have an amber, pink, gray-white or bluish color, usually moves poorly.

A chronically draining ear may be observed with *histiocytosis. Rhabdomyosarcoma* arising in the ear may present with ear pain, chronic aural discharge, granulation tissue or polyp in the canal and facial paralysis.

Schwartz, R. H., Movassaghi, N., and Marion, E. D.: Rhabdomyosarcoma of the middle ear: A wolf in sheep's clothing. Pediatrics 65:1131, 1980.

Purulent conjunctivitis in infants and young children may be accompanied by otitis media.

Bodor, F. F.: Conjunctivitis—otitis syndrome. Pediatrics 69:695, 1982.

Chronic otitis media, an inflammatory process lasting more than three months, may be accompanied by a perforation or retraction pockets. In the child with a central perforation, the discharge is intermittent and usually associated with upper respiratory tract infections. With a retraction pocket or perforation in the posterosuperior portion or pars flaccida of the drum, a cholesteatoma may appear as a mass with ill-defined borders. White greasy flakes may be visualized in the perforation, and an intermittent foul-smelling discharge may be present. Hyperimmunoglobulinemia recurrent infection (Job's) and the immotile cilia syndromes may be characterized by recurrent or chronic otitis media.

In addition to their occurrence in patients with persistent otitis with effusion, *cholesteatomas* may occur with an intact tympanic membrane. Using a halogen-illuminated otoscope, the mesotympanic cholesteatoma is seen as a whitish or golden mass medial to the translucent ear drum. The intramembranous type, which has the appearance of a pearl-like cyst in the tympanic membrane, needs to be differentiated from a scar, prominent lateral process of the malleus or a posterosuperior retraction pocket.

Bluestone, C. D.: Recent advances in the pathogenesis, diagnosis and management of otitis media. Pediatr. Clin. North Am. 28:727, 1981.

Klein, J. O.: Middle ear disease in children. Hosp. Pract. 11:45, 1976.

Paradise, J. L.: Otitis media in infants and children. Pediatrics 65:917, 1980.

Rowe, D. S.: Acute suppurative otitis media. Pediatrics 56:285, 1975.

Schwartz, R. H., Grundfast, K. M., Feldman, B., Linde, R. E., and Hermansen, K. L.: Cholesteatoma medial to intact tympanic membrane. Pediatrics 74:236, 1984.

Tetzlaff, T. R., Ashworth, C., and Nelson, J. D.: Otitis media in children less than 12 weeks of age. Pediatrics 59:827, 1977.

OTHER EAR FINDINGS

Hemorrhage over the mastoid, bleeding from the ear or cerebrospinal otorrhea may indicate a basal skull fracture.

Tinnitus or *ringing* in the ears occurs with salicylism, the uveomeningoencephalitic syndrome, chronic otitis media with effusion, cerebellopontine tumors and basilar artery migraine. Tinnitus may precede eighth nerve damage secondary to prolonged kanamycin therapy.

Temporomandibular joint dysfunction or *myofascial pain dysfunction* may cause unilateral pain in the ear with radiation to contiguous areas.

Hyperacousia, or hyperreactivity to sound, is frequent in Tay-Sachs Type I, GM_1 gangliosidosis and Sandhoff's diseases. Opisthotonus, flexion of the upper extremities and extension of the lower extremities, occurs when these patients respond to a loud sound. Patients with tetanus or strychnine poisoning are also hyperreactive to sound.

GENERAL REFERENCES

Bluestone, C. D., and Stool, S. E.: Disorders of the Ear, Nose and Throat in Children. Philadelphia, W. B. Saunders Co., 1978.

5 / THE NOSE

Immediately after birth, the newborn's nose is frequently misshapen and flattened, with a septal deviation or subluxation. The columella is tilted, the tip of the nose is deviated, and the nasal alae are asymmetrical. Usually the normal shape is regained within a short time, either spontaneously or with gentle manipulation. Deformity of the nose and a short columella are frequent in the infant with a cleft lip.

Sneezing, a common occurrence in newborn infants, is generally interpreted as the infant's only method of effectively clearing his upper respiratory tract. Intractable sneezing may have a psychogenic etiology.

Bergman, G. E., and Hiner, L. B.: Psychogenic intractable sneezing in children. J. Pediatr. 105:496, 1984.

Flaring or movement of the alae nasi with respiration may occur in patients with pneumonia, peritonitis, hyperpyrexia, chest pain, acidosis, paralysis of the respiratory musculature and other causes of respiratory failure characterized by hyperpnea, tachypnea and dyspnea.

NASAL OBSTRUCTION

Obstruction of the nasal airway may be attributable to unilateral or bilateral *congenital closure of the posterior choanae.* A wisp of cotton held below the involved side does not move with respiration. Obstruction may be confirmed by attempting to pass a No. 8 French rubber catheter through the nose. Skull roentgenograms after instillation of a liquid contrast medium may confirm the clinical impression. Since infants are obligate nose breathers, sleeping with their mouths closed and breathing through their nose, patent nasal airways are important for normal respiration. Bilateral choanal atresia precipitates respiratory distress immediately after birth; unilateral choanal atresia causes few symptoms. The nasal obstruction may lead to irritability, cyanosis, dyspnea and difficulty in feeding. A persistent nasal discharge may be present, and a large amount of glairy, translucent, mucoid secretion may be removed from the involved nostril.

Nasal congestion may persist for several days in newborn infants whose mothers have received reserpine. A stuffy nose and rhinorrhea are characteristics of neonatal drug withdrawal. Hypothyroidism has also been reported as a cause of difficulty in infants' nasal breathing. Allergic rhinitis is a common cause of nasal obstruction in children. A horizontal nasal crease over the bridge of the nose occurs in children with allergic rhinitis or other chronic nasal congestion. Nasal congestion occurs in the immotile cilia syndrome. Stuffiness may be an adverse effect of beta-blockers and antidepressants.

Fibrous dysplasia of the facial bones is an unusual cause of bony nasal obstruction. Nasal obstruction may also be caused by an encephalocele or nasal glioma.

NASAL DISCHARGE

A unilateral, persistent nasal discharge accompanied by obstruction of the airway and, at times, a fetid odor may be caused by a foreign body or an imperforate choana. *Snuffles* is the term applied to the persistent and profuse mucopurulent or bloody nasal discharge in infants with congenital syphilis.

Persistent rhinorrhea occurs early in the Hurler syndrome. The differential diagnosis of persistent rhinitis includes vasomotor rhinitis, allergic rhinitis, recurrent viral infection and eosinophilic nonallergic rhinitis.

Meltzer, E. O., Zeiger, R. S., Schatz, M., and Jalowayski, A. A.: Chronic rhinitis in infants and children: Etiologic, diagnostic, and therapeutic considerations. Pediatr. Clin. North Am. 30:847, 1983.
Rupp, G. H., and Friedman, R. A.: Eosinophilic nonallergic rhinitis in children. Pediatrics 70:437, 1982.
Simons, F. E. R.: Chronic rhinitis. Pediatr. Clin. North Am. 31:801, 1984.

Wegener's granulomatosis or idiopathic lethal midline granuloma of the nose and face is a progressively destructive process characterized by persistent nasal discharge, crusted and pustular lesions, swelling, induration and, finally, ulceration of midline structures of the face, such as the nasal septum, inferior choanae, lip and hard palate.

CONGENITAL ANOMALIES

A flat, *depressed nasal bridge* or *saddle nose* may be noted with syphilis, Down's syndrome, congenital ectodermal dysplasia, craniometaphyseal dysostosis, congenital hypothyroidism, Conradi's syndrome, chondrodystrophy, Larsen's syndrome, osteopetrosis, cleidocranial dysostosis, Hurler's syndrome and Stickler syndrome.

The nose in chondrodystrophy and Hurler's syndrome may be somewhat large and *turned up* at the end with relatively large nostrils. The Smith-Lemli-Opitz syndrome is also characterized by a broad nose with upturned nares. The fetal alcohol and fetal hydantoin syndrome include a low nasal bridge with a short or upturned nose. A small nose and anteverted nares occur in the Aarskog syndrome. Wide, anteverted nostrils occur in 3-M slender-boned nanism. Hypoplastic alae nasi and a broad nasal tip occur in the femoral hypoplasia syndrome in some infants of diabetic mothers. Anteverted nostrils also are seen in patients with the DiGeorge syndrome.

A thin, *beaklike nose* occurs in patients with progeria and craniofacial dysostosis, including Apert's syndrome and pycnodysostosis. In the Hallermann-Streiff syndrome, the nose is thin, curved and pointed, giving a parrot-like facial profile. A beak nose is also seen in patients with Pfeiffer's syndrome, the Rubinstein-Taybi syndrome and with craniofacial dysostosis. The

Saethre-Chotzen syndrome is characterized by a beaked nose, craniosynostosis, ptosis of eyelids, brachydactyly and syndactyly.

Holoprosencephaly (arhinencephaly) may be characterized by a proboscis-like structure instead of a nose or a rudimentary nose that resembles that of the platyrhine monkey (cebocephaly).

Anosmia, or absence of smell, occurs in Kallman's syndrome along with hypogonadotropic hypogonadism and in some patients with the immotile cilia syndrome.

A *dermoid* may appear in the newborn period, infancy or during later development as a persistent small nodule, cystic swelling or dimple in the midline of the nose. A sinus tract may be present, and sebaceous material may be expressed.

An *encephalocele* may appear as a nasofrontal or nasoethmoid swelling over the bridge of the nose.

SINUSES

Although the sphenoid sinuses are present at birth, the ethmoid and maxillary sinuses are the clinically important ones during childhood. The frontal sinuses are usually not involved until ten years of age. During infancy, the ostia of the sinuses are relatively larger than later in life, so the sinuses usually become infected during an episode of acute rhinitis. This complication usually clears spontaneously.

Acute sinusitis is commonly characterized by a mucopurulent or serous nasal discharge, fever, headaches, facial or dental pain and malodorous breath. Cough, which may be of a barking quality, is present during the day and worse at night. Swelling of the upper eyelids may occur, most prominently on awakening. Acute ethmoid sinusitis may cause swelling of the periorbital region, especially medially. This swelling may initially be minimal and easily overlooked. Frontal sinusitis occasionally may be complicated by osteomyelitis of the frontal bone producing localized pitting edema.

Chronic sinusitis, unusual in children unless some other problem exists, may occur secondary to diving into water feet first, nasal allergy, cystic fibrosis, cleft palate, Kartagener's or the immotile cilia syndrome, choanal atresia, immunodeficiency disorders and Hurler's syndrome.

Veerman, A. J., VanDelden, L., Feenstra, L., and Leene, W.: The immotile cilia syndrome: Phase contrast light microscopy, scanning and transmission electron microscopy. Pediatrics 65:698, 1980.

Chronic sinusitis is associated with obstruction and a persistent or recurrent yellow, clear, mucoid, mucopurulent or purulent nasal discharge from above or below the middle turbinate. The inferior turbinates may be so engorged as to obscure the middle turbinates. Tenderness and swelling may be present over the affected sinus during acute exacerbations. Digital pressure over the sinus does not produce pain in chronic infections. Slight puffiness of the eyelids and dark circles about the eyes may be noted in children with chronic sinusitis. On gagging, a postnasal drip may be observed coming from the nasopharynx. Sinusitis may also be present without evidence of a nasal discharge.

Wald, E. R., Pang, D., Milmoe, G. J., and Schramm, V. L., Jr.: Sinusitis and its complications in the pediatric patient. Pediatr. Clin. North Am. 28:777, 1981.

Wald, E. R.: Acute sinusitis in children. Pediatr. Infect. Dis. 2:61, 1983.

EPISTAXIS

Epistaxis most commonly arises from Kiesselbach's area, the anastomotic site for a number of terminal arterioles, on the nasal septum about 0.5 cm within the nose and above the nasal floor. Varicosities that develop here under the thin mucous membrane are easily traumatized by nose picking and excessive drying of the mucous membrane, the most common causes of epistaxis.

Other causes of epistaxis include rheumatic fever, infectious mononucleosis, sickle cell anemia, systemic hemorrhagic disorders and prolonged instillation of phenylephrine. Hemangiomas and hereditary telangiectasis are more unusual etiologies. A chronic bloody nasal discharge may be caused by nasal diphtheria or a foreign body. Following an acute head injury, epistaxis or cerebrospinal fluid rhinorrhea may occur secondary to a basal skull fracture.

Juvenile angiofibroma of the nasopharynx, which usually develops after the age of ten years almost exclusively in boys, is characterized by progressive unilateral or bilateral nasal obstruction, mucoid or mucopurulent discharge and recurrent, severe epistaxis. The tumor may protrude into the nasal passages anteriorly or behind the soft palate. Olfactory neuroepithelial tumors may also cause nasal obstruction and recurrent epistaxis.

Sessions, R. B., Zarin, D. P., and Bryan, R. N.: Juvenile nasopharyngeal angiofibroma. Am. J. Dis. Child. 135:535, 1981.

Lymphoepithelioma, an uncommon malignant nasopharyngeal tumor, is characterized by unilateral, tender, cervical lymphadenopathy; epistaxis; trismus; and painful torticollis.

Pick, T., Mauer, H. M., and McWilliams, N. B.: Lymphoepithelioma in childhood. J. Pediatr. 84:96, 1974.

TURBINATES

The turbinates may be pale and boggy in children with *allergic or vasomotor rhinitis.*

Rhinitis medicamentosa, owing to chronic abuse of topical nasal decongestants, may cause a thickened, reddened and edematous nasal mucosa.

Nasal polyps are soft, glistening, smooth, pinkish-gray and movable. These may occur in children with sinusitis, allergic rhinitis or Kartagener's (immotile cilia) syndrome. Multiple, recurrent polyps frequently obstruct the nasal airways in children with *cystic fibrosis. Woake's syndrome* is characterized by nasal polyposis and bronchiectasis. A syndrome of nasal polyps, aspirin sensitivity and asthma may also occur. A nasal *glioma* may simulate a polyp.

Septal deviation and injury may result from trauma, even in the absence of epistaxis, edema or ecchymosis. Nasal trauma requires a careful examination for widening, hematoma, deviation or dislocation of the septum, mucosal tear, or protrusion of bone or cartilage.

Olsen, K. D., Carpenter, R. J., III, and Kern, E. B.: Nasal septal trauma in children. Pediatrics 64:32, 1979.

6 / THE MOUTH, PHARYNX, AND LARYNX

THE MOUTH

EXAMINATION

For young children, inspection of the oral cavity and pharynx is usually an unpleasant part of the physical examination. Consequently, it should be performed quickly, yet completely, and with minimal discomfort. Before examining the throat, one may ask to see the patient's teeth. A tongue depressor may then be introduced, and after examining the teeth, one may say, "Let's look way back there," and then examine the throat. Many children are able to open their mouths so widely and protrude their tongues so far that a tongue depressor is unnecessary. The procedure need not gag the patient, although gagging, at times, may be necessary to allow satisfactory visualization. Gagging may be avoided by asking the older child to breathe through his mouth during the examination. Some children have extremely active gag reflexes and tend to gag, and even vomit, when a tongue blade is placed on the back of their tongues. At times, the examination of the pharynx may be facilitated by first depressing one side of the base of the tongue and then the other. Examination of an infant's pharynx may be difficult because the infant often keeps his mouth tightly closed. In such event, one should wait until the infant relaxes his clenched jaws or cries. Actually, one may obtain a fair view of the mouth and part of the pharynx while the infant is crying. The posterior pharynx is not easily visualized in young infants. Forcing the mouth open or holding the infant's nose shut is both unnecessary and undesirable. During the examination of the pharynx, infants and young children may have to be held by a parent or nurse. The child's arms may be extended above and held tightly against his head. This may be accomplished best if the parent cups her fingers around the child's elbows and uses her thumbs to rest on and control the infant's head. In this position the child cannot move his head. After examination of the pharynx, the head may be turned to either side for the examination of the ears.

Good intraoral lighting is essential. A pocket flashlight or a large flashlight with a condensing or spotlight lens is satisfactory. Usually the otoscope light is not bright enough to permit good visualization. A small tongue blade may be used to facilitate inspection of various areas of the mouth. A compact, combined spotlight and tongue blade holder may be substituted for the otoscope head during the examination of the mouth. This attachment is helpful in that one hand is free to hold the child or to take a throat culture under direct vision.

In children with epiglottitis, examination of the pharynx using a tongue depressor is contraindicated because it may precipitate a respiratory arrest.

ORAL DEVELOPMENT

The *sucking and swallowing* reflexes are present in the term newborn infant but are poorly developed or absent in some premature infants. Failure to suck well and difficulty in swallowing may suggest cerebral injury or an inborn error of metabolism. Infants with oropharyngeal incoordination owing to neuromuscular impairment feed slowly, gag easily and choke. The extensor postures of the neck and trunk, which may occur in infants with cerebral palsy during breast or bottle feeding, may make feeding difficult. Frantic sucking behavior is noted in infants of drug-addicted mothers. In infantile botulism, sucking and swallowing may be impaired with resultant pooling of saliva.

During early infancy, semisolid food introduced into the anterior part of the mouth is often pushed out by the tongue. By two and one-half to three months, and sometimes earlier, neuromuscular maturation has reached the point at which pureed foods can be carried back from the anterior part of the mouth to the pharynx and swallowed. At eight or nine months of age or later, licking and chewing motions are noted, and the infant enjoys chewing on toast or a crust of bread.

Infants normally sleep with their mouths closed. Nasal obstruction owing to an upper respiratory tract infection or atresia of the posterior choanae may lead to respiratory distress, difficulty in sucking and cyanosis.

Little salivation occurs in the newborn infant and is minimal until two to four months of age, at which time drooling may occur. Babies often drool excessively when teething.

OTHER ORAL FINDINGS

Excessive saliva and mucus coming from the mouth of a newborn infant always sug- *gest esophageal atresia.* When an esophageal atresia is suspected, a No. 8 or 10 French soft rubber catheter should be passed into the esophagus. If the catheter passes into the stomach, as verified by fluoroscopy, esophageal atresia is ruled out.

Drooling may be excessive and abnormally persistent in children with cerebral palsy because of oropharyngeal incoordination, mental retardation and familial dysautonomia, especially when the child is excited. Increased salivation and drooling occur with Wilson's disease, acute epiglottitis, scorpion stings, organophosphate insecticide poisoning, peritonsillar abscess, dysphagia, esophageal injury owing to caustic ingestion and pseudodiverticulum of the newborn.

Yawning, frequent swallowing movements and facial grimacing may be signs of nausea in infants. Neonatal narcotic withdrawal is also characterized by yawning.

Hiccups in young infants possibly are a reflection of neuromuscular immaturity and the gastric distention that frequently follows feeding. They also occur in neonatal narcotic withdrawal.

Brouillette, R. T., Thach, B. T., Abu-Osba, Y. K., and Wilson, S. L.: Hiccups in infants: Characteristics and effects on ventilation. J. Pediatr. 96:219, 1980.

Sucking pads, which produce a fullness of the cheeks anterior to the masseter muscle, become prominent in malnourished infants.

The loss of subcutaneous fat, which occurs gradually from the upper half of the body in patients with *progressive lipodystrophy,* is especially noticeable in the cheeks.

Mouth breathing in older children may be associated with sinusitis, hypertrophy of adenoid tissue or other nasopharyngeal obstruction. Snoring and cogwheel breathing may occur when the child sleeps on his back. Sleep apnea may occur. Chronic mouth breathing may lead to an "adenoid facies" with an open mouth, narrow pinched nose, short upper lip, a high palate and a dull facial expression. The upper incisors may be spaced and protrude beneath the lip. Mouth breathing may also occur with a retropharyngeal abscess, pneumonia or weakness of the respiratory musculature.

Risus sardonicus occurs in some patients with tetanus. The corners of the mouth are pulled outward and downward, and the lip is stretched across the upper incisors to produce a sardonic grin. The eyebrows may also be drawn upward and the palpebral fissures narrowed.

A large, *fishlike mouth* occurs in congenital myotonic dystrophy and in these syndromes: idiopathic hypercalcemia, oculoauriculovertebral dysplasia, Treacher-Collins and Williams. Patients with the fetal hydantoin syndrome have a wide mouth with prominent lips. *Microstomia* is characteristic of the following syndromes: femoral hypoplasia, Hallermann-Streiff, otopalatodigital, Robinow's and whistling face. A pursed mouth with a fixed smile occurs in the Schwartz-Jampel syndrome.

Children with the athetoid form of cerebral palsy often "tuck in" their chin when they walk. The mouth may also remain open because of depression of the lower jaw.

Failure of one corner of the mouth to move downward and outward, especially noticeable when the child cries, may be attributable to *congenital absence or hypoplasia of the depressor anguli oris muscle,* a disorder that must be differentiated from congenital facial palsy. The lateral part of the lower lip may feel thinner on the involved side.

Nelson, K. B., and Eng., G. C.: Congenital hypoplasia of the depressor anguli oris muscle: Differentiation from congenital facial palsy. J. Pediatr. 81:16, 1972.

"Bad breath," or halitosis, may be attributable to the following causes:
Poor oral hygiene
Vomiting
Dry mouth owing to dehydration
Tonsillitis
Blood in the mouth
Nasal foreign body
Sinusitis
Hypertrophy and infection of adenoid tissue
Herpetic and Vincent's stomatitis
Typhoid fever and other enteric infections
Ingestion of strong-smelling, volatile foods that produce odors because of pulmonary excretion
Acetone odor to the breath occurs with ketoacidosis.

LIPS

In *cleft lip* the unilateral or bilateral defect may range from a simple notching to a complete separation of the maxillary and premaxillary processes and an extension of the cleft into the nostril. Cleft palate is often an associated defect.

Congenital lip pits or fistulas are bilateral, blind sinuses, usually on the vermilion border of the lower lip or at the corners of the mouth, which occur with or without an associated cleft lip and/or palate, popliteal pterygia and genital anomalies.

Fusion of the upper lip to the underlying gum occurs in some patients with *chondroectodermal dysplasia* (Ellis-van Creveld syndrome).

The *labial or sucking tubercle* in the middle of the upper lip in young infants disappears after weaning. Sucking plaques are also frequently noted along the edges of the upper and lower lips, particularly in infants who suck vigorously.

The *philtrum,* the distance between the columella of the nose and the upper lip, is long in Hurler's syndrome, femoral hypoplasia, unusual facies, slender-boned nanism, generalized gangliosidosis, Wagner-Stickler, Weaver, Robinow, fetal alcohol and fetal hydantoin syndromes. A short philtrum is present in the DiGeorge, orofaciodigital and Williams' syndromes.

Herpes simplex lesions may appear on the lips either singly or grouped. Beginning as a small erythematous macule, the lesion rapidly progresses to a papule and then to a minute, painful vesicle. Rupture of the vesicle, crusting and secondary infection follow.

Cheilitis with drying, wrinkling, cracking and scaling of the lips may occur during acute febrile illnesses or with contact sensitivity or chapping.

Acrodermatitis enteropathica is characterized by an erythematous, moist skin eruption, fissuring around the mouth and other orifices; vesiculobullous or crusted lesions on the buttocks, elbows, knees, hands and feet; alopecia; and stomatitis.

Perlèche, characterized by fissuring, scaling, maceration and crusting of the angles of the mouth, is usually caused by a candidial or, at times, streptococcal infection. *Cheilosis* is a form of fissuring caused by a nutritional deficiency. *Rhagades,* moist, radiating lesions about the corners of the mouth, are a sign of congenital syphilis. Fissuring may also be noted in children who drool excessively.

Erythema of the lips occurs early in the *Kawasaki syndrome,* followed later by cracking, fissuring and bleeding.

Carbon monoxide poisoning may cause a cherry-red color of the mucous membranes and lips.

In the *Peutz-Jeghers syndrome,* discrete bluish-black or brown pigmented spots may occur around the eyes, nose and mouth, lips and oral mucosa.

Angioedema may cause an acute, nonpitting, perhaps pruritic, massive swelling of the lip or face.

The *Melkersson-Rosenthal syndrome* is characterized, in part, by painless, nonpitting, sudden and recurrent swelling of the lips, especially the upper, and adjacent regions of the face. Peripheral facial paralysis and a fissured tongue are associated findings.

Wadlington, W. B., Riley, H. D., Jr., and Lowbeer, L.: The Melkersson-Rosenthal syndrome. Pediatrics 73:502, 1984.

The *mucosal neuroma* or *multiple endocrine neoplasia syndrome* may present early with neuromas of the lips, the anterior part of the tongue and the conjunctiva. The lips are protuberant with a "blubbery" appearance. Medullary carcinoma of the thyroid and a pheochromocytoma may appear later. The patient has a Marfan-like habitus.

Schimke, R. N.: Phenotype of malignancy: The mucosal neuroma syndrome. Pediatrics 52:283, 1973.

The *fetal alcohol* and the *femoral hypoplasia* syndromes are characterized by a thinned, upper vermilion border of the lip.
Electrical burns of the mouth, usually caused by the child chewing on an electrical cord, initially cause a painless, white, parchment-like lesion of the skin followed in a few hours by considerable edema. Because the burn is always more extensive than it initially appears to be, serious bleeding may ensue one day to three weeks later from erosion of the labial artery.

Gifford, G. H., Jr., Marty, A. T., and MacCollum, D. W.: The management of electrical mouth burns in children. Pediatrics 47:113, 1971.

Self-mutilative behavior with a section of the lip or part of a finger bitten away occurs in the Lesch-Nyhan syndrome.

BUCCAL MUCOSA

Thrush, caused by *Candida albicans,* is characterized by white, raised, membranous patches that resemble milk curds on the buccal surfaces, lips, tongue and pharynx. The patches are removed with some difficulty and leave mucosal lesions slightly oozing with blood. Chronic oral pharyngeal candidiasis, which occurs in acquired immunodeficiency syndrome and other disorders characterized by T-lymphocyte deficiency, is usually the presenting complaint in severe combined immunodeficiency.
Acute necrotizing ulcerative gingivitis or *Vincent's stomatitis* (trench mouth) is characterized by crater-like ulcerated lesions on the gingival margins. These are covered by a white pseudomembrane and surrounded by a zone of erythema. The gums are severely tender, painful and bleed easily. The breath has a fetid odor. Submaxillary lymphadenopathy may be present.
Ulcerative stomatitis may occur in *chronic granulomatous disease.*

In *pachyonychia congenita* the buccal mucosa and the dorsum of the tongue are thick and white or gray-white.
Herpetic gingivostomatitis is characterized by fever, irritability and small vesicles that rupture, leaving shallow ulcers on the gums, tongue and buccal mucous membrane. The lesions, which are irregular and 0.3 to 1.0 cm in diameter, have a gray center and a red, elevated edge.
Canker sores appear as pinhead-sized vesicles which rupture quickly to leave small grayish or yellowish ulcers that may be encircled by a reddish areola and covered by a greenish or yellowish-gray membrane. Removal of the membrane leaves a raw area. Apthous ulcers often occur in children with inflammatory bowel disease.
Recurrent stomatitis and mouth ulcers may occur in patients with *cyclic neutropenia.*
Diffuse erythema of the oropharynx occurs in the *Kawasaki syndrome.*
Behçet's syndrome consists of recurrent oral and genital ulcerations, uveitis, meningoencephalitis, arthritis or arthralgia and erythema nodosum. The oral lesions, which may be single or multiple, are usually less than 1 cm in diameter and have a yellow center surrounded by erythema.

Mundy, T. M., and Miller, J. J., III: Behçet's disease presenting as chronic aphthous stomatitis in a child. Pediatrics 62:205, 1978.

Herpangina is a manifestation of an acute, epidemic, febrile disease caused by coxsackie viruses A and B, echoviruses and enteroviruses. This disorder, which occurs in the summer, is characterized by dysphagia, a mildly sore throat, and papulovesicular lesions that range in size from 1 to 4 mm. The vesicles are surrounded by a zone of intense erythema, and their rupture results in grayish-yellow or white ulcers. The lesions, usually few but at times numerous, appear chiefly on the anterior tonsillar pillars, occasionally on the tonsils and soft palate, and more unusually on the tongue. The pharynx may be diffusely injected. In contrast to herpetic gingivostomatitis, the buccal mucosa and gingivae are not involved.
Hand-foot-and-mouth disease is characterized by vesiculo-ulcerative lesions of the oropharynx accompanied by a maculopapular exanthem on the palms, soles, heels and, at times, the knees and legs.
One or a few small white or yellow follicles on an erythematous base may be seen on the anterior tonsillar pillars on the second or third day of life. These benign lesions disappear in two to four days.

Leukemia and *chemotherapeutic agents* such as methotrexate, actinomycin-D or adriamycin may cause buccal mucosal ulcerations.

Koplik spots occur during the prodromal phase of measles as grayish-white, opalescent specks surrounded by a light red, blotchy areola. Best seen in natural light, they appear first on the buccal mucosa opposite the lower molars. They are occasionally extensively distributed in the mouth.

Chickenpox lesions may occur on the palate as well as elsewhere in the mouth and pharynx.

Epidermolysis bullosa lesions may involve the buccal mucosa.

Brown or blue-black pigmented areas may occur on the buccal mucous membrane in *Addison's disease.* Similar pigmentation may also be observed in the *Peutz-Jeghers syndrome.*

Small submucosal hemorrhages or grayish-white plaques in the region of the molars may be of traumatic origin owing to malocclusion or jagged teeth. A bluish, translucent retention cyst of a labial or buccal mucous gland may develop on the lower lip secondary to trauma.

Popsickle panniculitis caused by exposure to cold is characterized by a deep, movable, firm, slightly elevated, red nodule on the cheek.

Epstein, E. H, Jr., and Oren, M. E.: Popsickle panniculitis. N. Engl. J. Med. 282:966, 1970.

Papillomas may arise from the buccal epithelium as pedunculated, smooth or verrucous tumors with a whitish surface.

Bulging cheeks occur in the whistling face syndrome.

GINGIVAE; ALVEOLAR PROCESSES

Epulis is a nonspecific term for any of the benign neoplasms or hyperplasias of the gingiva. Congenital epulis of the newborn is a benign, pedunculated, smooth, soft tissue growth arising from the maxillary or mandibular gingival edge.

Occasionally the midline membranous labial frenum from the upper lip to the labial surface of the upper alveolar process may extend between the central incisors to the lingual side of the arch as an *alveolar frenum,* producing a space between the central incisors.

In the orofaciodigital syndrome, a median notching of the upper lip extends through the vermilion border. Multiple fibrous bands course from the lower lip and cheeks onto the mandibular alveolar process and cause clefting of the process.

The gingival mucosa in the region of the unerupted molars is often pale or nearly colorless. Occasionally a pearly white *retention cyst* persists for months on the gingival margin in infants. Blue-domed, fluid-filled, raised lesions consistent with the microscopic findings of lymphangioma may occur along the posterior alveolar ridges in black newborns.

Levin, L. S., Jorgenson, R. J., and Jarvey, B. A.: Lymphangiomas of the alveolar ridges in neonates. Pediatrics 58:881, 1976.

Pyogenic gingival cysts in infants, to be differentiated from simple hemorrhagic pre-eruptive dentigerous cysts, are accompanied by fever, irritability, leukocytosis and elevated sedimentation rates. Bacteremia may occur.

Patamusucon, P., Wientzen, R. L., and Schwartz, R. H.: Group A beta-hemolytic streptococci causing pyogenic gingival cyst in infancy. Am. J. Dis. Child. 134:617, 1980.

An *eruption hematoma* may occur with trauma to an eruption cyst.

Histiocytosis X may cause gingivitis, swelling of the palate and loss of teeth.

Hydantoin therapy may cause extensive, painless, firm and lobulated *gingival hypertrophy.* Hypertrophy and injection of the gingivae may occur in persistent mouthbreathers. Poor dental hygiene may be contributory.

Periapical abscesses or "gum boils" occasionally occur at the base of a tooth, either lingually or labially. Localized areas of swelling and redness usually indicate a periapical infection. Pus may be noted to escape around the tooth which is usually nonvital and loose.

Pyogenic granuloma may occur on the gingiva secondary to trauma as a red, lobulated, prone to bleed and, perhaps, ulcerated lesion.

The gingivae of black children are brownish-red and the marginal aspects of the gingivae and the interdental papillae bluish-gray.

Gingivitis may be noted in adolescent children. The margin of the gum is red, edematous and bleeds easily. Gingivitis also occurs in patients with neutropenia or myelomonocytic leukemia when the absolute granulocyte count is less than 1000 cu mm and in the hyperimmune E recurrent infection (Job's) syndrome.

Jorgenson, R. J., Shapiro, S. D., Salinas, C. F., and Levin, L. S.: Intraoral findings and anomalies in neonates. Pediatrics 69:577, 1982.

Polson, A. M.: Gingival and periodontal problems in children. Pediatrics 54:190, 1974.

PALATE

Characteristics of the four chief types of cleft palate are as follows:
1. Involvement is limited to the soft palate.
2. The cleft extends through both the soft and hard palates up to the alveolar process.
3. The soft and hard palates are both involved, and a unilateral cleft of the alveolar process exists.
4. The soft and hard palates are both involved, and a bilateral cleft of the alveolar process exists.

Patients with a *submucous cleft* have no overt cleft, but the midline of the palate on palpation seems to be very thin. The palate may also be foreshortened and velopharyngeal closure incomplete. The uvula is bifid, and a notch in the posterior border of the hard palate is palpable. The speech has a prominent nasal quality owing to excessive nasal resonance. A submucous cleft of the primary and secondary palate occurs in the orofaciodigital syndrome. A bifid uvula may occur in patients with a submucous cleft or with the Apert, DiGeorge, orofaciodigital, Robin, Stickler or Treacher-Collins syndrome.

Shprintzen, R. J., Schwartz, R. H., Daniller, A., and Hoch, L.: Morphologic significance of bifid uvula. Pediatrics 75:553, 1985.

Cleft palate may occur as an isolated defect or as a component of these syndromes: congenital lip fistulas, diastrophic dysplasia, Larsen's, mandibulofacial dysostosis, orofaciodigital, popliteal pterygium, trisomy 13, trisomy 18 and Wolf-Hirschhorn.

The *Pierre Robin syndrome* is characterized by a posterior cleft of the palate, micrognathia and glossoptosis. These findings may also occur in the Beckwith-Wiedemann, diastrophic dysplasia, fetal hydantoin and Stickler syndromes.

Schreiner, R. L., McAlister, W. H., Marshall, R. E., and Shearer, W. T.: Stickler syndrome in a pedigree of Pierre Robin syndrome. Am. J. Dis. Child. 126:86, 1973.

Palatopharyngeal incompetence occurs when the soft palate and related pharyngeal musculature does not effectively separate the nasopharynx from the oropharynx. Associated symptoms include hypernasal speech, escape of fluid through the nose when swallowing, and inability to hiss, whistle, gargle, blow out a candle or inflate a balloon.

The palate should elevate when a tongue blade is gently applied to each pillar of the palatal arch. This *gag reflex*, which tests for function of cranial nerves IX (afferent) and X (efferent), is clinically significant only if one side persistently does not respond. It is absent in *botulism*. Patients with diphtheria may have paralysis of the palate.

In newborn infants, small, localized accumulations of epithelial cells or cysts are common on each side of the median raphe of the hard palate *(Epstein's pearls)* or along the alveolar ridge *(Bohn's nodules)*. Dental lamina cysts are present on the crest of the alveolar ridges, more commonly on the maxilla than the mandible. The lesions, which are white, firm and raised, range from pinhead to 3 mm in size.

Petechial spots are occasionally observed on the soft palate with pharyngitis or other respiratory diseases.

A *high, arched palate* may occur in mouth breathers and with these syndromes: cerebral gigantism, Ehlers-Danlos, Marfan's, Rubinstein-Taybi and Treacher-Collins.

In young infants, two reddened or yellow-gray, slightly eroded lesions, sometimes called *Bednar's aphthae,* may occur far back on the hard palate on each side of the midline. These lesions are usually caused by trauma from the nipple or, perhaps, overvigorous cleansing of the mouth at the time of birth.

Palatal groove formation may occur in newborn infants who have required an orotracheal tube, especially when the tube has been in place for more than 15 days.

Erenberg, A., and Nowak, A. J.: Palatal groove formation in neonates and infants with orotracheal tubes. Am. J. Dis. Child. 138:974, 1984.

THE TONGUE

Since it follows the neural growth curve, the tongue may appear relatively large at birth and during early infancy. Occasionally, slight protrusion of the normally large tongue may suggest macroglossia.

Functional or neurologic impairment of tongue movements may interfere with feeding and speech. The movements of the tongue necessary for normal feeding and speech include the ability to extend the tongue forward between the lips and teeth, retract it back into the mouth, move it laterally and elevate its base or tip.

The dorsal surface of the tongue is covered with conical, filiform, fungiform and vallate papillae. The fungiform papillae, which appear as red, pinhead sized elevations clustered near the tip of the tongue among the gray-white filiform papillae, are absent in *familial dysautonomia*.

Enlargement of the tongue or *macroglossia* may be associated with congenital hypothyroidism, cystic hygroma, Down's syndrome, ectopic thyroid, enteric duplication, glycogenosis Type II (Pompe's disease or acid maltase deficiency), hemangioma, Hurler's syndrome, lymphangioma, mannosidosis, neurofibromatosis and rhabdomyoma. Enlargement of the tongue may also occur in amyloidosis type I, congenital muscular hypertrophy, generalized gangliosidosis and Sandhoff's disease. At times, the cause of the hypertrophy is unknown. Hemihypertrophy of the tongue may also occur.

The *Beckwith-Wiedemann syndrome* consists of macroglossia, omphalocele, increased birth weight, hepatomegaly, ear lobe anomalies and, at times, hypoglycemia and hemihypertrophy.

Filippi, G., and McKusick, V. A.: The Beckwith-Wiedemann syndrome. Medicine 49:279, 1970.

Lobulations, bifurcation or multi-furcation of the tongue and a shortened frenulum occur in the orofaciodigital syndrome.

Microglossia or aglossia occurs in the aglossia-adactylia and Möbius' syndromes.

A *thyroglossal duct cyst* at the base of the tongue may lead to its enlargement and protrusion and to airway obstruction. The base of the tongue should be palpated in infants with otherwise unexplained stridor or dysphagia.

Glossoptosis, or posterior positioning of the tongue, is usually associated with hypoplasia of the mandible. Because of the resultant small airway and the tendency to hypoxia, infants with glossoptosis have great difficulty in feeding, fail to thrive, and have episodes of respiratory distress and cyanosis. The respiratory difficulty may be greatest when the infant is supine.

Glossoptosis occurs along with cleft palate in the Pierre Robin syndrome.

Although the frenulum of the tongue may occasionally be short and cause a notch at the tip of the tongue, true *tongue-tie* or congenital ankyloglossia is extremely rare. Hypermobility and hyperextensibility of the tongue may occur in the Ehlers-Danlos syndrome.

Ranula is a translucent, bluish retention cyst of the sublingual glands, usually on one side of the frenulum beneath the tongue.

Frequent *protrusion of the tongue* occurs in infants with mental retardation, Down's syndrome, congenital hypothyroidism, and Niemann-Pick disease. In the newborn, Foote's sign, a rhythmic protrusion of the tongue, suggests intracranial hemorrhage or cerebral edema. A kind of tongue thrust-ing may occur in children with familial dysautonomia. Tongue protrusion occurs in the puppet-like syndrome of Angelman. Tongue thrusting is often noted in infants who later demonstrate athetosis.

In Sydenham's *chorea*, the tongue is often undulating and cannot be held still on protrusion. When the child is asked to smile, the smile is fleeting. Tremor of the protruded tongue is also noted in hyperthyroidism. *Werdnig-Hoffmann disease* is characterized by fasciculations and atrophy of the tongue, best observed with the infant asleep.

Dryness of the tongue may be caused by dehydration or mouth breathing.

White, grayish or brownish-white *coating of the tongue* occurs commonly in febrile illnesses and in the early stages of scarlet fever, measles and other exanthemata. The coating consists of desquamated cells, food debris and bacteria.

The *white strawberry tongue* is characterized by red, congested and edematous fungiform papillae present against a white-coated background produced by the smaller filiform papillae. Such coating may occur between the second and fifth days in patients with scarlet fever, occasionally in patients with measles and, at times, in patients who have other febrile illnesses.

In patients with a *red strawberry or raspberry tongue,* desquamation of the white coating and filiform papillae has occurred, leaving the red, swollen fungiform papillae against a raw, beefy-red background. This finding occurs on or about the sixth or seventh day in scarlet fever. A strawberry tongue may also accompany other severe febrile illnesses, including Kawasaki disease and toxic shock syndrome. Acute bacterial glossitis has also been reported with *Haemophilus influenzae, type B.*

In *ariboflavinosis*, the tongue is purplish-red and has a smooth to pebbly surface. In pellagra, redness and induration of the edges of the tongue occur early. With a more advanced deficiency, a beefy-red color and swelling of the papillae develop, followed by atrophy and matting.

Pernicious anemia is a rare cause of glossitis in childhood.

Fissured tongue is characterized by irregular fissures or grooves in a leaflike, cerebriform or scrotal pattern.

In *geographic tongue,* annular, smooth, red patches with slightly raised gray margins begin posteriorly on the dorsum and spread anteriorly and laterally. Somewhat similar but more transient patches may be noted in acute febrile illnesses.

Furrowed tongue occurs with recurrent facial nerve palsy and edema of the lips in the *Melkersson-Rosenthal syndrome.*

Venous congestion occurs under the tongue in congestive cardiac failure, constrictive pericarditis and the superior vena cava syndrome.

Premonitory symptoms of *basilar artery migraine* may include numbness and tingling of the lips and the tongue.

THE TEETH

Deciduous Teeth

Eruption. Although the eruption of teeth follows a developmental pattern, much individual variation occurs. Deciduous teeth tend to erupt in three groupings with an interval of one and one-half to three months between each group:

2 lower central incisors	5-10 months
2 upper central incisors	8-12 months
2 upper lateral incisors	9-13 months
2 lower lateral incisors	10-14 months
2 lower anterior molars	13-16 months
2 upper anterior molars	13-17 months
4 canines	12-22 months
4 posterior molars	24-30 months

Rarely, one or two teeth are prematurely present at birth. These supernumerary teeth are usually loosely held and easily removed. The tooth buds of the deciduous teeth are readily evident in the gums of the young infant. Eruption of the deciduous teeth may be delayed normally until the end of the first year. Further delay may occur in infants with hypothyroidism or hypopituitarism. All 20 deciduous teeth should be present before the end of the third year. The lower central incisors are usually the first deciduous teeth to be lost. The last deciduous tooth is shed by about 12 years of age. During the preschool period, spacing between the anterior deciduous teeth is normal. Prolonged retention of deciduous teeth may be noted in pycnodysostosis and cleidocranial dysostosis.

Permanent Dentition

The permanent teeth usually erupt in the following order:

First molars	6-7 years
Incisors	7-9 years
Premolars	9-11 years
Canines	10-12 years
Second molars	12-16 years
Third molars	17-25 years

During the first years after their eruption, the permanent teeth appear relatively large and may be irregularly spaced and aligned. With further growth of the face, however, the teeth no longer appear disproportionately large. Under the influence of muscular forces exerted by the lips, cheeks and tongue, the malalignment usually does not persist, and the spacing between the upper permanent incisors customarily disappears after eruption of the canine teeth.

The incisal margin of the newly erupted anterior permanent teeth have three sawtoothed projections or mamelons, remnants of the developmental lobes of the teeth, which are worn down after a time.

The first (sixth-year) molar of the permanent dentition erupts behind the baby molars. This tooth has an extremely important role in the positioning of other teeth and is the keystone of the dental arch.

Malocclusion

Malocclusion may be categorized as malpositioning of the teeth with normal relation of the jaws; retrusion of the mandible with accompanying protrusion or retrusion of the upper incisors; and protrusion of the mandible. Vigorous and persistent thumb sucking may lead to malpositioning, especially if continued after the age of five or six years.

Normally, alignment of the teeth is maintained by the muscular forces of the lip, cheeks and tongue. The upper lip in children who breathe through their mouths becomes shortened and slack and, therefore, does not exert its normal molding action on the upper dental arch. The lower lip may also become flaccid and everted and with retrusion of the mandible may be held behind the upper incisors. Spacing and protrusion of the upper incisors result.

Protrusion and spacing of the teeth may occur in children with *thalassemia major*.

Disturbances of the Teeth

Total or partial *anodontia,* or absence of teeth, may occur with hypohidrotic ectodermal dysplasia, Marfan's syndrome and cleidocranial dysostosis. In congenital ectodermal dysplasia, the upper lateral incisors, and occasionally other teeth, are cone- or peg-shaped. Deformity of the teeth may also occur in children with chondroectodermal dysplasia.

Premature loss of teeth or "floating teeth" may occur in patients with histiocytosis X, vitamin D–resistant rickets, cyclic neutropenia, hypophosphatasia and neoplasms, such as reticulum cell sarcoma or Ewing's sarcoma. In histiocytosis X, the gingivae are friable, swollen and ulcerated, especially on the lingual or palatal side of the erupting molars. Juvenile periodontitis in adolescents is accompanied by extensive bone loss around the permanent first molars and lower incisors with resultant tooth mobility. Premature loss of the deciduous teeth may occur with palmar-plantar hyperkeratosis.

Enamel hypoplasia, characterized by pitting or grooving of the enamel surface, may occur owing to tetracycline administration, rickets, hypoparathyroidism, oculodentoosseous dysplasia, congenital syphilis, malnutrition, diarrhea and severe systemic disease in early life. Enamel hypoplasia, hypodontia and other dental malformations occur in *Rieger's syndrome* along with aniridia and glaucoma.

During the period of tooth development, from the latter half of pregnancy to eight years of age, *tetracycline* causes yellow-gray-brown permanent discoloration of the teeth, occasionally accompanied by enamel hypoplasia.

Brown teeth, or amelogenesis imperfecta, results from malfunctioning of the ameloblasts or enamel-forming cells. The brown dentin is not covered by an adequate coating of enamel.

Grooving and pitting of the enamel may occur in chronic idiopathic hypoparathyroidism.

Opalescent dentin, or dentinogenesis imperfecta, may occur with osteogenesis imperfecta. The deciduous and permanent dentition may be characterized by a browning opalescence and rapid attrition.

In *congenital syphilis* the upper central permanent incisors may be peg-shaped and notched on their distal border. These so-called Hutchinson teeth are shaped like the tip of a screw driver. "Mulberry" molars, which have irregularly formed crowded cusps on a dwarfed occlusal surface, are another stigma of congenital syphilis.

Infection of a tooth bud, usually that of the first molar, in newborn infants causes inflammatory changes in the lip, cheek, orbital region and the underlying alveolar process. A purulent nasal discharge may also develop.

Grinding of the teeth or bruxism occurs chiefly during sleep but may be diurnal as well. A grating, rasping sound is produced, and the teeth may be worn down rapidly.

Greenish-black discoloration near the gingival margin of the teeth in children is caused by tartar and *calculus deposits.*

Nursing bottle caries with rampant decay, especially on the labial aspect of the primary canine and incisor teeth, may occur in infants over one year of age with prolonged bottle feeding of milk or a carbohydrate-containing solution when placed down to sleep.

Shelton, P. G., Berkowitz, R. J., and Forrester, D. J.: Nursing bottle caries. Pediatrics 59:777, 1977.

Erosion of the dental enamel may occur in adolescents with bulimia.

Neonatal jaundice may cause a permanent greenish color (the *green neonatal ring*) in the enamel being formed at birth. As a result, the portion of the deciduous teeth formed prenatally is completely green.

Erythrodentition with pink or reddish-brown coloration of the teeth may occur with chronic porphyria.

THE PHARYNX

The tonsils are normally large in childhood, an expression of the luxuriant lymphoid growth characteristic of this age period. When tonsillar enlargement occurs during an infection, normal size is usually regained two or three weeks later. Marked tonsillar hypertrophy may produce sleep apnea owing to obstruction of the airway.

Tonsillitis and pharyngitis are discussed on page 372. During the first few days of life the infant's pharynx may normally appear red.

The patient who has a *peritonsillar abscess* is unable to open his mouth wide and may hold his head tilted toward the involved side. Frequent swallowing movements may be noted. Because swallowing is very painful, drooling may occur. The limited pharyngeal examination that is possible reveals anterior and superior displacement of the involved tonsil, bulging of the soft palate and movement of the uvula toward the opposite side.

Retropharyngeal abscess occurs largely in infants. Patients with a retropharyngeal abscess tend to lie with their head either tilted to one side or retracted. Cervical adenopathy is usually present on the ipsilateral side. Stiffness of the neck, mouth breathing and stridor may also occur. Extreme caution is indicated in the examination of the pharynx in these patients, since forceful depression of the tongue with a blade may precipitate a respiratory arrest. Lateral soft tissue x-rays of the neck should be obtained. Palpation of the retropharyngeal abscess should be performed quickly, gently and without pressure. Standing at the head of the patient, the examiner may insert his finger dorsally along the roof of the mouth and posterior pharyngeal wall until the abscess is palpated, or the tongue may be gently depressed with a tongue blade and the examining finger introduced at the corner of the mouth and passed over the base of the tongue to the posterior pharyngeal wall. The abscess is felt as a smooth, tense and, perhaps, fluctuant swelling, sometimes more prominent laterally than in the center of the pharynx.

Lymphosarcoma may rarely involve a tonsil. Unilateral enlargement of a tonsil is an indication for a tonsillectomy-biopsy.

Rhabdomyosarcoma in the nasopharynx may cause denasalized speech, a persistent nasal discharge, enlargement of the cervical lymph nodes in the upper third of the neck and cranial nerve palsies.

Ulceration of the pharynx may occur in patients with leukemia or agranulocytosis.

Infectious mononucleosis may cause a thick, dull, white pseudomembrane over the tonsils and lymphoid tissue on the posterior pharyngeal wall but not extending beyond the lymphoid tissue.

Tangier disease is characterized by huge, lobulated or honeycombed yellowish-gray tonsils, hepatosplenomegaly, lymphadenopathy and transient neuropathy.

Hyperplasia of lymphoid follicles on the posterior pharyngeal wall may occur in children who have chronic sinusitis or recurrent pharyngitis. The mucosa of the posterior pharynx becomes granular and pebbled with small glistening islands of lymphoid tissue.

In children with sinusitis or chronic nasopharyngitis, a yellowish, glairy, mucopurulent curtain may hang down or drain from the nasopharynx.

The *gag reflex* should be checked in patients thought to have cranial nerve palsies. Pharyngeal pooling of saliva may occur in patients with bulbar palsy or botulism.

Edema of the uvula (Quincke's disease) may occur acutely. Swelling of the uvula may also accompany tonsillitis or pharyngitis. Isolated *uvulitis*, occurring in the absence of pharyngitis or epiglottitis, may be caused by *Haemophilus influenzae, type b.* Findings include fever, irritability, drooling, pain on swallowing and a large, erythematous uvula.

Li, K. I., Kiernan, S., Wald, E. R., and Reilly, J. S.: Isolated uvulitis due to *Haemophilus influenzae type b.* Pediatrics 74:1054, 1984.

Epiglottitis is characterized by the acute onset of fever, sore throat, dysphagia, drooling and muffled voice. The patient sits upright and leans forward with his mouth open and tongue extended. The child may be able to open his mouth wide enough to permit visualization of a swollen, cherry-red epiglottitis, but the use of a tongue depressor is contraindicated because it may precipitate a respiratory arrest.

7 / SPEECH

SPEECH DEVELOPMENT

Crying is largely an undifferentiated noise in the neonatal period, but in a few weeks many mothers are able to identify the type of cry, depending upon its cause. During the second month of life, the baby may begin to make cooing sounds; and in the third month, the mother may report that her baby "talks" to her. This is the "babbling" stage of vocalization. At first, most of the sounds produced are vowels, with consonants appearing later.

In the latter half of the first year, the infant enters the period of vocal verbal play. He enjoys squealing and making other sounds of varying frequency and intensity, listening and then repeating the sounds. Infants with severe hearing impairment do not spontaneously progress beyond the babbling stage. Blind children may also demonstrate a prolonged babbling period.

Toward the end of the first year, the infant begins to repeat the speech of his parents. During the eighth month most infants can say "da-da." At the end of the first year, their vocabulary may consist of one to three words in addition to "ma-ma" and "da-da." At the age of about one year or, possibly, sooner, the child begins to attach a definite meaning to words. By 18 months, the infant's vocabulary includes 6 to 50 words. Children between the ages of 21 and 24 months may begin to use two or three word phrases. Between two and three years, they may begin to speak in sentences. Of course, the time at which these stages of language development normally occur varies greatly.

Referral to a speech and language consultant is indicated if a child has no words by 20 months of age or no two-word phrases by 30 months of age or fails to use sentences by 36 months of age. Other indications for referral are obvious echolalia; speech that is unintelligible to parents after two years of age; failure to understand appropriately for his age the speech of others; and speech that is unintelligible to strangers after three years of age.

Instruments that may be used for the office evaluation of language development include the Denver Developmental Screening Test, the Peabody Picture Vocabulary Test, the Utah Test of Language Development and the Mecham Verbal Language Development Scale.

Resnick, T. J., Allen, D. A., and Rapin, I.: Disorders of language development: Diagnosis and intervention. Pediatr. Rev. 6:85, 1984.

DELAYED SPEECH

Mental retardation is the major cause of language delay. Emotional disturbance and family turmoil are other common etiologies. Speech retardation also occurs in the deaf or hearing impaired child, including impairment that is secondary to prolonged otitis media with effusion. Lack of appropriate environmental stimulation results in speech delay. Infants with psychosocial failure to thrive are frequently very quiet and do little or no cooing, babbling, squealing or laughing. The overdependent child may also be slow to talk. Twins and the children of deaf and mute parents may show delayed speech, as may the neurologically injured child. Autistic children are frequently first seen because of failure to speak or noncommunicative speech.

Speech retardation occurs with histidinemia.

Teele, D. W., Klein, J. O., Rosner, B. A., et al.: Otitis media with effusion during the first three years of life and development of speech and language. Pediatrics 74:282, 1984.

DYSFLUENCY

Repetitive or mildly dysfluent speech occurs transiently in most preschool children. Some hesitation or uneveness in speech may be present and repetitiveness may occur with syllables, words or combinations of words. This normal developmental process should not be labeled as stuttering.

Stuttering, much more common in boys than in girls, is a type of speech dysfluency that is accompanied by secondary manifestations such as blocking, apprehension about speaking, mannerisms, and avoidance of troublesome sounds and words. Other secondary manifestations include tic-like movements of the face and changes in breathing when the child tries to speak fluently.

Rosenfield, D. B.: Stuttering. Cur. Prob. Pediatr. 12:4, 1982.

Cluttering is an unusual type of speech characterized by repetition of words or phrases, repeated false starts, changes in context in the middle of the sentence and general verbal confusion.

OTHER ABNORMAL SPEECH PATTERNS

Echolalia may occur in association with blindness, autism and Gilles de la Tourette's syndrome.

Elective mutism is the clinical situation in which the child speaks to members of his family or close friends but not to strangers or school acquaintances. *Traumatic mutism* occurs after a psychological shock.

Kolvin, I., and Fundudis, T.: Elective mute children: Psychological development and background factors. J. Child Psychol. Psychiatry 22:219, 1981.

Rote repetition of songs, commercials or various lists may be a splinter skill in some autistic children.

SPEECH IN HEARING-IMPAIRED CHILDREN

The child who has a hearing impairment may also have retarded speech; an articulatory speech defect; or an abnormality in pitch, loudness or other vocal quality. Cooing, crying and babbling occur in children with impaired hearing, as well as in those who hear normally. An infant's ability to babble and, perhaps, say "da-da" does not necessarily mean that his hearing is adequate for speech perception. The infant with serious hearing impairment is handicapped in advancing to the next stage of speech development because such progress depends upon verbal-vocal play and the imitation of sounds made by himself and others.

ARTICULATORY SPEECH DISORDERS

The time at which distinct speech is achieved varies. Although some children demonstrate correct articulation relatively early, more frequently it is not perfected until the late preschool or early elementary school period. Some articulatory speech defects are minor and, in time, disappear. In extreme disorders of articulation, speech is largely or completely unintelligible.

Four types of articulatory speech defects are usually considered: *substitution*, in which one sound is substituted for the correct sound, as w for r (*run* becomes *wun*); *omission*, in which a sound is omitted; *insertion*, in which an extra sound is added to a word; and *distortion*, in which the sound is made incorrectly and, therefore, is indistinct. *Lisping* is characterized by the use of the "th" sound for the "s" sound. Speech consultation is desirable for an articulatory speech defect if a three-year-old child talks in a jargon unintelligible to strangers. If speech is intelligible, the decision as to speech therapy may be delayed until school entrance.

Dyslalia is the term applied to an articulatory disorder for which no organic basis can be found. Children with cerebral palsy or central neurologic damage may have articulatory difficulty owing to a poorly functioning tongue, paralysis of the palate or incoordination of the pharyngeal muscles. A cleft palate, submucous cleft, severe malocclusion, malalignment of the teeth or other oral deformity may be etiologic. Intellectual retardation or a hearing loss are other important considerations.

Persistence of infantile speech in an otherwise normal child may reflect social and emotional immaturity or overdependence. Some functional difficulty in the use of the structures involved in speech must also be considered. Office assessment may be based on the Denver Articulation Screening Examination.

Dysarthria is the term applied to difficulty in articulating the individual sounds of speech secondary to an organic motor defect in the speech mechanism, to cerebellar dysfunction and to Wilson's disease. *Dysphasia*, a language disturbance owing to damage or dysfunction of those areas in the brain involved in symbolic formulation, is characterized by motor or expressive difficulty in using speech, defective perception with an inability to understand the meaning of words or both. Speech may be completely lacking or primitive and unintelligible.

SPEECH QUALITY

Hyponasal speech, which sounds about the same whether the nostrils are open or pinched shut, may occur secondary to nasal allergy or enlarged adenoids. *Hypernasality* may be associated with complete or submucous cleft palate with velopharyngeal insufficiency or neurogenic dysfunction of the palate.

Normal speech depends upon unimpaired respiratory movements, since a relatively long and sustained expiratory phase is needed. In the child with *cerebral palsy* the respiratory excursions may be rapid, irregular, spasmodic or non-synchronized; consequently, the speech may be halting, strained and dysrhythmic, with short, irregular spurts. The pitch of the speech may also be abnormal. Patients with Friedreich's ataxia or chorea may have similar speech.

Slurred speech occurs in Wilson's disease, in impending hepatic coma and in children or adolescents who sniff leaded gasoline or other solvents.

Children with paralysis of the palatal and pharyngeal muscles have a nasal twang to their voice. Sinusitis and adenoid hypertrophy cause the so-called adenoid voice owing to impairment of nasal resonance.

Differential diagnosis of *hoarseness* or huskiness includes vocal abuse through excessive shouting, screaming or singing. Between five and ten years of age, such abuse may cause vocal cord nodules with hoarseness or a husky voice. *Papilloma of the larynx*, the most common cause of persistent hoarseness in children, occurs most frequently between the ages of one and four years. Progressive airway obstruction may develop. Direct laryngoscopy is required. Other causes of hoarseness include:

Chronic or acute sinusitis with hoarseness, sometimes present on arising

Laryngitis or croup (Acute epiglottitis produces a muffled voice.)

Laryngeal foreign body

Unilateral paralysis of the recurrent laryngeal nerve

Ectodermal dysplasia

Lipoid proteinosis

Measles

Thyroid malignancy; Hashimoto's thyroiditis

Ninth and tenth cranial nerve paresis associated with the Arnold-Chiari malformation

Hoarseness may be noted at birth in infants with disseminated lipogranulomatosis.

Hoarseness may be caused by laryngeal

involvement in patients with chronic mucocutaneous candidiasis.

Paroxysms of inappropriate laughter occur in the puppet-like syndrome of Angelman.

Deepening of the voice occurs in boys during adolescence. Premature deepening and coarsening of the voice appear with precocious sexual development or masculinization.

A patient's speech may give an impression of his affect, e.g., the slow, monotonal and, at times, almost inaudible speech of the chronically ill or depressed child; or the whisper, stuttering or aphonia of the child with a conversion disorder.

Aphonia with coughing and wheezing suggests a laryngeal foreign body.

Aphonia or hoarseness may occur as a sequela in patients who survive Reye's syndrome.

Reitman, M. A., Casper, J., Coplan, J., Weiner, L. B., Kellman, R. M., and Kanter, R. K.: Motor disorders of voice and speech in Reye's syndrome survivors. Am. J. Dis. Child. 138:1129, 1984.

CRY

Infants with hypothyroidism may have a weak, low-pitched, hoarse cry.

Some infants with congenital heart disease have a weak or hoarse cry owing to pressure of enlarged pulmonary vessels on the left recurrent laryngeal nerve.

A weak cry occurs with infant botulism.

In the *cri du chat syndrome,* the cry during the first year of life is weak, high-pitched, mewing and plaintive, similar to that of a distressed kitten. The characteristic cry may disappear by two years of age.

A high-pitched, persistent cry occurs in neonatal drug withdrawal.

The cry in neurologically impaired newborn infants may be feeble, whiny, plaintive or intermittent, shrill, sharp and piercing.

8 / THE JAW AND SALIVARY GLANDS

The mandible, which appears relatively small in newborn infants, grows forward and downward during early life. But by the latter half of the first year, the mandible has become more proportionate to the face. *Micrognathia* or hypoplasia of the mandible may be accompanied by glossoptosis. The *Pierre Robin syndrome* consists of a cleft palate, micrognathia and glossoptosis. The cerebro-costo-mandibular syndrome is characterized by cerebral maldevelopment, multiple posterior rib gaps, micrognathia, cleft palate and glossoptosis.

Silverman, F. N., Strefling, A. M., Stevenson, D. K., and Lazarus, J.: Cerebro-costo-mandibular syndrome. J. Pediatr. 97:406, 1980.

A small mandible with the typical *vogelgesicht* (bird facies) may occur in juvenile rheumatoid arthritis owing to interference with growth at the temporomandibular joint. Ankylosis of the temporomandibular joint may also be caused by birth injury, postnasal trauma or infection. The involved side of the mandible fails to grow normally, and the midpoint of the jaw is displaced toward the ipsilateral side.

Micrognathia may be noted in the *Treacher-Collins syndrome* along with hypoplasia of the facial bones. The malar bones, the zygomatic arch and the infraorbital ridges are either absent or defective. In hemifacial microsomia, the mandibular ramus and condyle do not develop on the involved side.

The *Hallermann-Streiff syndrome* is characterized by a hypoplastic mandible, birdlike facies, scaphocephaly, brachycephaly, beaked nose, hypotrichosis, skin atrophy, dental anomalies, congenital cataracts and understature.

Micrognathia also occurs in these syndromes: arteriohepatic dysplasia, cri du chat, Di George, fetal alcohol, pycnodysostosis, Rubinstein-Taybi, Russell-Silver's,

Schwartz-Jampel, Smith-Lemli-Opitz, trisomy 13, trisomy 18, Wagner-Stickler and Warkany.

Prominence of the mandible, or *prognathism,* may be noted in chondrodystrophy, Crouzon's disease and the fragile X syndrome. Soft-tissue prognathism occurs in the mucosal neuroma syndrome.

Mandibular involvement occurs in *infantile cortical hyperostosis* as a soft tissue swelling that may simulate mumps.

Grooves in the chin occur in the whistling face syndrome.

Cherubism is a hereditary, hard, painless, symmetrical swelling of the jaw that begins in early childhood. This disorder is accompanied by abnormal dentition in the mandible and regional lymphadenopathy. Fibrous dysplasia may also cause a prominent mandible.

A *draining fistula* in the submandibular area may arise from a periapical dental abscess. Actinomycosis is an unusual etiologic possibility.

Disorders to be considered in the differential diagnosis of *tumors of the jaw* in childhood include osteomyelitis, eosinophilic granuloma, giant cell tumor, Ewing's tumor, fibrosarcoma, osteogenic sarcoma and odontogenic tumors. Tender, localized, swelling of the jaw, fever and inability to open the mouth may occur in association with mandibular cyst formation in patients with the nevoid basal cell carcinoma syndrome.

Burkitt's lymphoma may present as a soft tissue tumor or swelling in the mandible or maxilla.

Trismus, an inability to open the mouth, most commonly occurs in patients with tetanus but may be noted in patients with phenothiazine toxicity; encephalitis; brain tumors; primary hypoparathyroidism; the infantile form of Gaucher's disease; and tumors of the jaw, such as rhabdomyosarcoma.

Dislocation or subluxation of the temporomandibular joint may be caused by the intermittent extensor thrust of the jaw in patients with athetosis.

Familial, perpendicular, rhythmic *trembling of the chin,* may occur during periods of emotional stress. Newborn and young infants demonstrate some trembling of the chin during periods of crying.

Myofascial pain dysfunction is characterized by dull, aching pain that is usually worse in the morning. The pain may be referred to the ear, face, neck or mandibular angle. The patient may also have a history of bruxism, painful chewing, jaw clicking and "locking." Jaw movement may be limited, and muscle tenderness may be present.

Belfer, M. L., and Kaban, L. B.: Temporomandibular joint dysfunction with facial pain in children. Pediatrics 69:564, 1982.

Mumps causes a tender, somewhat painful, unilateral or bilateral enlargement of the parotid and, rarely, the submaxillary glands. The swelling, present below and anterior to the ear lobe, extends onto the face, below the mandible and toward the mastoid. Because of the swelling, the ear lobe may be pushed out from the face, and the angle of the mandible may not be palpable. Swelling, greatest during the second and third days of the illness, persists for a week to 10 days. A brawny, gelatinous edema surrounds the swelling, and the overlying skin may be slightly erythematous and shiny. Presternal edema may occur. The orifice of Stensen's duct opposite the upper second molar tooth may be injected and puffy. Submaxillary or sublingular mumps may occur without parotid involvement.

Lymphadenopathy in the parotid area may require differentiation from mumps. With lymphadenopathy, the angle of the mandible can be palpated and the swelling, which is mostly submandibular, except for preauricular adenopathy, is usually more discrete.

Purulent parotitis may occur in newborn infants or in older children. The gland is enlarged and tender, and the overlying skin is red and warm. With fluctuation, pus may be expressed from Stensen's duct. Similar involvement of the submaxillary glands may occur.

David, R. B., and O'Connell, E. J.: Suppurative parotitis in children. Am. J. Dis. Child. 119:332, 1970.

Leake, D., and Leake, R.: Neonatal suppurative parotitis. Pediatrics 46:203, 1970.

Recurrent swelling of the parotid gland usually begins after two years of age and continues intermittently throughout childhood. Tenseness and erythema of the skin occur over the parotid area. A sense of fullness and pain may be present, but no systemic symptoms occur. Attacks usually persist for two or three weeks. Spontaneous remission is the rule, but suppuration occasionally develops. Salivary gland involvement, including recurrent parotitis, has been reported with *mixed connective tissue disease.* Chronic parotid swelling occurs in some patients with acquired immunodeficiency syndrome. Chronic or recurrent enlargement of the salivary glands, usually the parotid, but, at times, the submaxillary, occurs in *Sjögren's syndrome*, along with keratoconjunctivitis sicca and dry mouth. This syndrome may occur with juvenile rheumatoid arthritis or sarcoidosis. Chronic enlargement of the parotid glands causes a chipmunk appearance.

Athreya, B. H., Norman, M. E., Myers, A. R., and South, M. A.: Sjögren's syndrome in children. Pediatrics 59:931, 1977.

Parotid enlargement may rarely be caused by a calculus in Stensen's duct.

Hemangioma, probably the most common of parotid tumors and frequently present at birth, enlarges rapidly in the first few weeks and months of life. Discoloration of the overlying skin may be present. The tumor feels compressible, elastic and lobulated. *Lymphangiomas* may also be present at birth or appear during the first year. The benign *mixed tumor* of the parotid gland presents as a round, firm, painless mass beneath and just anterior to the ear. Burkitt's lymphoma may involve the salivary glands.

Submandibular gland enlargement occurs in most children with cystic fibrosis over two years of age.

Parotid gland enlargement is an uncommon finding in acute histoplasmosis. It may also occur with the acquired immunodeficiency syndrome.

Mikulicz's syndrome is characterized by bilateral, firm, painless enlargement of the parotid, lacrimal and, at times, submaxillary glands, with resultant dryness of the mouth and an absence of tears. The syndrome may be associated with tuberculosis, lymphoma or leukemia.

The *auriculotemporal syndrome*, which follows injury to the auriculotemporal nerve near the parotid gland, is characterized by a sense of warmth, sweating, flushing, erythema and, occasionally, pain involving the cheek when the patient eats.

Davis, R. S., and Strunk, R. C.: Auriculotemporal syndrome in childhood. Am. J. Dis. Child. 135:832, 1981.

Uveoparotid syndrome is characterized by uveitis along with an indurated, painless, unilateral or bilateral enlargement of the parotid glands. The patient may complain of dryness of the mouth. Facial nerve paralysis may be an associated finding.

Hypertrophy of the masseter and/or temporalis muscles owing to excessive chewing or malocclusion may be confused with swelling of the parotid glands. Enlargement of the masseter muscle occurs anterior to the ramus of the mandible, whereas hypertrophy of the temporalis muscle is present anterior to and above the tragus.

Kalish, G. H., and Gellis, S. S.: Hypertrophy of the masseter or temporalis muscles or both. Am. J. Dis. Child. 121:346, 1971.

Kwashiorkor may be characterized by a chipmunk appearance with pendulous cheeks owing to edema, hypotonic facial muscles and well-preserved fat in the sucking pads.

9 / THE NECK

The neck is normally short in infants. Abnormally short necks occur in patients with these syndromes: chondrodystrophia calcificans congenita, hypothyroidism, Goldenhar, Hunter, Hurler, Klippel-Feil, Morquio, Noonan, platybasia, pterygium colli, spondyloepiphyseal dysplasia congenita, bilateral Sprengel's deformity and Turner's.

CERVICAL MASSES

Cervical adenopathy is a common cause of neck enlargement.

A *thyroglossal duct cyst* appears as a round, smooth, firm swelling, ¼ to 1½ inches in diameter. It is usually located in or near the midline of the neck between the foramen cecum of the tongue and the suprasternal notch, usually at or about the level of the thyroid cartilage. The cyst, which moves upward in the neck when the patient protrudes his tongue or swallows, may become apparent during a respiratory infection as a painful, tender and rapidly increasing mass. Differentiation between a thyroglossal cyst above the hyoid bone and enlargement of a submandibular lymph node may be difficult. Inflammatory changes may be intermittently present in both.

A *thyroglossal duct sinus*, which may present anywhere along the midline, from the level of the hyoid bone to the suprasternal notch, retracts on protrusion of the tongue. Occasionally, a few drops of a clear, mucoid or purulent discharge may drain from the sinus and produce a local inflammatory reaction. Rarely, an ectopic thyroid gland in the midline may simulate a thyroglossal duct cyst.

Kaplan, M., Kauli, R., Lubin, E., Grunebaum, M., and Laron, Z.: Ectopic thyroid gland. J. Pediatr. 92:205, 1978.

Dermoid or sebaceous cysts in the midline of the neck are attached to the overlying skin; thyroglossal duct cysts, unless infected, are attached to underlying structures.

A *first branchial cleft anomaly* may present as a sinus or cyst at or above the level of the hyoid bone about halfway between the midline of the neck and the anterior border of the sternocleidomastoid muscle. A fistulous tract opening into the external auditory canal may cause a chronic aural discharge. Small, subcutaneous *cartilaginous tags* or remnants rarely occur in the neck, most commonly anterior to the sternocleidomastoid muscle. The tags may be pedunculated or extend into the tissues of the neck.

Branchial cleft cysts are slightly movable, smooth, tense, nontranslucent, unilocular subcutaneous swellings from 1 to 5 cm in diameter that appear in late childhood along the anterior border of the sternocleidomastoid muscle. The overlying skin is freely movable. A sticky, clear mucoid secretion may occasionally drain from an opening along the anterior border of the sternocleidomastoid muscle between the hyoid bone and the suprasternal notch.

An enlarging, firm, usually painless mass in the neck in a child with Horner's syndrome suggests a *neuroblastoma* of the cervical sympathetic chain.

A *cystic hygroma* may occur just above the clavicle or elsewhere in the neck as a soft, diffuse, poorly demarcated cystic mass that is moderately movable, translucent and multilocular. In some instances, the tumor does not seem lobulated. The overlying skin may be thin and bluish.

Lipomas rarely appear as lobulated masses in the neck.

Edema of the neck may occur in diphtheria, infections of the deep cervical spaces, herpetic stomatitis, superior vena cava syndrome and anasarca.

Rapidly enlarging lumps or swellings in the neck, neck pain or trismus raise the possibility of a rhabdomyosarcoma or neuroblastoma.

Jaffe, B. F., and Jaffe, N.: Head and neck tumors in children. Pediatrics 51:732, 1973.
Pratt, C. B., Smith, J. W., Woerner, S., Mauer, A. M., Hustu, H. O., Johnson, W. W., and Shanks, E. C.: Factors leading to delay and affecting survival of children with head and neck rhabdomyosarcoma. Pediatrics 61:30, 1978.

A hernia of the lung may present in the midline above the sternum as a soft, spongy, lemon-shaped mass. The apices of the lungs above the clavicles may rarely appear to puff out in infants during crying.

Jones, J. G.: Cervical hernia of the lungs. J. Pediatr. 76:122, 1970.

Crepitation on palpation of the neck along with neck or shoulder pain is diagnostic of subcutaneous air secondary to pneumomediastinum.

TORTICOLLIS

The *Klippel-Feil syndrome*, caused by a fusion of two or more cervical vertebrae, is characterized by limitation of movement, shortening of the neck, a low posterior hairline and torticollis.

Congenital torticollis occurs in the first weeks of life. Tilting of the head is usually the presenting complaint. A circumscribed, firm or hard, fusiform mass, ¾ to 1½ inches in diameter, is palpable in the sternocleidomastoid muscle. The tumor, which may be demonstrated most readily when the infant's shoulders are elevated so that his head falls backward, is usually not present at birth. The mass may enlarge for two to four weeks, then regress with complete disappearance between four and eight months of age. Unresolved torticollis leads to asymmetry of the face and skull. Growth on the involved side is diminished.

Infants and children with *strabismus* or *disorder of ocular motility* may tilt their heads to one side to avoid a double visual image (ocular torticollis).

Patients with an astrocytoma or other *tumor of the cerebellar hemispheres* or *tonsillar herniation* may rotate or tilt the occiput toward the shoulder on the involved side. Tumors of the cervical spine and syringomyelia may cause torticollis.

Paroxysmal torticollis of infancy, the infantile form of benign paroxysmal vertigo, is characterized by episodes of head tilting that recur two or three times a month and last from 10 minutes to three days. Other symptoms are vomiting, pallor and restlessness.

Snyder, C. H.: Paroxysmal torticollis in infancy. A possible form of labyrinthitis. Am. J. Dis. Child. 117:458, 1969.

Torticollis owing to muscle spasm may accompany *acute cervical adenitis.* Cervical Pott's disease and retropharyngeal space abscesses also cause torticollis.

Rarely, torticollis may occur as a somatic symptom of an emotional problem.

Eosinophilic granuloma is a possibility in a child with neck pain, torticollis and a cervical vertebral lesion.

Davidson, R. I., and Shillito, J., Jr.: Eosinophilic granuloma of the cervical spine in children. Pediatrics 45:746, 1970.

An *osteoid osteoma* in the cervical spine may cause torticollis.

Acquired torticollis may be caused by a nontraumatic *subluxation of the atlantoaxial joint* associated with inflammatory processes about the neck, such as pharyngitis and cervical adenitis. Clinical manifestations include pain and tenderness at the base of the skull and limitation of head rotation. With bilateral anterior subluxation, the head is held rigidly in the midline and tilted forward with the chin depressed. With an anterior unilateral subluxation, the head is tilted forward and toward the involved side, and the neck is rotated away from the affected side. In a unilateral posterior subluxation, tilting of the head and rotation of the neck occur toward the involved side. Careful roentgenographic examination, including stereoscopic views, is indicated.

Atlantoaxial subluxation may occur in Down's syndrome, juvenile rheumatoid arthritis, Morquio syndrome, pseudoachondroplasia, spondyloepiphyseal dysplasia and cartilage-hair hypoplasia.

Dislocation secondary to atlantoaxial instability may cause neck pain, torticollis, deterioration of gait and fatigue in walking, increased clumsiness, changes in bowel or bladder function, hyperactive reflexes, clonus and intermittent or progressive weakness of the extremities.

Hreidarsson, S., Magram, G., and Singer, H.: Symptomatic atlantoaxial dislocation in Down's syndrome. Pediatrics 69:568, 1982.

Occipitalization, in which the bony ring of the atlas is partially or completely fused to the base of the occiput, is manifested by torticollis, a low posterior hairline, a short neck and limitation of motion.

Basilar impression of the skull may account for the sudden onset of neck stiffness, head tilting, headache and neurologic findings. Appropriate skull films and CT scan are diagnostic.

Teodori, J. B., and Painter, M. J.: Basilar impression in children. Pediatrics 74:1097, 1984.

Congenital *anomalies of the odontoid* may cause torticollis or subtle neurologic symptoms. Patients with a mucopolysaccharidosis or spondyloepiphyseal dysplasia often have odontoid anomalies.

Hensinger, R. H.: Orthopedic problems of the shoulder and neck. Pediatr. Clin. North Am. 24:889, 1977.

Sandifer's syndrome, characterized by bizarre movements of the head and neck, usually during or immediately after eating, occurs in some children with a hiatus hernia or gastroesophageal reflux with severe esophagitis. Usually the neck is extended and the head rotated to one side.

Hyperextension of the head and neck may occur in infants with a *vascular ring.*

NUCHAL RIGIDITY

Meningitis, cerebral abscess and other central nervous system disorders accompanied by nuchal rigidity are listed on page 119.

Tetanus is characterized by progressive stiffness of the neck muscles.

Nuchal rigidity may occur in infants with *hypernatremia* and in the *toxic shock syndrome.*

Cervical and posterior auricular adenopathy associated with rubella, infectious mononucleosis or acute cervical lymphadenitis may cause slight stiffness of the neck. Nuchal rigidity may also occur with a retropharyngeal abscess. Lyme disease may cause marked neck stiffness and pain.

Neck pain, stiffness and limitation of motion may be early symptoms of *rheumatoid arthritis.*

Calcification of the cervical intervertebral disc may cause localized pain, limitation of motion, muscle spasm, tenderness and torticollis.

Stretching of the cervical dura owing to herniation of the brainstem or cerebellum secondary to increased intracranial pressure may cause neck stiffness and pain.

VASCULAR MANIFESTATIONS

Venous engorgement in the neck, best seen with the patient sitting up, is observed in congestive cardiac failure, constrictive pericarditis, enlarged mediastinal nodes and pneumomediastinum.

Superior vena cava syndrome is characterized by venous engorgement of neck and chest veins; edema and cyanosis or plethora of the face, neck and upper trunk; stridor; cough; chest pain; and dyspnea. This disorder may occur secondary to congenital heart disease surgery, malignant lymphoma, mediastinal fibrosis secondary to histoplasmosis, cystic hygroma and other obstructive mediastinal lesions. Swelling of the face, especially periorbitally in the morning, may be the initial sign.

Issa, P. Y., Brihi, E. R., Janin, Y., and Slim, M. S.: Superior vena cava syndrome in childhood: Report of ten cases and review of the literature. Pediatrics 71:337, 1983.

A *cervical aortic arch* presents as a pulsating mass in the suprasternal region or above the clavicle. It is best seen when the patient is seated with his head retracted. A systolic murmur and thrill may be present. Symptoms owing to compression of the trachea and esophagus may be reported.

Mullins, C. E., Gillette, P. C., and McNamara, D. G.: The complex of cervical aortic arch. Pediatrics 51:210, 1973.

Unusual pulsation of the carotid arteries may occur with aortic insufficiency. Pulsation of the neck vessels also occurs with a large patent ductus arteriosus.

Takayasu's aortitis may be characterized by a bruit in the neck, carotid tenderness and neck pain.

The hepatojugular reflex is present with congestive heart failure. With the patient recumbent, venous distention in the neck becomes accentuated when pressure is applied over the liver.

CONGENITAL ANOMALIES

Pterygium colli, webbed neck or "sphinx neck," is characterized by a thick web of skin that extends from behind the ears to the distal portion of the clavicle and to the acromial process. Pterygium colli is sometimes seen in trisomy 18 and in *Turner's* and *Noonan's syndromes*. Redundant, loose longitudinal folds of skin may also occur over the neck. Nuchal webbing and a low hairline may be present in the *fetal hydantoin syndrome*.

Redundancy and laxity of the skin about the neck occur in *Down's, Zellweger* and *Klippel-Feil* syndromes.

THYROID

The size and other characteristics of the isthmus and lobes of the thyroid may be determined by standing behind the patient, hyperextending his head, and palpating the gland with the fingers of both hands as it moves upward during swallowing. Another approach is to face the patient, place one's thumbs along the upper border of the isthmus, position the fingers along the posterior border of the sternocleidomastoid muscle, and ask the patient to swallow. Moderate enlargement of the thyroid is, of course, readily evident on inspection. Normally, the right lobe may be larger than the left.

Gas, A., and Reiter, E.: The thyroid. Recent advances in normal and abnormal physiology. Adv. Pediatr. 26:441, 1979.
Reiter, E. O., Root, A. W., Rettig, K., and Vargas, A.: Childhood thyromegaly: Recent developments. J. Pediatr. 99:507, 1981.

Neonatal goiters, characterized either by a slightly nodular or a soft, diffuse enlargement, usually disappear in a short time. A large goiter may cause tracheal compression, respiratory difficulty and hoarseness. Babies whose mothers received propylthiouracil or methimazole during pregnancy may have a goiter at birth. An enlarged thyroid may also appear a few days after birth in babies whose mothers received iodides prenatally. Maternal iodine deficiency may be associated with neonatal goiter. The cause for some neonatal goiters is unknown.

Senior, B., and Chernoff, H. L.: Iodide goiter in the newborn. Pediatrics 47:510, 1971.

A soft, diffuse and usually transitory increase in size of the thyroid may occur physiologically during or immediately after puberty, especially in rapidly growing girls. The gland is smooth with indistinct edges.

Simple or endemic goiter owing to iodine deficiency, a rare occurrence in North

America, is characterized by a diffuse, smooth, compressible enlargement of the thyroid gland. A bruit and thrill may be present.

Doland, T. F., Jr., and Gibson, L. E.: Complications of iodide therapy in patients with cystic fibrosis. J. Pediatr. 79:684, 1971.

Chronic lymphocytic thyroiditis and Grave's disease account for more than 90 per cent of goiters in children and adolescents. Children with insulin-dependent diabetes mellitus have an increased frequency of autoimmune thyroid disease. Patients with hyperthyroidism, toxic thyroiditis, a pituitary adenoma or inappropriate secretion of TSH have a diffuse, symmetric, smooth, and nontender, soft enlargement of the thyroid. A continuous bruit and a palpable thrill are often present over the gland. The thyroid is usually very prominent but, occasionally, may be only slightly enlarged.

Vaidya, V. A., Bongiovanni, A. M., Parks, J. S., Tenore, A., and Kirkland, R. T.: Twenty-two years' experience in the medical management of juvenile thyrotoxicosis. Pediatrics 54:565, 1974.

Hashimoto's thyroiditis or *chronic lymphocytic thyroiditis* is a common cause of goiter in children and adolescents, especially girls. Usually the thyroid enlargement in these patients is asymptomatic, but occasionally the patient may complain of local pressure, sore throat, dysphagia, and hoarseness. Symptoms and signs of hypo- or hyperthyroidism may also be present. Nontender, coarsely granular or pebbly and firm in consistency, the gland may be asymmetrically or symmetrically enlarged. Rarely, a single nodule may be palpable. The delphian node may be felt above the isthmus.

An irregular, *nodular enlargement* of the thyroid may be neoplastic, especially if the lesion is hard, rapidly growing, fixed and accompanied by hoarseness or cervical adenopathy. Enlargement of the delphian and other cervical lymph nodes may be the presenting finding of a thyroid neoplasm. A unilateral thyroid mass may be caused by Hashimoto's thyroiditis, ectopic thyroid, cyst or adenoma.

In the *mucosal neuroma* or multiple endocrine neoplasia syndrome, *medullary carcinoma* of the thyroid gland may be accompanied by a Marfan-like body habitus and multiple nodularities of the tongue and lips. Pheochromocytoma and ganglioneuroma may also be present.

Levin, D. L., Perlia, C., and Tashjian, A. H., Jr.: Medullary carcinoma of the thyroid gland: The complete syndrome in a child. Pediatrics 52:192, 1973.

Acute and subacute thyroiditis, either of a viral or a bacterial etiology, is characterized by fever and exquisite tenderness and pain that is referred, at times, to the angle of the jaws.

Familial goiters or *familial dyshormonogenesis* is caused by a defect in thyroid hormone synthesis. Hypothyroidism appears in infancy or early childhood with a soft, diffuse goiter apparent late in the first decade or adolescence.

Goitrogen or *drug-induced goiter,* e.g., owing to iodides or lithium, is rare in childhood.

Foley, T. P., Jr.: Goiter in children. Pediatr. Rev. 5:259, 1984.

GENERAL REFERENCES

Ferguson, C. F., and Kendig, E. L.: Pediatric Otolaryngology. Vol. II: Disorders of the Respiratory Tract in Children. Philadelphia, W. B. Saunders Co., 1972.
Strome, M.: Differential Diagnosis in Pediatric Otolaryngology. Boston, Little, Brown and Co., 1975.

10 / THE CHEST

RESPIRATIONS

During early infancy, and especially in prematures, respiratory movements may be irregular, intermittent and variable in rate and depth. Breathing may be almost imperceptible during sleep. *Periodic breathing* with brief respiratory pauses of up to 10 seconds without cyanosis is common during sleep in normal infants, especially premature infants, and in the early weeks of life. Brief apneic periods may follow a sigh.

Breathing during infancy is characteristically abdominal or diaphragmatic. A thoracic respiratory component in young infants suggests pulmonary disease, unless abdominal distention or disorder is present. The thoracic type of respiration, more prominent as the child grows older, becomes predominant at about seven or eight years of age.

In full-term newborn infants the respiratory rate averages about 45 per minute when awake and 35 per minute when asleep, with a considerable normal range on either side of these averages. The rate also tends to be higher in premature infants. An increase to a rate of 70 or 80 may occur with very little excitation. Because of this, accurate respiratory rates are best obtained during sleep. The rate is around 30 per minute at one year of age, 20 to 25 per minute during the preschool period and about 20 per minute at 10 years of age. Table 10–1 lists the respiratory rates for children of various ages.

A *rapid respiratory rate* may occur with pulmonary infections, paroxysmal atrial tachycardia, myocarditis, congestive heart failure, neonatal narcotic withdrawal, meningitis, fever, pain, severe anemia, metabolic acidosis, hyperammonemia, shock and acute anxiety. Tachypnea ranging from 50 to 100 per minute during sleep may be the first sign of left heart failure. Abdominal distention may be an important cause of respiratory difficulty in infants, producing respiratory distress, tachypnea and even cyanosis, especially in the presence of patchy atelectasis or pneumonitis. Because of the pain, respiratory movements in patients with peritonitis are rapid, chiefly thoracic, rather than abdominal, and accompanied by grunting. Expiratory grunting may also be noted with pneumonia, heart failure, pulmonary edema and the neonatal respiratory distress syndrome. Gasping respiration occurring continuously for several hours to a week is caused by benzyl alcohol poisoning in premature infants.

Gershanik, J., Boecler, B., Ensley, H., McCloskey, S., and George, W.: The gasping syndrome and benzyl alcohol poisoning. N. Engl. J. Med. 307:1384, 1982

Because salicylate poisoning may cause an increase in the respiratory rate, a blood salicylate level should be obtained in all young children with hyperpnea, even if aspirin ingestion is denied.

Intermittent hyperventilation and irregular, sighing respiration occur with *subacute necrotizing encephalomyelopathy* (Leigh's syndrome).

Neurogenic hyperventilation may be caused by midbrain-pontine herniation secondary to increased intracranial pressure.

Kussmaul breathing owing to metabolic acidosis and characterized by deep respiratory movements and use of the accessory respiratory musculature may occur in diabetic ketoacidosis, renal failure, salicylism, inborn errors of metabolism, lactic acidosis and Reye's syndrome.

Hypoxic states in infants and children are usually accompanied by apprehension, anxiety, restlessness and tachypnea.

Orthopnea occurs with asthma, pulmonary edema, epiglottitis, croup and cystic fibrosis.

Bulbar or central involvement of the respiratory center may lead to irregular and shallow respiratory movements characterized by spasmodic or jerky, hiccup-like inspirations and intervals of apnea. The early diagnosis of *intercostal or diaphragmatic paralysis* permits prompt use of assisted ventilation to prevent fatigue and hypoxia. Early signs of respiratory insufficiency include irregular, shallow respirations with, perhaps, an increase in respiratory rate; use of the accessory muscles of respiration; dilatation of the alae nasi; slight grunting; unwillingness to talk; frequent interruptions in speech; monosyllabic speech; restlessness; anxiety; fear of falling asleep; mental confusion; headache; and, occasionally, euphoria. Decreased vital capacity can be demonstrated by asking the patient to count rapidly to 10. Patients with respiratory difficulty cannot do this. Cyanosis and unresponsiveness are *late* signs, as is forced use of the accessory muscles of respiration with gasping and opening of the mouth for each breath.

Intercostal and diaphragmatic paralysis may occur simultaneously or independently. In young children it may be possible to localize paralysis of the intercostals or diaphragm by splinting the chest and then the abdomen while observing the action of the alternate group of muscles. With paralysis of the intercostals, the patient is able to exhale but cannot inhale. The converse is true with diaphragmatic involvement. When the intercostal muscles are paralyzed, abnormal expansion of the abdomen occurs on inspiration, unaccompanied by enlargement of the chest or by unilateral or bilateral pulling in of the chest wall. When the diaphragm is paralyzed, the chest expands on inspiration, and the upper part of the abdomen retracts. With unilateral paralysis of the diaphragm, wide flaring of the ribs on

TABLE 10–1. Respiratory Rates per Minute of Normal Children,
Both Sexes, Sleeping and Awake*

Age	Sleeping			Awake			Mean Difference Between Sleeping and Awake
	No.	Mean	Range	No.	Mean	Range	
6–12 months	6	27	22–31	3	64	58–75	37
1– 2 years	6	19	17–23	4	35	30–40	16
2– 4 years	16	19	16–25	15	31	23–42	12
4– 6 years	23	18	14–23	22	26	19–36	8
6– 8 years	27	17	13–23	28	23	15–30	6
8–10 years	19	18	14–23	19	21	15–31	3
10–12 years	11	16	13–19	17	21	15–28	5
12–14 years	6	16	15–18	7	22	18–26	6

*From Waring, W. W. *In* Kendig, E. L., Jr., and Chernick, V. (eds.): Disorders of the Respiratory Tract in Children. 3rd ed. Philadelphia, W. B. Saunders Co., 1977, p. 84.

the ipsilateral side occurs if the intercostals are intact.

Respiratory difficulty may occur in patients with the Guillain-Barré syndrome. Diaphragmatic paralysis may be a manifestation of diphtheritic neuritis. Patients with chorea may have paradoxical respiration with retraction instead of abdominal expansion at the beginning of a deep inspiration (*Czerny's sign*).

Respiratory difficulty and irregular duration and amplitude may occur in children with spastic cerebral palsy owing to incoordination of the respiratory musculature. The respiratory excursions may be jerky and halting.

Unequal expansion and respiration lag suggest pneumonia, pleurisy, pneumothorax, empyema, hydrothorax, diaphragmatic hernia or atelectasis. Flattening of the involved side of the chest and narrowing of the intercostal spaces may occur with massive atelectasis.

RETRACTIONS AND BULGING

When expansion of the lungs lags behind the forced expansion of the thoracic cage during labored breathing, increased negative intrathoracic pressure results and retractions occur. The sternum and ribs are lifted during inspiration, while the soft tissues in the suprasternal, infrasternal, intercostal, subcostal and supraclavicular spaces move inward.

Slight retractions are normal. More marked retractions occur with atelectasis, pneumonia, bronchiolitis, cystic fibrosis, asthma and respiratory tract obstruction, especially laryngeal. Mild retractions may occur in young infants when the nasal airway is blocked by a purulent discharge or in infants with congenital choanal atresia. With congenital hypoplasia of the mandible and glossoptosis, compromise of the airway may cause retractions.

Because of the poorly developed and yielding thoracic skeleton in prematures and in some term infants, retraction of the thoracic cage, especially over the anterior chest wall and along the line of diaphragmatic attachment, may occur when the diaphragm contracts during inspiration. During infancy the sternum may demonstrate paradoxical motion on respiration, moving inward rather than outward on inspiration. Retraction of the sternum during inspiration does not always imply insufficient pulmonary aeration, particularly in small premature infants. Inspiratory collapse of the thoracic wall in such infants is also not necessarily the cause or result of atelectasis.

Intercostal bulging may occasionally be noted with a large pleural effusion or exudate or with a marked expiratory effort.

Precordial bulging may occur in patients with pneumomediastinum or with right ventricular hypertrophy.

STRUCTURAL ANOMALIES OR CHANGES

Funnel chest or pectus excavatum is characterized by a depression of the sternum and costal cartilages, most prominent during inspiration. The defect usually begins at about the second interspace and becomes more prominent toward the xiphoid. The apex of the depression may be in the midline, over or slightly lateral to the xiphoid. Lateral funnel chest may be associated with absence of the pectoralis major and minor. Pectus excavatum occurs with the Marfan's and Noonan's syndromes.

Pigeon breast or pectus carinatum is characterized by a prominent, protruding sternum with vertical depressions along the costochondral junctions lateral to the sternum. Patients with the Morquio's, spondyloepiphyseal dysplasia congenita, Marfan's, Noonan's and Schwartz-Jampel syndromes have notable pigeon breast deformities.

Harrison's groove, a horizontal depression of the rib cage along the attachment of the diaphragm extending from the lower end of the sternum to the midaxillary line, may be congenital or a sequela of rickets. Some flaring of the costal margins occurs below this groove.

A *barrel-shaped chest*, in which the sternum appears to be pushed out and the ribs are more horizontal than normal, may develop as a result of chronic obstructive pulmonary diseases such as asthma, cystic fibrosis and bronchopulmonary dysplasia.

Asphyxiating thoracic dystrophy, a generalized skeletal abnormality, causes a narrow, fixed thorax. The circumference of the chest at the nipple line is decreased. Respiratory distress and cyanosis occur when the abnormality is severe.

Oberklaid, F., Danks, D. M., Mayne, V., and Campbell, P.: Asphyxiating thoracic dysplasia: Clinical, radiological and pathological information on 10 patients. Arch. Dis. Child. 52:758, 1977.

The *cerebro-costo-mandibular syndrome* is characterized by multiple, bilateral, posterior rib gaps; micrognathia; cleft palate; and glossoptosis. In infants with the Pierre Robin syndrome, diagnosis of this disorder may be made by obtaining a chest radiograph.

In *Morquio's disease* the vertical length of the chest is decreased, and the anteroposterior diameter and width are increased. Protrusion of the sternum develops during early childhood.

The costochondral junctions are palpable in many normal infants but not to the extent that they are with rickets or scurvy. The *rachitic rosary* consists of rounded, knoblike prominences or beading at the costochrondral junctions. *Scorbutic beading* is characterized by sharp, angular deformities of the costochondral junctions. The sternum and the adjacent cartilage may be displaced inwardly or dorsally at the costochondral junction to produce the so-called bayonet deformity. Enlargement of the costochondral junctions may also occur in chondrodystrophy and hypophosphatasia.

Agenesis or hypoplasia of the pectoralis major and minor muscles is accompanied by hypoplasia or absence of the breast and nipple. Lack of a well-developed anterior axillary fold is evident on inspection. In Poland's syndrome, ipsilateral hypoplasia of the upper extremity and syndactyly may occur, along with defects in the ribs and costal cartilages.

Brooksaler, R. S., and Graivier, L.: Poland's syndrome. Am. J. Dis. Child. 121:263, 1971.

Tietze's syndrome is characterized by a firm, tender and painful fusiform swelling of one or more of the upper four costal cartilages. Although it is usually localized to the involved cartilage, the pain may radiate elsewhere.

Both *blunt* and *penetrating* thoracic trauma may occur in children.

Meller, J. L., Little, A. G., and Shermeta, D. W.: Thoracic trauma in children. Pediatrics 74:813, 1984.

PERCUSSION AND TRANSILLUMINATION

Percussion is performed in infants and children much as in adults, either indirectly, by striking the middle phalanx of one middle finger with the tip of the other middle finger; or by percussing the chest wall directly with the finger tips. Because of the thinness of an infant's chest wall, the percussion findings in that age group differ from those in older children. Tactile sensations, such as a feeling of resistance or fullness, may be more informative than the percussion note.

In the examination of the lung fields in infants and children, light percussion over the interspaces may be used, beginning in the supraclavicular spaces and proceeding downward, comparing the percussion notes obtained on both sides of the chest. Physical findings related to the upper lobes are represented over the upper half of the chest anteriorly, the upper axillae laterally and the upper third of the back posteriorly. The lower lobes largely account for pulmonary findings over the rest of the thorax except in the nipple and midaxillary areas on the right.

Liver dullness in infants usually extends up to the lower border of the sixth rib anteriorly. The dullness shades off above this point to about the region of the fourth rib. An impaired percussion note may be present over the left lower hemithorax anteriorly when the stomach of an infant is distended with fluid. Usually, however, a tympanitic percussion note is elicited on the left side below the sixth rib owing to the gastric air bubble.

Preferably, the child should sit or stand erect during percussion of the chest; however, in infants and children too ill or disinclined to sit up, the patient should lie as straight as possible so that flexion of the trunk and uneven contact with the bedclothing do not produce misleading percussion notes.

Impairment of the percussion note with dullness or flatness may be noted in lobar pneumonia during consolidation, massive atelectasis, pleural thickening, an intrathoracic neoplasm or diaphragmatic hernia. Patchy atelectasis may be characterized by areas of impaired resonance, but the percussion note is usually modified by the compensatory emphysema. In the presence of pleural effusion, empyema, or chylothorax, the percussion note over the involved area is flat. If the effusion is only moderate in amount, a tympanitic percussion note may be found above the area of dullness. Except in the presence of massive effusion, shifting dullness may be noted when the patient changes from a sitting to a recumbent position.

Hyperresonance may be noted in pneumothorax, lobar emphysema, asthma, bronchiolitis, cystic fibrosis or bronchopulmonary dysplasia. Tympany on percussion may be obtained in some infants with a diaphragmatic hernia.

Transillumination of the affected side occurs with massive pneumothorax in the neonate.

Kuhns, L. R., Bednarek, F. J., Wyman, M. L., Roloff, D. W., and Borer, R. C.: Diagnosis of pneumothorax or pneumomediastinum in the neonate by transillumination. Pediatrics 56:355, 1975.

AUSCULTATION

In auscultating an older child's chest, the examiner may have the child breathe deeply through his mouth ("pant like a dog"), after demonstrating what is desired, then follow the child's respirations by saying "In" and "Out" as auscultation proceeds. Since forced respiration may be tiring, the child should be given a brief respite during the examination. The choice of a bell or a diaphragm type of stethoscope is a matter of individual preference and experience. Either should be small enough, however, to fit closely over the interspaces.

In prenasal and preoral auscultation, the examiner listens to the breath sounds with the bowl of the stethoscope held ½ to 1 inch in front of the infant's nose or mouth. This permits an evaluation of the infant's respiration and air movement without awakening or causing him to cry.

In infancy the breath sounds are relatively louder and harsher than in adults. This relative increase in the intensity of breath sounds is present up to the age of five or six years. The breath sounds over the medial and upper portions of the chest are characterized by a relatively prolonged expiratory phase as compared to the same areas in adults. These sounds, which resemble the adult's bronchovesicular breathing, have been called puerile breathing. In young infants no noticeable pause may occur between expiration and the next inspiration; on the other hand, expiration may be quiet, and a brief pause may be noted before the inspiratory phase.

Breath sounds may be classified as vesicular, tracheal (bronchial, tubular) and bronchovesicular.

In older children *vesicular breath sounds* are heard over most of the chest, except for those limited areas characterized by tracheal or bronchovesicular breathing. Inspiration is louder, higher-pitched and longer in duration than expiration. The latter may be so brief and faint as to be almost imperceptible in the older child. Vesicular breath sounds are most intense over the upper part of the chest and axillae. As in percussion, one begins with the examination of the supraclavicular fossae and proceeds downward, an interspace at a time, comparing findings on both sides of the chest. Slight variations in the sounds on the two sides of the chest may be present, but with experience one learns the normal limits of this variation. As noted earlier, the breath sounds are more intense and harsh in early life, and puerile or bronchovesicular breath sounds with relative prolongation of the expiratory phase are present medially and over the upper portion of the chest.

Diminished or suppressed vesicular breathing, characterized by a decrease in intensity, may occur early in pneumonia. In infants and young children the transmission of breath sounds through an area of pleural effusion may be only slightly diminished, although the percussion note is dull. Diminished vesicular breathing may also be noted with hydrothorax, pneumothorax, lobar emphysema, pleurisy, patchy atelectasis, massive atelectasis if the associated bronchus is closed, pulmonary edema, bronchitis, and paralysis of the respiratory musculature.

Tracheal breath sounds are normally heard over the trachea, larynx, and upper part of the sternum, and along the vertebral column above the first thoracic vertebra.

These breath sounds are louder and more tubular and have a much higher pitch than the vesicular breath sounds. The expiratory phase is also longer and louder. A brief pause may occur between inspiration and expiration. *Tubular breathing* may be heard in pneumonia during consolidation; tuberculosis; atelectasis, if the bronchus to the atelectatic area remains open; massive pericardial effusion; and in some instances of pleurisy with effusion.

In infants and young children, *bronchovesicular breath sounds* are heard parasternally and over the upper part of the chest. In older children these findings are limited to the area of the larger bronchi—over the manubrium, along the sternal angle of Louis and posteriorly in the upper interscapular area. Usually, the expiratory phase is longer, louder and higher-pitched than the inspiratory phase.

In patients with a *congenital diaphragmatic hernia*, breath sounds may be distant or absent on the involved side. Bowel sounds may be heard in the chest; however, bowel sounds occasionally can be heard over the left anterior lower hemithorax in normal infants.

Rhonchi are musical, continuous sounds, wheezes and vibrations.

Rales are crackling or bubbling, discontinuous sounds or vibrations. Rales of the medium or fine variety may be heard in a number of disease states, such as bronchitis, pneumonia, atelectasis, pulmonary edema, heart failure, bronchiectasis and tuberculosis.

Wheezing is discussed on page 369.

A *pleural friction rub* causes a grating, jerky, leathery, creaking, rubbing sound that seems close to the examiner's ear. It can be intensified by slight pressure with the stethoscope on the chest wall. The rub is usually most distinct at the end of inspiration but may be present in both phases and disappear when the patient holds his breath. A pleuropericardial rub has auscultatory features of both pleural and pericardial rubs.

GENERAL REFERENCES

Waring, W. W.: The history and physical examination. In Kendig, E. L., Jr., and Chernick, V. (eds.): Disorders of the Respiratory Tract in Children. 3rd ed. Philadelphia, W. B. Saunders Co., 1977, p. 71.

THE BREASTS

Breast examination is helpful in assessing the newborn's gestational age. In the premature the areola and nipple are barely visible, and breast tissue is not palpable. The areola becomes evident at about 34 weeks. The term infant has 5 to 6 mm of palpable breast tissue, and the areola is raised. The postmature infant has 10 to 12 mm of breast tissue.

Unilateral or bilateral *engorgement of the breasts* may appear in both male and female term newborn infants on the second to fourth day, gradually increase for a time and persist in some for several weeks. A colostrum-like secretion from the breasts may be noted. Engorgement does not occur in prematures. *Mastitis* or infection of the breast in the newborn infant characterized by local redness, heat and swelling, is usually caused by *Staphylococcus aureus*, or, more rarely, gram-negative organisms. A benign bloody nipple discharge may occur in the first week of life.

Berkowitz, C. D., and Inkelis, S. H.: Bloody nipple discharge in infancy. J. Pediatr. 103:755, 1983.

Supernumerary nipples may occasionally occur in the axillary line or below and medial to the nipple. Although increased internipple distance may be associated with the Noonan's or Turner's syndromes, it is not a diagnostic finding.

Collins, E.: The illusion of widely spaced nipples in the Noonan and the Turner syndromes. J. Pediatr. 83:557, 1973.

Breast development or *thelarche*, generally the earliest of the secondary sexual characteristics to appear, usually begins in adolescent girls at 11.2 years with a range between 8 and 14.8 years. Onset of thelarche under 8 years of age is premature; absence of breast development beyond 15 years of age represents delayed puberty. Normal progression of breast development occurs over two to four years. Menarche usually occurs within three years after thelarche but in some cases may not develop until five years later. A considerable difference in the status of breast development, size and contour exists among girls of the same chronologic age. In the individual girl, one breast may develop chronologically somewhat in advance of the other.

The Tanner stages of breast development are as follows:

Stage I.   Preadolescent. Only the papilla is elevated.

Stage II. The breast bud stage. The breast and the papilla are both elevated as a small mound, and the diameter of the areola is enlarged. Peak height velocity often occurs between Stages II and III.

Stage III.   Further enlargement and eleva-
             tion of the breast and areola oc-
             cur with no distinct separation
             of their contours.
Stage IV.   Projection of the areola and the
             papilla to form a secondary
             mound above the level of the
             breast.
Stage V.   The mature stage, in which only
             the papilla projects because of
             the recession of the areola to the
             general contour of the breast.

In some girls, breast development does
not progress beyond Tanner Stage III until
late adolescence or during pregnancy and
lactation.

Breast examination should be routinely
included in the general physical examination of adolescent girls. A simple explanation of the importance of such examination
helps allay embarrassment.

Occasionally, unilateral or bilateral *precocious breast development (premature
thelarche)* may be noted in the absence of
other signs of sexual maturation. Although
this enlargement usually does not proceed
beyond the bud stage, continued observation
for other signs of precocious development is
indicated. Children who proceed to complete
sexual precocity usually demonstrate advanced height and bone age and estrogen
effects on the vaginal mucosa.

Precocious breast development has also
been reported in young children owing to
accidental ingestion of diethylstilbestrol. Intense, dark brown areolar pigmentation in
a girl with pseudoprecocious puberty suggests exogenous estrogen as a cause for the
precocity. Other drugs reported to cause enlargement of the breasts include cimetidine,
digitalis, spironolactone and phenothiazines.

During the prepubertal period, a unilateral or bilateral, transient, indurated, *discoid swelling*, 1 or 2 inches in diameter,
may occur behind the areola in both boys
and girls. The swelling may be painful, and
secretion of a colostrum-like substance may
occur.

Breast swelling and tenderness occur in
the *premenstrual syndrome*.

Enlargement of the breast and nipple and
an underlying disclike mass occurs in patients with *leprechaunism*.

Some degree of unilateral or bilateral
breast enlargement or simple *adolescent gynecomastia* is common in adolescent boys,
especially those 13 to 14 years of age. In
some instances the enlargement may be
moderate. Most instances of gynecomastia
in adolescent males are of nonendocrine
etiology. Spontaneous regression should occur within a few months to two or three

years. Gynecomastia is present in 1.6 per
cent of 17-year-old males. Obese children
may seem to have enlarged breasts, but this
appearance is usually due to adipose rather
than glandular tissue.

August, G. P., Chandra, R., and Hung, W.: Pub-
    ertal male gynecomastia. J. Pediatr. 80:259,
    1972.
Latorre, H., and Kenny, F. M.: Idiopathic gyneco-
    mastia in seven preadolescent boys. Am. J. Dis.
    Child. 126:771, 1973.

Klinefelter's syndrome is characterized
by postpubertal, bilateral gynecomastia,
which may be prominent. Other secondary
sexual characteristics are normal, but the
testes are small and spermatogenesis does
not occur.

Pathologic causes for gynecomastia in adolescence are rare, but they include severe
liver disease, congenital virilizing adrenal
hyperplasia, thyrotoxicosis, feminizing tumors of the adrenal, true hermaphroditism,
interstitial cell tumor of the testis, congenital anorchia, mixed gonadal dysgenesis,
Reifenstein's and Rosewater's syndromes,
chorionepithelioma, exogenous estrogen,
heroin, marijuana, tricyclic antidepressants, cimetidine and spironolactone. Gynecomastia may be a result of Leydig cell
dysfunction in adolescent boys secondary to
chemotherapy for malignant disease.

Sherins, R. J., Olweny, C. L. M., and Ziegler, J.
    L.: Gynecomastia and gonadal dysfunction in
    adolescent boys treated with combination che-
    motherapy for Hodgkin's disease. N. Engl. J.
    Med. 299:12, 1978.

Breast development does not generally occur in a girl with Turner's syndrome unless
cyclic estrogen treatment is used. Slight
breast development may occur in XO/XX
mosaics.

Occasionally, unilateral or bilateral massive *virginal breast hypertrophy* may occur
in an otherwise normal adolescent girl.

In girls with scoliosis, the size of one
breast may appear smaller because of ipsilateral flattening of the ribs.

The most common adolescent female
breast tumor is the benign *fibroadenoma*,
which is palpable as a rubbery, firm, mobile,
2.5 × 3.0 cm mass with a smooth or slightly
irregular surface. Multiple bilateral and
tender breast masses suggest benign intra-
ductal hypertrophy.

Turbey, W. J., Buntain, W. L., and Dudgeon, D.
    L.: The surgical management of pediatric breast
    masses. Pediatrics 56:736, 1975.

Galactorrhea, a rare occurrence in adolescent males, may be caused by a hypothalamic or pituitary tumor, usually a prolac-

tinoma. In adolescent girls, galactorrhea, with either a spontaneous discharge or one occurring upon manipulation of the nipple accompanied by amenorrhea, may occur with hypothalamic or pituitary abnormalities or tumor, especially a craniopharyngioma. Prolactin determinations are indicated in such instances. Galactorrhea may also occur as a side effect of a variety of drugs, including tranquilizers, oral contra-ceptives, steroids, tricyclic antidepressants and antihistamines.

GENERAL REFERENCES

Dewhurst, J.: Breast disorders in children and adolescents. Pediatr. Clin. North Am. 28:287, 1981.
Dudgeon, D. L.: Pediatric breast lesions: Take the conservative approach. Contemp. Pediatr. 2:61, 1985.

11 / THE HEART AND BLOOD PRESSURE

THE HEART

APEX BEAT

The apex beat—usually not apparent in infants and young children unless the heart is enlarged or the subcutaneous fat over the chest is minimal—may be palpable, although not as well-localized as in older children. Because of the heart's relatively horizontal position, the apex beat in children up to three years of age is usually present in the fourth interspace outside the mammary line. In children aged four to seven years, the apex beat is usually in the fifth to sixth interspace within the mammary line. The heart's right border normally extends to the right sternal margin, and the left border is usually within the mammary line. The apex beat is best palpated with the child sitting and leaning forward.

The apical impulse may be diffuse and almost inapparent in patients with pneumomediastinum, pericarditis with effusion and pleurisy with effusion. In the presence of hyperthyroidism, excitement or anxiety, the apex beat may be prominent.

When the heart is enlarged, the apex beat is displaced to the left. Location of the apex beat more than 1 cm lateral to the midclavicular line in the fourth interspace in young children and outside this line in the fifth interspace in older children suggests cardiomegaly. In the presence of pleurisy with effusion, pneumothorax or lobar emphysema, the apex beat shifts toward the uninvolved side. With atelectasis, the apex beat shifts toward the involved side. The apex beat is present on the right in dextrocardia.

THRILLS

The palm or finger tips may be used in palpating for a thrill. Light palpation is usually best, although, at times, a thrill is more readily detected by firm palpation. Differentiation between an active but normal cardiac thrust and a thrill may be difficult, especially in the patient with a thin chest wall. Other than reflecting the loudness of a murmur (at least Grade IV), a thrill has no significance.

Systolic Thrill. Aortic stenosis is almost always accompanied by a thrill over the base of the heart to the right of the sternum, over the carotid arteries and at the suprasternal notch. A systolic thrill may be present in the second and third left interspaces in atrial septal defects, especially if another anomaly such as pulmonary stenosis or interventricular septal defect is also present, and over the third and fourth left interspaces in interventricular septal defects. Pulmonary stenosis, either isolated or present in the tetralogy of Fallot, may be accompanied by a thrill in the second and third left interspaces and in the suprasternal notch. A venous hum may be accompanied by a thrill.

Continuous Thrill. About half of the patients with a patent ductus arteriosus have a systolic or continuous thrill at the base of the heart, parasternally along the first and second left interspaces, and below the left clavicle.

PULSE

Because it is unaffected by exercise, anxiety or excitement, the sleeping pulse represents the baseline heart rate in infants and children. Tachycardia during sleep is of diagnostic interest in relation to rheumatic fever and hyperthyroidism. It is difficult to determine the pulse rate in infants by radial palpation, so auscultation of the heart must be used. The approximate rate at various ages is given in Table 11–1. An increase in rate occurs in patients with fever, severe anemia, hypoxia, hyperthyroidism and myocarditis. Asymmetric pulses may be present in Takayasu's arteritis.

Tachycardia, with a rate of 150 to 200 in infants and 100 to 150 in older children, is a constant finding in children in congestive cardiac failure and is an early manifestation of dehydration. A rapid heart rate and palpitations may also occur paroxysmally in pheochromocytoma. In sinus tachycardia, the rate varies some 10 to 15 beats a minute, in contrast to paroxysmal atrial or supraventricular tachycardia, in which the onset and termination of tachycardia are abrupt; the rate, almost uncountable but always greater than 200 beats a minute, remains constant during an episode. Supraventricular tachycardia in the older child may be associated with the Wolff-Parkinson-White syndrome.

Myocarditis accompanies many viral diseases. The initial symptoms of interstitial myocarditis in children may simulate those of a severe pneumonia or a mild gastroenteritis. The patient, however, soon exhibits tachycardia, a change in the quality of heart sounds, gallop rhythm, cardiac enlargement, dyspnea, hepatomegaly, edema and possibly cyanosis.

Bradycardia in the presence of fever suggests a salmonella infection. Sinus bradycardia may be associated with severe systemic disease, acidosis and increased intracranial pressure. Rheumatic fever patients treated with cortisone may also have bradycardia. A slow heart rate is noted in trained athletes and in patients with hypothyroidism or anorexia nervosa.

The heart rate is an important diagnostic and prognostic sign in neonatal asphyxia. Rates under 100 warrant special concern. The occurrence of bradycardia at birth may follow poisoning by local anesthetics administered to the mother during labor. Bradycardia may also be caused by congenital or acquired complete atrioventricular heart block. Infants with neonatal lupus erythematosus may exhibit bradycardia owing to a congenital atrioventricular heart block.

Pinsky, W. W., Gillette, P. C., Garson, A., Jr., and McNamara, D. G.: Diagnosis, management and long-term results of patients with congenital complete atrioventricular block. Pediatrics 69:728, 1982.

Patients with aortic insufficiency have a bounding pulse with a quick rise and fall. Capillary pulsations may be noted in the fingernails.

Palpation of the femoral pulse should be routinely performed in infants and young children as well as in infants with cardiac enlargement. An absent or weak femoral pulse suggests coarctation of the aorta and is an indication for blood pressure determination; however, the presence of a palpable femoral pulse does not exclude coarctation.

TABLE 11–1. AVERAGE PULSE RATES AT REST*

Age	Lower Limits of Normal		Average		Upper Limits of Normal	
Newborn	70		120		170	
1–11 months	80		120		160	
2 years	80		110		130	
4 years	80		100		120	
6 years	75		100		115	
8 years	70		90		110	
10 years	70		90		110	
	Girls	Boys	Girls	Boys	Girls	Boys
12 years	70	65	90	85	110	105
14 years	65	60	85	80	105	100
16 years	60	55	80	75	100	95
18 years	55	50	75	70	95	90

*From Behrman, R. E., and Vaughan, V. C., III (eds.): The Nelson Textbook of Pediatrics. Philadelphia, W. B. Saunders Co., 1983, p. 1100.

Simultaneous palpation of both the radial and femoral pulses may be helpful. Normally, both impulses are felt at the same time, but in coarctation, the femoral pulse wave may be slightly delayed.

In *Takayasu's arteritis,* the carotid, brachial and radial pulses may be absent or diminished.

Although an *arrhythmia* may be noted clinically, a specific diagnosis depends on an electrocardiograph. Arrhythmia may occur in patients with Guillain-Barré syndrome, Rocky Mountain spotted fever and mitral valve prolapse.

Gillette, P. C.: Cardiac dysrhythmias in children. Pediatr. Rev. 3:190, 1981.
Guntheroth, W. G.: Disorders of heart rate and rhythm. Pediatr. Clin. North Am. 25:869, 1978.

In *sinus arrhythmia* the pulse rate increases during inspiration and slows during expiration. A normal finding in most children above the age of three years, this arrhythmia is prominent during later childhood and puberty and infrequent during infancy. In older children sinus arrhythmia may superficially suggest dropped beats or premature contractions.

Pulsus paradoxus, characterized by a diminution or disappearance of the pulse during inspiration, may occur in patients with cardiac tamponade owing to pericardial effusion or bleeding, purulent pericarditis, constrictive pericarditis, severe asthma, pleural effusion and pneumothorax. Pulsus paradoxus is more clearly demonstrated by use of the sphygmomanometer. A significant drop in systolic pressure is noted at the end of a full inspiration compared to expiration. A difference of over 20 mm is highly suggestive of cardiac tamponade, whereas values between 10 and 20 mm are suspicious.

Extrasystoles, premature cardiac contractions without a compensatory pause, occur in normal children and are insignificant unless associated with rheumatic carditis or congenital heart disease. Extrasystoles occurring in normal children usually disappear after exercise, while those associated with cardiac lesions may become more pronounced.

Premature contractions followed by compensatory diastolic pauses may cause cardiac irregularity. The compensatory pauses may suggest dropped beats. Premature contractions that disappear after exercise are benign.

Jacobsen, J. R., Garson, A., Jr., Gillette, P. C., and McNamara, D. G.: Premature ventricular contractions in normal children. J. Pediatr. 92:36, 1978.

Dropped beats occurring with a partial heart block also cause irregularity of the cardiac rhythm. Cardiac arrhythmias and bradycardia may be caused by digitalis toxicity.

Patients with acute carditis may demonstrate a *"tic-tac" rhythm* in which the interval between the first and second sounds is equal to or even longer than diastole. Instead of the normal 1:2 relation between the systolic and diastolic intervals, the ratio becomes more nearly 1:1.

During episodes of *paroxysmal tachycardia,* which may last for minutes, hours or days, the heart rate may be too rapid to count. In infancy the symptoms include restlessness, irritability, cyanosis or pallor, tachypnea, anorexia, vomiting, fever and, in some patients, hepatomegaly and other signs of congestive heart failure. Episodes of paroxysmal tachycardia may occur in infants with endocardial fibroelastosis or congenital heart disorders such as coarctation.

Palpitation may occur with hyperventilation syndrome, paroxysmal supraventricular tachycardia, pheochromocytoma, hypochondriasis and anxiety.

PERCUSSION

Light indirect or direct percussion along the interspaces from the periphery toward the midline may be used to estimate heart size. Although moderate or marked enlargement may be detected by this technique, the determination of heart size by percussion is of limited accuracy, especially in infants. The position of the apex beat may be a better reflection of heart size.

In patients with massive atelectasis, the area of cardiac dullness shifts toward the involved side. In the presence of pleurisy with effusion or pneumothorax, this area shifts to the contralateral side.

Pericarditis with effusion may cause an increased area of dullness over the precordium.

Enlargement of the heart in infants may be caused by congestive heart failure, endocardial fibroelastosis, glycogenosis Type II (Pompe's disease), idiopathic cardiomyopathy, rhabdomyoma, coarctation of the aorta, anomalous origin of the coronary arteries, aortic stenosis, septal defects and a large patent ductus. Cardiomegaly is also present in some infants of diabetic mothers. Cardiac enlargement in older children may be caused by rheumatic fever, severe anemia or hypertension.

With *pneumomediastinum,* the area of cardiac dullness may be reduced with hyperresonance present over the precordium, especially when the patient is supine. Hyperresonance may not be present when the patient leans forward in the sitting position.

AUSCULTATION

The preferred stethoscope for cardiac auscultation in children is one with a combined bell (for murmurs of low frequency) and diaphragm (for murmurs of high frequency) of small diameter. The room should be quiet and the child helped to be as cooperative as possible.

The rate, rhythm, regularity, intensity and quality of heart sounds should be assessed with the patient in the supine, upright and left lateral positions and leaning forward. Because of the thinness of the chest wall in infants, cardiac murmurs are widely transmitted and heard over a wider area than in older children and adults. Their location and transmission, therefore, is not always as significant in infants as in older children.

In childhood, except in young infants, the intensity of the first apical heart sound (S_1) is greater than that of the second (S_2). The converse is true in the pulmonic area. The first heart sound is louder when cardiac output is increased owing to factors such as hyperthyroidism, fever and anemia. This difference in loudness facilitates timing of the cardiac cycle. *Splitting of the pulmonary second sound*, heard best in the second left intercostal space with the stethoscope diaphragm, is a normal finding. The sounds are widely split during inspiration but almost synchronous during expiration. Accentuation of the aortic second sound may accompany hypertension, and diminution may be noted in congenital aortic stenosis. Absence of or a quiet, unsplit pulmonary second sound is characteristic of valvular pulmonary stenosis, whereas pulmonary hypertension is suggested by a loud, high-pitched, booming pulmonic second sound. A single, loud pulmonic second sound is heard in primary pulmonary hypertension and in the Eisenmenger syndrome. An incomplete bundle branch block accompanying an atrial septal defect may be suspected when the second pulmonic sound is widely split and remains fixed during both inspiration and expiration. In the newborn infant, the pulmonary second sound is either single or minimally split.

In patients with pericardial effusion, the intensity of heart sounds may be so diminished that they are difficult to hear. The pulse, however, usually remains full and strong. Myocarditis should be considered when the heart sounds are of poor quality

and difficult to hear. Feeble heart tones and a weak, rapid pulse occur in infants with 10 per cent dehydration. Pneumothorax may also cause the heart sounds to be distant and weak.

With pneumomediastinum, subcutaneous emphysema may appear, and a concomitant pneumothorax, usually on the left, is often present. *Hamman's sign*, the occurrence of crackling, bubbling, crunching and churning sounds, may occasionally be heard over the precordium with pneumomediastinum. Although these sounds may be present through the entire cardiac cycle, they are usually most apparent during systole in the left lateral recumbent position and during the expiratory phase of respiration.

A *pericardial friction rub* is a rough and grating or soft and scratchy, superficial, to-and-fro or inconstant sound, similar to the rustling of hair. It is usually heard best in the third and fourth left interspaces parasternally and over the sternum. Transient and easily missed, the rub may occur synchronously with the heart beat and be intensified by firm pressure of the stethoscope on the chest. Except for the time relation with the respiratory movements, a pleural friction rub may simulate a pericardial rub. With the development of a purulent or serous effusion, the rub usually disappears except, perhaps, at the base of the heart. Echocardiography is a useful diagnostic tool when pericardial effusion is suspected.

Purulent pericarditis, often secondary to a primary infection elsewhere, is a pediatric and surgical emergency. Diagnostic pericardiocentesis should be done promptly and the purulent effusion drained.

Vanreken, D., Strauss, A., Hernandez, A., and Feigin, R. D.: Infectious pericarditis in children. J. Pediatr. 85:165, 1974.

Pericarditis may be associated with rheumatic fever, viral infections, systemic-onset rheumatoid arthritis, systemic lupus erythematosus, uremia, thalassemia, metastatic malignancy, histoplasmosis and Kawasaki disease.

Bernstein, B., Takahashi, M., and Hanson, V.: Cardiac involvement in juvenile rheumatoid arthritis. J. Pediatr. 85:313, 1974.

In the *postpericardiotomy syndrome*, which may occasionally occur after cardiac surgery, pericardial and pleural reactions and effusion accompanied by the abrupt onset of fever and chest pain appear during or after the second postoperative week. The pain, which frequently radiates from the precordial region to the neck and shoulder unilaterally or bilaterally, may be accentuated by a deep breath. A pericardial friction rub may be heard, especially with the patient supine.

A *third heart sound* is often heard during diastole in normal children. This low-pitched, short sound, best heard at the apex, is thought to occur at the end of rapid filling of the left ventricle. A number of differences exist between a split second and a third heart sound. The interval between the split second sound is less than that between the beginning of the second and third heart sounds. The duplicate second sounds have identical quality and pitch, whereas the third heart sound has a quiet, dull, lump- or thud-like quality. Split second sounds are most frequent at the base of the heart and parasternally on the left. The third heart sound is usually heard best at the apex or just medial to and above the apex after exercise or with the slowing of the heart rate that occurs during the expiratory phase of respiration, with the child in the left recumbent position and the stethoscope bell lightly applied. In active rheumatic fever, differentiation of a third heart sound from an early diastolic murmur may be difficult, especially when the heart rate is rapid. A *fourth heart sound* at the apex in late diastole is an abnormal finding.

Differentiation is required, at times, between a third heart sound and a *gallop rhythm*. As a general rule, if other evidences of carditis are present, the three sounds usually represent a gallop rhythm; on the other hand, if no evidence of cardiac disease exists, the diastolic sound may be considered to be a third heart sound. A protodiastolic gallop may be a manifestation of carditis, severe anemia, thyrotoxicosis, mitral and aortic insufficiency, patent ductus and septal defects that cause ventricular diastolic overloading. Presystolic gallops may be associated with systolic overloading caused by lesions such as moderately severe aortic stenosis, coarctation of the aorta or pulmonary stenosis. *Protodiastolic gallop* is generally best heard in the apical region or between that area and the lower portion of the sternum. *Presystolic gallop* is heard best along the left sternal border and the base of the heart. Gallop sounds are faint and heard best in a quiet room with the stethoscope bell lightly applied.

MURMURS

Verifying the presence of a murmur and identifying it as *innocent* or *organic* may be difficult. Whereas some murmurs have diagnostic characteristics, others require correlation with additional clinical findings.

Their significance may not be evident until the child has been further observed.

Each murmur may be described according to the following characteristics:

Position in the cardiac cycle (i.e., systolic [early, middle or late] or diastolic [early, middle, late or presystolic]). Although location of the murmur and its point of maximal intensity is of diagnostic interest, murmurs of specific lesions may be variable. Systolic murmurs are usually best heard with the stethoscope diaphragm.

Ejection or regurgitant. *Ejection murmurs* occur during the ejection phase of ventricular systole. A short interval is present between the first heart sound and the onset of the murmur. Many have a crescendo-decrescendo (diamond) quality, end before the second heart sound and are usually heard best with the stethoscope bell. They may occur in normal patients as well as in those with lesions such as aortic stenosis. *Regurgitant systolic murmurs* have an organic etiology and are caused by an abnormal flow of blood from a ventricle, as in mitral insufficiency or ventricular septal defect. The regurgitant murmur is holosystolic. Regurgitant diastolic murmurs may also occur in aortic or pulmonic insufficiency.

Transmission

Duration. Holosystolic murmurs are caused by an organic lesion.

Quality. Blowing, rasping, rumbling

Pitch

Intensity

Response to exercise and change of position

The intensity of murmurs may be graded from I to VI for systolic and I to IV for diastolic murmurs. A grade I murmur, just barely audible after careful auscultation for a time, is clinically insignificant in the absence of other findings. Grade II is also faint but heard immediately. Grade III is a moderate murmur; grade IV, a loud murmur; grade V a very loud murmur. Grade VI can be heard without a stethoscope. Although this classification may be helpful in describing what is heard, the intensity of a murmur, in itself, is not diagnostic.

Murmurs may be produced or intensified by an increase in cardiac output owing to hypermetabolic states such as fever, exercise, hyperthyroidism, anemia (hemic murmur) or anxiety. Because of changes in blood flow, vigorous crying may cause murmurs to diminish or disappear.

During the neonatal period, *transient* systolic ejection *murmurs* may be heard, especially in the third and fourth interspaces parasternally. These murmurs usually disappear after a few days. If they persist, a congenital defect is probably present; on the other hand, the murmur associated with a congenital defect, such as a patent ductus arteriosus or a ventricular septal defect, may initially be almost inaudible but become moderately loud in a few days or weeks. Harsh murmurs heard on the first day of life are often caused by pulmonic or aortic stenosis.

Innocent murmurs occur frequently in normal children at the base of the heart or along the left parasternal or pulmonic areas, especially during a febrile illness. Although they can often be readily recognized as nonorganic, differentiation from organic murmurs is occasionally difficult and may require further observation and study. Innocent murmurs are systolic, of short duration and usually soft and blowing, although occasionally loud and harsh. Almost all systolic murmurs in otherwise asymptomatic children are either innocent or caused by a ventricular septal defect. The intensity of a murmur does not permit its categorization as either innocent or organic. Innocent murmurs may diminish in intensity or disappear after exercise, but they may also become more prominent and may be heard in the back. The nature of the murmur may vary according to the phase of the respiratory cycle. Innocent murmurs usually have a lower pitch than the blowing murmur of mitral insufficiency, which is heard maximally at the apex and transmitted to the axilla.

Moss, A. J.: The "incidental" systolic murmur. Pediatrics 45:687, 1970.

The *vibratory murmur* is the most common innocent murmur, especially between the ages of three and seven years. It is about grade II or III in intensity, brief in duration, early to mid-systolic in time and maximal at the third or fourth left interspace or medial to the apex and transmits to the apex. Vibratory murmurs are usually heard best with the bell of the stethoscope and with the patient recumbent. Such murmurs decrease or disappear when the patient is sitting or standing. Their vibratory, buzzing, low-pitched, "twanging-string" or groaning quality is usually diagnostic. The location of maximal intensity of the innocent murmur medial to the apex helps differentiate it from the murmur of mitral insufficiency. At times, differentiating the innocent murmur from that caused by a ventricular septal defect or cardiomyopathy is difficult.

The *pulmonic ejection murmur*, another innocent murmur, especially common in young adolescents, is well-localized parasternally in the second and third left interspaces. Grade I to III, short, early to mid-systolic, and blowing, this murmur is transmitted along the sternum and toward the apex. The murmur may be caused by an increase in pulmonary blood flow associated with fever, anxiety, exercise or anemia. A similar murmur may be caused by mild pulmonic stenosis or an atrial septal defect. The latter may be suggested by a pulmonary second sound that remains widely split in both inspiration and expiration.

The pulmonic ejection murmur in the *straight back syndrome* is an innocent murmur heard in children who do not have the normal thoracic curvature. This syndrome has its highest incidence in infants up to two years of age. Although not readily apparent clinically, it is easily recognized roentgenographically when the ratio of the anteroposterior diameter to the transverse diameter of the thorax is determined. Functional murmurs may also occur in patients with scoliosis, kyphoscoliosis and pectus excavatum.

The *cardiorespiratory murmur*, a benign finding occasionally encountered in children, may be heard over the precordium, the apex or the cardiopulmonary borders. Characteristically mid- or late systolic in time and sharply localized, the murmur begins and ends suddenly, diminishes during inspiration, and sounds like a high-pitched, short squeal close to the examiner's ear. Sometimes called the "*systolic whoop*," it may begin with a systolic click. This murmur may be heard in patients with chest deformities.

Isolated *systolic clicks* may be heard infrequently in normal children. Ejection clicks, important findings with aortic or pulmonic stenosis, may be difficult to hear.

Mitral valve prolapse, usually asymptomatic in children, may cause a mid-systolic click; a high frequency, usually loud intensity sound with a scratchy quality; a mid-late grade II-III systolic murmur heard best with the diaphragm of the stethoscope in a small area near the apex in the left lateral decubitus or standing positions; and whoops or whistles audible even without a stethoscope. The click may be thought to be normal splitting of the first heart sound. In late adolescence, arrhythmias and precordial discomfort may occur. The prevalence of mitral valve prolapse is increased in children with Duchenne's muscle dystrophy and in the Willebrand, Ehlers-Danlos and Marfan syndromes.

McNamara, D. G.: Idiopathic benign mitral valve prolapse. Am. J. Dis. Child. 136:152, 1982.

A *carotid bruit* may be heard as a well-localized early or mid-systolic grade II to III murmur over the neck vessels supraclavicularly on the right but not in the aortic area.

In *rheumatic carditis* the murmurs and heart sounds are inconstant, varying in quality from one examination to the next. The sounds may appear muffled and dull. Impaired quality of the first heart sound and shortening of diastole produce a "tic-tac" rhythm characteristic of acute carditis. A gallop rhythm may also be present. Occasionally, a high-pitched, vibrant, somewhat raucous murmur is heard at the apex, in addition to the murmur of mitral insufficiency. A transient, low frequency, proto-diastolic murmur may also be heard at the apex.

Systolic Murmurs

Mitral insufficiency is characterized by a soft to moderately loud (usually not over Grade III in intensity), high-pitched, generally holosystolic and blowing apical murmur, best heard with the diaphragm during expiration with the patient in the left lateral recumbent position. The murmur, which is maximal at the apex and transmitted toward the left axilla, the base of the heart and, at times, to the back, may eventually become loud and harsh and replace or muffle the first sound.

Aortic stenosis is characterized by a harsh, very loud, systolic ejection, crescendo-decrescendo murmur maximal in the second right interspace and widely transmitted to the right shoulder, clavicle, up the vessels of the neck and toward the apex. Occasionally, in infants and young children the murmur may be loudest at the apex. With subvalvular aortic stenosis, the murmur is heard maximally over the upper sternum. With supravalvular aortic stenosis, the maximal intensity may be at the suprasternal notch. Diastolic murmurs are also heard in some patients. Aortic ejection clicks are common. A systolic thrill is present along the base of the heart and over the neck vessels.

Pulmonic stenosis of mild degree may produce a holosystolic murmur in the second and third left interspaces identical to that of the innocent pulmonary ejection murmur or an atrial septal defect. The pulmonic second sound is decreased with severe but not mild stenosis. *Peripheral pulmonary stenosis* is characterized by a soft systolic murmur over one or both lung fields.

A *ventricular septal defect* causes a grade III or IV, harsh, widely transmitted holosystolic murmur along the left parasternal area at the third and fourth interspaces and over the xiphoid process. The murmur, which obscures the first sound, may not be noted until days or weeks after birth. A systolic thrill is also often present. With a very large defect, a low-pitched, early diastolic murmur may be heard at the apex. With very small defects, the murmur may be grade I to II, soft and blowing. If the septal defect closes, the murmur gradually diminishes, becomes confined to early systole and then disappears. The murmur may also diminish in intensity and duration if pulmonary hypertension develops. In the latter event, the murmur may be accompanied by a loud, single, pulmonary second sound. The murmur of an AV canal simulates that of a ventricular septal defect.

An *atrial septal defect*, more commonly the secundum type, is usually characterized by a relatively soft, less than grade III, blowing systolic ejection murmur maximal in the second and third left interspaces and well transmitted. A systolic thrill may be present. The pulmonic second sound demonstrates a wide splitting with the second component louder than the first. A low-pitched, early diastolic murmur may be heard over the end of the sternum. The murmur of an atrial septal defect may not be noted for several months or years after birth. In defects of the ostium primum type with a split mitral valve, the murmur may be lower in position and accompanied by a prominent holosystolic apical murmur. The murmur accompanying an ostium primum defect is harsh, loud and well-transmitted. An atrial septal defect murmur is often indistinguishable from an innocent functional pulmonic ejection murmur.

Patients with *isolated pulmonary stenosis* may have a loud, harsh and widely transmitted murmur or a soft, scratchy and localized systolic murmur in the second or third left interspace parasternally. The murmur may be transmitted toward the left clavicle and posteriorly to the interscapular area. A systolic thrill may be present. The pulmonary second sound may be normal but is usually diminished in intensity or absent. Increased splitting of the second sound occurs in mild to moderate pulmonic stenosis. In the tetralogy of Fallot, the pulmonic murmur is maximal in the third left interspace along the sternum. Duplication of the second sound, heard best in the third and fourth interspaces, does not occur in patients with tetralogy. With mild stenosis of the pulmonic valve, an ejection click may be heard just before the murmur. A pulmonic murmur may be absent in some infants who have severe, isolated pulmonic stenosis.

When a murmur occurs with *coarctation of the aorta*, it is usually a soft or moderately loud, systolic or, rarely, continuous murmur, especially prominent at the base in the left infraclavicular area and transmitted to the left interscapular area. In a few patients, the murmur is more prominent posteriorly than precordially.

Diastolic Murmurs

Mitral stenosis is characterized by a soft to loud, harsh, rumbling, though occasionally blowing, low-pitched mid-diastolic or crescendo presystolic murmur that may terminate in an accentuated and snapping first sound. Not widely transmitted, the murmur is heard best with the stethoscope bell in a limited area just medial to and above the apex after exercise and with the patient in the left lateral recumbent position. The patient should be asked to hold his breath in moderate expiration. During active rheumatic carditis, a brief, blowing apical murmur may be audible in proto- or mid-diastole. Probably related to myocardial disease and cardiac dilatation, this murmur disappears as the rheumatic heart process becomes quiescent. The murmur of mitral stenosis usually does not appear until a number of years later.

Aortic insufficiency is characterized by a soft to loud, high-pitched, blowing, decrescendo diastolic murmur, usually maximal along the left sternal border in the second and third interspaces and heard best with the stethoscope diaphragm firmly applied. The murmur, which is usually not transmitted to the apex, becomes most prominent when the patient leans slightly forward and holds his breath in expiration. The Austin Flint murmur, a presystolic or protodiastolic apical murmur, may accompany that of aortic insufficiency.

Diastolic murmurs may also be heard in some patients with atrial or ventricular septal defects, Eisenmenger's syndrome, patent ductus arteriosus, pulmonary hypertension and cardiomegaly.

Continuous Murmur

Diagnosis of a *patent ductus arteriosus* can be made on the basis of the physical examination in almost every instance. The murmur of a patent ductus is present in the second and third left interspaces and transmitted to the precordium, the vessels of the neck, the left axilla and the interscapular area, especially on the left. Since the systolic component is more widely transmitted than the diastolic, the double murmur is not heard in all areas. Characteristically harsh, rumbling, rasping, humming or machine-like, the murmur is usually continuous throughout the heart cycle, loudest during systole and softest in mid- or late diastole. A systolic thrill is usually palpable.

A continuous murmur may be present in newborn infants in association with prematurity and the respiratory distress syndrome. In other infants, the murmur is absent or only the systolic component is noted at this time. Before one year of age, absence of the diastolic component does not rule out a patent ductus. An apical systolic murmur may also occur. The diastolic component is usually best heard with the child supine. Rarely, no murmur may be present. In a small number of patients with a patent ductus, only a systolic component is present, even after the age of three or four years. This finding has been noted in patients with either a very small shunt or an extremely large ductus with a high pulmonary artery pressure. Patients with large shunts sometimes have a diastolic murmur in the mitral area and a systolic murmur in the aortic area in addition to the classic continuous murmur.

The sudden onset of a continuous precordial murmur, maximal on the right, is observed with a ruptured congenital aneurysm of the sinuses of Valsalva. Chest pain, dyspnea and a widened pulse pressure are accompanying features. High interventricular septal defects may be difficult to differentiate from a patent ductus. Some of these patients also have an atrioventricular conduction defect and a low diastolic pressure.

A continuous murmur may be heard over a *pulmonary arteriovenous fistula*.

A continuous, loud *venous hum* may frequently be heard over the upper sternum, clavicle, and vessels of the neck, especially on the right, but occasionally also along the left parasternal border in normal children. The intensity of the hum varies greatly with changes in position of the head and neck. It is loudest during diastole with the patient in the upright position, especially with the neck extended or stretched, and diminishes or disappears in the recumbent position or with compression over the neck vessels. The murmur may be accompanied by a thrill.

GENERAL REFERENCES

Liebman, J.: Diagnosis and management of heart murmurs in children. Pediatr. Rev. 3:321, 1982.

Moss, A. J., Adams, F. H., and Emmanouilides, G. C. (ed.): Heart Disease in Infants, Children, and Adolescents. 2nd ed. Baltimore, The Williams and Wilkins Co., 1977.

Nadas, A. S., and Fyler, D. C.: Pediatric Cardiology. 3rd ed. Philadelphia, W. B. Saunders Co., 1972.

BLOOD PRESSURE

Children three years of age and above should have an annual determination of blood pressure. In children under three years of age, pressures need be taken only when hospitalized or when a specific indication is present. Except for infants, the blood pressure should be taken with the child sitting and the manometer at the examiner's eye level. Only mercury manometers should be used.

Figures 11–1 and 11–2 give the percentiles of blood pressure measurements for children over the age of two years.

From the Report of the Task Force on Blood Pressure Control in Children. Prepared by the National Heart, Lung, and Blood Institutes Task Force. Pediatrics 59:797, 1977.

DETERMINATION

The use of a proper-sized cuff is important in the determination of children's blood pressure. The greater the length of the arm, the wider the blood pressure cuff should be. An appropriately sized cuff usually covers about two thirds of a child's upper arm. The largest size cuff that will fit the arm or thigh should be used without overlying the ante-

cubital or popliteal fossae. In addition, the inflatable bladder within the cuff should completely and snugly encircle the arm without overlapping itself. In the obese child, this may require the use of a thigh-sized cuff on the arm. The stethoscope diaphragm should be applied lightly over the brachial artery. A 2.5-cm cuff is available for newborns and infants under one year of age, but the 5-cm cuff is often preferred. For children under 8 years of age, the 9-cm cuff may be used and a 12.5-cm cuff for older children. A false elevation of the blood pressure reading is obtained if the cuff is too narrow; on the other hand, with too wide a cuff, the reading is spuriously low. In patients being followed because of borderline or elevated blood pressure, the conditions of the determination should be recorded, e.g., the patient's position, arm used and cuff size.

The cuff should be inflated rapidly but deflated slowly at the rate of 2 to 3 mm per second. The first sound heard (Korotkoff Phase I) signifies the systolic pressure. The point at which the sounds become low-pitched and muffled (Korotkoff Phase IV) is regarded as the best index of diastolic blood pressure in children, whereas the fifth phase, characterized by disappearance of sound, is the best criteria for diastolic pressure in adults. Both the fourth and fifth

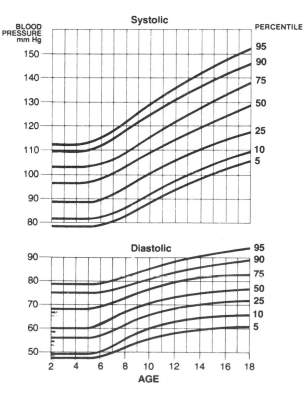

FIGURE 11–1. Percentiles of blood pressure measurements in boys (right arm, seated). (From the Report of the Task Force on Blood Pressure Control in Children. Prepared by the National Heart, Lung and Blood Institute's Task Force. Pediatrics 59:797, 1977.)

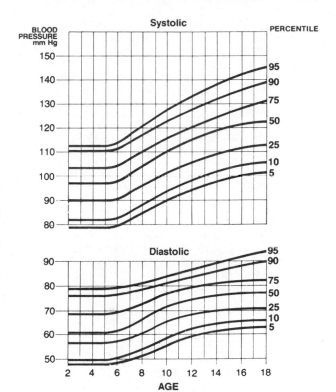

FIGURE 11–2. Percentile of blood pressure measurements in girls (right arm, seated). (From the Report of the Task Force on Blood Pressure Control in Children. Prepared by the National Heart, Lung and Blood Institute's Task Force. Pediatrics 59:797, 1977.)

phase readings should be recorded, e.g., 100/60/0.

> Moss, A. J.: Criteria for diastolic pressure: Revolution, counter revolution, and now a compromise. Pediatrics 71:854, 1983.

The auscultatory method of determining blood pressure is used in older infants and children. In small infants, the palpatory, flush or Doppler method must usually be used, since the Korotkoff sounds are almost inaudible on auscultation. If the baby is given a bottle or pacifier, one may, however, be able to use the auscultatory method. In the flush method, a 2.5-cm cuff is wrapped around the ankle or wrist in the customary manner. The infant may be given a bottle or a pacifier so that he does not cry during the procedure. Before the cuff is inflated, rubber sheeting or a rubber glove is wrapped around the foot or hand, beginning at the distal portion of the extremity and proceeding proximally toward the cuff. The cuff is then inflated above the expected systolic pressure, and the rubber wrapping is removed. The pressure within the cuff is permitted to fall slowly, not faster than 6 to 7 mm per second. Good lighting is necessary. The systolic pressure is that at which the blanched foot or hand suddenly becomes flushed. This value usually approximates

the mean arterial pressure. The flush method usually requires two examiners.

The Doppler ultrasound method, now widely employed, permits the determination of both systolic and diastolic pressures in the newborn or older infant.

Whenever the blood pressure is elevated in one arm, determinations should be made in the other arm and in the lower extremities. To obtain the pressure in the lower extremities, a large cuff is wrapped around the thigh with the patient in the prone position. The sounds are then noted over the popliteal artery. The diastolic pressure is about the same in both the upper and the lower extremities; however, the intra-arterial pressure in the lower extremities ranges from 10 to 40 mm Hg higher than that in the upper extremities.

> Moss, A. J.: Indirect methods of blood pressure measurement. Pediatr. Clin. North Am. 25:3, 1978.

In the term newborn, hypertension may be defined as systolic pressure over 90 mm Hg and diastolic pressure over 60 mm Hg. Similar values for the premature infant are 80 mm and 45 mm respectively.

When the blood pressure is unexpectedly elevated in an adolescent and no related complaints or findings are present, the parents and the adolescent should be informed that a high normal blood pressure was recorded; and return visits must be scheduled to determine whether the elevation is transient, perhaps owing to anxiety, or sustained.

Julius, S.: Clinical and physiologic significance of borderline hypertension at youth. Pediatr. Clin. North Am. 25:35, 1978.

Rames, L. K., Clarke, W. R., Connor, W. E., Reiter, M. A., and Lauer, R. M.: Normal blood pressures and the evaluation of sustained blood pressure elevation in childhood: The Muscatine study. Pediatrics 61:245, 1978.

Elevation of blood pressure above the 95th percentile on three separate occasions is abnormal. Once an elevation of blood pressure is established, the following possibilities may be considered:

ETIOLOGIC CLASSIFICATION OF HYPERTENSION

I. RENAL

A. Acute post-streptococcal glomerulonephritis. Sudden elevation of the pressure in these patients may cause hypertensive encephalopathy. Restlessness, irritability, vomiting, nausea, headache or visual disturbances are danger signs in the presence of a rising blood pressure. Acute post-streptococcal glomerulonephritis may present with hypertensive encephalopathy as its only clinical manifestation.
B. Congenital dysplastic kidney
C. Hydronephrosis and obstructive uropathy
D. Wilm's tumor may infrequently be associated with hypertension.
E. Polycystic kidney
F. Chronic pyelonephritis; chronic glomerulonephritis
G. Henoch-Schönlein purpura with nephritis
H. Acute renal failure
I. Hemolytic-uremic syndrome
J. Unilateral or bilateral fibromuscular dysplasia or stenosis of renal arteries; anomalous renal artery. Renal artery stenosis may cause hypertension in patients with neurofibromatosis. A bruit may be noted over the flanks in fibromuscular dysplasia.

Makker, S. P., and Moorthy, B.: Fibromuscular dysplasia of renal arteries; an important cause of renovascular hypertension in children. J. Pediatr. 95:940, 1979.

Mena, E., Bookstein, J. J., Holt, J. F., and Fry, W. J.: Neurofibromatosis and renovascular hypertension in children. Am. J. Roentgenol. 118:39, 1973.

K. Membranoproliferative glomerulitis. Hypertension is an early finding.
L. Nephrotic syndrome
M. Renal vein thrombosis
N. Renal tubular acidosis with nephrocalcinosis
O. Idiopathic hypercalcemia
P. Post–renal transplantation
Q. Fabry's disease
R. Familial nephritis
S. Cystinosis

Leumann, E. P., Bauer, R. P., Slaton, P. E., Biglieri, E. G., and Holliday, M. A.: Renovascular hypertension in children. Pediatrics 46:362, 1970.

Robson, A. M.: Special diagnostic studies for the detection of renal and renovascular forms of hypertension. Pediatr. Clin. North Am. 25:83, 1978.

II. CEREBRAL

A. Increased intracranial pressure may cause an elevation of blood pressure.
B. Diencephalic disorders; hypothalamic tumors
C. Pontine tumors
D. Encephalitis
E. Guillain-Barré syndrome

Stapleton, F. B., Skoglund, R. R., and Daggett, R. B.: Hypertension associated with the Guillain-Barré syndrome. Pediatrics 62:588, 1978.

F. Anxiety
G. Closed head trauma
H. Meningitis

Eden, O. B., Sills, J. A., and Brown, J. K.: Hypertension in acute neurological diseases of childhood. Dev. Med. Child. Neurol. 19:437, 1977.

III. CARDIOVASCULAR

A. Coarctation of the aorta. If the systolic pressure determined in the upper extremities is high and that in the lower extremities is low, coarctation of the aorta probably exists. When the coarctation is proximal to the point of origin of the left subclavian artery or an atresia of the proximal portion of the left subclavian artery is present, a difference of 30 or 40 mm Hg may be found in the blood pressure readings between the two upper extremities, that in the left arm being lower than the right. The blood pressure values in the upper extremities are the converse if there is stenosis of the right subclavian artery or an anomalous right subclavian artery that originates from a left aortic arch distal to the coarctation. Differences in pressure in the two arms may also be present when the coarctation is distal to the origin of the left subclavian artery. In instances in which the coarctation is not severe or there is an accompanying subaortic or aortic stenosis, the blood pressure in the upper extremities may be only slightly elevated, while that in the lower extremities is relatively decreased. In the presence of a patent ductus arteriosus with the ductus distal to the coarctation, the femoral pulses may be palpable. The *mesenteric arteritis syndrome* is an unusual complication that may occur on the third postoperative day, predominantly in males, following surgical repair of a coarctation. Symptoms and signs include hypertension, abdominal pain, abdominal tenderness, vomiting, intestinal hemorrhage, fever and leukocytosis. At long-term follow-up after corrective surgery, recurrence of hypertension may be noted in some patients.

Beermann, L. B., Neches, W. H., Patnode, R. E., Fricker, F. J., Mathews, R. A., and Park, S. C.: Coarctation of the aorta in children. Am. J. Dis. Child. 134:464, 1980.
Ho, E. C. K., and Moss, A. J.: The syndrome of "mesenteric arteritis" following surgical repair of aortic coarctation. Pediatrics 49:40, 1972.

B. Periarteritis nodosa
C. Lupus erythematosus
D. Idiopathic arterial calcification of infancy.

Milner, L. S., et al.: Hypertension as the major problem of idiopathic arterial calcification of infancy. J. Pediatr. 105:934, 1984.

E. Takayasu's arteritis

Wiggelinkhuizen, J., and Cremin, B. J.: Takayasu arteritis and renovascular hypertension in childhood. Pediatrics 62:209, 1978.

IV. HORMONAL

A. Pheochromocytoma. This lesion may occur in association with neurofibromatosis, von Hippel-Lindau disease and multiple endocrine neoplasia. The triad of paroxysmal perspiration, headaches and palpitations, perhaps associated with tachycardia in the presence of hypertension, is highly suggestive of pheochromocytoma. Although the hypertension may be persistent, it is often paroxysmal, occurring several times a day or month and usually lasting less than one hour. The patient is asymptomatic between episodes.

Bravo, E. L., and Gifford, R. W., Jr.: Pheochromocytoma: Diagnosis, localization and management. N. Engl. J. Med. 311:1298, 1984.

B. Cushing's syndrome
C. Neuroblastoma
D. Primary aldosteronism may be characterized by hypertension in the absence of muscle weakness or polyuria.
E. Adrenal virilizing tumors
F. 11-Beta-hydroxylase deficiency associated with congenital adrenal hyperplasia
G. 17-hydroxylase deficiency with hypogonadism and male pseudohermaphroditism
H. Turner's syndrome when accompanied by coarctation of the aorta
I. Hyperthyroidism (systolic only)
J. Hyperparathyroidism with hypercalcemia
K. Gonadal dysgenesis
L. Corticosteroid administration
M. Vasoactive intestinal peptide-secreting ganglioneuroma or ganglioneuroblastoma

V. ESSENTIAL HYPERTENSION

VI. MISCELLANEOUS

A. Psychological factors may produce transient blood pressure elevation.
B. Familial dysautonomia may be characterized by a transient blood pressure elevation. Postural hypotension is also a frequent finding. A fall in systolic and diastolic pressures of 10 to 60 mm Hg may occur over several minutes following standing from the supine position.
C. Vitamin D poisoning
D. Burns. About 30 per cent of children with burns are hypertensive. Convulsions owing to hypertensive encephalopathy may occur.
E. Lead or mercury poisoning
F. Acute porphyria
G. Oral contraceptives
H. Post–umbilical artery catheterization arterial abnormalities
I. Hallucinogens (LSD, psilocybin, phencyclidine ["angel dust"], mescaline), jimson weed abuse
J. Mydriatic drugs in neonates and prematures
K. Immobilization by orthopedic traction or casts
L. Hypertension has been reported in the newborn following closure of abdominal wall defects.
M. Scorpion envenomation
N. Cockayne syndrome

A *fall in blood pressure* may occur in patients with shock, pericardial effusion, Addison's disease, hyponatremic dehydration, toxic shock syndrome and hypothyroidism. The systolic pressure may fall to between 60 and 80 mm Hg with severe cardiac failure. The systolic blood pressure in neonatal hypotension is under 40 mm Hg in prematures and under 50 mm Hg in term newborn infants. Disorders causing neonatal shock include blood loss; sepsis, especially group B *Streptococcus*; asphyxia; hypoplastic left heart; and cytomegalovirus infection.

The onset of a narrow pulse pressure is a worrisome finding in patients with pericarditis with effusion. The pulse pressure may be decreased in chronic constrictive pericarditis, hypothyroidism, shock or severe aortic stenosis. An increase in the pulse pressure may occur with a patent ductus arteriosus, aortic insufficiency, hyperthyroidism, ruptured congenital aneurysm of the sinuses of Valsalva, complete heart block, peripheral arteriovenous fistula, anemia and fever. The diastolic pressure may not be decreased with a small patent ductus; however, the diastolic pressure may fall to 50 to 40 mm Hg if the fistula is large.

GENERAL REFERENCES

Adelman, R. D.: Neonatal hypertension. Pediatr. Clin. North Am. 25:99, 1978.

Gill, D. G., Medes de Costa, B., and Cameron, J. S.: Analysis of 100 children with severe and persistent hypertension. Arch. Dis. Child. 51:951, 1976.

Goldring, D., and Hernandez, A.: Hypertension in children. Pediatr. Rev. 3:235, 1982.

Hediger, M. L., Schall, J. I., Katz, S. H., Gruskin, A. B., and Eveleth, P. B.: Resting blood pressure and pulse rate distributions in black adolescents: The Philadelphia blood pressure project. Pediatrics 74:1016, 1984.

Lieberman, E.: Blood pressure and primary hypertension in childhood and adolescence. Curr. Probl. Pediatr. 10:4, 1980.

Londe, S.: Causes of hypertension in the young. Pediatr. Clin. North Am. 25:55, 1978.

Report of the Task Force on Blood Pressure Control in Children. Prepared by the National Heart, Lung, and Blood Institute's Task Force on Blood Pressure Control in Children. Pediatrics 59:797, 1977.

12 / THE ABDOMEN

EXAMINATION

Abdominal examination in infants and children requires gentleness and patience. If the infant or young child becomes overly apprehensive or cries, an adequate examination may be difficult or impossible. The approach to the child with an acute abdominal problem must be especially well considered, since accurate diagnostic appraisal is possible only with the child's cooperation. It is often well to have the mother undress the child so that the physician need not chance resistance in uncovering him. The examination may also begin with the child on his mother's lap. If the child seems especially apprehensive, it is best to leave the otoscope and other diagnostic instruments out of sight until the abdominal examination has been completed. An opportunity must also be allowed for mutual inspection, perhaps at some distance. The amount of time required for this varies considerably with different children. Once the physician has been accepted, however, valid physical findings can be elicited within a relatively short time.

When an immediate and exact examination is essential for diagnosis and therapy, and cooperation cannot be obtained, the rectal administration of a rapidly acting barbiturate provides sufficient relaxation for examination. The rectal dose of Seconal is 6.4 mg or 0.1 grain per pound of body weight up to a maximum of 200 mg or 3 grains. This is mixed with 8 cc of water and administered rectally through a catheter with an attached funnel. After administration of the sedative, the buttocks are taped together with a strip of 1-inch tape to prevent escape of the medication. In the presence of an upper respiratory tract infection or anemia, this dose should be reduced by one half.

INSPECTION

Inspection is of great value in the clinical assessment of the child with an acute abdominal complaint. In the presence of peritoneal irritation, the child lies almost immobile on his back, and movement of the abdominal wall on inspiration is greatly restricted. Localized fullness in the right lower quadrant owing to an appendiceal abscess may sometimes be noted on inspection.

Visible *peristaltic waves* usually indicate obstruction in the gastrointestinal tract, more commonly at the pylorus or in the duodenum. Gastric peristaltic waves, passing across the abdomen from left to right, are classically present with pyloric stenosis. Peristaltic waves and projectile vomiting may also occur with malrotation of the bowel, duodenal stenosis or atresia, duodenal ulcer, gastrointestinal allergy, urinary tract infection and adrenal insufficiency.

The *superficial abdominal veins,* normally prominent in infancy, become increasingly conspicuous with abdominal distention. Normally the venous flow is downward in the veins below the umbilicus. With obstruction of the inferior vena cava or hepatic venous outflow (Budd-Chiari syndrome), dilatation of the abdominal veins and reversal of venous flow may occur. The direction of venous flow may be determined by stripping the vein, first placing one's index fingers together and then pushing in opposite directions along the vein. Filling of the vein from below should not occur when the pressure exerted by the lowermost finger is released. Pushing one's index finger upward along the course of the vein does not empty the vessel if the venous flow is reversed because the vein continues to fill from below.

The abdomen normally bulges at the beginning of inspiration. In patients with chorea, retraction of the abdomen may occur at this time (*Czerny's sign*).

A *scaphoid abdomen* in the newborn infant may imply a diaphragmatic hernia.

Diaphragmatic flutter may occur in clinical tetany.

ABDOMINAL ENLARGEMENT

A prominent, "potbelly" contour is normal in infants and young children. Pathologic enlargement of the abdomen may be caused by ascites, tympanites, enlargement of an organ, the presence of a neoplasm or cyst or an abnormality of the abdominal wall. Since the respiratory pattern of infants is chiefly abdominal, such enlargement creates a serious problem in infants with pneumonia or atelectasis.

Ascites is accompanied by a tense abdominal wall, shifting dullness (unless the amount of fluid present is large) and a fluid wave. The mechanisms involved in ascites formation and the differential diagnosis are

discussed on page 408. Chylous ascites is characterized by the collection of lymph within the peritoneal cavity. Paracentesis may be diagnostically helpful, especially if it reveals bile, blood, chyle or evidence of infection.

High *intestinal obstruction* may lead to epigastric or right upper quadrant distention, whereas jejunal or ileal obstruction causes generalized distention.

Intestinal patterning may occur with intestinal obstruction or distention. Because of the thin abdominal wall in normal premature and some term infants, intestinal patterning is occasionally observed. The rectus muscles may also be clearly outlined in these infants.

Other causes for *tympanites* include:
  Peritonitis
  Paralytic ileus
  Chronic idiopathic intestinal *pseudo-obstruction syndrome* consists of symptoms of intermittent intestinal obstruction and abdominal distention owing to a disturbance in intestinal motility.

Byrne, W. J., Cipel, L., Euler, A. R., Halpin, T. C., and Ament, M. E.: Chronic idiopathic intestinal pseudo-obstruction syndrome in children—clinical characteristics and prognosis. J. Pediatr. 90:585, 1977.

Pneumonia and other acute infectious diseases may be accompanied by paralytic ileus, especially in infants.
Celiac syndrome
Meconium ileus
Megacolon may be accompanied by gaseous distention.
Lactobezoars in low birth weight infants

Erenberg, A., Shaw, R. D., and Yousefzadeh, D.: Lactobezoar in the low-birth-weight infant. Pediatrics 63:642, 1979.

Fecal impaction
Aerophagia may accompany crying, faulty feeding techniques and comatose states. Air swallowing, which occurs as a habit in some normal or tense children, may cause intermittent marked abdominal distention and excessive flatus.
Bloating may occur in the premenstrual syndrome.
Abdominal distention occurs in newborn infants undergoing phototherapy.
A tracheo-esophageal fistula is frequently accompanied by abdominal distention owing to forcing of air into the stomach and alimentary tract.

Pneumoperitoneum
Gastric perforation in the newborn
Withdrawal in the fetal alcohol syndrome
Interposition of the colon between the liver and the diaphragm (Chilaiditi's syndrome)
Hypopotassemia may cause abdominal distention, in part owing to hypotonia of the abdominal musculature.
Viral diarrhea in the newborn
Acute enteritis
Inflammatory bowel disease, especially with toxic megacolon
Intestinal perforation

Hardy, J. D., Savage, T. R., and Shirodaria, C.: Intestinal perforation following exchange transfusion. Am. J. Dis. Child. 124:136, 1972.

Disseminated fungal infection in very low birth weight infants
Necrotizing enterocolitis in premature infants. Abdominal distention is an early sign.

Kliegman, R. M., and Fanaroff, A. V.: Neonatal necrotizing enterocolitis: A nine year experience. I. Epidemiology and uncommon observations. Am. J. Dis. Child. 135:603, 1981.

Enlargement of an Organ. Occasionally a distended urinary bladder is mistaken for an abdominal tumor. With high intestinal obstruction, abdominal distention is chiefly present over the upper abdomen. Distention is more generalized with obstruction of the lower intestinal tract. Other causes of organ enlargement are:
Malrotation with or without midgut volvulus
Volvulus without malrotation
Congenital peritoneal bands
Gastric dilatation
Aganglionic megacolon
Intussusception
Renal enlargement. Hydronephrosis and congenital multicystic kidney with or without atresia of the ureteropelvic juncture account for one half of the abdominal masses found in newborn infants.
Hepatomegaly. Subcapsular hemorrhage of the liver in the newborn may cause an abdominal mass, shock and respiratory distress.

French, C. E., and Waldstein, G.: Subcapsular hemorrhage of the liver in the newborn. Pediatrics 69:204, 1982.

Splenomegaly
Duplication of the bowel
Hydrops of the gallbladder may cause a right upper quadrant mass.

Hydrocolpos may cause a large mass in the lower abdomen.
Pregnancy
Adrenal hemorrhage in the newborn infant
Torsion of a fallopian tube and ovary may cause a freely movable, midabdominal mass in the newborn.

Neoplasms and Cysts. Transillumination of the abdomen with a bright light in a dark room is a valuable technique in differentiating between solid and cystic masses. The transillumination that occurs in normal infants with abdominal distention is easily differentiated from that with a large cyst.
Wilms' tumor
Neuroblastoma
Embryonal rhabdomyosarcoma
Lymphomas, including Hodgkin's disease and non-Hodgkin's lymphomas
Ovarian cyst or tumor
Mesenteric cyst or tumor
Omental cyst
Choledochal cyst
Duplication of the bowel
Urachal cyst
Vitelline duct cyst
Retroperitoneal sarcoma
Retroperitoneal teratoma
Pancreatic pseudocyst is a diagnostic possibility in children with abdominal fullness and a history of abdominal trauma.
Hepatic cyst or tumor
Dermoid cyst
Teratoma
Polycystic kidneys
A large hydronephrotic kidney may transilluminate well.

THE ABDOMINAL WALL

The atonic musculature in patients with anemia, rickets, hypothyroidism, hypokalemia or Down's syndrome may predispose to abdominal distention.
Omphalocele, a defect of the umbilical ring covered by both peritoneum and amnion and containing eviscerated organs such as the liver and the intestines, is more likely to occur in premature infants, in the Beckwith-Wiedemann syndrome, in trisomies and in association with other congenital gastrointestinal, genitourinary and cardiac anomalies.
Gastroschisis occurs lateral to the umbilicus and between the rectus muscles, with evisceration of the bowel through the defect. A chemical peritonitis is present. Intestinal atresia occurs in 10 to 15 per cent of patients.

Abdominal wall abscess

Abdominal wall neoplasms such as a hemangioma, lipoma, teratoma, fibroma or desmoid tumor

Obesity

Edema, erythema and tenderness of the abdominal wall may occur with necrotizing enterocolitis, perforation of the stomach or peritonitis in the newborn.

With complete or partial *absence of the abdominal muscles* (prune belly or Eagle-Barrett syndrome) the abdominal wall is flabby, balloons out in the flanks and does not contract during crying. Skin creases may radiate laterally and downward from the umbilicus. Genitourinary tract anomalies, undescended testes, enlargement of the bladder, hydroureter and hydronephrosis may be associated findings.

Thinning of the abdominal wall may occur in infants secondary to fetal ascites (idiopathic or XO Turner's syndrome) or organ enlargement (Beckwith-Wiedemann syndrome, polycystic kidneys, or bladder obstruction).

Pagon, R. A., Smith, D. W., and Shepard, T. H.: Urethral obstruction malformation complex: A cause of abdominal muscle deficiency and the "prune belly." J. Pediatr. 94:900, 1979.

HERNIAS AND HYDROCELES

Umbilical Hernia. An umbilical hernia appears as a soft, bulging, but easily reducible mass that becomes especially prominent during crying. A hernial ring is palpable around the abdominal defect. Umbilical hernias are most common in black infants and in those with Down's syndrome, hypothyroidism, chondrodystrophy, and Hurler's syndrome or other mucopolysaccharidoses. An abdominal neoplasm or organomegaly may cause an acquired umbilical hernia owing to increased intra-abdominal pressure. Flattening or a slight protrusion of the umbilicus occurs with abdominal distention.

A *linea alba hernia* may be characterized by abdominal pain and the finding of a small, tender, fixed, subcutaneous nodule on light palpation with the finger tips along the linea alba in the region of the umbilicus.

Bugenstein, R. H., and Phibbs, C. M., Jr.: Abdominal pain in children caused by linea alba hernias. Pediatrics 56:1073, 1975.

Inguinal Hernia. Congenital inguinal hernias may not be evident until the second or third month of life. The parent may first notice a bulge at the internal ring, along the inguinal canal or in the scrotum when the infant cries, coughs or strains. The history is diagnostically important as the hernia may not be evident at the time of consultation. Inspection for a hernia should be made with the patient in both the supine and erect positions. Hernias are usually readily reducible and slip back into the abdominal cavity rapidly with a swishing or gurgling sensation. In general, hernias do not transilluminate well unless the herniated loop is empty and distended. An expansile impulse on coughing or straining may be noted in older children. In children, one does not invaginate the scrotum and palpate the external inguinal ring, as in adults.

At times, an ovary, along with a fallopian tube, may be palpated in an inguinal hernia sac as a bean-sized movable nodule. Femoral or direct inguinal hernias may rarely cause an inguinal mass. In the *testicular feminization syndrome,* the external genitalia appear unambiguously female, but the uterus and fallopian tubes are absent. These children are often seen because of an inguinal hernia or a labial lump.

Children initially presenting with a left inguinal hernia have about a 50 per cent chance of a hernia developing on the right. Those with a right inguinal hernia usually do not develop one on the left. Bilateral hernias occur frequently in patients with exstrophy of the bladder. Unrecognized inguinal hernias in infants may account, at times, for irritability. With incarceration, the parent is unable to reduce the hernia, and the infant is fretful and in pain. Tachypnea, abdominal distention and vomiting may occur. The herniated loop in the inguinal canal or scrotum may become firm and tender.

Spigelian Hernias. These hernias may rarely occur in the anterior abdominal wall along the spigelian semilunar line, which extends from the eighth or ninth costal cartilage to the pubic tubercle. The usual finding is a mass in the lower abdominal wall which disappears on external pressure or in the supine position. Congenital lumbar hernia in the newborn period may cause a large, compressible, soft, usually unilateral, lumbar mass.

Graivier, L., and Alfieri, A. L.: Bilateral spigelian hernias in infancy. Am. J. Surg. 120:817, 1970.

Hydroceles. Hydroceles, caused by an accumulation of fluid in the tunica vaginalis, may be congenital or acquired, acute or chronic, unilateral or bilateral. Swelling may be limited to the cord or encircle both the cord and testis. The former represents a hydrocele of the cord, whereas the latter is a hydrocele of the tunica vaginalis testis. Depending upon the presence or absence of a communication with the peritoneal cavity through an incompletely closed processus funicularis, the hydrocele may be communicating, noncommunicating or encysted.

A *hydrocele of the tunica vaginalis testis* appears as an elastic, fluctuating, smooth, occasionally tense and usually translucent scrotal swelling. The testis is displaced posteriorly and somewhat upward, and fluid in the hydrocele sac may make palpation of the testis difficult. In the communicating type, the swelling can sometimes be reduced by pressure and is less evident after sleep. This type of hydrocele, which occurs frequently at birth, usually resolves in a few weeks or months.

A *hydrocele of the cord* causes a small, elastic, translucent, usually irreducible, sausage-shaped swelling above the testis or within the inguinal canal. The testis is in its normal position.

An *abdominoscrotal hydrocele* represents an extension of the scrotal hydrocele into the abdomen as a mass.

Acquired hydroceles are usually caused by trauma or infection and epididymitis. The cause of the chronic hydrocele that may occur in older boys usually cannot be determined.

Differentiation between a hydrocele and a hernia may be difficult, and they may coexist. Unless the tunica vaginalis is considerably thickened, hydroceles usually transilluminate well. Although hernias may not, they are translucent in some instances, especially in infants. Hernias are usually readily reducible with a swish, but hydroceles commonly are irreducible or reduce slowly. Except in the communicating type, the top of the scrotal swelling caused by a hydrocele can be palpated, in contrast to that of a hernia.

Occasionally a *hydrocele of the canal of Nuck* may occur in a girl as a firm, cystic, nonmovable and nontranslucent swelling, 1 to 2 cm in diameter, along the inguinal canal.

The finding of firm masses in the inguinal regions of patients with normal female genitalia should raise the possibility of *testicular feminization*. This disorder may require differentiation from prolapse of a normal ovary into an inguinal hernia.

UMBILICUS

Normally the umbilical cord is pearly white. Green or yellow staining suggests pathology. Mummification occurs during the first week, and the cord usually separates in the latter part of the first or early part of the second week. A moist, pink to bright red, small nubbin of friable granulation tissue with a grayish mucoid or mucopurulent discharge may then appear. This usually heals within a few days with scab formation and epithelialization.

Delayed separation of the cord until three weeks of age, the occurrence of multiple abscesses and polymicrobial infections along with abnormal leukocyte adherence and chemotaxis may be associated with absence of a granulocyte membrane glycoprotein.

Normally the umbilical cord contains one large vein, usually centrally placed, and two smaller umbilical arteries. A number of congenital defects, including renal anomalies, have been associated with a *single umbilical artery*.

In infants with an *amniotic navel,* the thin, transparent amniotic membrane that normally covers the umbilical cord extends beyond the cord to the surrounding abdominal wall. If the defect is small, umbilical healing occurs without event, except for a flat scar.

Omphalocele is a rare anomaly, 3 to 4 inches in diameter, in which the anterior abdominal wall around the umbilicus consists solely of thin amniotic membrane. The abdominal viscera may protrude, covered only by the translucent or opaque amniotic membrane.

Ravitch, M. M.: Omphalocele. Pediatr. Clin. North Am. 51:1383, 1971.

The *Beckwith-Wiedemann syndrome* consists of an omphalocele or umbilical hernia, macroglossia, enlargement of the kidneys and liver, nevus flammeus over the forehead, ear lobe grooves and, at times, symptomatic hypoglycemia. Complications may include hemihypertrophy and intra-abdominal malignancies, e.g., adrenocortical carcinoma, Wilms' tumor, hepatoblastoma and gonadoblastoma.

Cohen, M. M., Jr., Gorlin, R. J., Feingold, M., and tenBensel, R. W.: The Beckwith-Wiedemann syndrome. Am. J. Dis. Child. 122:515, 1971.

In infants with a *cutis or skin navel,* the skin of the abdominal wall extends up the cord for an inch or more, and a long, protruding stump remains after separation of the cord.

Gastroschisis is a para-umbilical, full-thickness abdominal wall defect, usually a few centimeters in diameter and situated to the right of the umbilicus, through which the herniated abdominal viscera, usually the small and large bowel, present as an adherent, dark purple mass covered by a thick, gelatinous or fibrinous material. A normal umbilicus and umbilical cord are present, and there is no covering membrane.

Children with *exstrophy of the bladder* have a flattened umbilicus without the usual depression.

Diastasis recti, or separation of the abdominal rectus muscles especially above the umbilicus, occurs in infants and small children. A bulge may be present when the intra-abdominal pressure is raised by crying or defecation. Diastasis recti commonly accompanies exstrophy of the bladder.

A *patent omphalomesenteric duct* may open into the center of a moist and glistening, red umbilical polyp. Serous, mucoid or fecal discharge from the duct may excoriate the surrounding skin. Prolapse of the duct may occur when the infant strains or cries. Peristaltic movements in the walls of the duct have also been reported. A *vitelline cyst* in the intermediate part of the omphalomesenteric duct may present as an umbilical mass.

In infants with a *patent urachus*, urine may leak from the umbilicus, especially with pressure on the bladder. A *urachal cyst* may occur as a deep swelling in the midline between the umbilicus and the bladder. A *urachal rest* may be palpated as a cordlike structure that extends from the umbilicus to the bladder.

Omphalitis is characterized by a red, warm, moist, periumbilical inflammation and a foul, purulent discharge.

The *Cruveilhier-Baumgarten syndrome* is characterized by prominent collateral circulation around the umbilicus, a localized venous hum and thrill, portal hypertension and splenomegaly.

AUSCULTATION

In patients with peritonitis, the bowel sounds, which at first may be increased, later diminish and disappear. Bowel sounds are increased in the presence of hyperperistalsis, and tumultuous bowel sounds may be heard with diarrhea. With obstruction of the intestine, the sounds at first are high-pitched and tinkling but later disappear. Bowel sounds are diminished or absent with paralytic ileus.

A persistent epigastric or flank bruit in a child with diastolic hypertension suggests the need for renal aortography.

PALPATION

Before palpating the abdomen, it is a good practice to talk quietly with the child about topics such as pets, school, siblings or television and to continue the conversation in a relaxed fashion through the examination. Palpation is greatly facilitated if the child is distracted by conversation. Light palpation should initially be used in the abdominal examination of infants and children because deep probing may evoke muscle guarding. If necessary, deeper palpation may be used later. The examiner's hand should be warm. With the examining hand flat on the abdominal wall, palpation is performed with the finger cushions rather than the tips. The examiner's fingernails should be trimmed. Flexion of the patient's knees and placement of a pillow beneath the child's head may promote abdominal relaxation. The physician can usually best perform the examination of the abdomen seated at the bedside, rather than standing above the child. If the child is lying quietly on his parent's lap, it is often wise to begin the abdominal examination there, rather than chance upsetting him.

In the presence of abdominal tenderness, the nontender areas are palpated first, and the tender area is approached *slowly* and *gently.* The child's facial expression is a sensitive indicator of tenderness and should be watched for wincing, squinting or other signs of distress. The child may stop talking or abruptly cry out. Muscle guarding may also be noted. It is not necessary to ask the child whether it hurts. The examiner can tell by watching his face. If the abdominal wall is not relaxed, the examiner may hold his hand gently in place until voluntary muscle tenseness is gradually overcome. The physician may also have the child palpate his own abdomen under the examiner's hand when there is a question of tenderness. The child will often palpate his abdomen much more vigorously than the physician!

Palpation of Masses. Position, size, surface configuration, consistency, tenderness and mobility may be noted in the palpation of abdominal masses. If an abdominal mass is suspected to be neoplastic, palpation should be performed only by the persons immediately concerned with management. Detection of intra-abdominal masses is difficult in the presence of ascites. Ballottement of the mass may be attempted by quickly dipping one's finger tips into the abdomen in the hope that enough fluid is displaced to permit palpation.

Wilms' tumor is a firm, smooth, but occasionally irregular abdominal mass. Usually unilateral, the tumor does not extend across the midline in most cases.

The abdominal *neuroblastoma* is firm but not as hard as a Wilms' tumor. The surface is finely nodular and irregular. Neuroblastomas frequently extend across the midline.

D'Angio, G. J.: Wilms' tumor and neuroblastoma in children. Pediatr. Rev. 6:10, 1984.

Burkitt's lymphoma may appear as an abdominal tumor or ovarian mass.

Embryonal rhabdomyosarcoma, the third most common malignant abdominal tumor in childhood, usually arises in the genitourinary tract. It presents as a hard, immobile mass in the pelvis, bladder or vagina; retroperitoneally; or elsewhere in the abdomen.

The *choledochal cyst* (cystic dilatation of the common bile duct) may infrequently be palpable as an ill-defined mass in the right upper quadrant immediately below the liver. Because its cystic nature is often not apparent on palpation, differentiation from a localized enlargement of the liver may be difficult. Colicky, right upper quadrant abdominal pain, vomiting and intermittent obstructive jaundice may also occur, but the triad of pain, mass and jaundice is infrequent. In the young infant, obstructive jaundice may be the presenting symptom, with the patient often appearing to have biliary atresia. Abdominal distention and hepatomegaly may be other presenting signs. Ultrasonography may be diagnostically useful.

Barlow, B., Tabor, E., Blanc, W. A., Santulli, T. V., and Harris, R. C.: Choledochal cyst: A review of 19 cases. J. Pediatr. 89:934, 1976.

Localized abdominal tenderness and a mass in the right upper quadrant may occur with *cholecystitis. Acute hydrops of the gallbladder,* which causes a palpable right upper quadrant mass, can be readily diagnosed by sonography. Gallbladder hydrops may occur in Kawasaki disease, leptospirosis, scarlet fever, familial Mediterranean fever and with a vasoactive intestinal peptide secreting tumor such as a ganglioneuroma or a ganglioneuroblastoma. A normal gallbladder may also present as a right upper quadrant abdominal mass in the newborn.

Andrassy, R. J., Treadwell, T. A., Ratner, I. A., and Buckley, C. J.: Gallbladder disease in children and adolescents. Am. J. Surg. 132:19, 1976.
Magilavy, D. B., Speert, D. P., Silver, T. M., and Sullivan, D. B.: Mucocutaneous lymph node syndrome: Report of two cases complicated by gallbladder hydrops and diagnosed by ultrasound. Pediatrics 61:699, 1978.

A *pseudocyst of the pancreas* may present as a tender, firm, globular, upper abdominal mass. Ascites may also be present.

Large, hard, *fecal masses* can often be palpated along the large bowel in patients who are chronically constipated. The masses in some cases may be large enough to suggest an intra-abdominal neoplasm.

Fecal retention in children with cystic fibrosis may cause a right lower quadrant abdominal mass and intestinal obstruction. Palpable, hard fecal masses, 3 to 5 cm in diameter in the right lower quadrant, may cause obstructive symptoms and abdominal pain (*meconium ileus equivalent*).

The intestinal loops of newborn infants with *meconium ileus* are rubbery or hard and easily outlined.

The *abdominal aorta* is palpable in many normal children.

An *anterior meningomyelocele* can sometimes be palpated through the abdominal wall.

A *duplication of the bowel* may occasionally be palpable as a movable, smooth, round, nontender mass.

In *endometriosis,* a pelvic mass may be palpable on abdominal examination.

In *superior mesenteric artery thrombosis,* the gangrenous proximal bowel may cause a palpable mass.

In *chronic ulcerative colitis* the ascending and sometimes the descending and sigmoid colons may be palpable as tender tubes. *Crohn's disease* may cause a palpable abdominal mass owing to matted loops of thickened bowel, particularly in the right lower quadrant.

A *sausage-shaped tumor* or an unusual fullness may be palpated in the upper abdominal quadrants in some infants and children with *intussusception.*

A *lactobezoar* in a low birth weight infant may be palpated as an abdominal mass.

Palpation of a *pyloric tumor,* possible in 95 to 98 per cent of infants with *hypertrophic pyloric stenosis,* is diagnostic. The tumor can best be felt immediately after the infant has vomited because of the relaxation of the abdominal wall at that time. The examiner stands or sits on the infant's left side, places his hand on the infant's abdomen and palpates with his middle finger flexed at nearly a right angle. Usually the tumor is found, at times moderately deep in the abdomen, between the edge of the rectus muscle and the costal margin on the right. Occasionally, the pyloric tumor is present below this, and, rarely, even underneath the costal margin. It is usually moderately firm and olive-shaped and sized but may be smaller and harder. Persistent or repeated examinations may be necessary.

A palpable pyloric mass may occur in some infants with duodenal obstruction owing to malrotation of the intestine or to other causes. Such a mass appears and disappears, depending upon the pressure within the distended first portion of the duodenum.

Peritonitis. Abdominal pain, tenderness and constant involuntary, broadlike rigidity or spasm of the abdominal wall along with rebound tenderness is characteristic of peritonitis in older children. Young infants may not demonstrate abdominal rigidity but distention, a doughy feel, and tenderness. Edema and a reddish-blue discoloration of the abdominal wall, flanks and genital region may be present. Patients with peritoneal irritation lie very still.

The abdominal wall may have a doughy, inelastic feel in some patients with tuberculous peritonitis, but this finding is also present in dehydrated or malnourished patients. In fibrinous tuberculous peritonitis, irregular masses may be palpable. Chylous peritonitis may occur following rupture of a mesenteric cyst. Localized erythema of the abdomen may develop with neonatal necrotizing enterocolitis. Peritonitis owing to *Streptococcus pneumoniae* may occur in children with the nephrotic syndrome. Continuous, ambulatory peritoneal dialysis may also be complicated by peritonitis.

Clark, J. H., Fitzgerald, J. F., and Kleiman, M. B.: Spontaneous bacterial peritonitis. J. Pediatr. 104:495, 1984.

Bile ascites, owing to spontaneous rupture of the bile duct may present with pain, distention and toxicity as an acute surgical abdomen (bile peritonitis) in young infants. A greenish-yellow discoloration of the scrotum or umbilicus may be noted.

Hansen, R. C., Wasnich, R. D., DeVries, P. A., and Sunshine, P.: Bile ascites in infancy: Diagnosis with I[131]-rose bengal. J. Pediatr. 84:79, 1974.

Appendicitis. Abdominal tenderness, especially *localized or point tenderness,* is the finding of greatest diagnostic significance in children with acute appendicitis and is almost always present. Before palpation, the child may be asked to point to the "spot where it hurts the most." Young children, unable to localize this very well, almost invariably point to their umbilicus. Because the appendix is relatively long and mobile, the point of maximal tenderness is often not localized at McBurney's point but rather in the right upper quadrant, in the flank, near the inguinal canal or, rarely, even on the left side. Tenderness in the right flank may indicate an inflamed retrocecal appendix. Instead of localization to one point, the abdominal tenderness may be diffuse.

Abdominal rigidity, usually in the right lower quadrant, indicates that extension of the inflammatory process to the parietal peritoneum has occurred. Although often present when the patient is first seen, rigidity is not necessary for diagnosis, which optimally is made before much peritoneal involvement has occurred. Abdominal rigidity or spasm may be present if the inflamed appendix is pelvic, retrocecal or surrounded by the omentum so that it does not contact the peritoneum. Infants often demonstrate no abdominal resistance.

Differentiation between voluntary and involuntary muscle spasm is important, since many extra-abdominal disease processes are accompanied by the former. Such differentiation may, however, be difficult. The examiner's hand is gently placed on the abdominal wall and permitted to rest there for a time before gradually increasing the pressure. Simultaneously, the patient should be distracted by conversation. Spasm of the abdominal muscles owing to extra-abdominal causes may diminish or disappear with this gentle, but continued, pressure or on a repeated examination; however, that caused by peritonitis persists. The child may wince, cry out, shift position or try to push the examiner's hand away. Occasionally a young child is too irritable to permit an adequate abdominal examination. Rectal administration of a rapidly acting barbiturate may permit such appraisal without masking tenderness and involuntary muscle spasm.

The diagnosis of appendicitis is often difficult to establish and may require repeated examinations over a few hours, especially when abdominal tenderness is minimal and rigidity absent.

Rebound tenderness, elicited by the sudden release of manual pressure on the abdominal wall, denotes peritoneal involvement. Besides being painful, this sign has limited reliability in the young child and is best omitted.

When firm pressure is exerted along the descending colon, the patient with appendicitis may experience pain in the right lower quadrant (*Rovsing's sign*). This sign is also of limited reliability in young children.

The child with appendicitis may walk with a limp and lie with the right thigh flexed. When the psoas muscle is involved in the inflammatory process, hyperextension of the right leg, e.g., having the child drop his right leg off the bed, may be very painful (*psoas sign*). This finding may also be found with a perinephritic abscess. Flexion and internal rotation of the right thigh may also cause abdominal pain (*obturator sign*).

With rupture of the appendix, the abdomen may become soft and nontender, and the child may complain less of pain for an hour or two. The pulse rate, however, usually increases during this time, and extreme abdominal tenderness and board-like rigidity soon appear. Localization and abscess formation may lead to a palpable abdominal mass.

The rectal examination in children with appendicitis is discussed on page 106.

Savrin, R. A., and Clatworthy, W., Jr.: Appendiceal rupture: A continuing diagnostic problem. Pediatrics 63:37, 1979.

OTHER CAUSES OF ABDOMINAL TENDERNESS

Other disease processes characterized by abdominal pain, tenderness and muscle spasm include pleurisy, right lower lobe pneumonia, acute pyelonephritis, rheumatic fever, diabetic ketoacidosis, torsion of an ovarian cyst, gastroenteritis, inflammatory bowel disease, primary peritonitis, Meckel's diverticulitis and sickle cell anemia. Boardlike abdominal rigidity is also seen in tetanus and may be present with primary hypoparathyroidism and black widow spider poisoning. Diffuse, generalized abdominal tenderness, often accompanied by muscle guarding, occurs in the *toxic shock syndrome*.

Patients with Addison's disease or acute adrenal insufficiency may demonstrate pain and tenderness in the costovertebral angles.

Upper abdominal tenderness may occur in patients with *pancreatitis*.

Iliac adenitis may cause constant lower abdominal pain. Physical findings include deep lower abdominal tenderness, a positive psoas sign and limp. Localized edema, induration and a palpable mass below and medial to the anterior superior spine may develop later.

Acute salpingitis is characterized by sudden, bilateral, lower abdominal pain accompanying menstruation, a vaginal discharge, fever and chills. Palpation reveals bilateral lower abdominal tenderness. Right upper quadrant tenderness may also be noted if perihepatitis is present.

PERCUSSION

The abdomen is usually tympanitic on percussion, especially in patients with intestinal obstruction, aerophagia and ileus. Occasionally, a distended bladder may be detected by percussion. Shifting dullness may be noted in patients with ascites, unless the large amount of fluid causes generalized dullness.

THE SPLEEN

EXAMINATION

Palpation of the spleen may be performed from the patient's right by placing the examining hand flat on the abdomen and feeling for the edge of the spleen with the finger tips. By placing the left hand under the child's left flank and pressing up, the edge of the spleen may be felt to slip under the examiner's fingers, palpating the abdomen as the patient breathes normally or inspires deeply. Another method is to stand on the patient's left, place the right hand flat on the lower left hemithorax, and slip the fingers under the costal margin from above as the patient breathes deeply. In infants and children with apparent abdominal enlargement, the edge of the spleen should first be sought below the level of the umbilicus; otherwise, one may palpate on top of the spleen and miss the edge. Palpation of the spleen may be facilitated with the patient in the right recumbent position. The tip of the spleen is usually palpable in prematures and can be felt, at times, in normal term infants. In children with a thin abdominal wall, the tip may be just palpable on deep inspiration. An enlarged spleen seems to lie superficially, immediately under the abdominal wall. The spleen edge is firm, usually sharp, and notched. Rarely, ptosis of the spleen ("floating" spleen) has to be differentiated from splenomegaly. The spleen and liver are transposed in situs inversus.

Congenital absence of the spleen may be accompanied by congenital heart disease and Howell-Jolly bodies on the peripheral blood smear.

Careful examination of the left upper quadrant is important after blunt trauma. Traumatic *rupture of the spleen* may be accompanied by tenderness and muscle spasm in the left upper quadrant and by abdominal distention. Pain may be reported in the left shoulder or neck with pressure over the left upper quadrant. Rarely, the child may present in a state of shock. Palpation of the spleen in patients with infectious mononucleosis should be gentle, since spontaneous rupture sometimes occurs. The finding of a ruptured spleen in a child under the age of three years suggests child abuse.

Sinal, S. H.: Splenic trauma. Pediatr. Rev. 1:203, 1980.

Splenomegaly. Enlargement of the spleen is usually but one manifestation of a systemic disease. Hepatomegaly and other symptoms and signs are often also present. On the other hand, splenomegaly may be the sole finding. The following is a partial list of diseases in which enlargement of the spleen may occur.

ETIOLOGIC CLASSIFICATION OF
SPLENOMEGALY

I. INFECTIOUS DISEASES

A. Bacteremia
B. Subacute bacterial endocarditis
C. Salmonella infections
D. Abscess of the spleen
E. Brucellosis
F. Tuberculosis
G. Syphilis
H. Toxoplasmosis
 I. Histoplasmosis
J. Malaria
K. Infectious mononucleosis
L. Q fever
M. Leptospirosis
N. Congenital infectious diseases
O. Cytomegalovirus infection
P. Other infectious diseases

II. BLOOD DISEASES

A. Hemolytic disease of the newborn owing to blood group incompatibility
B. Congenital hemolytic anemia
C. Acute, acquired hemolytic anemia. Splenomegaly is not a constant finding.
D. Thalassemia
E. Sickle cell anemia. Splenomegaly occurs in most infants with homozygous sickle cell disease. Fibrosis of the spleen gradually occurs in these patients so that the spleen is nonpalpable after about the age of six years. In sickle cell disease, functional asplenia occurs in the first two years of life. Acute enlargement may be caused by splenic sequestration of erythrocytes accompanied by severe anemia and shock.
F. Other hemoglobinopathies, such as sickle cell-hemoglobin C disease or hemoglobin C disease
G. The spleen may be enlarged in children with iron deficiency anemia.
H. Thrombocytopenic purpura may be accompanied by splenomegaly.

III. CONGESTIVE SPLENOMEGALY—PORTAL HYPERTENSION

A. Splenic vein thrombosis
B. Cavernous transformation of the portal vein

C. Hepatic cirrhosis
D. Congenital hepatic fibrosis
E. Chronic aggressive hepatitis
F. Galactosemia
G. Chiari's disease—thrombosis of the hepatic vein
H. Congestive heart failure
 I. Constrictive pericarditis
J. Cystic fibrosis

IV. METABOLIC DISEASES

A. Gaucher's disease
B. Niemann-Pick disease
C. Sandhoff's disease
D. Histiocytosis X
E. Hyperlipoproteinemia
F. Multiple sulfatase deficiency
G. Familial hemophagocytic reticulosis
H. Hemosiderosis
 I. Mucopolysaccharidoses
J. Amyloidosis
K. Cystinosis
L. Porphyria
M. Wolman's disease
N. Fucosidosis
O. Mannosidosis
P. Mucolipidoses
Q. GM_1 gangliosidosis type 1 (generalized gangliosidosis)

V. NEOPLASTIC DISEASES

A. Leukemia
B. Lymphosarcoma
C. Hodgkin's disease
D. Hamartomas

VI. CYSTS

VII. MISCELLANEOUS

A. Serum sickness
B. Sarcoidosis
C. Rheumatoid arthritis. Occasional patients with polyarticular, seropositive juvenile rheumatoid arthritis develop Felty's syndrome with splenomegaly and leukopenia.
D. Lupus erythematosus
E. Osteopetrosis
F. Infant of a diabetic mother
G. Chronic granulomatous disease
H. Acquired immune deficiency syndrome
 I. Gianotti-Crosti syndrome (papular acrodermatitis)

THE LIVER

EXAMINATION

The methods described for palpation of the spleen may also be used in palpation of the liver. Riedel's lobe, a congenital hepatic anomaly, may be felt extending downward on the right. Except for its more medial location, an enlarged left lobe of the liver may be mistaken for an enlarged spleen. In patients with situs inversus, the liver edge is palpable on the left. Absolute liver dullness is usually present on percussion below the sixth rib on the right anteriorly and at about the level of the ninth rib posteriorly. Relative dullness is present for one or two interspaces above this. Apparent enlargement of the liver as detected by abdominal palpation should be confirmed by percussion of the upper and lower borders of hepatic dullness. Rarely, seeming hepatomegaly may, in fact, be attributable to downward displacement of the liver secondary to thoracic deformity or pulmonary hyperinflation.

Table 12–1 lists the expected liver span of infants and children determined by percussion of the upper and lower borders in the midclavicular line with the child supine. The liver edge is usually palpable in premature infants. In full-term infants, the liver may be palpated from 1.6 to 4.4 cm below the costal edge at the midclavicular line. Determination of liver size by abdominal palpation alone is unreliable. Younoszai and Mueller, who based their measurements on palpation rather than percussion of the lower border, found the mean liver span to increase from about 7 cm at 5 years to about 9 cm at 12 years, with a standard deviation of 1.0 to 1.3.

Ashkenazi, S., Mimowi, F., Merlob, P., Litmanovitz, I., and Reisner, S. H.: Size of liver edge in full-term, healthy infants. Am. J. Dis. Child. 138:377, 1984.

Lawson, E. E., Grand, R. J., Neff, R. K., and Cohen, L. F.: Clinical estimation of liver span in infants and children. Am. J. Dis. Child. 132:474, 1978.
Younoszai, M. K., and Mueller, S.: Clinical assessment of liver size in normal children. Clin. Pediatr. 14:378, 1975.

Systolic *pulsation* of the liver may occur with tricuspid insufficiency or congestive failure. Presystolic hepatic pulsation may be caused by tricuspid stenosis, constrictive pericarditis and pulmonary stenosis.

Hepatic tenderness may occur with infectious hepatitis, infectious mononucleosis, leptospirosis, passive congestion secondary to cardiac failure and liver abscess. In the first year of life, liver size is important in assessing cardiac failure; however, liver tenderness is uncommon. Gonococcal perihepatitis (Fitz-Hugh–Curtis syndrome), characterized by right upper quadrant tenderness, hepatomegaly and elevated SGPT, may be accompanied by gonococcal salpingitis.

Litt, I. F., and Cohen, M. I.: Perihepatitis associated with salpingitis in adolescents. JAMA 240:1253, 1978.

Hepatomegaly is often but one manifestation of a generalized disease process and is frequently accompanied by splenomegaly.

ETIOLOGIC CLASSIFICATION OF HEPATOMEGALY

I. INFECTIONS

A. Bacteremia
B. Infectious hepatitis
C. Infectious mononucleosis

TABLE 12–1. EXPECTED LIVER SPAN OF INFANTS AND CHILDREN*

Males			Females		
Age, yr	Mean Estimated Liver Span	SEM	Age, yr	Mean Estimated Liver Span	SEM
6 mo	2.4	2.5	6 mo	2.8	2.6
1	2.8	2.0	1	3.1	2.1
2	3.5	1.6	2	3.6	1.7
3	4.0	1.6	3	4.0	1.7
4	4.4	1.6	4	4.3	1.6
5	4.8	1.5	5	4.5	1.6
6	5.1	1.5	6	4.8	1.6
8	5.6	1.5	8	5.1	1.6
10	6.1	1.6	10	5.4	1.7
12	6.5	1.8	12	5.6	1.8
14	6.8	2.0	14	5.8	2.1
16	7.1	2.2	16	6.0	2.3
18	7.4	2.5	18	6.1	2.6
20	7.7	2.8	20	6.3	2.9

*From Lawson, E. E., Grand, R. J., Neff, R. K., and Cohen, L. F.: Am. J. Dis. Child. 132:475, 1978.

D. Syphilis
E. Leptospirosis
F. Histoplasmosis
G. Brucellosis
H. Toxoplasmosis
 I. Tuberculosis
J. Ascariasis
K. Amebiasis or amebic abscess

Meritt, R. J., Coughlin, E., Thomas, D. W., Jariwala, L., Swanson, V., and Sinatra, F. R.: Spectrum of amebiasis in children. Am. J. Dis. Child. 136:785, 1982.
Harrison, H. R., Crowe, C. P., and Fulginiti, V. A.: Amebic liver abscess in children: Clinical and epidemiologic features. Pediatrics 64:923, 1979.

L. Pyogenic abscess of the liver may cause fever, abdominal pain and hepatomegaly. Scintillation scanning is diagnostically useful to detect lesions larger than 2 cm.

Chusid, M. J.: Pyogenic hepatic abscess in infancy and childhood. Pediatrics 62:554, 1978.

M. Visceral larva migrans
N. Congenital infections

Ballard, R. A., Drew, L., Hufnagle, K. G., and Riedel, P. A.: Acquired cytomegalovirus infection in preterm infants. Am. J. Dis. Child. 133:482, 1979.

O. Cytomegalic inclusion disease
P. Q fever
Q. Reye's syndrome
R. Gonococcal or chlamydial perihepatitis (Fitz-Hugh–Curtis syndrome) is characterized by slight hepatomegaly, tenderness in the right upper quadrant and, at times, a hepatic friction rub.
S. Acquired immune deficiency syndrome
T. Neonatal enteroviral infection

II. ANEMIAS

A. Hemolytic disease of the newborn owing to blood group incompatibility
B. Other hemolytic anemias
C. Sickle cell anemia
D. Thalassemias

III. PASSIVE CONGESTION

A. Congestive cardiac failure
B. Constrictive pericarditis
C. Chiari's disease—thrombosis of the hepatic vein
D. Mulibrey nanism, secondary to constrictive pericarditis

IV. METABOLIC DISEASES

A. Glycogenosis Type 1 (glucose-6-phosphate deficiency). Hepatomegaly may be present at birth or appear soon thereafter. Other symptoms in early infancy include hypoglycemia, ketosis and lactic acidosis. Glycogenosis Type III (debrancher enzyme deficiency) and glycogenosis Type VI (phosphorylase deficiency) are also characterized by hepatomegaly. Glycogenosis Type IV is characterized by an enlarged, nodular liver; splenomegaly; and cirrhosis. Glycogenosis Types IX, XI and XII present with hepatomegaly.
B. Mucopolysaccharidoses, e.g., Hurler's and Hunter's syndromes
C. Hereditary fructose intolerance; fructose-1,6-diphosphatase deficiency
D. Galactosemia. Enlargement of the liver is usually present early in infancy.
E. Cystinosis. Hepatomegaly is a late manifestation.
F. GM_1 gangliosidosis type I (generalized gangliosidosis)
G. I cell disease
H. Niemann-Pick disease
 I. Sandhoff's disease
J. Gaucher's disease
K. Lipogranulomatosis
L. Wolman's disease
M. Hyperlipoproteinemia
N. Hereditary tyrosinemia is characterized by hepatomegaly, failure to thrive, vomiting, diarrhea, rickets and cirrhosis.
O. Tangier disease is a familial disorder characterized by hepatosplenomegaly, tonsillar hypertrophy, lymphadenopathy and hypocholesterolemia.
P. Wilson's disease
Q. Congenital porphyria
R. Methylmalonic acidemia; propionic acidemia
S. Lysosomal acid phosphatase deficiency
T. Ornithine transcarbamoylase deficiency
U. Argininosuccinic aciduria; citrullinemia
V. Fucosidosis
W. Mannosidosis
X. Mucolipidoses

V. CHOLESTATIC DISORDERS

VI. NEOPLASTIC DISEASE

A. Hepatoma
B. Hepatic cell carcinoma
C. Infantile choriocarcinoma is characterized in young infants by hepatomegaly, anemia and hemorrhage (hemoptysis, hematemesis, hematuria or melena). Urine chorionic gonadotropin is elevated.
D. Hepatoblastoma or embryonal cell carcinoma

E. Hemangioma, hemangioendothelioma. Multiple cutaneous hemangiomas, hepatomegaly and high output cardiac failure owing to arteriovenous shunts may occur. An epigastric systolic bruit may be present.

Gates, G. F., Miller, J. H., and Stanley, P.: Scintiangiography of hepatic masses in childhood. JAMA 239:2667, 1978.
Rocchini, A. P., Rosenthal, A., Issenberg, H. S., and Nadas, A. S.: Hepatic hemangioendothelioma: Hemodynamic observations and treatment. Pediatrics 57:131, 1976.

F. Leukemia
G. Hodgkin's disease
H. Metastatic neuroblastoma; especially type IVa

VII. Cysts

A. Congenital cysts
B. Echinococcus cyst
C. Traumatic cyst
D. Inflammatory cyst

VIII. Miscellaneous Diseases

A. Congenital hepatic fibrosis. In addition to firm hepatomegaly, especially of the left lobe, and polycystic kidneys, portal hypertension may develop.

Alvarez, F., Bernard, O., Brunelle, F., Hadchouel, M., Leblanc, A., Odievre, M., and Alagille, D.: Congenital hepatic fibrosis in children. J. Pediatr. 99:370, 1981.

B. Fatty infiltration of the liver may occur in patients receiving cortisone therapy.
C. Fatty infiltration may occur secondary to protein calorie malnutrition (Kwashiorkor), poorly controlled diabetes and systemic carnitine deficiency.
D. Hepatic cirrhosis
E. Alpha-1-antitrypsin deficiency
F. Juvenile rheumatoid arthritis, especially the systemic onset type
G. Sarcoidosis
H. Subcapsular hematoma owing to trauma may occur in the newborn or older child.
I. Lupus erythematosus
J. Infants born to diabetic mothers
K. Cerebro-hepato-renal syndrome

Patton, R. G., Christie, D. L., Smith, D. W., and Beckwith, J. B.: Cerebro-hepato-renal syndrome of Zellweger. Am. J. Dis. Child. 124:840, 1972.

L. Chronic, aggressive hepatitis
M. Histiocytosis X; Letterer-Siwe disease; xanthomatosis
N. Familial hemophagocytic reticulosis
O. Cystic fibrosis
P. Vitamin A poisoning
Q. Poisons and toxins including acetaminophen intoxication
R. Hemosiderosis
S. Amyloidosis
T. Osteopetrosis
U. Gianotti-Crosti syndrome (papular acrodermatitis of childhood)
V. Chronic granulomatous disease

THE KIDNEYS

Examination

The kidneys in premature and term infants may be felt on deep palpation; however, they are usually not palpable in older infants and children, although occasionally a lower pole may be felt, especially on the right. To palpate for the left kidney, the examiner stands on the patient's left and presses anteriorly with his right hand in the posterior flank. The left hand, placed laterally to the rectus muscle and immediately below the thoracic cage, is used for abdominal palpation. When the patient takes a deep breath, an enlarged kidney may be felt to move between the examiner's hands. Ballottement may also be helpful in determining renal size. At the end of a deep inspiration, the kidney is quickly pushed upward against the upper hand pressed deeply into the abdomen.

In newborn infants, abdominal muscular relaxation may be obtained by flexing the baby's knees on the abdomen, supporting the infant in a 45-degree upright posture with one hand under the occiput and cervical region and flexing the infant's head. The fingers of the examining hand support the flank posteriorly while the thumb palpates the abdomen.

Mims, L. C.: Palpation of the kidneys in the newborn. Letter to the Editor. Pediatrics 47:1097, 1971.
Museles, M., Gaudry, C. L., Jr., and Bason, W. M.: Renal anomalies in the newborn found by deep palpation. Pediatrics 47:97, 1971.
Perlman, M., and Williams, J.: Detection of renal anomalies by abdominal palpation in newborn infants. Br. Med. J. 2:347, 1976.

RENAL ENLARGEMENT

Hydronephrosis, which causes an intermittent or constant cystic enlargement in the flanks, may require differentiation from a Wilms' tumor or other abdominal neoplasm. A large hydronephrotic kidney often transilluminates well, especially in infants and young children.

Congenital polycystic disease of the kidneys may occasionally account for renal enlargement in young infants. The lobulated and cystic character of the kidneys may be apparent on careful palpation.

Wilms' tumor is a primary consideration in the differential diagnosis of an intra-abdominal mass in infants and young children. When a Wilms' tumor is suspected, the work-up should be accomplished within a few hours. Usually unilateral, the Wilms' tumor has a hard consistency and a smooth or gently lobulated surface. It may range in diameter from a few inches to a mass that fills over half the abdomen. Unless very large, the tumor does not extend across the midline as frequently as an abdominal neuroblastoma. Differentiation from an enlarged liver or spleen should not be difficult, since these organs do not extend far back into the flank. Wilms' tumors may occur in patients with congenital hemihypertrophy, nonfamilial aniridia, and the Drash syndrome.

A *perinephritic abscess* is characterized by tenderness and spasm in the costovertebral area and by systemic symptoms such as fever and chills. The patient splints his back when walking and lies with the thigh on the ipsilateral side flexed. Diffuse swelling, cutaneous inflammatory changes and fluctuation may occur in the flank.

Costovertebral and flank tenderness and muscular rigidity following blunt abdominal *trauma* suggest renal damage. A perirenal hematoma or extravasation of urine after renal trauma may cause a palpable flank mass.

Unilateral or bilateral *thrombosis of the renal vein* may occur in severely dehydrated infants with diarrhea, bacteremia, burns, hypoxia, microangiopathic hemolytic anemia and the nephrotic syndrome. It may also occur in infants born to mothers with diabetes mellitus and in those who have received thiazide medication. Symptoms include sudden renal enlargement, shock, thrombocytopenia, hematuria and oliguria or anuria.

Oliver, W. J., and Kelsch, R. C.: Renal venous thrombosis in infants. Pediatr. Rev. 4:61, 1982.

Rarely, a *pelvic kidney* may be palpated as a pelvic mass.

Megaloureters can sometimes be palpated through the abdominal wall.

BLADDER

Distention of the urinary bladder may be evident on inspection, percussion or palpation, especially during infancy and early childhood when the bladder is essentially an intra-abdominal organ. A distended bladder may reach the level of the umbilicus. Although a distended bladder may occasionally be confused with some other suprapubic mass, spontaneous voiding or catheterization quickly permit differentiation. Distention of the bladder may be present with meningitis, the Guillain-Barré syndrome and transverse myelitis; in patients who are comatose or stuporous; and postoperatively. Children with chronic bladder distention may dribble constantly or intermittently. *Investigation for posterior urethral valves or other partial urethral obstruction is indicated in these children.* When urethral obstruction is suspected, it may be well to observe the patient's urinary stream.

Neurogenic bladder dysfunction may occur in myelodysplasia and the caudal regression syndrome. In addition to bladder distention, dribbling may occur spontaneously or with external bladder compression.

Colodny, A. H.: Evaluation and management of infants and children with neurogenic bladders. Radiol. Clin. North Am. 15:71, 1977.

Exstrophy of the bladder is characterized by absence of the anterior abdominal wall over the bladder area with complete or partial exposure of the bladder mucosa. The mucosa, which is bright red, moist and raised in irregular folds, may be hypersensitive to touch. One may visualize the trigone, and urine may drip intermittently from the elevated ureteral orifices. Usually the testes are undescended, the penis is short and there is a complete epispadias. In girls, the clitoris and vulvar area are cleft and the uterine cervix exposed. Bilateral inguinal hernias are commonly present. The child has a waddling gait owing to separation of the symphysis pubis.

Exstrophy of the cloaca, accompanied by an omphalocele, is characterized by a stoma or prolapsed terminal ileum over the opening of the colon.

13 / GENITALIA

Inspection of the genitalia is an important aspect of the examination of infants, children and adolescents. In the newborn infant, this examination permits early detection of the genital anomalies that characterize patients with pseudohermaphrodism, congenital adrenocortical hyperplasia and other developmental defects. Additional discussion of normal and abnormal genital development is presented in Chapter 32.

FEMALE GENITALIA

In addition to inspection of the female external genitalia, a rectal examination, a bimanual abdominal-rectal or abdominal-vaginal, digital vaginal or vaginoscopic examination may be performed, depending upon the presenting complaint. Vaginal, pelvic or rectal examinations are not routine parts of the physical appraisal in normal girls, although some physicians recommend a pelvic examination for adolescents over the age of 18 years. A rectal examination may give considerable information about the presence of a vaginal foreign body or other vaginal or pelvic pathology; however, the small size of the pelvic organs in children makes it difficult to be sure about their normality when palpated through the rectum. In the young child, the adnexa are not palpable unless they are abnormal. Tenderness and nodularity may be present in the uterosacral ligaments in adolescent girls with endometriosis. In the bimanual abdominal-rectal examination of the adolescent girl, one can palpate the cervix and uterus. In the sexually immature child, the small mass palpable in the midline on rectal examination is usually the uterine cervix, rather than the fundus. The ratio of fundus to cervix increases from 1:3 in the infant to 1:1 at puberty to 3:1 in the mature female.

Inspecting the vagina for vaginitis by opening the hymen may be accomplished by a gentle lateral and posterior movement of the examiner's fingers placed on each side lateral to the labia majora and posterior fourchette with the child supine; or the examiner may ask the child to separate the labia herself. When examination of the pre-pubertal vagina is necessary, veterinary otoscope specula may be used with the operating otoscope head to visualize the vagina and cervix, if the girl is cooperative and not frightened. The 7-mm speculum is satisfactory for a 5-year-old patient. Some examiners prefer to conduct the examination with the prepubertal girl in the knee-chest position: knees 6 to 8 inches apart, head on one side on her arm, abdomen relaxed as the child takes several deep breaths. With the nurse gently holding the child's buttocks apart laterally and dorsally, the vagina may open sufficiently to permit visualization of the vagina and cervix with the magnification light provided by an otoscope; use of a speculum may be unnecessary. Other physicians find that young girls are less threatened if they are asked to flex their hips in the supine frog leg position with the soles of their feet approximated.

Pelvic examination is indicated in adolescents with menstrual disorders, history of maternal use of diethylstilbestrol, vaginal discharge, persistent lower abdominal pain and before prescription of contraceptives.

Gynecologic examination in girls should be performed by a skilled physician. Children who are old enough to understand should be told the reasons for the examination and prepared for what is to be done. Depending upon the girl's preference, either her mother or a nurse should be present if the examination is done by a male physician. The examination should proceed slowly and gently.

Vaginoscopy should be preceded by gentle digital examination of the vagina and localization of the cervix. A bimanual abdominal rectal examination may be used. Instruments recommended (Cowell) for vaginoscopy include: for the child under age 6, the Cameron Miller vaginoscopy kit, the Mueller vaginoscope, the Killian nasal speculum or the Stortz fiberoptic telescope with vaginoscope sheath; for the 6 to 12 year-old girl, the Pedersen bivalved children's speculum; and, for adolescents, the Huffman-Graves virginal bivalved speculum. A disposable plastic speculum is also available. Painful stretching of the hymenal ring should be avoided when the speculum is opened. Because the vulva is sensitive, it is a good practice for the examiner to touch the thigh or lower abdomen with the hand or the speculum blade before separating the labia majora. A cotton-tipped applicator causes discomfort, especially in the prepubertal child, so vaginal secretions for smear and culture should be obtained with a bacteriologic loop or a sterile medicine dropper moistened with saline.

Billmire, M. E., Farrell, M. K., and Dine, M. S.: A simplified procedure for pediatric vaginal examination: Use of veterinary otoscope specula. Pediatrics 65:824, 1980.

Capraro, V.: Gynecologic examination in children and adolescents. Pediatr. Clin. North Am. 19:511, 1972.

Cowell, C. A.: The gynecologic examination of infants, children and young adolescents. Pediatr. Clin. North Am. 28:247, 1981.

Emans, S. J. H., and Goldstein, D. P.: Pediatric and Adolescent Gynecology. Boston, Little, Brown and Co., 1977.

DEVELOPMENT

The external genitalia are not fully developed in premature and in some term infant girls. The labia minora are relatively prominent and protrude between the labia majora as a red, taglike cuff around the hymen and vaginal orifice. The greater the immaturity of the infant, the more prominent the protrusion. Normally, the edges of the labia minora in premature and full-term newborn girls are darkly pigmented. Turgescence and swelling of the external genitalia may be present during the early neonatal period. Clitoral width is normally less than 5 mm. In the older girl, a clitoral width greater than 10 mm represents virilization. The clitoris may also appear relatively prominent in the premature girl, in leprechaunism and, rarely, in neurofibromatosis. A small clitoris and hypoplastic labia are present in female infants with the Prader-Willi syndrome. Inflammatory enlargement of the clitoris may be caused by herpes simplex vulvovaginitis.

Riley, W. J., and Rosenbloom, A. L.: Clitoral size in infancy. J. Pediatr. 96:918, 1980.

If the clitoris is abnormally large, the possibility of virilization is to be considered. Occasionally, an isolated congenital hypertrophy of the clitoris occurs. In girls with *congenital adrenocortical hyperplasia*, varying degrees of masculinization of the external genitalia are noted. These findings are discussed on page 293. Virilizing adrenal hyperplasia should also be considered a diagnostic possibility in seriously ill infants with anomalies of the external genitalia.

An inguinal mass in a phenotypic female may represent a testis associated with the testicular feminization syndrome.

Small cysts ranging in size from 0.5 to 1.0 cm in size may be present on the hymen or below the urethral meatus in newborn girls.

Pubic hair normally appears at an average age of 12 ± 1.1 years in girls. Its appearance before the age of 8.5 years is precocious.

Adhesion of the labia minora with a thin, semitransparent membrane may occur in infant girls. Posterior labial fusion with clitoromegaly is a rare presenting finding in congenital adrenal hyperplasia.

VAGINAL DISCHARGE; VAGINITIS

During the first week or two of life, and especially on the second and third days, a tenacious or thin, mucoid or glairy, grayish or milky and occasionally blood-tinged *vaginal discharge* may be present between the labia in term infants.

Nonspecific vaginitis is common with a slight discharge that stains the girl's underpants. Pruritus, frequency and dysuria may also be reported. Predisposing factors include poor hygiene, obesity, use of bubble bath powders and tight nylon leotards or jeans. Often no specific cause is evident. Mixed bacterial flora are found on culture. A nonirritating physiologic leukorrhea may occur for several months before menarche.

In patients with *bacterial vulvovaginitis*, the profuse discharge causes inflammation of the vulva. The etiologic agent may be the *Pneumococcus, Streptococcus* or *Haemophilus vaginalis*. Gonococcal vaginitis is characterized by reddening of the vulva and genital mucosa along with a thick, yellow, creamy discharge. A bloody discharge may occur with *Shigella* vaginitis. Gonorrhea, though commonly associated with dysuria or a vaginal discharge, is frequently asymptomatic and, therefore, diagnosed only by culture. *Chlamydia trachomatis* may occur concurrently with gonococcal genital infections.

Chacko, M. R., and Lovchik, J. C.: Chlamydia trachomatis in sexually active adolescents: Prevalence and risk factors. Pediatrics 73:836, 1984.

Rettig, P. J.: Pediatric genital infection with Chlamydia trachomatis: Statistically nonsignificant, but clinically important. Pediatr. Infect. Dis. 3:95, 1984.

In *toxic shock syndrome*, vaginal erythema may occur, along with tenderness and hyperemia of the external genitalia.

In *acute salpingitis*, a purulent vaginal and urethral discharge is present. Movement of the cervix on palpation causes severe pain. The adnexa are very tender. Abdominal muscle guarding and rebound tenderness are signs of general or pelvic peritonitis.

Primary *herpetic vulvovaginitis* owing to herpes type II is characterized by painful vesicular lesions on an erythematous base that appear on the vulva, in the vagina, around the anus and on the surrounding skin. The lesions may progress to ulceration.

Vaginitis may be caused by *Mycoplasma hominis*.

Vulvovaginitis may also be associated with pinworm, ascaris or whipworm infestations. *Trichomonas* may also cause vaginitis in infants and children. Vaginitis and vulvitis with redness and edema may also be caused by a *Candida* infection.

Al-Salihi, F. L., Curran, J. P., and Wang, J-S.: Neonatal *Trichomonas vaginalis*. Pediatrics 53:196, 1974.

Altchek, A.: Vulvovaginitis, vulval skin disease and pelvic inflammatory disease. Pediatr. Clin. North Am. 28:397, 1981.

Davis, T. C.: Chronic vulvovaginitis in children due to *Shigella flexneri*. Pediatrics 56:41, 1975.

Emans, S. J.: Vulvovaginitis in children and adolescents. Pediatr. Rev. 2:319, 1981.

Emans, S. J., and Goldstein, D. P.: The gynecologic examination of the prepubertal child with vulvovaginitis: Use of the knee-chest position. Pediatrics 65:758, 1980.

Litt, I. F., Edberg, S. C., and Finberg, L.: Gonorrhea in children and adolescents: A current review. J. Pediatr. 85:595, 1974.

Wald, E. R.: Gynecologic infections in the pediatric age group. Pediatr. Infect. Dis. 3:510 (suppl.), 1984.

OTHER FINDINGS

A vaginal *foreign body*, e.g., wadded toilet tissue, may account for an otherwise unexplained, profuse and, perhaps, foul-smelling or sanguineous vaginal discharge.

Paradise, J. E., and Willis, E. D.: Probability of vaginal foreign body in girls with genital complaints. Am. J. Dis. Child. 139:472, 1985.

Hydrocolpos, caused by the retention of vaginal secretions in newborn girls owing to an imperforate hymen, may present as a midline, lower abdominal mass or as a small, cystic and somewhat displaceable swelling between the labia. Spontaneous release of the retained secretions may occur, or surgical drainage may be necessary.

Hydrometrocolpos in newborn or young infants may cause a lower abdominal mass that may extend above the umbilicus and cause urinary retention. Hydrometrocolpos is often caused by an atresia of the vagina or a transverse vaginal septum not immediately evident. The Kaufman syndrome is characterized by polydactyly, congenital heart disease and hydrometrocolpos.

Hematocolpos, owing to retention of menstrual discharge in adolescent girls with an imperforate hymen, is characterized by lower abdominal pain and a suprapubic mass. The hymen may appear bluish and may bulge outward.

Verrucae acuminatae (condylomata acuminata) are filiform, papular, clustered or soft and multidigitated lesions in the perineal and genital areas. Sexual abuse is to be considered as an etiologic possibility in the presence of these lesions. Moist, flat plaques (condylomata lata) occurring in the genital area may be caused by syphilis.

DeJong, A. R., Weiss, J. C., and Brent, R. L.: Condylomata acuminata in children. Am. J. Dis. Child. 136:704, 1982.

Sarcoma botryoides arise from beneath the vaginal epithelium and appear at the vulva as moist, grapelike, fleshy masses. The history may indicate bleeding or hematuria. *Clear cell adenocarcinoma of the genital tract* in adolescent girls may be associated with prenatal intrauterine exposure to diethylstilbestrol. The patient may present with abnormal vaginal bleeding or discharge, but often the tumor is asymptomatic and found only on the periodic pelvic examinations indicated in these patients.

Soyka, L. F.: Prenatal exposure to stilbestrol and adenocarcinoma of the female genital tract: The pediatrician's responsibility. Pediatrics 55:456, 1975.

Chickenpox lesions may occasionally occur on the genital mucous membranes.

Genital ulcers on the vulva and vagina may be one of the findings in *Behçet's disease*.

Edema of the vulva may occur in Schönlein-Henoch purpura and in osteomyelitis of the pelvis.

Lichen sclerosus et atrophicus, a rare disorder in premenarchal girls, is characterized by atrophied, thin, white, wrinkled and excoriated skin of the perineum and vulva. Moderate pruritus may be present.

Prolapse of the urethra in young girls is characterized by an abnormal protrusion around the urethra, pain on urination, hematuria and vaginal bleeding.

Klaus, H., and Stein, R. T.: Urethral prolapse in young girls. Pediatrics 52:645, 1973.

Chlamydial urethritis may cause urinary frequency and dysuria.

Epispadias in girls is characterized by a

midline division of the mons and clitoris and a dorsal opening of the urethra.

MALE GENITALIA

NORMAL DEVELOPMENT

Growth and development of the penis, scrotum and prostate commensurate with the patient's age is a reflection of normal androgenic activity. During adolescence the penis doubles in length and diameter. The prostate, which usually cannot be felt earlier, may become palpable.

In *Tanner* maturational stages for genital development, *stage 1* represents preadolescence. In *stage 2* the scrotum and testes enlarge, and the skin of the scrotum becomes reddened and altered in texture. With *stage 3* the penis enlarges, initially in length, and further growth of the testes and scrotum is noted. *Stage 4* is characterized by further growth of the penis in width, increased darkening of the scrotum and continued growth of the scrotum and testes. Progress from stage 2 to stage 4 requires about two years, as does development from stage 4 to 5. The adult genital size is referred to as *stage 5*. The maturation of pubic hair is described on page 181.

EXAMINATION OF THE PENIS

During early infancy, adhesions between the prepuce and glans of the penis may prevent retraction of the prepuce so that the urethral meatus and glans cannot be uncovered.

Paraphimosis occurs when the foreskin has been retracted behind the corona of the glans and cannot be slipped forward. Swelling and discoloration of the glans develop rapidly.

Small, white epithelial pearls or *inclusion cysts* may be transiently present on the distal portion of the prepuce in the newborn boy. *Ectopic sebaceous glands* may cause slightly elevated, discrete yellow papules on the shaft of the penis from which a sebaceous material may be expressed.

Pink, pearly papules are a benign, uniformly sized lesion, 1 to 3 mm in diameter, present in many adolescents on the penile corona, especially the anterior border, in one to five rows. These lesions are not to be confused with venereal warts.

Neinstein, L. S., and Goldenring, J.: Pink pearly papules: An epidemiologic study. J. Pediatr. 105:594, 1984.

Balanitis refers to an inflammation of the glans. *Posthitis* refers to an inflammation of the prepuce.

Enlargement of the penis, prostate and scrotum in boys with *congenital virilizing adrenocortical hyperplasia* may be noted at birth or not appear until months or years later. The scrotum is darkly pigmented in infants with virilizing adrenal hyperplasia.

Micropenis refers to a small penis. The normal stretched penile length in young infants is 3.9 ± 0.8 cm. Micropenis may occur in patients with hypogonadotropic hypogonadism (Kallmann's, Prader-Willi, Rud's and septo-optic dysplasia); primary hypogonadism (Klinefelter's or testicular degeneration during fetal life); and partial androgen insensitivity. A small penis may occur in boys with the Noonan's, Robinow's, Carpenter's, Cornelia de Lange's, Down's, Fanconi's anemia, Hallermann-Streiff, long-arm 18 deletion and Williams syndromes. Hypoglycemia may accompany micropenis in newborns with hypopituitarism. A small phallus also occurs in the syndrome of X-linked hypogammaglobulinemia with growth hormone deficiency. Parents should be reassured about the normalcy of the genitalia in very obese infants or children.

Lee, P. A., Mazur, T., Danish, R., Amrhein, J., Blizzard, R. M., Money, J., and Migeon, C. J.: Micropenis. I. Criteria, etiologies and classification. Johns Hopkins Med. J. 146:156, 1980.
Lovinger, R. D., Kaplan, S. L., and Grumbach, M. M.: Congenital hypopituitarism associated with neonatal hypoglycemia and microphallus: Four cases secondary to hypothalamic hormone deficiencies. J. Pediatr. 87:1171, 1975.

Transitory erection of the penis occurs commonly during infancy. Priapism or persistent erection may be associated with local irritation, urethritis, urethral or bladder calculi, spinal cord lesions, leukemia, sickle cell anemia, thrombosis of the corpora cavernosa and Fabry's disease.

In boys with *epispadias*, the urethral opening is on the dorsal surface of the penis. The balanitic type of epispadias involves the glans. In the penile form, a groove is present along the shaft and glans of the penis. The penopubic type is characterized by complete epispadias and the urinary opening beneath the symphysis. Urinary incontinence and separation of the pubic rami may also be present.

In *hypospadias*, the urethral meatus opens on the ventral surface of the penis. The meatus in these patients usually occurs near the glans, but it may be anywhere along the shaft of the penis or, rarely, in the perineum in association with a bifid scrotum. The various types of hypospadias include glandular or balanitic; penile; penoscrotal, perineal; and pseudovaginal. A hooded prepuce may cover the dorsal but not the ventral surface of the glans, and the penis may be otherwise malformed or rudimentary. Cryptorchidism is a frequent finding. Pseudohermaphroditism is a diagnostic possibility in infants with a small penis and a hypospadias. Hypospadias occurs in the Smith-Lemli-Opitz syndrome. Because of the frequency of associated urinary tract abnormalities, renal ultrasonography is indicated.

Stenosis of the urethral meatus, a rare condition, cannot reliably be diagnosed by inspection but may be inferred if the urinary stream is impeded or deflected.

Urethral meatal stenosis in males. Statement of the Urology Section of the American Academy of Pediatrics. Pediatrics 61:778, 1978.

Superficial *ulceration of the urethral meatus* occurs frequently in infant boys, especially those who have been circumcised. The meatus is reddened and inflamed, with excoriation and ulceration of the surrounding glans. Frequently, a serous crust interferes with urination. Urinary retention results because of pain on micturition. Irritant diaper dermatitis is often contributory. Meatitis also occurs in the Kawasaki and the Stevens-Johnson syndromes.

Urethritis may be caused by *Chlamydia trachomatis* infections. Findings include pain on urination, frequency or urgency and meatal irritation.

Feiman, Y. M., and Nikitas, J. A.: Nongonococcal urethritis. JAMA 245:381, 1981.
Rosenberg, A. M., and Petty, R. E.: Reiter's disease in children. Am. J. Dis. Child. 133:394, 1979.

Ulcers of the penis and scrotum may be findings in Behçet's disease.

EXAMINATION OF THE SCROTUM AND TESTES

Hydroceles and inguinal hernias are discussed on page 87.

Torsion of the spermatic cord, which may occur from the neonatal period through adolescence, is a surgical emergency. Examination may be difficult because of the swelling and pain. Characteristically, swelling and ipsilateral bluish or erythematous discoloration of the involved side of the scrotum and testis occur with severe testicular pain and tenderness. Pain may be referred to the inguinal region, thigh or the lower abdomen. The epididymis usually cannot be palpated. A shock-like state may be present.

Differentiating testicular torsion from epididymitis or other cause of acute swelling of the scrotum may be difficult. A scan to measure testicular perfusion may be diagnostically helpful. If equivocal, surgical exploration may be required.

In patients with *orchitis*, the scrotum is swollen, painful and tender. The skin overlying the involved testicle may be reddened and shiny. Viral orchitis may be caused by the coxsackie, mumps, echo or rubella viruses.

Leukemic infiltration of the testes may occur during complete bone marrow remission with relapse restricted to this site. Firm enlargement of the testes and testalgia may occur, or the child may be asymptomatic.

Wong, K. Y., Ballard, E. T., Strayer, F. H., Kisker, C. T., and Lampkin, B. C.: Clinical and occult testicular leukemia in long-term survivors of acute lymphoblastic leukemia. J. Pediatr. 96:569, 1980.

Epididymitis is characterized by painful swelling and redness of the scrotum and enlargement and tenderness of the epididymis. Fever, dysuria, frequency and pyuria may be present. The testes are usually not involved, but the symptoms and signs may simulate those of testicular torsion. In young boys, epididymitis may be related to major urologic anomaly or disorder.

Amar, A. D., and Chabra, K.: Epididymitis in prepubertal boys. Presenting manifestation of vesicoureteral reflux. JAMA 207:2397, 1968.

Torsion of the appendix testis or epididymis is characterized by the sudden onset of severe pain followed within hours by edema of the involved side of the scrotum. A "blue dot" discoloration may be visible through the skin. An extremely tender mass may be palpated near the superior pole of the testis.

Scrotal edema, bleeding into the scrotum, and acute, severe testicular pain, swelling or both may occur in boys with *Schönlein-Henoch purpura*. Acute scrotal edema may also occur in infant boys with peritonitis.

Sahn, D. J., and Schwartz, A. D.: Schönlein-Henoch syndrome: Observations on some atypical clinical presentations. Pediatrics 49:614, 1972.

Varicocele involving the pampiniform plexus occurs not infrequently in pubertal boys, usually on the left side, as a palpable ("bag of worms") or visible mass above the testicle. The varicocele is particularly distended on standing and diminishes in size in the recumbent position. An acutely appearing varicocele may be caused by intraabdominal venous compression.

Berger, O. G.: Varicocele in adolescence. Clin. Pediatr. 19:810, 1980.

UNDESCENDED TESTES

In the premature infant, few scrotal rugae are present and the testes are in the inguinal canal. Normally the testes are in the scrotum at birth in term infants. Frequently, however, one or both are in the inguinal canal but can be easily drawn into the bottom of the scrotum. Repeated, gentle examinations are indicated in evaluating the presence of undescended testes. Placing the child in a warm bath for a time may cause the testes to descend into the scrotum. Most undescended testes are of the migratory or retractile type in which spontaneous descent may be expected before or during adolescence. The retractile testis may be moved medially along the inguinal canal, grasped at the external ring and pulled into the scrotum.

Another method of differentiating pseudo- from true cryptorchidism is to have the child sit on a straight-back chair and flex his knees tightly against his chest so that his feet rest on the seat of the chair. The pressure thus exerted on the inguinal canal may cause a migratory testis to appear in the upper part of the scrotum. The boy may also be asked to sit in the cross-legged tailor or the catcher position so that an active cremasteric reflex is prevented from causing upward retraction of the testis.

Testes that cannot be palpated along the inguinal canal or in the scrotum may be intra-abdominal or absent. Rarely a testis may lie ectopically above and superficial to the external inguinal ring, in the femoral area, at the base of the penis or in the perineum. These areas should be palpated for a testis in children with cryptorchidism. An extrascrotal migratory testis can sometimes be brought down into the scrotum by gentle traction. If not, the testis may be considered anatomically fixed, perhaps by adhesions or bands. Unusual shortness of the spermatic cord, which may prevent full descent, usually undergoes spontaneous correction with growth of the cord during adolescence. Extrascrotal testes that have been present in the scrotum previously may be expected to redescend spontaneously.

Allen, T. D.: Cryptorchidism. Pediatr. Rev. 5:317, 1984.

Buccal smears for nuclear chromatin pattern should be obtained in all patients with true cryptorchidism, since a phallic urethra and a normal-appearing scrotum and penis may occasionally occur in female pseudohermaphrodites. Cryptorchidism occurs in males with the Prader-Willi syndrome.

An inguinal hernia is frequently present in patients with an incompletely descended testis.

Before the age of 11 years the testis is between 1.5 and 2.0 cm in length. If the testes are less than 1 cm in length during this prepubertal period, a buccal smear or karyotype is indicated. Little growth of the testis occurs before this time. The rapid growth of the testis, which begins from 9.5 to 13.8 years with a mean of 11.64 years, is accompanied by thinning and reddening of the scrotum. By the end of the eighteenth year, its length has increased to between 3.5 and 5.0 cm. Testicular size, which may be determined by the use of the Prader orchiometer, reflects pubertal status. The exact measurement of testicular size is, therefore, clinically important. Failure of testicular enlargement to occur by 14 years of age is a significant delay. Pubic hair in boys normally appears at 13.5 ± 1.2 years; its appearance before 10 years is precocious.

The testes in boys with neurogenic or idiopathic isosexual precocity are abnormally enlarged for chronologic age. This enlargement does not usually occur, however, if the precocity is caused by an adrenal cortical carcinoma or hyperplasia. The rare occurrence of aberrant cortical tissue in the testes is an exception to this generalization. These patients demonstrate stimulation of the Leydig cells, which add little to the growth in size of the testes, but no spermatogenesis. When sexual precocity is caused by a testicular tumor, the involved testis is abnormally enlarged, but the other testis remains normal for chronologic age. During adolescence the testes in boys with adrenocortical hyperplasia develop normally; however, testicular tumors have been reported in some of these adolescents. Precocious testicular enlargement may occur with hypothyroidism.

Laron, Z., Karp, M., and Dolberg, L.: Juvenile hypothyroidism with testicular enlargement. Acta Paediatr. Scand. 59:317, 1970.

Macro-orchidism is a nearly universal finding in postpubertal males with the *fragile-X syndrome*, especially if the testicular volume is measured with an orchidometer. Macro-orchidism, which is not specific to the fragile-X syndrome, may be detected by meticulous measurement in the prepubertal child, even in infancy. Testicular length that exceeds 2 cm or a volume greater than 2 ml is an indication for cytogenetic studies.

Carmi, R., Meryash, D. L., Wood, J., and Gerald, P. S.: Fragile-X syndrome ascertained by the

presence of macro-orchidism in a 5-month-old
infant. Pediatrics 74:883, 1980.
Turner, G., Daniel, A., and Frost, M.: X-linked
mental retardation, macroorchidism, and the
X₉27 fragile site. J. Pediatr. 96:837, 1980.

The testes are small in *Klinefelter's syndrome* and relatively small in patients with
hypopituitarism, the size attained depending upon the level of gonadotropins.

The possibility of a *testicular malignancy*
must be considered when a generalized,
firm, nonpainful enlargement of a testis is
noted or a hard or cystic nodule is palpated
within a testis. Adolescent males should be
instructed in self-examination of the testes.
Careful palpation for a testicular teratoma
or an interstitial cell tumor is indicated in
boys with isosexual precocity. Sarcoidosis
may present as a scrotal mass.

Brosman, S. A.: Testicular tumors in prepubertal
children. Urology 13:581, 1979.

PSEUDOHERMAPHRODITISM

Infants who are *male pseudohermaphrodites* may have external genitalia resembling those of a female. Anatomic features
vary widely, and it is usually impossible to
differentiate between a male and female
pseudohermaphrodite by examination of the
external genitalia alone. In some instances
these children resemble those with female
pseudohermaphroditism owing to congenital virilizing adrenal hyperplasia, except
that testes are present in the male pseudohermaphrodite. The scrotum may be cleft
and resemble labia. Examination of infants
with pseudohermaphroditism should include careful palpation of the inguinal region and labia or scrotum for testes. The
Drash syndrome consists of male pseudohermaphroditism, nephritis and Wilms' tumor.

14 / ANUS AND RECTUM

CONGENITAL ANOMALIES

Inspection of the anus after birth is usually sufficient to determine its patency. Digital examination is not necessary if meconium stools are passed and signs of intestinal
obstruction are absent.

The various types of *imperforate anus* are
discussed in Chapter 21. Because anomalies
of the urinary tract and vertebral column
occur frequently in association with an imperforate anus or other anorectal anomaly,
a renal ultrasound is indicated early. Rectovesical, rectourethral, rectoperineal or
rectovaginal fistulas occur in over 50 per
cent of these patients. Meconium or flatus
may be passed from the urethra or vagina
in the presence of such fistulas. The urine
may contain meconium. A rectoperineal fistula in a baby with an imperforate anus has,
at times, been misinterpreted as a normal
anus.

The *VATER association* consists of Vertebral defects, Anal atresia, T-E (tracheoesophageal) fistula with esophageal atresia,
Radial and Renal dysplasia. Ventricular
septal defects and single umbilical artery
are associated anomalies. The *cat's eye syn-*

drome consists of imperforate anus, ocular
colobomata, preauricular pits/tags, congenital heart disease and renal malformation.

Anorectal stenosis may be palpable on
rectal examination as a fibrous ring or diaphragm about ¾ to 1 inch above the anus.
High-grade rectal stenosis that fails to respond to conservative dilatation raises the
question of a presacral teratoma, anterior
sacral meningocele or bony anomaly as the
cause for the stenosis.

Malangoni, M. A., Grosfeld, J. L., Ballantine, T. V.
N., and Kleiman, M.: Congenital rectal stenosis:
A sign of a presacral pathologic condition. Pedi-
atrics 62:584, 1978.

Anterior displacement of the anus may
be associated with constipation.

Reisner, S. H., Sivan, Y., Nitzan, M., and Merlob,
P.: Determination of anterior displacement of the
anus in newborn infants and children. Pediatrics
73:216, 1984.

Anomalous anal papillae may appear as
small, smooth and rounded anal tags. Fissures at their base may cause severe pain
on defecation and bright red blood in the
stools.

ACQUIRED LESIONS

Rectal prolapse appears as a bright red, tubelike protrusion of the rectum. There may be a history of bright red blood on the stools. Prolapse may occur in patients with constipation, chronic diarrhea, chronic ulcerative colitis, infravesicular urinary tract obstruction, pertussis, malnutrition, cord lesions, polyps, and hypothyroidism. Prolapse of the rectum may be the initial complaint in patients with cystic fibrosis.

Acquired anorectal fistulas, which usually open on the perineum near the anus, may develop from a recurring, exquisitely painful and deep perianal abscess. Perianal abscesses may occur in children with chronic ulcerative colitis and in infants with severe and prolonged diarrhea. Anal tags, perirectal and perianal fistulas and abscesses often occur in Crohn's disease and may precede the occurrence of diarrhea and abdominal pain by a period of months. Perirectal cellulitis, abscesses and rectal fistulae may also occur in children with neutropenia, leukemia and chronic granulomatous disease. Anorectal ulcerating lesions may occur in patients with leukemia.

Ament, M. E., and Ochs, H. D.: Gastrointestinal manifestations of chronic granulomatous disease. N. Engl. J. Med. 288:382, 1973.

Enberg, R. N., Cox, R. H., and Burry, V. F.: Perirectal abscess in children. Am. J. Dis. Child. 128:360, 1974.

Anal fissures or excoriations are an important cause for otherwise unexplained crying in infants. A careful examination for these lesions is indicated in infants who cry excessively. Bright red blood may also be present on the stools. A fissure near the mucocutaneous junction may not be evident unless the infant is placed in the knee-chest position, the buttocks are spread widely apart and a bright light is used for the examination. A well-lubricated anoscope or otoscope speculum may be used to visualize lesions not seen on external inspection. Constipation in the early months of life is a common cause of persistent anal fissures and excoriations.

Fecal incontinence occurs only when the somatic innervation of the external striated muscle anal sphincter is impaired.

Occasionally, the external anal sphincter may not function well after surgical repair of an imperforate anus, resulting in *fecal incontinence*. Incontinence may occur with the caudal regression syndrome, myelodysplasia and intraspinal tumors. In these patients, sphincter tone may be lacking, the anus may gape open during crying, and

perineal sensation may be absent. Children with myelodysplasia often have some anal sphincter tone.

Hemorrhoids are extremely rare in children.

Pruritus ani may be caused by poor perianal hygiene or pin worms.

Perianal cellulitis owing to group A streptococci is characterized by a marked erythema of the perianal tissues and a history of painful defecation.

An *ischiorectal abscess* is characterized by local pain, swelling and warmth.

DIGITAL EXAMINATION OF THE RECTUM

Digital examination of the rectum is not routinely performed in the physical examination of infants and children. When indicated, a rectal examination may often be substituted for a vaginal examination. If a child is old enough to understand, he should be told briefly, in words intelligible to him, what the physician is going to do in the examination and why it is necessary. He should also be informed that he will experience some discomfort and, if true, some pain. Unless the child is cooperative, one cannot be certain about the finding of tenderness.

The child is placed or lies on his back in the lithotomy position. For the rectal examination, the little finger is used in infants and the index finger in older children. With a well-lubricated finger cot or glove, the examining finger is placed flat along the perineum with the finger tip touching the sphincter. Once the sphincter relaxes, the finger is introduced slowly and gently. If the child cries or complains of pain, one should pause a moment before attempting to palpate adjacent structures. At times a combined abdominal-rectal palpation may be informative.

In the absence of anorectal stenosis, the little finger can be easily inserted into the rectum of newborn infants. In newborn female infants a relatively large uterus may be palpated. In young boys the flat and small prostate, about 1 cm in diameter, is usually not palpable unless inflammatory changes have occurred.

Rectal examination in infants with aganglionic megacolon reveals a normal sphincter, a well-formed anal canal and a small, empty or nearly empty rectal ampulla. In patients with encopresis secondary to chronic constipation, rectal examination reveals a patulous anal sphincter, a short anal canal and a large amount of feces in the rectal ampulla.

A mass resembling the uterine cervix may be palpable on rectal examination in some patients who have an *intussusception.* Rarely, the mass may protrude from the anus. Such protrusion can be differentiated from a rectal prolapse by inserting the examining finger between the presenting invaginating bowel and the anal ring.

A *duplication of the rectum* may be palpable on digital examination. Occasionally a rectal polyp may also be detected in this manner.

Although *appendicitis* can often be diagnosed on the basis of abdominal findings and history, the findings of right-sided tenderness on rectal examination may be helpful, especially if other signs are equivocal or the appendix is pelvic in position. An appendiceal abscess is often not evident on abdominal examination but may be palpable as bogginess or a tender mass anterior to and pressing on the rectum. A diffuse boggy feel and tenderness may be noted if generalized pelvic peritonitis has developed.

In girls with right-sided abdominal pain owing to torsion of an ovarian pedicle, rectal examination may reveal a small, firm mass on the right or left side. An ovarian tumor may also be palpated by rectal or a combined abdominal-rectal examination.

15 / THE NERVOUS SYSTEM

GENERAL APPROACH

The neurologic examination of infants and young children requires patience and flexibility. For an accurate appraisal it may be necessary to see the child on a number of occasions. Observation of spontaneous behavior and play may be a revealing part of the appraisal. A few simple toys such as a ball, blocks and crayons are facilitative. Young children may be examined best, at least in part, while sitting in their mothers' laps. Children should be asked to walk, perhaps down a hall, while the examiner observes for asymmetrical use of the upper or lower extremities and presence of truncal ataxia on turning. Children over five years should be able to walk on their toes and hop. The ability to skip occurs by seven years of age and tandem walking by nine years. Evaluation of a gait is often best accomplished if the child is unaware of being watched.

NEURODEVELOPMENTAL AND BEHAVIORAL ASSESSMENT OF THE INFANT AND YOUNG CHILD

Assessment of the newborn's neurologic status is based upon observation of spontaneous behavior and response to external stimulus. Brazelton's Neonatal Behavior Assessment Scale includes observations of behavior and the introduction of specific stimuli through six states, from deep sleep to fully awake and crying. Reactions to stimuli may vary markedly as the infant passes from one state to another. The examiner may evaluate the infant's ability to react toward the human voice, fix on and follow a human face and watch a red ball or other brightly colored object.

Amiel-Tison, C.: A method for neurologic evaluation within the first year of life. Curr. Probl. Pediatr. 7:3, 1976.
Anders, T. E.: State and rhythmic process. J. Am. Acad. Child Psychiatry 17:401, 1978.
Brazelton, T. B.: Neonatal Behavioral Assessment Scale. Clinics in Developmental Medicine. No. 88. London, Spastics International Medical Publications. Philadelphia, J.B. Lippincott Co., 1984.
Prechtl, H.: The Neurological Examination of the Full Term Newborn, 2nd ed. Clinics in Developmental Medicine. No. 63. London, Spastics International Medical Publications. Philadelphia, J.B. Lippincott Co., 1977.

DEVELOPMENTAL ACHIEVEMENTS IN THE FIRST 5 YEARS OF LIFE

2 to 4 Weeks

1. Raises his head slightly when lying prone

2. Fixes on a face or object and follows its movements with his eyes

2 Months

1. Holds his head temporarily erect when held upright, but head control is unsteady until 3 months of age
2. Grasps a rattle when placed in hand and holds it transiently
3. Smiles socially
4. Coos reciprocally, vocalizes
5. Regards one's face when it is in his direct line of vision, begins to distinguish his parents and others and responds more to them
7. Looks at the person talking to him
8. Brightens up when given appropriate visual, auditory or tactile stimuli

4 Months

1. Holds his head high and raises his body on his hands when lying prone
2. Can maintain steady head control when held upright
3. Rolls from prone to supine
4. Can assume a symmetrical posture
5. Has hands open while at rest; his hands engage in midline
6. Plays with his hands
7. Looks at a mobile and his arms activate
8. Holds a rattle
9. Follows his parent with his eyes; his eyes follow object through 180 degrees
10. Smiles, coos, laughs, squeals and gurgles
11. Initiates social contact by smiling or vocalization; may be displeased or cry when the adult moves away
12. Shows excitement when parent appears
13. Recognizes preparations for feeding and is able to wait a short time

6 Months

1. Rolls over
2. Shows no head lag when pulled to a sitting position
3. Sits with support or leans forward on his hands when placed in a sitting position; begins to demonstrate right- and left-side parachute reflex
4. Bears some weight on the lower extremities
5. Reaches for and grasps objects; by the end of six months, transfers objects from hand to hand
6. May be able to hold his own bottle to feed

7. Approaches tiny objects with a raking movement
8. Plays with his feet
9. Turns to sounds that originate from out of his immediate sight and changes his activity
10. Shows the first signs of stranger anxiety; distinguishes between angry and friendly voice patterns
11. Laughs, squeals, takes the initiative in vocalizing and babbling at others; blows bubbles and imitates things such as a cough or "raspberry"
12. Shows displeasure at loss of toy

9 Months

1. Sits well
2. Crawls, creeps on his hands or hitches on his bottom
3. Pulls to a stand; cruises
4. Uses inferior pincer grasp; pokes with the index finger
5. Bangs two toys together
6. Can finger feed partially
7. May have one or two meaningful vocalizations, imitates vocalizations and demonstrates monosyllabic and possibly polysyllabic babbling
8. Responds to his own name, "No," "Where is mama (or dada)?," to familiar objects when named; understands a few words: "no-no," "bye-bye"
9. May say "dada" or "mama" in a nonspecific way
10. Enjoys social games with adults: peek-a-boo, pat-a-cake
11. Reacts to strangers with soberness, anxiety or even fear
12. Shows emotions through facial expressions
13. Imitates simple gestures
14. In most cases, has a concept of object permanence; retrieves a toy hidden by a cloth

12 Months

1. Pulls to stand
2. Cruises
3. Walks with support and may take a few steps alone
4. Shows a precise pincer grasp; points
5. Bangs two blocks together
6. Puts one object inside another
7. May say one to three words or meaningful sounds, besides using "mama" and "dada" correctly; imitates vocalization
8. Has a concept of object permanence: looks for a dropped or hidden object
9. Plays social games: e.g., peek-a-boo, pat-a-cake, so-big; waves bye-bye

10. May cooperate in dressing and in feeding himself; uses a cup

15 Months

1. Walks alone, stops and starts, stoops, walks backward, explores
2. Is able to crawl up stairs
3. Builds tower of two cubes; inserts a raisin in a bottle
4. Uses his fingers in self-feeding; drinks well from a cup
5. Has a three- to six-word vocabulary; uses jargon and gestures (If the child fails to say any recognizable words by the age of 18 months, referral should be made for hearing evaluation.)
6. Scribbles spontaneously and demonstrates incipient imitative strokes
7. Points to one or two body parts on request
8. Understands simple commands: "No," "Give me," "Come here"
9. Shows a shoe on request
10. Pats a picture in a book and attends to a story being read to him
11. Recognizes himself in the mirror
12. Indicates his wants by pulling, pointing, grunting or vocalizing
13. Finds an object placed out of sight
14. Rolls a ball and anticipates its return; may roll it again with great joy if the parent waits
15. Can remove a garment; tries to put on a hat
16. Gives and takes a toy
17. Hugs

18 Months

1. Walks fast, may run stiffly, walks up stairs with one hand held, walks backwards, sits in a small chair, climbs into an adult chair, kicks a ball
2. Stacks three or four blocks; may place rings on a cone, then dump them and try again
3. Turns single pages in book or magazine
4. Uses a vocabulary of 4 to 10 words with specificity; may combine two-word phrases; understands and follows some simple directions; may voice two or more wants; shows an imitative vocabulary greater than his vocabulary of spontaneously used words; identifies (points to) some body parts on request; names picture
5. Pulls a toy
6. Throws a ball
7. Feeds himself, uses a spoon appropriately, holds and drinks from a cup adequately

8. Looks selectively at pictures in a book and identifies one
9. Imitates a crayon-stroke on paper
10. May dump a raisin from a bottle without previous demonstration
11. Holds and "loves" a doll or stuffed animal; may use a household-type toy (e.g. toy telephone) functionally
12. Can pucker his lips and kiss his parent on the cheek

2 Years

1. Climbs and descends steps alone, one step at a time, holding the stair rail or the parent's hand
2. Jumps off the floor with both feet; stands on one foot momentarily; runs with ease
3. Opens doors
4. Climbs on furniture
5. Stacks five to six cubes and aligns two to three blocks after demonstration
6. Uses a spoon and cup well
7. Has a vocabulary of 50 or more single words; makes two-word phrases with pronouns such as "I," "me," "you"; refers to himself by name. (If speech is not intelligible to parents or is delayed, the child should be referred for diagnostic speech and hearing evaluation.)
8. Kicks a ball; throws overhand
9. Asks frequent questions: "What's that?"
10. Responds to two-part verbal commands
11. Spontaneously makes or imitates horizontal and circular strokes with a crayon
12. Shows incipient interest in bowel and bladder control
13. Enjoys imitating adult domestic activities and work
14. Shows interest in helping the parent dress him; washes and dries his hands
15. Is beginning the formation of gender identity
16. Selects and uses a toy appropriately (e.g., hammering pegs in a cobbler's bench)

3 Years

1. Jumps in place, kicks a ball, balances and stands briefly on one foot
2. Pedals a tricycle
3. Alternates feet in ascending stairs
4. Can open doors
5. Builds a tower of nine cubes; imitates a bridge made of three cubes
6. Demonstrates speech that is 50 per cent intelligible. (The child who fails to speak in sentences or whose speech is unintelligible to strangers should be referred

for speech, language and hearing evaluation.)

7. May give his full name, knows his age and sex, counts to three

8. May comprehend "cold," "tired," "hungry," and may understand the prepositions "on" and "under"; differentiates "bigger" and "smaller"; can convey the use of a ball, scissors, key and pencil; understands "two" or "three" when applied to objects

9. Copies a circle, may imitate a cross and begins to recognize colors

10. Describes action in picture books

11. Puts on some clothing; dresses with supervision

12. Feeds himself

13. Washes and dries his hands

4 Years

1. Alternates his feet in descending stairs; hops; jumps forward; can stand on one foot for three to five seconds

2. Can climb a ladder

3. Can ride a tricycle

4. Can walk on tip-toes

5. Holds and uses a pencil with good control

6. Builds a tower of 10 or more cubes

7. Has the ability to cut and paste

8. Engages in conversational give-and-take; correctly uses the pronoun "I"

9. Asks why? when? how? and inquires about the meaning of words

10. May name and match three or four primary colors

11. Can count from 1 to 10; can sing a song

12. Enjoys jokes

13. Washes and dries his hands and brushes his teeth

14. If allowed sufficient time, can dress and undress with supervision except for handling laces and buttons in the back; may begin to be selective about clothes

15. Initiates dramatic make-believe and dress-up play in which he assumes a specific role

16. Is imaginative and intensely curious

17. Has formed gender identity

18. Copies a cross, a circle, and possibly a square

19. Draws a person with a face and with arms

20. Enjoys the companionship of other children, plays cooperatively and shows interest in other children's bodies

5 Years

1. Skips, can walk on tip-toes, broad-jumps

2. Throws a ball overhand

3. Washes and dries his hands and brushes his teeth

4. Can cut and paste

5. Identifies coins

6. May name four or five colors

7. Can state his age

8. Can tell a simple story

9. Defines at least one word, e.g., "ball," "show," "chair," "table," "dog"; can name materials of which objects are made

10. Can dress and undress without supervision

11. Knows several nursery rhymes

12. Copies a triangle from an illustration

13. Draws a person with a head, body, arms and legs

14. Beginning to understand right and wrong, fair and unfair

15. Understands that games have rules

NEUROLOGIC INJURY IN THE NEWBORN INFANT

Brachial Plexus Injuries. The *Erb-Duchenne* type of brachial plexus injury involves the fifth and sixth cervical cords. The fingers can be used for grasping, but the arm is flaccid and lies in a position of adduction and internal rotation with pronation of the forearm. Extension of the elbow and flexion of the wrist (waiter's tip position) occurs. Extension of the arm at the elbow may be possible, but the shoulder is functionless. Movements of the fingers and wrist are unaffected. Most of the function that is destined to return will have done so by the age of three months; however, slow improvement may continue up to two years of age. Concomitant injury to the *phrenic nerve* may occur with resultant unilateral paralysis of the diaphragm.

Brachial plexus neuropathy may occur secondary to osteomyelitis of the proximal humerus.

The *Klumpke type* of paralysis, secondary to involvement of C-8 and T-1 vertebrae, does not have as favorable a prognosis as the Erb-Duchenne type. The arm is held flexed at the elbow and the musculature of the hand is paralyzed so that the infant is unable to grasp objects with his fingers. Edema of the involved hand may occur. The first thoracic vertebra and its accompanying sympathetic fibers may also be injured with a resultant Horner's syndrome. Rarely, the entire arm is paralyzed.

Molnar, G.E.: Brachial plexus palsy in the newborn infant. Pediatr. Rev. 6:110, 1984.

Spinal Cord Injury. Spinal cord injury in the newborn infant is characterized by flaccid paralysis, loss of deep tendon reflexes, and absence of sweating below the site of the lesion. Although all extremities may be involved, some function is frequently retained in the upper extremities. Abdominal breathing with intercostal retraction may be noted. Flaccidity persists in these infants and is not replaced by spasticity.

Byers, R.K.: Spinal-cord injuries during birth. Dev. Med. Child Neurol. 17:103, 1975.

Paralysis of the Facial Nerve. Facial nerve paralysis occasionally occurs in newborn infants. Birth injury, abnormal intrauterine position or a congenital absence of the nucleus of the facial nerve may be etiologic.

Periventricular/Intraventricular Intracranial Hemorrhage. Intracranial hemorrhage in the newborn is a common complication in premature infants but also in those at term. Predisposing factors include hypoxia, acidosis, hypotension, dehydration and hypernatremia. The course may be asymptomatic, catastrophic, intermittent or subtle. Findings include seizures, opisthotonus, bulging fontanel, coma, decerebrate posturing, bradycardia, apnea, hypotension, acidosis, fall in hematocrit, decrease in spontaneous activity and hypotonia. Abnormal eye signs include staring, persistent nystagmus, anisocoria, lack of normal pupillary responses to light and absence of the doll's eyes reflex. Diagnosis requires ultrasound and a CT scan.

Lazzara, A., Ahmann, P., Dykes, F., Brann, A.W., Jr., and Schwartz, J.: Clinical predictability of intraventricular hemorrhage in preterm infants. Pediatrics 65:30, 1980.

Mitchell, W. and O'Tuama, L.: Cerebral intraventricular hemorrhages in infants: A widening age spectrum. Pediatrics 65:35, 1980.

Volpe, J. J.: Intraventricular hemorrhage in premature infants. Pediatr. Rev. 2:145, 1980.

Cerebral Damage. Predicting the newborn infant's future neurologic status based on an assessment made in the first days of life is an uncertain prophecy; however, the rapidity with which a baby demonstrates recovery from an impaired neurologic status over the first days or weeks of life seems to be of prognostic significance. Findings in the neurologic examination depend on the infant's gestational age and state of arousal as well as the examiner's skill and experience.

Clinical manifestations of brain damage may not be evident at birth, especially in premature infants. It is also usually not possible to differentiate the clinical picture caused by cerebral hemorrhage from that caused by anoxia or a developmental defect.

Cerebrally injured infants may be pale or cyanotic. The fontanel may be tense and bulging. Ocular palsies, unequal pupil size, nystagmus, failure of the pupils to react to light and a wandering gaze may occur. The Moro reflex may disappear, and the grasp reflex may be absent or weak. The infant may be apathetic and sleep almost constantly, or may be constantly or intermittently restless and irritable. Term newborn infants lie in a position of flexion. With hypotonia, the extremities are extended; with hypertonia they are excessively flexed.

Intracranial damage should be suspected in newborn infants who have a persistent, open-eyed stare. The normal tremulousness of the newborn may be increased. While hypertonicity, localized muscular twitchings, tremors and reflex extension or flexion of the extremities may occur, muscle tone and resistance may be diminished or absent. In addition to the mass type of reflex response which may occur after tapping of the patellar tendon, a jumping jack response may be noted in infants who are cerebrally injured. This response consists of a sudden and simultaneous jerk of all extremities when the sternum or the muscles of the chest or thigh are tapped sharply. Nuchal rigidity, retraction of the head and opisthotonus are also characteristic. A rhythmic protrusion of the tongue, the so-called Foote's sign, may occur. Cerebral injury is the most important cause of convulsions in the newborn infant. The cry may be feeble, plaintive and whiny, or intermittent, shrill, sharp and piercing.

The respiratory rhythm may be abnormally irregular and similar to Cheyne-Stokes respiration in character. The pulse rate may be either increased or decreased. Hyperpyrexia may result from impairment of temperature control. The cerebrally damaged infant often does not feed well since his sucking and swallowing reflexes are either poorly developed or absent. Feeding proceeds slowly. The somnolence of the baby, the protrusion of the tongue and gagging may make feeding difficult. Vomiting, at times forceful, may also occur.

In the *placing reaction*, normally present from birth through the first year of life, the infant is held upright around his chest, and, with one lower extremity flexed, the anterior tibial surface or the dorsum of the foot of the other extremity is lightly touched to the edge of a table. The normal baby brings his foot up to the top of the table. This response is absent in the presence of brain-damage, infantile spinal atrophy and spinal cord injury and is asymmetrical in hemiplegia.

Kernicterus is a complication of neonatal hyperbilirubinemia. In premature infants with severe respiratory problems, hypoxia and acidosis, kernicterus may occur with bilirubin levels under 20 mg/dl. Low serum bilirubin and kernicterus have been described with bacterial sepsis in the newborn. During the first week of life, affected infants may be listless, unresponsive, feed poorly, have a high-pitched cry and regurgitate or vomit. Opisthotonus, irritability and seizures may occur. In patients who survive beyond the first week, athetosis may appear in the latter half of the first or in the second year. Neurosensory deafness is commonly present. An inability to move the eyes upward or downward may also be noted.

The *Crigler-Najjar syndrome* is a congenital, familial disorder characterized by nonhemolytic jaundice. Kernicterus usually develops in the Type I syndrome but is unusual in the Type II. The infants may be persistently jaundiced from a few days after birth. Rigidity, athetosis and an expressionless facies may appear between two weeks and three months of age.

CEREBRAL PALSY

Usually the term *cerebral palsy* implies abberations in motor behavior that arise from central nervous system damage. Hearing impairment, visual problems, mental retardation, speech defects, convulsive disorders and psychological problems may be accompanying handicaps.

The clinical manifestations of cerebral palsy may not be apparent until the latter half of the first year or later, so it is difficult to establish a firm diagnosis of cerebral palsy before one year of age. Careful developmental and neurologic appraisal, however, may permit the diagnosis to be suspected before that time. Cerebral palsy is a consideration with an abnormal persistence of primitive reflex patterns, such as the asymmetric tonic neck reflex; an obligatory tonic neck reflex; delayed gross motor performance; or atypical developmental patterns, such as preferential use of one hand before the age of one to two years, atypical crawling patterns or alterations in muscle tone. The obligatory asymmetric tonic neck reflex, an abnormal finding, is elicited by turning and holding the infant's head to one side for thirty seconds. Failure of a baby who is awake and crying to reverse the asymmetric tonic neck reflex posture is a positive sign.

The *parachute reaction* or anterior propping reaction, normally present by seven to nine months of life, may be delayed or abnormal in infants with cerebral palsy. In this maneuver, the infant held in ventral suspension, is abruptly tilted forward toward the floor. Normally, protective abduction of the arms, extension of the elbows, wrists and spreading of fingers occur. The response is asymmetric in infants with hemiparesis with the affected arm remaining flexed at the elbow. Absence of the parachute reaction is not a significant finding until after eight to nine months of age.

TYPES OF NEUROMUSCULAR DISABILITY

Spasticity. Muscle stiffness is the chief clinical feature of spastic cerebral palsy. Occasionally this is preceded or accompanied by muscular hypotonia and flaccidity. Spasticity usually becomes apparent within the first six months of life, somewhat later if hypotonia has been extensive. Early findings related to motor development appear as either retardation or alteration in normal patterns. The normal extremities are used preferentially, and the affected parts participate less in such activities as kicking, reciprocation and grasping. The parent may report that it is difficult to spread the infant's thighs when changing diapers. Spasticity of the adductors and internal rotators of the thighs and of the flexors of the hip accounts for this limitation of abduction and for the tendency of the lower extremities to scissor or cross over when the child is supported erect, stands or begins to walk. Infants with spastic diplegia usually keep the knees in flexion when supine. In the supported standing position with the soles touching a table surface, the lower extremities are usually rigidly extended and adducted internally with the feet in an equinovarus position. The affected child stands or walks on the toes. Spasticity of the gastrocnemius muscle is demonstrated by resistance to dorsiflexion of the foot, which should be grasped by the toes to avoid causing a reflex plantar flexion, and loss of full range of motion at the ankle joint in infants under six months of age.

When held upright under the axilla, flexion of the lower extremities occurs in normal babies up to four months of age; however, with spastic diplegia, the lower extremities either remain extended, or adduct and scissor. Involvement of the upper extremities may be characterized by adduction of the arm, pronation of the forearm and flexion of the elbow, wrist and interphalangeal joints. The lower extremities are more commonly and severely involved than are the upper. The normal seven- to nine-month-old infant, when suspended by his heels and lowered so that his head touches the examining table, drops his arms below his head. With spasticity or athetosis, this does not occur. Instead, the involved arm is rigidly extended outward, and the forearm is pronated. With spasticity of the hip extensors, the baby cannot be pulled to sit but rather is lifted boardlike directly to standing from a supine position without flexion of the hips or knees. Increased extensor tone is also reflected in opisthotonic posturing of the baby. In the presence of increased extensor tone in the musles of the neck and back, an infant under three to four months of age raises his head higher than his trunk when held in ventral suspension with the examiner's hand under the abdomen. Such hyperextension does not occur in normal infants until four months of age.

A *positive crossed extensor reflex* after four months of age is indicative of an upper motor neuron lesion. When one lower extremity is held extended with the infant in the supine position and the sole of the ipsilateral foot is stimulated, the contralateral leg is flexed and withdrawn, followed by extension and adduction.

The *stretch reflex* is pathognomonic of spasticity. Rapid passive stretching of a spastic muscle leads to a powerful muscle contraction and a sudden resistance to and blocking of the movement. The reflex is not elicited if the motion is performed slowly. This increased resistance (clasp-knife spasticity) is transient, however, and the movement can then be completed. If the child cries or voluntarily tenses his muscles, it may be difficult to be sure about a stretch reflex. Although often delayed in patients with mild spasticity or hypotonia, the stretch reflex usually appears within the first year of life. With severe involvement, it may be present within the first month.

Voluntary motor acts that require coordination may be accompanied by an "overflow" with participation by muscles not primarily concerned. This may be manifested by facial contortions, lip compression, increased extension of the lower extremities, an increase in respiratory rate and the production of guttural sounds. Such manifestations may simulate athetosis.

Children with spastic cerebral palsy may also have hyperactive deep tendon reflexes, ankle clonus, muscle clonus when a muscle is quickly stretched and positive Babinski's reflexes. In infancy, however, the patellar tendon reflexes are difficult to interpret if the infant is crying, tense or his head is not in the midline. Tapping over the shins and moving proximally to the patellar tendon may elicit a knee jerk response. Strabismus, convulsive seizures and mental retardation occur more commonly than in other types of cerebral palsy. Contractures may develop in the absence of preventive measures.

Hypotonia, often an early finding in infants with cerebral palsy, is replaced over a period of months by spasticity. Muscle tone is dynamic and varies with the position of the baby and turning of the head. The *scarf* and *hip* signs seen with hypotonia are discussed on page 112.

The terms *atonic spastic diplegia* and *atonic cerebral palsy* may be applied to muscular hypotonia and weakness without a true flaccid paralysis. Hypotonia may be limited to the muscles that oppose the action of the spastic muscles or may be so generalized as to simulate the "floppy" baby syndrome. The presence of normal or increased deep tendon reflexes, however, is a differentiating feature. Good muscle tone is apparent when voluntary motor activity is attempted. Another difference is demonstrated by lifting the infant with muscular hypotonia by his armpits. The lower extremities of patients with benign muscular hypotonia remain extended while those of patients with atonic spastic diplegia are flexed at the hips and knees. A positive Babinski reflex and ankle clonus are present in some of these children. Muscle stiffness, spasticity and a stretch reflex may appear later and the hypotonia becomes less evident. But some children remain hypotonic and hyperreflexic. Though hyperflexibility of the joints may be present early, many of these patients eventually have flexion contractures.

Dyskinesias. Dyskinesias are characterized by involuntary, nonpurposeful, incoordinated movements often accompanied by increased muscle tone. The movements decrease during sleep or periods of motor in activity and increase during voluntary activity. The manifestations of the dyskinesias are more distinct in the upper than in the lower extremities. The following subgroups frequently overlap. Other causes of dyskinesia are discussed on page 120.

CHOREA. Chorea is characterized by spasmodic, involuntary, nonpurposeful, quick and jerky movements.

ATHETOSIS. Athetosis is manifested by continuous or spasmodic, bizarre, twisting, writhing and wormlike muscular movements that are slower and more tortuous than in chorea. Athetosis is usually most evident in the fingers and wrists. Occasionally, both types of dyskinesia are present in an individual patient (choreoathetosis). When the motions are of large amplitude, athetosis is readily apparent. In many patients, however, findings may be evident only when voluntary efforts are made. This is especially true in patients with muscular hypotonia. In reaching for an object, involuntary extension of the wrist and extension of the fingers may occur. Athetoid movements may be accentuated by asking the child to lie quietly on the examining table in the supine position. Although it may be suspected earlier, athetosis is not fully apparent until the end of the first or during the second year. The appearance of increased muscular tension in infants during voluntary motor activities suggests incipient dyskinesia. Such tension may be manifested as intermittent stiffening spells or extensor spasms which occur spontaneously or in response to minimal stimuli. When the extensor thrust reflex occurs, the involved portion of the body, commonly the trunk, is suddenly thrust into extension.

Attempts to suppress involuntary athetoid movements result in tension, which is misinterpreted, at times, as spasticity. The heightened muscle tone in patients with tension athetosis disappears with passive motion. The converse may occur in the patient with spasticity. The stretch reflex is absent in the former but present in the latter. Tension decreases in the athetoid child when the involved extremity is rapidly shaken but increases in the child with spasticity. Some intermittent resistance may, however, be encountered upon slow joint movement in the patient with tension athetosis. When voluntary motor activity of one extremity is attempted, athetoid movements may overflow into other parts of the body. Non-persistent scissoring of the lower extremities and ankle clonus may occur.

RIGIDITY. The musculature in patients with rigidity is stiff, hypertonic and plastic. Rigidity may be constant, variable or intermittent. The affected child usually lies in an opisthotonic position. Passive movement of a joint, especially when slowly performed, may meet with a constant "lead pipe" or an interrupted "cogwheel" resistance, findings less notable with rapid movement. Deep tendon reflexes are not increased. Other causes of rigidity are discussed on page 118.

Ataxia. In children with ataxia, the movements of the extremities are incoordinated and clumsy. The patient walks late and with a wide-based, unsteady gait. Muscular atony or hypotonicity with hyperactive deep reflexes is characteristic. Nystagmus may be present. Other causes of ataxia are discussed on page 119.

Mixed Forms. Many patients present features characteristic of more than one category.

LOCALIZATION OF INVOLVEMENT

Diplegia is the term used in patients whose major involvement is in the lower extremities but who also have some involvement in the upper extremities. Early hypotonia, rather then hypertonia of the lower extremities, is present. Infants with spastic diplegia, often prematurely born, may be seen because of their delay in sitting up or atypical crawling patterns, e.g., using the arms to propel themselves forward, bunny-hopping on the knees or pushing along on the buttocks.

Hemiparesis indicates involvement of one half of the body, usually spastic in type, and more pronounced in the upper than in the lower extremities. In infants with congenital hemiparesis, a definite hand preference may be noted by six months of age, and the parent may report that the infant reaches out with the same hand each time. At this age, a normal infant will use both hands to pull off a cover placed over his face. If the baby uses only one hand, that extremity should be momentarily restrained by the examiner to see if the other hand is used appropriately. The crawling pattern is also abnormal. While walking, the involved lower extremity may be dragged along or circumducted, and the child may walk on his toes. Mild hemiparesis may be detected by observing asymmetric associated movements of the upper extremities when the child walks or runs. The involved arm is carried in more of a hemiparetic posture while running than while walking. An asymmetric response to the lateral propping reaction also occurs in which the infant over six months of age is held by the trunk in the sitting position and then abruptly tilted to one side and then the other. The normal response is for the ipsilateral arm to extend and the hand to open in order to prevent the child from falling. This reaction is asymmetric in spastic hemiparesis. Absence of the lateral propping reflex is abnormal after eight or nine months. Growth retardation, perhaps more extensive in the upper extremity, may occur on the involved side. Sensory modalities such as two-point discrimination and stereognosis are often impaired. Other causes of hemiparesis are discussed on page 125.

Molnar, G. E., and Taft, L. T.: Pediatric rehabilitation. Part I: Cerebral palsy and spinal cord injuries. Curr. Probl. Pediatr. 7:3, 1977.
Taft, L.T.: Cerebral palsy. Pediatr. Rev. 6:35, 1984.

EXAMINATION OF THE CRANIAL NERVES

I. The olfactory nerve may be tested by eliciting the recognition of odors such as peppermint and cloves. Each nostril is tested separately. Anosmia occurs along with hypogonadotropic hypogonadism in the Kallmann's and Rud's syndromes and in some patients with the immotile cilia syndrome.

II. In the functional examination of the optic nerve, the eyes are tested individually and then together for visual acuity, color perception and ability to follow objects. An ophthalmologic examination and delineation of the visual fields are also indicated.

III, IV and **VI.** These cranial nerves control eye movement. Defects in this innervation may be detected by having the patient follow objects up and down and from side to side while the head is held in a fixed position. Paralysis of the eye muscles and paralytic strabismus are discussed on page 34.

III. The oculomotor nerve supplies the levator palpebrae superioris, so a peripheral lesion of this nerve causes ptosis of the eyelid and narrowing of the palpebral fissure. The sphincter of the pupil and the ciliary muscle are also supplied by the oculomotor nerve; consequently, dilatation of the pupil and failure to react to light and accommodation are additional findings. Divergent strabismus is also noted. The ptosis and pupillary changes may not occur in patients who have a nuclear lesion of the oculomotor nerve.

IV. The trochlear nerve is rarely affected alone but usually along with the oculomotor nerve.

V. The sensory division of the trigeminal nerve is responsible for sensation over the face and tongue. The *corneal reflex* is elicited by touching the cornea with a wisp of cotton after the patient has been directed to look away from the examiner. The normal response is bilateral blinking, the motor component of the reflex being mediated through the facial nerve. If the lesion involves the trigeminal nerve, neither eye blinks. With a lesion affecting the ipsilateral facial nerve, the other eye blinks. The corneal reflex is absent in comatose and anesthetized patients. It may also be absent in conversion disorder and familial dysautonomia. Involvement of the motor division of the trigeminal nerve causes the jaw to deviate to the paralyzed side when the patient opens his mouth. With clenching of the teeth, contraction of the masseter and temporal muscles on the involved side is feeble.

VI. When the abducens nerve is involved, lateral eye movement is not possible, so internal strabismus and diplopia result. Because paralysis of the abducens nerve is often caused by a generalized increase in intracranial pressure, its presence may not help localize intracranial disease. Abducens paralysis developing in the absence of signs of increased intracranial pressure suggests a pontine tumor, especially if other cranial nerves are involved. An isolated, benign VI nerve palsy may also occur in some children.

Robertson, D. M., Hines, J. D., and Rucker, C. W.: Acquired sixth-nerve paresis in children. Arch. Ophthalmol. 83:574, 1970.

VII. *Peripheral or nuclear paralysis of the facial nerve.* Asymmetry of the face owing to peripheral facial paralysis is especially noticeable when the patient laughs or cries. The involved side is flat, drooped and expressionless. The angle of the mouth sags, and the nasolabial fold is obliterated or less prominent than normal. The patient cannot frown, wrinkle his forehead or close his eyelids tightly. When the child attempts to close the eyelids, the eye on the involved side rolls upward (*Bell's phenomenon*). The sense of taste on the anterior two-thirds of the tongue may be lost, and salivary secretion decreased. Facial paralysis may be demonstrated by asking the patient to talk, whistle, smile, inflate his cheeks or show his teeth.

Peripheral facial nerve paralysis is an occasional cause for facial asymmetry in the newborn. It also occurs acutely and unilaterally in children as Bell's palsy. Bilateral facial weakness may be present with the Guillain-Barré syndrome. The Ramsay Hunt syndrome, owing to herpetic involvement of the ear and the geniculate ganglion, is characterized by vesicles on the ear and in the external auditory canal, facial paralysis, tinnitus, vertigo, severe pain in the external auditory canal and pinna and impaired hearing. Facial diplegia also occurs in congenital myotonic dystrophy.

Partial facial paralysis involving only a single branch of the facial nerve may cause marked asymmetry of the lower lip when the child cries and pouting and drawing of the unaffected side downward and outward.

Pape, K. E., and Pickering, D.: Asymmetric crying facies: An index of other congenital anomalies. J. Pediatr. 81:21, 1972.

Melkersson-Rosenthal syndrome consists of recurrent peripheral facial paralysis, edema of the lips and face and a furrowed tongue.

Wadlington, W. B., Riley, H. D., Jr., and Lowbeer, L.: The Melkersson-Rosenthal syndrome. Pediatrics 73:502, 1984.

Möbius' syndrome, owing to incomplete or complete, unilateral or bilateral weakness of the facial musculature, is characterized by a masklike facial expression. Other cranial nerves, especially VI, may be involved. Anomalies of the brachial and thoracic muscles and the extremities may occur.

Facial nerve palsy may be caused by an *embryonal rhabdomyosarcoma of the middle ear cleft*. A conductive hearing loss, refractory otitis media and a mass in the external auditory canal may be present.

Leviton, A., Davidson, R., and Gilles, F.: Neurologic manifestations of embryonal rhabdomyosarcoma of the middle ear cleft. J. Pediatr. 80:596, 1972.

Facial paralysis may also occur in children with *hypertension* and in Henöch-Schonlein purpura.

Supranuclear paralysis of the facial nerve may be caused by cerebral hemorrhage or another central nervous system lesion. Because of their bilateral cortical innervation, the upper facial muscles are not affected in patients with unilateral supranuclear facial paralysis. The eye can usually be closed to some extent and the forehead wrinkled.

VIII. Testing of auditory acuity is discussed on page 39. Involvement of the cochlear branch of the auditory nerve causes neurosensory deafness. Lesions of the vestibular branch of the auditory nerve may be demonstrated by vestibular function tests. The rotational test can be performed with the child sitting in his mother's lap. The normal response after turning is a broad, roving type of nystagmus with fast and slow components. If nystagmus does not occur

after rotation, labyrinth damage is present. If nystagmus is not obtained on the rotational test, the caloric test, which provides a unilateral stimulus to the labyrinth, may be used. Absence of nystagmus in the caloric test indicates that the labyrinth being tested is not functioning. The sensitivity and reliability of the rotational test is greater than that of the caloric test.

IX. Difficulty in swallowing and loss of the pharyngeal reflexes may occur with lesions of the glossopharyngeal nerve. Usually, however, isolated involvement of this nerve does not occur.

X. Lesions of the vagus nerve may cause difficulty in swallowing and choking when feeding. Foods and liquids may be regurgitated through the nose. Pooling of mucus in the posterior pharynx may cause a loose, "bulbar" cough. The voice has a nasal quality. With a unilateral lesion of the vagus nerve, the uvula deviates to the uninvolved side. With bilateral paralysis, elevation of the palate does not occur during phonation, and the gag reflex may be absent.

XI. Contraction of the sternocleidomastoid and trapezius muscles may be impaired in patients with involvement of the spinal accessory nerve. The child may be unable to shrug his shoulders, and torticollis may be present.

XII. Deviation of the tongue toward the affected side occurs in patients with hemiplegia.

Bulbar involvement may be characterized by pooling of secretions in the posterior pharynx. The pharyngeal muscles may continue to contract in response to touch with a tongue blade. Poliomyelitis may cause paralysis of the ninth, tenth, eleventh and twelfth cranial nerves.

The infantile form of Gaucher's disease may be characterized by a pseudobulbar syndrome with dysphagia and laryngospasm.

Recurrent strokes in sickle cell anemia may lead to a pseudo-bulbar palsy.

Dysphagia, regurgitation, poor sucking ability and pooling of saliva may occur in infants with Pompe's disease or Type II glycogenosis. *Infant botulism* is characterized by bulbar dysfunction with feeding difficulty and dysphagia.

Long, S. S., Gajewski, J. L., Brown, L. W., and Gilligan, P. H.: Clinical, laboratory and environmental features of infant botulism in Southeastern Pennsylvania. Pediatrics 75:935, 1985.

Diphtheritic neuritis may cause pharyngeal paralysis or weakness with dysphagia and difficulty in coughing. Bulbar symptoms may also be noted in tick paralysis and with the Guillain-Barré syndrome.

toms may also be noted in tick paralysis and with the Guillain-Barré syndrome.

Bulbar symptoms may result from phenothiazine toxicity.

Cranial nerve involvement may also occur in patients with tuberculous meningitis, encephalitis and the demyelinating diseases.

Multiple involvement of the cranial nerves suggests a pontine glioma.

REFLEXES AND NEUROLOGIC SIGNS

Examination of Reflexes. Examination of reflexes in infants and children is performed much as in adults except that the response is more variable in infants. Unsustained ankle clonus is not a significant finding in infants. Abdominal reflexes may not be obtained in infants, especially during the first six months. When testing the patellar reflexes, the child's head should be in the midline, since the reflex is modified by the tonic neck reflex. Adduction of the thighs as an overflow of the knee jerk reflex is normal in the first six months of life. A slight increase or decrease in the deep tendon reflexes is not clinically significant. In infants it is often difficult to be certain as to whether or not brisk knee jerks are normal or abnormal.

In deep coma, all reflexes, muscle tone and meningeal signs are absent.

Kernig's sign, which denotes meningeal irritation, is elicited by extension of the knee with the patient in the supine position and the thigh flexed to 90 degrees. When Kernig's sign is positive, the knee can be extended only slightly and extension is painful. A positive sign is usually not present early in young infants with meningitis. Kernig's sign may also be elicited with transverse myelitis.

Brudzinski's sign is adduction and flexion of the lower extremities when an attempt is made to flex the child's head.

Plantar Reflexes. *Babinski's sign*, which may be positive in normal infants, perhaps as a reflection of immaturity of the nervous system, does not become clinically significant until the end of the second year. *Chaddock's sign* with extension of the big toe is elicited by stroking along the lateral malleolus and dorsolateral aspect of the foot. *Oppenheim's sign* is characterized by dorsiflexion of the toe when the examiner strokes downward along the medial aspect of the tibia. *Gordon's sign* consists of extension of the toe when the calf muscles are squeezed.

These signs indicate the presence of a pyramidal tract lesion.

ALTERATION OF TENDON REFLEXES

Diminished Tendon Reflexes. Although the deep reflexes may be diminished or absent in patients with the *Guillain-Barré syndrome*, the superficial reflexes are usually not affected.

In *pseudohypertrophic muscular dystrophy*, the deep reflexes gradually disappear.

The tendon reflexes in the lower extremities in *Friedreich's ataxia* gradually disappear.

Although the deep tendon reflexes may be hyperactive for a time in patients with *Werdnig-Hoffmann disease*, they eventually diminish.

Diminution or absence of the deep tendon reflexes is characteristic of patients with *peripheral neuritis*. Similar findings are present during episodes of *familial periodic paralysis*. The deep tendon reflexes may be absent or decreased in *familial dysautonomia*.

Cerebellar tumors are usually accompanied by a diminution in the deep tendon reflexes. Occasionally, increased tendon reflexes may occur with a medulloblastoma because of compression of the pyramidal tracts. Hyperactive tendon reflexes are commonly present with brain stem tumors.

Enhanced Tendon Reflexes. *Hyperactive deep tendon reflexes* are present with spastic cerebral palsy, Tay-Sachs disease, platybasia, demyelinating encephalopathies and neonatal narcotic withdrawal syndrome.

SENSORY CHANGES

Determination of sensory loss in infants and young children, two-point discrimination and temperature differences, is difficult. It is usually possible, however, to test for pain with a pin prick, since in the absence of paralysis, this stimulus causes withdrawal of the extremity.

Position and vibratory senses in the lower extremities are impaired with *Friedreich's ataxia*.

Hyperesthesia may occur in the Guillain-Barré syndrome, Rocky Mountain spotted fever and meningococcal meningitis. *Paresthesia* may occur with the Guillain-Barré syndrome, lupus erythematosus, transverse myelopathy, tick paralysis, Refsum's disease, reflex sympathetic dystrophy and peripheral neuropathy. The pain and burning sensation may be so marked that the child cannot tolerate the weight of the bedsheet or being touched.

Sensory changes ranging from anesthesia to hyperesthesia may occur with *conversion disorder* and require differentiation from a peripheral neuropathy.

In *congenital indifference to pain*, the children do not cry or demonstrate pain in response to painful stimuli or injury; however, other sensations are not lost. Bizarre skeletal lesions may occur. In *congenital sensory neuropathy,* pain, temperature and touch sensibility is absent or diminished in the extremities and parts of the trunk. A relative indifference to pain occurs with *familial dysautonomia*.

Axelrod, F. B., and Pearson, J.: Congenital sensory neuropathies. Am. J. Dis. Child. 138:947, 1984.

Sensory loss in the affected extremity may occur in children with hemiplegia.

TREMORS

Brief, coarse tremors of the jaw and the extremities, along with some stiffening of the extremities, often occur in normal newborn infants in response to being picked up, having their extremities moved or other sudden postural changes. Tremors may also occur in response to loud noises and chilling. The significance of these startle responses in infants with possible cerebral injury may be difficult to establish in the neonatal period. Since these findings normally disappear in a few weeks, their persistence probably indicates a cerebral lesion.

Tremors and jitteriness are almost a constant finding in newborns with *narcotic withdrawal* or *fetal alcohol syndrome*. Tremulousness is a manifestation of narcotic withdrawal syndrome in adolescents.

Sweet, A. Y.: Narcotic withdrawal syndrome in the newborn. Pediatr. Rev. 3:285, 1982.

Muscle twitching occasionally occurs in infants with hypernatremia.

Tetany of the newborn may cause a coarse tremor of the extremities.

A slow, involuntary, rhythmic tremor may be present in some children with *cerebral palsy*. This tremor may be present at rest, but it is most prominent during voluntary motor activity.

An *intention or action tremor* may occur in patients with cerebellar and brain stem tumors and with Wilson's disease. Tremor associated with lesions of the cerebellar hemispheres is absent at rest but evident with action (intention) and increases in amplitude as the object or end point is approached, e.g. in the finger-to-nose test.

Essential, hereditary or familial tremor usually begins in adolescence. Most noticeable in the fingers and hands when the upper extremities are extended in front of the patient, it increases in amplitude as the hand approaches an object. The tremor also becomes worse during attempts to write. An associated lateral tremor of the head may occur.

Shuddering attacks, at times accompanied by posturing and flexion of the large joints, may appear in infants or young children as an early clinical manifestation of essential tremor. The episodes may be precipitated by emotional stress. Tics may also be present.

Vanasse, M., Bedard, P., and Andermann, F.: Shuddering attacks in children: an early clinical manifestation of essential tremor. Neurology 26:1027, 1976.

The severity of the tremor in children with *hyperthyroidism* is variable. It may be fine or coarse and present in the hands, tongue and extremities. Usually the tremor is most prominent during voluntary motor activity and best demonstrated when the patient extends his upper extremities and spreads his fingers. The tongue may also show a fine tremor if protruded at this time.

Anxiety may cause a fine to coarse, rapid tremor of the forearms and hands. The tremor is present at rest and increases with voluntary movement. Nervousness and anxiety may be associated with a pheochromocytoma or hyperthyroidism. Bizarre tremors may be noted in children who live in stressful home environments.

Encephalitis, hypoglycemia, hypomagnesia, hypocalcemia, uremia or pheochromocytoma may cause tremors.

Wilson's disease may begin with an action tremor and poor coordination, especially apparent in fine motor performance such as handwriting. Although the tremor may be present at rest, it is usually accentuated with purposeful movements and emotional stress. The tremor varies from fine to coarse, slow or choreoathetoid. At times, it is localized to one hand, but it may be generalized, involving the head, tongue and upper extremities. Asterixis and cogwheel rigidity may occur. Other findings include awkwardness, slurred speech, difficulty in speaking or writing, excessive salivation, dystonia, dysphagia, an unusual laugh, and deterioration in school performance.

Slovis, T. L., Dubois, R. S., Rodgerson, D. O., and Silverman, A.: The varied manifestations of Wilson's disease. J. Pediatr. 78:578, 1971.

Involuntary movements, especially wing-beating tremors of the arms or *asterixis*, are seen in *hepatic, pulmonary and renal failure* and in Wilson's disease. When the patient is asked to touch his nose with his index finger, sudden movements of flexion and extension occur at the wrists, producing a flapping movement of the hands and, at times, the entire upper extremity.

Jerking, writhing, flailing and marked agitation occur in *scorpion envenomation*.

Thallium poisoning may cause tremor, ataxia, paresthesia and alopecia. Hydantoin toxicity is characterized by an intention tremor.

Tremor, rigidity, dystonia, oculogyric crises and fixed stare may be caused by *phenothiazine toxicity*. Antihistamines, amphetamines, theophylline, gasoline sniffing, salicylate toxicity and phosphate insecticide poisoning may cause a tremor.

Flapping, excited movements are made by some retarded children. Blind children may rub at their eyes or flutter their hands in front of their face (blindisms).

Parkinsonian-like involuntary movements of the hands may occur in patients with kwashiorkor.

Tetany may be characterized by laryngospasm, twitching, tremors, restlessness, muscular rigidity, unsteadiness and convulsions. *Carpopedal spasm* begins with flexion and adduction of the thumb across the cupped palm of the hand. The fingers then flex at the metacarpophalangeal joints and extend at the interphalangeal joints. Flexion and some ulnar deviation of the wrist may also occur. Plantar flexion of the feet in a varus or equinus position may appear along with cupping of the sole and flexion of the toes. Both the upper and lower extremities may be flexed and adducted. Carpopedal spasm may be a manifestation of conversion disorder as well as tetany. The *peroneal sign*, uncommon in infants, is obtained by tapping the peroneal nerve over the head of the fibula. Dorsiflexion and eversion of the foot occur when this sign is positive. *Chvostek's sign* is obtained by tapping over the facial nerve just anterior to the tragus. Contraction of the facial muscles occurs with blinking of the eyelids, twitching of the alae nasi and elevation of the

corner of the mouth. Although a common manifestation of tetany during infancy and early childhood, the sign can be elicited in normal newborn infants.

Sleep myoclonus refers to the abrupt jerk, either generalized or of the extremities, which may occur normally when some children fall to sleep.

RIDIGITY

Tetanus is characterized by muscle spasm and rigidity. Opisthotonus, clenching of the fingers and extension of the lower extremities and feet may occur.

The musculature in *cerebral palsy* of the rigid type is stiff, hypertonic and plastic. The rigidity may be constant or intermittent.

Decerebrate rigidity is characterized by the constant or paroxysmal occurrence of rigid extension of the extremities with hyperpronation of the forearms, flexion of the wrists, fingers, feet and toes, extension of the head and opisthotonus. Coma, pinpoint pupils and bilateral Babinski signs may also be present. Decerebrate rigidity may occur with tumors in the region of the midbrain or the third ventricle and as a result of increased intracranial pressure caused by other lesions, such as hemorrhage into the brain stem, extradural hematoma, severe hypoxemia owing to cardiorespiratory arrest, encephalitis and meningitis. Decerebrate rigidity occurs late in Schilder's disease and terminally in infants with Tay-Sachs disease.

Rigidity may be a finding in *Huntington's chorea* and is often an early sign of *malignant hyperthermia*.

Rigidity of the back, or "poker spine," owing to spasm of the muscles of the back, is common with poliomyelitis. To sit up from the supine position, the child first turns and raises one side on his elbow and forearm. He then places the other hand on the bed behind his back and raises himself into the so-called tripod position, still maintaining a stiff back. If the child is pulled from the supine to the sitting position and given some support beneath his head, the head, neck, and back move as an almost inflexible unit. Both maneuvers may be accompanied by pain owing to muscle spasm. If head support is not provided, the head may fall backward ("head-drop" sign). Sitting with his lower extremities flexed, the child cannot touch his knees with his forehead. Moderate stiffness of the neck may be present. Limited lateral movement of the head may be possible. It is difficult or impossible for the child to flex the neck so that his chin touches his chest.

Nuchal rigidity may occur with the following disorders:
Subarachnoid hemorrhage
Brain abscess
Poliomyelitis
Meningitis. Nuchal rigidity is often not present in young infants with meningitis.
Meningismus
Leptospirosis
Infantile Gaucher's disease
Spinal cord tumors
Intracranial tumors, especially cerebellar tumors with herniation. Nuchal rigidity is occasionally present in patients with supratentorial tumors.
Transverse myelopathy
Encephalitis
Aseptic meningitis
Phenothiazine toxicity. Severe retractional and rotational spasms of the neck may occur.
Arnold-Chiari malformation
Behçet's syndrome

In struggling infants, involuntary and voluntary nuchal rigidity may be differentiated by placing the supine infant with his shoulders at the edge of the table, with his head supported by the examiner's hand. Involuntary rigidity will persist in this position when an attempt is made to flex the head.

Opisthotonus may occur in
Tetanus
Meningitis
Encephalitis
Cerebral hemorrhage and anoxia
Acute infantile Gaucher's disease
Kernicterus
Tay-Sachs disease
1-Glutaric aciduria
Rabies
Miller-Dieker syndrome in the newborn with hypotonia and microcephaly
Withdrawal symptoms in the newborn with fetal alcohol syndrome or maternal narcotic addiction

HYPERACTIVITY

See Chapter 37.

SOFT NEUROLOGIC SIGNS

A number of so-called soft neurologic signs may occur during normal development. These include choreiform movements of the upper extremities, hyperactivity, short attention span, synkinesis (involuntary mirror movements of fingers on opposite hand), poor motor coordination, inability to hop or tandem walk, failure to appreciate simultaneous touch to face and hands, poorly performed alternating movements, mixed or confused laterality and inability to appreciate numbers drawn on the hand. These signs may have a statistical relationship to learning problems, but they are not clinically helpful in the individual child.

Barlow, C. F.: "Soft signs" in children with learning disorders. Am. J. Dis. Child. 128:605, 1974.
Page-El, E., and Grossman, H. J.: Neurologic appraisal in learning disorders. Pediatr. Clin. North Am. 20:599, 1973.

ATAXIA

Detection of ataxia in children under the age of two years may be difficult. Head wobbling may be noted in infants less than six months of age. Truncal ataxia with unsteadiness and swaying in the sitting position may be present in older infants. A history of a change in gait is significant, especially the parent's report that the child staggers, is unsteady or walks on a wider base than before. An important part of the neurologic examination is observation of the child's spontaneous activity, retrieval of a ball or approach to a toy. Patients old enough to cooperate should be asked to stand with their feet together, walk in tandem heel-to-toe fashion, hop on one foot and turn quickly while walking. In the older child, the finger-to-nose and heel-to-knee tests or picking up cubes or raisins may be used to evaluate coordination and balance. Vestibular ataxia owing to bilateral labyrinthine disease or secondary to disturbances in proprioception (sensory ataxia) is accentuated when the eyes are closed; with cerebellar ataxia, this is less marked. Muscle weakness of the lower extremities and pelvic girdle, e.g., associated with polymyositis, may be confused with ataxia.

The more common disease states characterized by ataxia include:
Primary cerebellar ataxia; cerebellar hypoplasia. In addition to ataxia, an intention tremor, dysdiadochokinesia, dysarthria and nystagmus may be present.
Acute, intermittent familial cerebellar ataxia
Ataxic cerebral palsy
Intracranial tumors, especially those involving the cerebellum
Cerebellar abscess

Encephalitis
Friedreich's ataxia and other degenerative
spinocerebellar disorders. A staggering
ataxic gait begins insidiously between the
ages of five and fourteen years. Later,
clumsiness in writing, nystagmus, dysar-
thria, pes cavus, kyphoscoliosis and loss
of position and vibratory senses are noted.
The deep tendon reflexes disappear early.
Tick paralysis
Pernicious anemia
Hydantoin sensitivity or intoxication
Lead poisoning
Sniffing of leaded gasoline

Seshia, S. S., Rajani, K. R., Boecky, R. L., and
Chow, P. N.: The neurological manifestations of
chronic inhalation of leaded gasoline. Dev. Med.
Child. Neurol. 20:323, 1978.

Guillain-Barré syndrome
GM_1 and GM_2 gangliosidosis
Schilder's disease, metachromatic leukodystrophy, Pelizaeus-Merzbacher and
other degenerative diseases
Hartnup syndrome causes intermittent
ataxia, diplopia and a pellagra-like rash.
Fisher's syndrome with ptosis, ophthalmoplegia and areflexia

Becker, W. J., Watters, G. V., and Humphreys, P.:
Fisher syndrome in childhood. Neurology
31:555, 1981.

von Hippel-Lindau syndrome with retinal
and cerebellar angiomas
Marinesco-Sjögren's syndrome with ataxia,
cataracts, mental retardation and skeletal
anomalies
Drug intoxication, including phencyclidine
Argininosuccinic aciduria
Maple syrup urine disease in older children
may be characterized by episodes of
ataxia.
Pyruvate decarboxylase deficiency may
cause intermittent cerebellar ataxia.
Metachromatic leukodystrophy
In children with chronic cholestatic hepatobiliary diseases, vitamin D deficiency is
associated with a progressive neurologic
disorder characterized by cerebellar
ataxia, posterior column dysfunction and
peripheral neuropathy.
Conversion disorder. In the Romberg test,
the patient with a conversion disorder is
more likely to sway from the hips than
from the knees. When asked to perform
another simultaneous task, e.g., finger-to-
nose, the patient may stop swaying,
whereas the child with a true ataxia
would not.
Acute labyrinthitis
Multiple peripheral neuropathy

Angelman's syndrome is characterized by
puppet-like ataxic movements, mental retardation, seizures, microcephaly, tongue
protrusion and paroxysms of laughter.
Ataxia-telangiectasia. Neurologic symptoms and signs usually first appear when
the child begins to walk. Choreiform and
athetoid movements, myoclonic jerks and
nystagmus may be present in addition to
ataxia.
Acute bacterial meningitis. Ataxia may be
a prominent presenting clinical finding or
appear as a complication.

Kaplan, S. L., Goddard, J., Van Kleeck, M., Catlin,
F. I., and Feigin, R. D.: Ataxia and deafness in
children due to bacterial meningitis. Pediatrics
68:8, 1981.

Occult neuroblastoma may present with
ataxia.

Solomon, G. E., and Chutorian, A. M.: Opsoclonus
and occult neuroblastoma. N. Engl. J. Med.
279:475, 1968.

Refsum's syndrome, along with neurosensory deafness, retinitis pigmentosa and
polyneuropathy
The myoclonic movements in *Kinsbourne's
myoclonic encephalopathy* are a mixture
of ataxia and tremor.
Acute cerebellar ataxia is characterized by
the sudden onset of ataxia in a young
child. Intention tremor, nystagmus and
other cerebellar signs may be present.
Perilymphatic fistula of the oval window
region may cause ataxia, neurosensory
hearing loss and episodic vertigo.

Healy, G. B., Friedman, J. M., and DiTroia, J.:
Ataxia and hearing loss secondary to perilymphatic fistula. Pediatrics 61:238, 1978.

Obstruction of cerebrospinal fluid shunts
Abetalipoproteinemia is characterized by
ataxia, retinitis pigmentosa, acanthocytosis (thorny red cells), celiac syndrome
and polyneuropathy.
Basilar artery migraine
Basilar impression of the skull. Other findings may include head tilt, headache,
neck stiffness, brain stem and pyramidal
signs.

DYSKINESIAS; CHOREA; CHOREOATHETOSIS; DYSTONIA

Patients with *Sydenham's chorea* demonstrate emotional lability. Their restlessness may be so marked that the child cannot
sit still. Involuntary movements are sudden,

jerking, irregular, asymmetrical, uncoordi-
nated and purposeless. Choreiform movements, especially notable in the upper extremities and face, cause grimacing and
twitching of the fingers and hands. In hemi-
chorea, the manifestations are predominantly unilateral. Occasionally, temporary
paresis of an extremity occurs. The movements decrease or disappear after rest and
during sleep and increase if the child is
aware of being observed or is instructed to
sit still. The patient has difficulty counting
up to ten and back again rapidly. Speech
and writing may be almost unintelligible. If
the child is asked to smile, the expression
fades rapidly. The patient is able to protrude
his tongue only for a short time and cannot
maintain a tight hand grasp. A "hung-up"
patellar reflex is occasionally observed.
When the arms are extended and the fingers
spread apart, flexion of the wrist and hyperextension of the fingers may occur (bayonet
or dinner fork position). When the arms are
extended above the head, pronation occurs
so that the backs of the hands touch. Chorea
may be a manifestation of rheumatic fever,
lupus erythematosus, hyperthyroidism, infectious mononucleosis, toxins or a side effect of oral contraceptives.

Herd, J. K., Medhi, M., Uzendoski, D. M., and
Saldwar, V. A.: Chorea associated with systemic
lupus erythematosus: Report of two cases and
review of the literature. Pediatrics 61:308, 1978.

The *Lesch-Nyhan syndrome* is a familial
disorder characterized by mental retardation, choreoathetosis, spasticity, opisthotonic spasms, dysphagia, self-mutilative biting of lips and fingers and aggressive
behavior. Hyperuricemia is a constant finding, and clinical gout may occur.

Nyhan, W. L.: Clinical features of the Lesch-Nyhan
syndrome. Arch. Intern. Med. 130:186, 1972.

Huntington's chorea becomes manifest
in childhood in about 1 per cent of patients.
The initial findings may include seizures,
articulatory speech defects, rigidity, slow
voluntary movements, propulsive gait, intention tremor, dystonic posturing, behavioral problems, parkinsonian tremor and
progressive dementia. Later, choreiform
movements appear with facial grimacing
and random jerks, which may initially simulate tics.
Other familial, non-progressive choreas
may occur.

Chun, R. W. M., Daly, R. F., Mansheim, B. J., and
Wolcott, G. J.: Benign familial chorea with onset
in childhood. JAMA 225:1603, 1973.

Familial paroxysmal choreoathetosis of
Mount and Reback occurs as severe, transient episodes (five minutes to four hours)
of choreoathetosis or tonic posturing, which
may be initiated by excitement, fatigue or
caffeine-containing beverages. Paroxysmal
kinesigenic choreoathetosis occurs as brief
paroxysms of dystonic posturing or choreoathetosis precipitated by sudden movement or startle. The episodes are almost
always preceded by a sensory prodrome
such as paresthesia or a sensation of tightness in the affected extremity.

Kinast, M., Erenberg, G., and Rothner, D.: Paroxysmal choreoathetosis: Report of five cases and
review of the literature. Pediatrics 65:1, 1980.
Lance, J. W.: Familial paroxysmal dystonic choreoathetosis and its differentiation from related
syndromes. Ann. Neurol. 2:285, 1977.
Tibbles, J. A. R., and Barnes, S. E.: Paroxysmal
dystonic choreoathetosis of Mount and Reback.
Pediatrics 65:149, 1980.

Choreoathetosis may be induced in infants by phenytoin administration.
Dystonia. The first symptom, usually appearing between 6 and 10 years of age, is
an intermittent, but eventually constant,
plantar flexion-inversion movement of the
foot and ankle while walking. This is followed by involuntary flexion or extension of
the wrist. The child may experience an involuntary flexion of the wrist and fingers
when attempting to hold a pencil. Later,
muscle contractions, torsion spasm and distortions of the neck and trunk may occur
while walking. These patients are often initially misdiagnosed as having a conversion
disorder.

TICS

Tics or nervous spasms usually present
no problem in differential diagnosis. The
characteristic repeated, rapid, involuntary
contractions of isolated muscles or muscle
groups include blinking of the eyelids, sniffing, wrinkling of the nose or forehead, twisting of the mouth, turning of the head to one
side, shaking or nodding of the head, coughing, clearing of the throat, twisting of the
neck, shrugging of the shoulders and jerking of the extremities. Although the involuntary facial grimacing of chorea may superficially resemble habit spasms, the two
are sufficiently dissimilar to permit ready
differentiation. Tics are most frequent between the ages of 6 and 10 years. Tic-like
mannerisms are also frequent in children
who stutter.

Gilles de la Tourette's syndrome, which usually begins before the age of 10 years, is characterized by both motor tics and vocalizations. Initially, tics involve the face or head with eye twitching and head jerking. Later, however, the rest of the body is affected with complex movements such as kicking and jumping. Involuntary noises are a central feature. They include barking, grunting, sniffing, coughing, yells, shrieks, cries, throat-clearing, hissing, and single words, including obscenities (coprolalia) and echolalia. A number of compulsive behaviors may occur, such as repeating the same word or phrase (palilalia), smelling, chewing, touching, obscene gestures (copropraxia), licking, jumping, or squatting. Ritualistic behaviors, such as handwashing or repeatedly rubbing the same area of skin, and obsessional thinking (e.g., of obscene words) may also be reported.

Golden, G. S., and Hood, O. J.: Tics and tremors. Pediatr. Clin. North Am. 29:95, 1982.

Hoder, E. L., and Cohen, D. J.: Tics. In Green, M., and Haggerty, R. J. (eds.): Ambulatory Pediatrics III. Philadelphia, W. B. Saunders Co., 1984, p. 336.

HYPOTONIA, MUSCLE WEAKNESS

See also discussion in Chapter 17.

Pathological hypotonia in infants may be documented by the *anterior scarf sign* and the *hip sign.* In a positive scarf sign, with the baby supine, head in the midline and shoulders firmly against the table, the infant's hands may be pulled across his chest, the elbow past his chin. A positive hip sign for hypotonia is present when the extended lower extremities can be abducted at the hip more than 160 degrees.

Taft, L. T., and Barabas, G.: Infants with delayed motor performance. Pediatr. Clin. North Am. 29:137, 1982.

The *"floppy" or hypotonic infant syndrome* has many specific etiologies. Accurate diagnosis often requires electromyographic and other sophisticated muscle studies.

Dubowitz, V.: Evaluation and differential diagnosis of the hypotonic infant. Pediatr. Rev. 6:237, 1985.

The term *benign congenital hypotonia* has been suggested for the clinical disorder in which symmetrical, generalized muscular weakness, hypotonia and flaccidity are apparent at birth or in the first year of life.

The tendon reflexes are normal. Although these findings are especially notable in the lower extremities, the trunk and the arms are also often involved. Muscular activity is decreased and motor development is delayed. Gradual improvement, at times complete, is the rule.

The neonatal form of *dystrophia myotonica* is characterized by severe hypotonia, facial diplegia and areflexia.

Werdnig-Hoffmann disease, or progressive spinal muscular atrophy, is characterized by generalized muscular hypotonia, weakness, fibrillation and atrophy. The onset may be prenatal, with generalized weakness present at birth. In another group, the onset is between the second and twelfth month, whereas other patients become symptomatic in the second year. The later the onset, the more localized the initial weakness and the longer the life span. Muscle fasciculation may be obscured by subcutaneous fat. Fibrillation and wasting may involve the muscles of the tongue and palate. Breathing becomes diaphragmatic, with paradoxical chest movement on inspiration owing to intercostal weakness. Joint contractures may also occur. Although hyperactive at first, the tendon reflexes gradually diminish. Tremor of the fingers, hands and arms may occur.

A number of metabolic and other disorders may cause hypotonia, such as hypercalcemia, Lowe's syndrome, hypothyroidism, fluid and electrolyte disturbances, mental retardation, propionic acidemia and other inborn errors of metabolism, rickets, infant botulism, malnutrition, Pompe's disease and cerebral degenerative disorders. Some infants who appear hypotonic have ligamentous relaxation and cutis hyperelastica. Hypotonia in infants commonly accompanies cerebral factors, such as hypoxia, hemorrhage, local anesthetic intoxication and the Down's, Zellweger and Prader-Willi syndromes. Many hypotonic infants later develop spasticity or athetosis.

Leigh's syndrome, or subacute necrotizing encephalomyelopathy, is characterized by exacerbations and remissions with hypotonia, ocular palsies, weakness, ataxia, convulsions, lethargy, feeding difficulties, failure to thrive, periodic acidosis, nystagmus and progressive motor deterioration. Intermittent hyperventilation, sobs, sighs and apnea may also occur.

Eisengart, M. A., Powers, J. M., and Rose, A. L.: Subacute necrotizing encephalomyelopathy. Am. J. Dis. Child. 217:730, 1974.

McCandless, D. W., and Hodgkin, W. E.: Subacute necrotizing encephalomyelopathy (Leigh's disease). Pediatrics 60:935, 1977.

Myasthenia gravis, characterized by muscular weakness and fatigability, may rarely be present at birth (congenital myasthenia gravis) or in infancy. Symptoms and signs include generalized hypotonia; weakness, especially of the facial muscles; feeble cry; cranial nerve palsies; and difficulty in sucking, swallowing and handling secretions. Infants born to affected mothers may demonstrate transient myasthenia. Sudden strabismus, diplopia or ptosis in an older child may be the initial manifestation of this disorder. Dysphagia and dysarthria may also occur. Muscular weakness, most marked late in the day and after activity, improves with rest. Weakness in the lower extremities, occasionally sudden in onset, may be the most prominent symptom in older children and adolescents. External ophthalmoplegia may also occur.

Drachman, D. B.: Myasthenia gravis. N. Engl. J. Med. 298:136, 186, 1978.

Familial periodic paralysis is characterized by recurrent episodes of flaccid paralysis, usually involving the extremities but, occasionally, generalized, that begin in adolescence. Death may result from respiratory paralysis. *Adynamia episodica hereditaria* or *hyperkalemic familial periodic paralysis* is characterized by episodes of paralysis accompanied by hyperkalemia.

NEUROPATHY

The *Guillain-Barré syndrome* may be characterized by acute, progressive, symmetrical, distal muscular pain, weakness or paralysis and by segmental paresthesia, hyperesthesia or anesthesia. Stocking or glove hyperesthesia with preservation of position sense may be noted. Tendon reflexes are diminished or absent. Muscle tenderness may be extreme. Symptoms often begin in the feet and progress steadily upward over a period of days. Paralysis of the respiratory musculature and bulbar involvement with difficulty in swallowing and speaking may occur. Some patients demonstrate unilateral or bilateral facial paralysis. Elevation of the optic disk may occur. *Fisher's syndrome,* which may be a variant of Guillain-Barré syndrome, is characterized by external ophthalmoplegia, ataxia, decreased or absent deep tendon reflexes, seventh nerve involvement and an increase in spinal fluid protein. *Tick paralysis* causes progressive motor neuropathy with possible involvement of bulbar and respiratory musculature.

An ascending paralysis may be caused by porphyria, heavy metal poisoning and rabies, especially when contracted through a bat bite.

Marks, H. G., Augustyn, P., and Allen, R. J.: Fisher's syndrome in children. Pediatrics 60:726, 1977.

The *floppy infant* syndrome may be caused by polyneuropathy.

Myeloradiculitis has occurred rarely after rubella vaccination. Brachial involvement causes paresthesias in the finger tips and shooting pains from the arms to the hands lasting from a few seconds to 30 minutes. Lumbosacral involvement causes aching and pain in the lower extremities that is worse on arising. The child walks on his toes with his hips and knees flexed.

Gilmartin, R. C., Jr., Jabbour, J. T., and Duenas, D. A.: Rubella vaccine myeloradiculoneuritis. J. Pediatr. 80:406, 1972.

In *infant botulism,* the child loses his ability to suck and swallow, and progressive weakness occurs within 24 to 48 hours following an initial period of constipation. The usual age of occurrence is two to six months. Within one to two weeks the infant has become profoundly weak, has no head control and only a feeble cry. The initial cranial nerve involvement is manifested by ptosis, pupils poorly reactive to light, facial weakness, a decreased or absent gag reflex and extraocular muscle palsies. Involvement progresses caudally in a symmetric fashion to involve the muscles of the trunk and extremities. Botulism in older children, which begins 18 to 36 hours after ingestion of the toxin, is characterized by diplopia, photophobia, blurred vision, dysphagia and generalized weakness.

Long, S.: Botulism in infancy. Pediatr. Infect. Dis. 3:266, 1984.

Tick paralysis is characterized by the sudden onset of irritability, weakness, an ataxic gait, paresthesia, an ascending symmetrical flaccid paralysis and disappearance of the deep reflexes. Bulbar involvement may also occur.

Peripheral neuritis, polyneuropathy or *multiple neuritis* is manifested by symmetrical muscular weakness, more marked distally than proximally; tenderness and progressive weakness or paralysis; hypotonia; hyporeflexia; sensory loss; and autonomic dysfunction. In some cases, proximal weakness affecting the shoulder or hip girdle and simulating muscular dystrophy may occur. Pain and tenderness along the nerves may be present. Paresthesia may also be a complaint. Wrist and foot drop often develop. Respiratory distress may be caused by intercostal or diaphragmatic involvement. Bulbar symptoms may follow pharyngeal paralysis. Involvement of the peripheral autonomic nervous system may be manifested by distal cutaneous redness, pallor, acrocyanosis and hyper- or hypohidrosis. Refsum's disease, metachromatic leukodystrophy, vincristine therapy, uremia, diabetes, lupus erythematosus, polyarteritis and rheumatoid arthritis may be accompanied by peripheral neuritis. Neuropathy rarely occurs in adolescents with diabetes. Rapidly developing multiple neuropathy occurs in botulism. Chronic interstitial polyneuropathy may become manifest in childhood and adolescence with palpable enlargment of peripheral nerves. Diphtheria toxin may cause palatal paralysis and blurred vision, owing to ciliary paralysis.

Evans, O. B.: Polyneuropathy in childhood. Pediatrics 64:96, 1979.

Neurogenic limb-girdle muscular atrophy syndrome (Kugelberg-Welander disease) is characterized by slowly progressive muscle atrophy, which simulates that in limb-girdle muscle atrophy. A form of neurogenic muscle atrophy simulating the facioscapulohumeral form of muscular dystrophy has also been described.

Furukawa, T., and Peter, J. B.: The muscular dystrophies and related disorders. II. Diseases simulating muscular dystrophies. JAMA 238:1654, 1978.

Brachial plexus neuropathy may be idiopathic or hereditary, unilateral or bilateral, acute or recurrent. A portion of or the entire brachial plexus may be involved. Shoulder pain is a prominent initial symptom, followed by rapid, progressive weakness; paresis; and atrophy of muscles of the shoulder, arm and, perhaps, the hand. In the young infant, brachial plexus neuropathy may occur secondary to osteomyelitis of the proximal humerus.

Clay, S. A.: Osteomyelitis as a cause of brachial plexus neuropathy. Am. J. Dis. Child. 136:1054, 1982.
Shaywitz, B. A.: Brachial plexus neuropathy in childhood. J. Pediatr. 86:913, 1975.

Pack or *rucksack paralysis,* owing to traumatic compression of the brachial plexus, is characterized by pain or sensory symptoms in the shoulder or arm followed by weakness or muscle atrophy in the shoulder girdle. The child may be unable to use the involved arm.

Rothner, A. D., Wilbourn, A., and Mercer, R. D.: Rucksack palsy. Pediatrics 56:822, 1975.

Sciatic nerve injury may be caused by antibiotic or other injections in the buttocks of infants. The risk is greatest in premature or small infants and with multiple injections. Findings include foot drop, sensory loss, absence of sweating over the distribution of the involved branches, change in the color and temperature of the foot and edema.

Gilles, F. H., and Matson, D. D.: Sciatic nerve injury following misplaced gluteal injection. J. Pediatr. 76:247, 1970.

Foot drop, with the child either dragging his foot or developing a steppage gait, may also be a symptom of lead poisoning.

Fabry's disease is characterized by acral pain, particularly in the hands and feet, and paresthesias.

Meralgia paresthetica causes numbness, burning, itching and paresthesia over the distribution of the lateral femoral cutaneous nerve on the anterior lateral aspect of the thigh.

Peroneal muscular atrophy (Charcot-Marie-Tooth disease), a familial disorder, may begin after age six with foot pain and deformity. Hyporeflexia, weakness and atrophy of the peroneal and anterior tibial muscles cause early instability of the foot. Foot drop, clawing deformity of the toes, pes cavus and inversion of the foot (stork-like foot) develop bilaterally. Involvement of the hands and forearms occurs later, with atrophy first of the thenar and then the hypothenar prominences.

Spinocerebellar degenerative disease presents with a progressive disturbance in gait, ataxia, weakness, hyporeflexia and sensory deficits in the lower extremities.

Reflex sympathetic dystrophy in an extremity is characterized by persistent burning or aching pain. Hyperesthesia, hypesthesia or paresthesia occurs in a glove, stocking or nerve distribution pattern along with discoloration, edema and hyperhidrosis.

Fermaglich, D. R.: Reflex sympathetic dystrophy in children. Pediatrics 60:881, 1977.

PARESIS; PARALYSIS

In infants and young children, the degree and extent of paralysis may be difficult to ascertain. The mother usually first notices that the child is not using his extremities normally. Failure to withdraw an extremity in response to appropriate stimuli is diagnostically helpful if sensation is unimpaired. When raised and then permitted to drop, a paralyzed extremity falls more rapidly than if it were normal. Paralysis secondary to central nervous system lesions is usually flaccid, with loss of tone in the affected muscles and loss of the tendon reflexes. A week or two later, spasticity develops and the reflexes become hyperactive.

Causes of Flaccid Paralysis

Poliomyelitis
Guillain-Barré syndrome
Neuromyelitis optica
Postdiphtheritic neuritis
Transverse myelitis
Familial periodic paralysis
Tick paralysis
Myasthenia gravis
Peripheral neuritis
Porphyria
Spinal cord injury at birth
Werdnig-Hoffmann disease
Platybasia
Organic phosphate poisoning
Idiopathic paroxysmal myoglobinuria
Rabies
Enterovirus 71

Infant botulism is characterized by profound weakness, hypotonia, ophthalmoplegia, ptosis, absent gag reflex and sluggish pupillary light reflex.

McKee, K. T., Jr., Kilroy, A. W., Harrison, W. W., and Schaffner, W.: Botulism in infancy. Am. J. Dis. Child. 131:857, 1977.

Muscle pain, weakness and paralysis are clinical features of *idiopathic myoglobinuria*. Acute episodes are characterized by muscle pain, weakness and red or burgundy-colored urine. Striated muscle anywhere in the body may be affected, and widespread motor impairment may occur. Involvement of the lower extremities is a constant feature. Swallowing, respiration and speech may be affected. Muscle pain usually precedes urinary findings by several hours.

Paralysis or weakness of the extremities may represent a *conversion reaction*.

HEMIPARESIS

Epidural, subdural, extradural and intracerebral hematomas
Sturge-Weber syndrome
Myxomas of the heart with embolization
Cerebral thrombosis and hemorrhage

Takayasu's arteritis
Acute infantile hemiplegia. Usually, no exact cause can be determined for an acute hemiplegia. Encephalitis owing to viral diseases such as herpes simplex, Coxsackie A-9 infection, herpes zoster, measles and rubella may be etiologic. The onset of acute hemiplegia is usually preceded by generalized or focal seizures, fever of 101° to 103° F (38.3° to 39.5° C), coma and hemiplegia. Status epilepticus may persist for hours or days.

Gold, A. P., and Carter, S.: Acute hemiplegia of infancy and childhood. Pediatr. Clin. North Am. 23:413, 1976.
Hilai, S. K., Solomon, G. E., Gold, A. P., and Carter, S.: Primary cerebral arterial occlusive disease. Part I: Acute acquired hemiplegia. Radiology 99:71, 1971.
Isler, W.: Acute Hemiplegias and Hemisyndromes in Childhood. Clin. in Dev. Med. Nos. 41/42. Philadelphia, J. B. Lippincott Co., 1971.

Todd's paralysis. Hemiparesis may follow a convulsive seizure.
Tuberculous meningitis
Fat embolism as a complication of a long bone fracture
Cerebrovascular insufficiency and stroke often occur in children and adolescents with *sickle cell anemia*. The peak incidence is in the early school years. One or more major cerebral arteries are occluded.

Huttenlocher, P. R., Moohr, J. W., Johns, L., and Brown, F. D.: Cerebral blood flow in sickle cell cerebrovascular disease. Pediatrics 73:615, 1984.
Portnoy, B. A., and Herion, J.C.: Neurological manifestations in sickle-cell disease. Ann. Intern. Med. 76:643, 1972.

Cyanotic congenital heart disease

Phornphutkul, C., Rosenthal, A., Nadas, A. S., and Berenberg, W.: Cerebrovascular accidents in infants and children with cyanotic congenital heart disease. Am. J. Cardiol. 32:329, 1973.

Brain abscess
Subacute bacterial endocarditis
Carotid artery thrombosis may cause an acute contralateral hemiparesis and an ipsilateral Horner's syndrome. Occlusion of the internal carotid artery may follow nonpenetrating trauma to the head or neck, e.g., blunt trauma to the peritonsillar area as a result of falling on an object carried in the mouth. A 24-hour delay may occur between injury and complication. Palpation of the carotid artery is indicated in these patients, and angiography is required for proof of arterial occlusion.
Moyamoya syndrome. This angiographic pattern is a nonspecific response that may

occur in neurocutaneous syndromes, sickle cell anemia, Down's syndrome and a variety of other disorders.

Carlson, C. B., Harvey, F. H., and Loop, J.: Progressive alternating hemiplegia in early childhood with basal arterial stenosis and telangiectasis. (Moyamoya syndrome). Neurology 23:734, 1973.

Hemolytic uremic syndrome.

Intermittent alternating hemiplegia may occur in early childhood as a familial migraine variant. Recovery occurs in hours to days. As the patient becomes older, a more characteristic pattern of migraine evolves. Although some patients do not experience headaches, a family history of migraine is usually obtained.

Verret, S., and Steele, J. C.: Alternating hemiplegia in childhood: A report of eight patients with complicated migraine beginning in infancy. Pediatrics 47:675, 1971.

Children with persistent familial lipoprotein abnormalities.

Glueck, C. J., Daniels, S. R., Bates, S., Benton, C., Tracy, T., and Third, J. H. C.: Pediatric victims of unexplained stroke and their families: Familial lipid and lipoprotein abnormalities. Pediatrics 69:308, 1982.

Schönlein-Henoch purpura.

Belman, A. L., Leicher, C. R., Moshê, S. L., and Mezey, A. P.: Neurologic manifestations of Schönlein-Henoch purpura: Report of three cases and review of the literature. Pediatrics 75:687, 1985.

BRAIN TUMORS

Brain tumors enter into the differential diagnosis of many symptoms and signs, including:
Vomiting
Headache
Enlargement of the head
Convulsions
Stupor, coma
Unsteady gait
Eyes
    Diplopia
    Ptosis
    Strabismus
    Papilledema
    Optic atrophy
    Nystagmus
    Failing vision
    Visual field defects
Endocrine disorders
    Precocious puberty
    Hypogenitalism
    Obesity
    Gigantism
    Understature
Cranial nerve palsies
Paresis of extremities
Tremor
Failure to thrive
Muscular hypotonia
Reflex changes
Abnormal neurologic signs
Stiffness of the neck
Torticollis
Behavioral disturbances—listlessness, irritability, change in behavior, deterioration in school performance

Some of the common diagnostic considerations are reviewed below.

Tumors of the Posterior Midline of the Cerebellum. An important clinical feature is a staggering, unsteady, swaying, wide-based, ataxic gait. The ataxia is more truncal than appendicular. Truncal ataxia is also manifested by swaying or gradual tilting of the trunk in the sitting position. Incoordination, although usually only mild or moderate in the upper extremities, is particularly prominent in the trunk and lower extremities. Adiadochokinesis and an intention tremor may be present. Muscular hypotonia and hypoactive tendon reflexes are usually found. Hyperactive reflexes and a positive Babinski sign occur with pressure on the pyramidal tracts. Nuchal rigidity is occasionally present. Nystagmus, usually horizontal but occasionally vertical, is seen in most patients. Strabismus is frequent. If the vermis of the cerebellum is symmetrically involved, nystagmus may not occur, and muscle tone may not change.

Tumors of Cerebellar Hemispheres. The initial symptom may be headache, vomiting, unsteady gait or a change in behavior. Pain in the neck, failing vision or strabismus may also be presenting complaints. Cerebellar signs may be absent early and demonstrated only on testing the gait. Truncal ataxia may become evident as unsteadiness when the child is asked to walk a straight line or change direction quickly. It is also manifested as swaying of the trunk when the child is sitting or standing still. The tendency to move or fall toward the involved side may be elicited by having the child walk around a chair or take a few steps forward and then backward. The ipsilateral shoulder may be hunched upward as the child walks, and the automatic swinging action of the ipsilateral arm may not occur. The finger-to-nose test, the heel-to-knee test and adiadochokinesis may all demonstrate incoordination. An intention tremor may also be noted. Nuchal rigidity and retraction of the head are occasionally seen, and the head may be tilted so that the occiput points toward the shoulder on the involved side. Muscular hypotonia and hypoactive reflexes are common, especially on the side of the tumor.

Nystagmus, especially on horizontal gaze, is common and usually evident when the patient focuses upon some point (fixation nystagmus). The nystagmus is slow and coarse on looking toward the side of the tumor; quick and minimal or absent when the gaze is to the opposite side. Headache, vomiting and paralysis of the lateral rectus muscles are also frequent.

Tumors of the Fourth Ventricle. Vomiting, the most frequent manifestation of tumors in this area, may persist for several months before other signs appear. Findings are similar to those with tumors of the cerebellar vermis.

Tumors of the Brain Stem. Cranial nerve involvement, especially of nerves V, VI and VII, is characteristic of tumors of the pons and medulla. Bulbar symptoms may include difficulty in swallowing. Nystagmus is often noted on horizontal and, occasionally, on upward gaze. Ptosis may also be present. The gait is often ataxic. Tendon reflexes are frequently hyperactive and ankle clonus and a Babinski's sign are commonly present. Cerebellar signs are often occur. Signs of increased intracranial pressure may be absent.

Panitch, H. S., and Berg, B. O.: Brain stem tumors of childhood and adolescence. Am. J. Dis. Child. 119:465, 1970.

Tumors involving the hypothalamus and optic chiasm cause headache, vomiting, and visual field defects owing to increased intracranial pressure. Hypothalamic disorders include obesity, diabetes insipidus, understature and sexual precocity or infantilism. Hyperthermia may also occur.

Increased intracranial pressure owing to cerebral edema, neoplasm, abscess or other cause is characterized by headache, vomiting, diplopia, personality changes and papilledema. Lethargy, stupor, coma and systolic hypertension may appear later.

Bell, W. E., and McCormick, W. F.: Increased Intracranial Pressure in Children. 2nd ed. Philadelphia, W. B. Saunders Co, 1978.
Rosman, N. P.: Increased intracranial pressure in childhood. Pediatr. Clin. North Am. 21:483, 1974.

Pseudotumor cerebri, or benign intracranial hypertension, is characterized by papilledema, abducens palsy, severe headache, vomiting and diplopia. Other symptoms of increased intracranial pressure may be present.

Brain abscess is to be considered in the differential diagnosis of localized neurologic findings, headache or fever. Patients with cyanotic congenital heart disease are at special risk.

Platybasia or basilar impression of the skull with congenital flattening of the base of the skull leads to a decreased size of the posterior fossa. A Klippel-Feil syndrome may also be present. Compression of the cerebellum, medulla and other structures in that area causes suboccipital pain, stiffness of the neck and hyperextension of the head and neck. Later, unsteady gait, weakness of the extremities, cerebellar ataxia, nystagmus and involvement of the cranial nerves may occur.

In the *Arnold-Chiari malformation,* the patient may present with dizziness, ataxia, syncope, infantile apnea, gait disturbance and poor coordination. The lower cranial nerves may also be involved. Spastic paraparesis may eventually occur.

SPINAL CORD

Spina bifida occulta, or incomplete closure of the vertebral laminae, is present, most commonly in the lumbosacral region, in about 25 per cent of children. While often asymptomatic, this defect may be found, along with myelodysplasia, in patients with an abnormal gait, urinary incontinence owing to impaired sphincter tone or motor and sensory changes in the lower extremities. Cutaneous lesions that occur along the midline of the back with spina bifida occulta, spinal dysraphism or diastematomyelia include tufts of hair, aplasia cutis, dimples, dermal sinuses, subcutaneous lipomas, pigmented nevi, hemangiomas, bony protrusion and scoliosis.

Occult spinal dysraphism or myelodysplasia represents developmental variants in the most caudal portion of the neural tube. Clinical manifestations include impaired urinary control, fecal incontinence, foot deformities and delay or awkwardness in walking. With a tight filum terminale (tethered cord syndrome), disturbances in gait such as limping and stumbling are common. Weakness and atrophy of muscles and aching pain occur in the lower extremities. Tightness of the hamstrings and the Achilles tendon is present. Urinary incontinence is frequent.

Anderson, F. M.: Occult spinal dysraphism: A series of 73 cases. Pediatrics 55:826, 1975.

The *meningocele* is a spherical, membranous or skin-covered, cystic protrusion along the spinal column, most commonly in the lumbar or lumbosacral area. Nervous tissue is not evident within the protruding sac of a meningocele, and signs of neurologic dysfunction, such as motor weakness or paralysis of the lower extremities, loss of sphincter tone and changes in cutaneous sensation are not seen. An anterior meningocele may be palpable on rectal or vaginal examination as a smooth, resilient pelvic mass. Persistent constipation may begin in infancy.

With a *myelomeningocele*, nervous tissue is involved and neurologic findings are present, including flaccid paralysis, sensory deficits and neurogenic bowel and bladder dysfunction. When fatty tissue accompanies these defects, the terms *lipomeningocele* and *lipomyelomeningocele* are used. The Arnold-Chiari malformation is frequently associated with a myelomeningocele.

Hoffman, H. J., Taecholarn, C., Hendrick, E. B., and Humphreys, R. P.: Management of lipomyelomeningoceles. Experience at The Hospital for Sick Children, Toronto. J. Neurosurg. 62:1, 1985.

The *myelocele* is the most extreme of these defects, with neural tissue directly exposed at the site of the lesion or covered by moist granulation tissue. *Encephaloceles* are meningoceles and myelomeningoceles that occur through bony defects in the skull (cranium bifidum) or at nasal, nasopharyngeal, frontal, parietal or occipital sites. The occipital location is the most common, and lesions there usually contain neural tissue. The Meckel syndrome, an autosomal recessive disorder, consists of an occipital encephalocele, polydactyly and polycystic kidneys, among other defects.

Hayden, P. W.: Adolescents with meningomyelocele. Pediatr. Rev. 6:245, 1985.
Molnar, G. E., and Taft, L. T.: Pediatric rehabilitation. Part II: Spina bifida and limb deficiencies. Curr. Probl. Pediatr. 7:3, 1977.
Shurtleff, D. B.: Myelodysplasia: Management and treatment. Curr. Probl. Pediatr. 3:7, 1980.

Syringomyelia and hydromyelia may accompany other developmental anomalies of the neuroaxis. Clinical manifestations, which are initially unilateral and later bilateral, include numbness of the fingers and weakness of the shoulder girdle, paravertebral, hand and finger muscles, muscle atrophy and thoracic scoliosis.

A congenital dermal sinus is an epithelium-lined tract that extends inward from the skin to the subcutaneous tissues, the meninges or into the spinal cord or brain anywhere along the midline of the scalp or back. An epidermoid or dermoid cyst along the course of the sinus may produce neurologic symptoms owing either to compression or to infection. Bacterial contamination may lead to meningitis or an abscess with *Staphylococcus aureus* as the most likely etiologic agent. The sinus opening, pinpoint or dimple-like and often surrounded by a small pigmented nevus or capillary hemangioma, may best be seen in bright light or through a plus ophthalmoscopic lens. A congenital dermal sinus in the scalp may not be evident unless the head is shaven. Hairs may project from the sinus, and a sebaceous or other discharge may occasionally cause local excoriation of the skin. Localized thickening of the scalp or a palpable subcutaneous mass may be present at the site. A skull roentgenogram demonstrates an underlying osseous defect.

Prompt recognition of an *epidural abscess* is of the utmost importance. The earliest clinical findings are back pain, tenderness on tapping over the spinous processes in the involved area and the patient's unwillingness to lie down. The presence of an accompanying pyogenic skin lesion makes the diagnosis presumptive. Sensory impairment, weakness, and paralysis of the lower extremities are *late* findings.

Spinal Cord Tumors. The early diagnosis of spinal cord tumors in children, especially in infants, is difficult. Intraspinal tumors occur most commonly in the first four years of life. Symptoms are often insidious with pain in the back, neck and extremities; weakness of the extremities, most commonly the lower; a disturbance of gait; urinary dysfunction; alteration of reflexes; and diminution in sensation below the involved level. Unexplained, intermittent or persistent pain in the neck, back, trunk or extremities always suggests an intraspinal tumor. Pain may be precipitated or accentuated by coughing, sneezing, jumping, flexion of the neck or back, straight leg raising or being picked up. The infant with a tumor may be unable to kick one of his lower extremities or move one hand. A history of constipation and urinary retention or incontinence may be elicited. Stiffness or rigidity of the neck and back is frequent owing to paraspinal muscle spasm. Torticollis, scoliosis or kyphosis may occur. Flexion of the back may be so restricted that the child will not bend over to pick up a toy. Instead, he keeps a poker spine and flexes his knees as he squats to retrieve the object. In some instances the onset may be sudden, with weakness of the extremities, stiff neck, fever and an increased number of cells in the cerebrospinal fluid. Roentgenograms should be taken of the *entire* spine when a spinal cord tumor is suspected.

Spinal cord injury at birth is discussed on page 110.

Cervical cord injury may cause quadriplegia.

Torg, J. S., and Das, M.: Trampoline-related quadriplegia: Review of the literature and reflections on the American Academy of Pediatrics' Position Statement. Pediatrics 74:804, 1984.

Transverse myelopathy may be characterized by back or nerve root pain with paresthesia or sensory loss below the level of the lesion. While in some patients paresis of the arms occurs first, in others the process begins in the lower extremities and moves upward. Although flaccid initially, the involved muscles may, in time, become spastic. Urinary and fecal incontinence or retention occasionally develops. Pain and dysesthesia may occur in a band at the level of the disorder. Motor and sensory impairment may demonstrate laterality. Transverse myelitis may be caused by accidental retrograde intra-arterial injection of penicillin. Sudden paraplegia is usually of a vascular etiology. A more gradual onset may be caused by a spinal cord tumor, epidural abscess or hematoma.

Freeman, J. M.: Diagnosis and evaluation of acute paraplegia. Pediatr. Rev. 4:327, 1983.

Neuromyelitis optica is characterized by impairment of vision and neurologic symptoms that may simulate transverse myelopathy or multiple sclerosis.

In *diastematomyelia,* a bony or fibrocartilaginous septum produces a sagittal division and transfixation of the spinal cord or cauda equina. The clinical picture includes delay or difficulty in walking, an abnormal gait, muscle atrophy and weakness, shortening of a lower extremity, absence of tendon reflexes, deformities of the feet and urinary incontinence.

The *caudal regression syndrome* consists of sacral agenesis with associated defects that may include a neurogenic bladder, paralysis of the lower extremities and defects of the feet, especially equinovarus deformities. The baby may lie in a frog-leg position.

Herniation of the lumbar intervertebral disc leads to back pain and sciatica. Findings include a slight scoliosis, decreased lumbar lordosis, paravertebral muscle spasm and a positive straight leg raising sign. Sensory and deep tendon reflex changes are variably present. A history of trauma is frequent.

MENINGITIS

Young infants with meningitis may not demonstrate the nuchal rigidity, extension of the head and neck, opisthotonus and positive Kernig's and Brudzinski's signs characteristically present in older infants and children. A tense or bulging fontanel is an especially important sign. Fever, vomiting and diarrhea may occur, or the infant may be unusually irritable or drowsy. A convulsion may be the initial symptom. Evaluation of hearing should be routinely accomplished on all patients on recovery from meningitis.

Symptoms of meningeal irritation may occur with leptospirosis.

The *Vogt-Koyanangi-Harada (uveomeningoencephalitic) syndrome* is characterized by meningoencephalitis, uveitis, depigmentation, alopecia and dysacousia.

Behçet's disease may cause a meningoencephalitis syndrome with stiff neck and headache or brain stem symptoms such as extraocular nerve palsies, nystagmus, ataxia and extensor toe signs.

Lyme disease may cause signs and symptoms of meningoencephalitis.

Reik, L., Steere, A. C., Bartenhagen, N. H., Shope, R. E., and Malawista, S. E.: Neurologic abnormalities of Lyme disease. Medicine 58:281, 1979.

MENINGISMUS

Infectious diseases such as pneumonia, pyelonephritis, salmonellosis, typhoid fever and bacillary dysentery may be accompanied by headache, nuchal rigidity, opisthotonus, a positive Kernig's sign and convulsions, even though a true meningitis may not be present. Since meningitis cannot be excluded clinically in these instances, a lumbar puncture is necessary. Central nervous system leukemia also causes meningismus.

GENERAL REFERENCES

Bell, W. E., and McCormick, W. F.: Neurologic Infections in Children. Philadelphia, W. B. Saunders Co., 1975.
Menkes, J. H.: Textbook of Child Neurology. 2nd ed. Philadelphia, Lea and Febiger, 1980.
Weiner, H. L., Bresnan, M. J., and Levitt, L. P.: Pediatric Neurology for The House Officer. Baltimore, Williams and Wilkins, 1977.

16 / THE SKELETAL SYSTEM

CONSTITUTIONAL DISEASES OF BONE

The skeletal dysplasias constitute several dozen distinct syndromes with a wide variety of clinical presentations. The International Nomenclature for Constitutional Diseases of Bone classifies these disorders into *osteochondrodysplasias* (abnormalities of cartilage or bone growth and development or both); *dysostoses* (malformation of individual bones, singly or in combination); *idiopathic osteolyses;* and *chromosomal aberrations: primary metabolic abnormalities.* The more common osteochondrodysplasias will be discussed in this section.

McKusick, V. A.: Heritable Disorders of Connective Tissue. 4th ed. St. Louis, The C V Mosby Co., 1972.
International nomenclature of constitutional diseases of bone. Revision–May, 1977. J. Pediatr. 93:614, 1978.
Sillence, D. O., Rimoin, D. L., and Lachman, R.: Neonatal dwarfism. Pediatr. Clin. North Am. 25:453, 1978.
Spranger, J. W., Langer, L. O., and Wiedemann, H-R: Bone Dysplasias: An Atlas of Constitutional Disorders of Skeletal Development. Philadelphia, W. B. Saunders Co., 1974.

OSTEOCHONDRODYSPLASIAS

Short-limb dwarfism may be *rhizomelic,* with shortening of the proximal segment, as in achondroplasia, hypochondroplasia, Langer's type of chondrodysplasia punctata and metaphyseal and spondyloepiphyseal dysplasias; *mesomelic* with shortening of the middle segment, as in mesomelic dysplasias; and *acromelic* as in short-rib polydactyly.

Sivan, Y.: Upper limb standards in newborns. Am. J. Dis. Child. 137:829, 1983.

Achondroplasia is usually diagnosed readily at birth by inspection when the characteristic skeletal features are present. Occasionally, however, the manifestations are incomplete or atypical. In the latter event, roentgenographic examination of the long bones may be helpful. The extremities, especially the thighs and upper arms, are short and wide, and their normal curvatures are exaggerated. The hands, often of the trident type, may not extend below the waist. Usually the patient cannot approximate his fingers when extended, especially the third and fourth. Enlargement of the epiphyses may limit extension at the shoulder, supination of the forearm and abduction of the hip. The head is relatively large, and the forehead and mandible are prominent. The bridge of the nose is depressed, the tip broad and turned up. The vertebral column is relatively normal in length. Lordosis, protrusion of the abdomen and prominent buttocks are additional characteristic features.

In *hypochondroplasia,* only a slight degree of rhizomelic (root of the extremities) dwarfism is present, and understature is not marked.

Metaphyseal chondrodysplasia type McKusick (cartilage-hair hypoplasia) is characterized by short-limbed dwarfism that simulates achondroplasia without the cranial enlargement or depressed nasal bridge. Additional features include ligamentous relaxation in the fingers and hands and sparse, fine, silky, light-colored scalp hair, eyebrows and eyelashes. The hair fractures easily, and the patient may be almost completely bald.

Diastrophic dysplasia is manifested by severe dwarfism with shortening of the limbs more proximally than distally, club feet, ulnar deviation of the hands, short fingers with extension contractures and fusion of proximal interphalangeal joints, hypermobile "hitchhiker" thumbs, scoliosis and, at times, kyphosis. Other manifestations include a tendency to subluxation and dislocation of the joints, limitation of motion of large joints with flexion contraction of knee and hip and cystic-like masses on the ears.

Walker, B. A., Scott, C. I., Hall, J. G., Murdoch, J. L., and McKusick, V.A.: Diastrophic dwarfism. Medicine 51:41, 1972.

Chondrodysplasia punctata (congenital stippled epiphyses) occurs as an autosomal dominant (Conradi's syndrome), a rhizomelic autosomal recessive or Langer's type, and an X-linked form. It is characterized by shortening of the extremities, most pronounced proximally in the rhizomelic type, and by other skeletal anomalies, such as joint contractures, dislocated hips and club feet. Involvement in the dominant form may be limited to one extremity or one side of the body. A flat face, saddle nose, optic atrophy and mental retardation are other findings. Congenital cataracts are frequently present. Failure to thrive may occur in the severe form of the disorder. Roentgenologic examination may reveal multiple punctate calcific deposits in the epiphyses.

Tasker, W. G., Mastri, A. R., and Gold, A. P.: Chondrodystrophia calcificans congenita (Dysplasia epiphysalis punctata). Am. J. Dis. Child. 119:122, 1970.

Chondroectodermal dysplasia (the Ellis-van Creveld syndrome) has features of both chondrodystrophy and ectodermal dysplasia. The extremities are decreased in length, relatively more distally than proximally. Genu valgum is regularly present, as is polydactyly with a sixth digit on the ulnar aspect of each hand. Ectodermal defects include fine, sparse hair; small, deformed nails; defective teeth; and fusion of the upper lip to the underlying gum. Congenital heart disease may be present.

Spondyloepiphyseal dysplasia congenita is characterized by a normal-shaped head, short neck, varus deformity of the feet, barrel-shaped chest, pectus carinatum, cleft palate, genu valgum, deformity of the knees, marked shortening of the spine, exaggerated lumbar lordosis and a waddling gait. Myopia and retinal detachment may also occur. As the child becomes older, the clinical appearance resembles Morquio's disease.

Spranger, J. W., and Langer, L. O., Jr.: Spondyloepiphyseal dysplasia congenita. Radiology 94:313, 1970.

In *pseudoachondroplasia,* sometimes considered a type of spondyloepiphyseal dysplasia and usually not diagnosed until one to two years of age, the extremities are more affected than the spine, the child is generally dwarfed, and mild kyphoscoliosis develops. The head and face are normal.

In *metaphyseal chondrodysplasia,* the joints are enlarged, the upper extremities are shorter than the lower, and the child is severely dwarfed. Marked anterior bowing of the legs may occur, along with a waddling gait.

Multiple epiphyseal dysplasia is characterized by epiphyseal dysgenesis, stubby digits and dwarfism. The patients experience joint pain, stiffness and difficulty in walking. A waddling gait is present if the hip joints are involved.

Enchondromatosis (Ollier's disease) becomes manifest early in life, owing to the presence of enchondromas near the end of the shafts. Usually unilateral in distribution, the lesions may be single or multiple. Minimal involvement may occur on the contralateral side. Shortening of the involved bones results, and facial asymmetry may develop. Rarely, a few cartilaginous exostoses may be present. Occasionally the localization of multiple enchondromata may be confined to the hands and feet, especially the phalanges, causing macrodactyly. *Maffucci's syndrome,* a variant, is characterized by deformities of the hands and feet, hypertrophy and cutaneous cavernous angiomas.

Multiple cartilaginous exostoses is a disorder characterized by single or multiple hard, irregular bony projections that grow from the epiphyseal region of the bone toward the diaphysis. Exostoses usually appear during the preschool age period or later. A familial incidence is present in most cases. The lesions, which are usually bilateral, vary considerably in form. Although most frequent around the knees, exostoses may involve the phalanges, ribs, vertebrae, scapulae and the base of the skull. Occasionally, some shortening in height occurs.

PRIMARY METABOLIC ABNORMALITIES

Hurler's syndrome (mucopolysaccharidosis IH) may first be suspected owing to a dorsolumbar kyphosis in a young infant. A similar kyphosis may occur in patients with fucosidosis, mannosidosis and the mucolipidoses. Other clinical characteristics become evident over a period of time. Physical findings include a large head with a broad, turned-up or pug-shaped nose; coarse facial features; bushy eyebrows; prominent supraorbital ridges; and a short neck. The fingers are held in partial flexion, and the hands are clawlike. The fourth and fifth fingers may be incurved. Both the hands and feet are relatively broad and short. Limitation of motion, chiefly of extension, may be noted at the shoulder, elbow, knee and other joints. Other manifestations include corneal clouding, mental retardation and hepatosplenomegaly.

Morquio's disease (mucopolysaccharidosis IV) usually does not become clinically manifest until the end of the first year of life or later. The head is relatively large, and the base of the nose may be flat and broad. The vertical height of the chest is shortened, and the anteroposterior diameter is elongated. The sternum bulges forward to an almost horizontal position. Thoracic kyphosis is prominent. Shortening of the extremities is not marked. Characteristically, the epiphyses are enlarged, and flexion deformities may be present at the hip and knees. Genu valgum and pes planus also occur. The child stands in a "jump" or crouching posture. Because of this position and the shortening of the trunk, the patient's hands extend to the level of the knees. Cataracts are a later complication.

EXTREMITIES

Amelia refers to a congenital absence of all extremities, *ectromelia* indicates absence of an individual extremity, and *hemimelia* denotes defects of the distal portions of the extremities. *Congenital constriction bands* (Streeter's dysplasia) and constrictions may encircle the digits, feet, hands or other parts of the extremities.

Baker, C. J., and Rudolph, A. J.: Congenital ring constrictions and intrauterine amputations. Am. J. Dis. Child. 121:393, 1971.

Higginbottom, M. C., Jones, K. L., Hall, B. D., and Smith, D. W.: The amniotic band disruption complex: Timing of amniotic rupture and variable spectra of consequent defects. J. Pediatr. 95:544, 1979.

Hemihypertrophy, characterized by enlargement of one half of the body, one or both extremities, parts of the face or other localized overgrowths, may be idiopathic or occur in the following syndromes: Beckwith-Wiedemann, Russell-Silver's, Klippel-Trenaunay-Weber and cutis marmorata telangiectatica congenita. Wilms' tumor, adrenocortical carcinoma and hepatocellular carcinoma may also occur. Neurofibromatosis may be associated with hypertrophy of a body part.

Congenital arteriovenous fistula may cause enlargement of an extremity, along with increased skin temperature, varices, pain and a local bruit.

Reflex neurovascular dystrophy is characterized by swelling, pain and exquisite tenderness in the involved extremities along with vasomotor instability, such as diminished peripheral pulses, perspiration and changes in color and skin temperature.

Patients with *arachnodactyly*, homocystinuria and the mucosal neuroma syndrome have long, thin extremities, hands, feet, fingers and toes.

Infantile cortical hyperostosis (Caffey's syndrome) is characterized by deep, diffuse, firm and, at times, exquisitely tender, nonpitting swelling of the face, especially over the mandible. The swelling is accompanied, at times, by involvement of the clavicles, ribs, scapulae and long bones. A similar clinical picture may occur in infants with *vitamin A poisoning*. Pressure over the long bones causes pain.

Congenital bowing deformities and thickening of the long bones, probably attributable to abnormal intrauterine positioning, may occur along with cutaneous dimpling over the center of the curvatures. Skin dimples may be present over the extremities with hypophosphatasia, over the knees in congenital rubella and on the thighs in the femoral hypoplasia syndrome.

Rickets, owing to familial hypophosphatemic vitamin D resistance, vitamin D dependency, chronic anticonvulsant therapy or inadequate vitamin D in the diet, causes epiphyseal enlargement at the wrists and ankles. Epiphyseal enlargement, angulation and deformity of the extremities along with costochondral beading may occur early with *hypophosphatasia*.

Epiphyseal enlargements also occur in Morquio's syndrome, chondrodystrophy and primary hyperparathyroidism.

Infants with *scurvy* experience severe pain when their extremities are handled, owing to exquisitely tender swellings over the femurs and other long bones. The infant lies in the frog-leg position with the lower extremities flexed at the knees and the hips and thighs abducted and externally rotated.

Osteochondritis owing to *congenital syphilis* may occur during the first three months of life. Physical findings include local swelling and pain on passive motion. The extremity is not moved voluntarily.

The early symptoms of *osteomyelitis* include pain and localized tenderness over the involved bone. Point tenderness, an especially suggestive diagnostic sign, is not always present. Occasionally, the pain and tenderness are diffuse, and actual bone pain is difficult to elicit. Muscle spasm may also be noted. Soft tissue swelling and redness may not be present initially but often develops within a short time. Tenderness on deep palpation between the ischial tuberosity and greater trochanter is an early finding in osteomyelitis of the femoral neck. Osteomyelitis of the pelvic bones may present with fever, abnormal gait, limitation of hip motion and point tenderness. Pain may be referred to the hip, abdomen, buttock or thigh. Swelling may occur in the inguinal region, perineum, labia or over the symphysis pubis. Multicentric osteomyelitis is a chronic disorder associated with the insidious appearance of local pain, swelling or limp. Multiple osteolytic lesions surrounded by sclerosis are evident on roentgenographic examination. Bone scanning is indicated if osteomyelitis is suspected.

Björksten, B., Gustavson, K-H., Eriksson, B., Lindholm, A., and Noroström, S.: Chronic recurrent multifocal osteomyelitis and pustular palmoplantaris. J. Pediatr. 93:227, 1978.

Dich, V. Q., Nelson, J. D., and Haltalin, K. C.: Osteomyelitis in infants and children. Am. J. Dis. Child. 129:1273, 1975.

Edwards, M. S., Baker, C. J., Granberry, W. M., and Barrett, F. F.: Pelvic osteomyelitis in children. Pediatrics 61:62, 1978.

Weissberg, E. D., Smith, A. L., and Smith, D. H.: Clinical features of neonatal osteomyelitis. Pediatrics 53:505, 1974.

Exquisitely painful, tense and slightly warm swellings, erythema and tenderness may occur over one or more long bones with vaso-occlusive bone involvement in patients with *sickle cell anemia*. An early osteomyelitis cannot be immediately excluded.

Keely, K., and Buchanan, G. R.: Acute infarction of long bones in children with sickle cell anemia. J. Pediatr. 101:170, 1982.

Traumatic separation of an epiphysis may occur in the newborn infant, causing tenderness and local swelling. The affected extremity is not used, and manipulation causes the infant to cry. Although the upper humeral epiphysis is most frequently involved, similar separation may occur at the elbow, wrist, knee or ankle. If the upper extremity is involved, the infant can still flex his arm, although this may be painful. This movement is not possible with a brachial plexus injury.

Subluxation of the head of the radius occurs frequently in preschool children, especially between the ages of two and four years. Traction on the extended arm of the child causes the head of the radius to be displaced distally. The child complains of pain, which may be localized in the wrist rather than in the elbow. The extremity is not used but is held, instead, at the side with the elbow slightly flexed and the hand pronated. Passive motion of the elbow joint is possible and is painless in all directions except supination. Limitation of supination is diagnostic. Roentgenographic examination of the elbow joint may rule in or out a fracture or dislocation but not a subluxation.

Subluxation or dislocation of the radial head occurs in the *nail-patella syndrome*. Pseudarthrosis of the radius may be associated with neurofibromatosis.

Madelung's deformity, usually bilateral, may appear in adolescent patients. Radial deviation of the hand occurs, along with dorsal bowing of the ulna and prominence of the ulnar styloid. Dorsiflexion of the wrist is limited. Dyschondrosteosis is the most common cause, but Madelung's deformity may also occur in Turner's syndrome or as a congenital deformity. Curving of the radius may be associated with multiple cartilaginous exostoses.

Cubitus valgus or increased carrying angle of the arm may be present in Turner's syndrome.

FRACTURES

When the humerus or femur is fractured during birth, local tenderness may occur without much swelling, and the infant does not move the extremity. Fractures in infants and young children always raise the possibility of *physical abuse*. With fractures of the extremities, the peripheral pulse and sensation should be carefully assessed. Most fractures in children are accompanied by local pain, swelling, ecchymosis and tenderness. Deformity, crepitation and a point of false motion are not present in greenstick fractures. Fractures through the distal femoral epiphysis without displacement are often overlooked. With fractures about the elbow, especially supracondylar or intercondylar fractures, a Volkmann's ischemic contracture is a possible complication.

Rang, M. C., and Willis, R. B.: Fractures and sprains. Pediatr. Clin. North Am. 24:749, 1977.

Osteogenesis imperfecta is characterized by frequent fractures. Intrauterine fractures account for the deformities present at birth. In osteogenesis imperfecta tarda, fractures do not occur during infancy. Fractures of the long bones are a complication of *hypophosphatasia*. *Fibrous dysplasia* is a diagnostic consideration when a pathologic fracture occurs in a patient with *cafe-au-lait* lesions.

The early findings in *wringer-arm injury* may be deceptively minimal. The injured extremity, which initially appears only mildly swollen or ecchymotic, may within hours become edematous owing to extensive subcutaneous and subfascial extravasation of blood.

HANDS AND FINGERS

During much of the first two months of life, the hands remain closed or fisted. In infants with hemiparetic cerebral palsy, the affected hand remains fisted at four months of age while the other hand is open. A palmar grasp reflex is present. During the third and fourth months both arms may be brought toward the midline, at first somewhat uncertainly, but later with enough coordination to grasp a rattle or other object placed in the midline (raking motions). With further maturation, the infant begins to use the radial aspect of his hand instead of a raking motion to grasp objects. He may then change from a somewhat simultaneous and bilateral approach to a more lateralized one. True handedness is not definitely established until the early preschool period. The development of more advanced prehensile ability with the use of the thumb and index finger occurs at about nine months. A little later, neuromuscular progress permits the infant to release and then to throw objects. The 15-month-old child can do this in the sitting position and a few months later while standing.

The use of the hands may be impaired in children with cerebral palsy. Because of spasticity, the clenched position of the fingers may be retained much longer than normal, and the fingers are not extended to grasp objects. Upper extremity function can be evaluated in an infant suspected to have a hemiparesis by placing a cloth over the baby's face (cover sign) and alternately restraining each extremity while observing the baby's ability to remove the cloth with the contralateral hand.

In *Hurler's syndrome* the hands are broad and short. The fingers are held in a clawlike position with limitation of extension. The fourth and fifth fingers are incurved. Broad hands and stubby fingers occur in Type I GM_1 gangliosidosis.

The whistling face syndrome or craniocarpotarsal dysplasia is characterized by contractures and ulnar deviation of the fingers.

Campodactyly, or flexure contractures of the fingers, may occur on a genetic or sporadic basis.

Goodman, R. M., Katznelson, M. B-M., and Manor, S.: Campodactyly: Occurrence in two new genetic syndromes and its relationship to other syndromes. J. Med. Genet. 9:203, 1972.

Eosinophilic fasciitis is characterized by flexion contractures of the small joints of the hands and feet preceded by arthralgia, swelling, stiffness and tenderness of peripheral joints.

Clinodactyly is the term applied to medial or lateral deviation of a finger.

Marchesani's syndrome is characterized by short, stubby fingers, thick palms and spade-like hands. Understature, spherophakia, severe myopia, glaucoma and ectopia lentis are other clinical features.

The *Aarskog syndrome* is characterized, in part, by brachydactyly with clinodactyly of the fifth fingers.

Patients with *chondrodystrophy* may have trident hands with spaces between the thumb and first finger and between the third and fourth fingers. The hands and feet are short and broad, and the index, middle and fourth fingers are about equal in length.

Clubbing of the fingers occurs most commonly in children with chronic pulmonary disease such as cystic fibrosis, interstitial pneumonia, bronchiectasis, immotile cilia syndrome, empyema and lung abscess; cyanotic congenital heart disease; chronic liver disease; juvenile polyposis; and long-standing gastrointestinal disorders characterized by diarrhea. Rarely, clubbing may be familial. Whereas advanced clubbing is readily evident, assessment of early changes may be difficult. One method for differentiation is the ratio of the distal phalangeal depth (DPD) of the index finger at the base of the nail to the distal interphalangeal joint depth (IPD). If by simple visual estimation from the side of one or both index fingers the DPD exceeds the IPD, the patient has clubbing.

Waring, W. W., Wilkinson, R. W., Wiebe, R. A., Faul, B. C., and Hilman, B. C.: Quantitation of digital clubbing in children. Am. Rev. Respir. Dis. 104:166, 1971.

Short, stubby fingers and toes with a drum-stick appearance and spoon-shaped nails along with short stature, osteopetrosis and bossing of the skull are seen in *pycnodysostosis*. When the distal phalanges are absent, the soft tissues appear telescoped. The fingers in *Pfeiffer's syndrome* may be short with absence or hypoplasia of the middle phalanges.

Infants with *Down's syndrome* have short digits, low-set thumbs, incurved little fingers and often a simian palmar crease.

Small hands and feet may be present in children with the *Prader-Willi* syndrome.

Shortening of the digits, particularly of the thumb and big toe, occurs in many patients with progressive myositis ossificans. The metacarpals are often shortened in patients with pseudohypoparathyroidism; pseudopseudohypoparathyroidism; the Turner's, Larsen's and nevoid basal cell carcinoma syndromes, and in some normal children. As a result, the thumb, the fourth and the fifth fingers also appear shortened. In the presence of a short fourth metacarpal, a dimple is present over the metacarpophalangeal joint (Albright's sign).

Slater, S.: An evaluation of the metacarpal sign (short fourth metacarpal). Pediatrics 46:468, 1970.

Distal hypoplasia of the digits and the nails, more marked on the ulnar aspect of the hands, may occur in the *fetal drug syndromes*. Chondroectodermal dysplasia and cleidocranial dysostosis may also be characterized by hypoplasia of the distal phalanges.

Short distal phalanges also occur in *arteriohepatic dysplasia*.

The "thumb sign," protrusion of the thumb beyond the palm when the hand is fisted, is characteristic of *Marfan's syndrome*.

Snapping or trigger thumb is usually fixed in flexion; however, it may be possible to force the thumb into extension. This maneuver is accompanied by a snapping sensation. Movement is limited by a nodular enlargement of the long flexor tendon of the thumb in the presence of a narrowed tendon sheath. A small swelling may be palpable on the palmar aspect of the metacarpophalangeal joint.

Proximally placed thumbs occur in the trisomy 22 and 10g+ syndromes and along with hypoplasia of the first metacarpal in the diastrophic dwarfism, 18q and Cornelia de Lange's syndromes. *Distally placed thumbs* occur with trisomy 18, partial trisomy 18, orocraniodigital and the Juberg-Hayward syndromes.

Merlob, P., Mimouni, F., Rosen, O., and Reisner, S. H.: Assessment of thumb placement. Pediatrics 74:299, 1984.

One or more extra creases on the fingers occurs in *Larsen's syndrome*. Extremely deep creases on the palms and soles in an infant with skeletal anomalies suggests mosaicism for trisomy 8.

Dactylitis, characterized by a painless, red, firm and spindle-shaped swelling of a digit, may be caused by tuberculosis, syphilis, coccidioidomycosis or sickle cell anemia.

Polydactyly with a sixth digit on the ulnar aspect of each hand occurs in the chondroectodermal dysplasia (Ellis-van Creveld syndrome), short-rib polydactyly dwarfism, and Lawrence-Moon-Biedl, Meckel's and trisomy 13 syndromes.

Syndactylism, fusion or webbing of the toes or fingers, may be an isolated defect or accompany other anomalies, such as premature synostosis of the cranial sutures.

When the three middle fingers are fused, a common nail may be present (mitten hand) as in Apert's syndrome. Syndactyly occurs in the Carpenter's, focal dermal hypoplasia, frontodigital, orofaciodigital, Pfeiffer's, Poland's and the Smith-Lemli-Opitz syndromes.

Macrodactyly, or enlargement of a digit, is usually idiopathic but may occur with neurofibromatosis, Ollier's disease, Mafucci's syndrome and congenital lymphedema. Large hands and feet occur in children with cerebral gigantism.

Arachnodactyly occurs in homocystinuria and the Marfan's, mucosal neuroma and Stickler syndromes. Congenital contractural arachnodactyly is accompanied by scoliosis and crumpled ears.

Anomalies of the hands and radius such as absence or hypoplasia of the thumb and the radius may be associated with cardiac lesions such as an atrial septal defect of the secundum type (Holt-Oram syndrome) or a ventricular septal defect. Fanconi's anemia may be accompanied by hypoplastic, absent or supernumerary thumbs. Radial aplasia may also occur when the thumbs are absent. Thrombocytopenia is present in patients with absence of the radii (TAR syndrome).

Carroll, R. E., and Louis, D.S.: Anomalies associated with radial dysplasia. J. Pediatr. 84:409, 1974.

Smith, A. T., Sack, G. H., Jr., and Taylor, G. J.: Holt-Oram syndrome. J. Pediatr. 95:538, 1979.

Short, broad terminal phalanges of the thumbs and great toes, mental retardation, prominent nose and high arched palate are seen in the *Rubinstein-Taybi syndrome*. Broad toes and thumbs may also occur in Leri's pleonosteosis and in Apert's, Carpenter's, frontodigital, Weaver, Pfeiffer's and Larsen's syndromes.

Marshall, R. E., and Smith, D. W.: Frontodigital syndrome: A dominantly inherited disorder with normal intelligence. J. Pediatr. 77:129, 1970.

Diastrophic dwarfism is characterized by broad, short hands with an ulnar deviation. The interphalangeal joints have contractures. The thumbs have a proximal insertion and are often subluxated in a "hitchhiker" position.

Flexion of the fingers with the index finger overlapping the third finger occurs in patients with *trisomy 18*. Flexion deformity of the fingers and retroflexed thumbs occurs in *trisomy 13*. The presence of a single flexion crease on the fifth finger is an indication for chromosome analysis.

In *symphalangism*, the first and second

phalanges of the fingers are ankylosed with the little finger always affected. If additional digits are involved, preference for those on the ulnar side of the hand occurs. Skin wrinkling over the involved joints is absent. The medial and lateral malleoli are prominent, and the patient may be unable to invert and evert the foot. Conduction deafness may be an associated finding.

Triphalangeal and other anomalies of the thumb may be associated with congenital hypoplastic anemia.

Alter, B. P.: Thumbs and anemia. Pediatrics 62:613, 1978.

Contractures of one or more fingers and variable limitation of active and passive flexion and extension of the metacarpophalangeal joints, wrists, elbows, toes, ankles, knees, hips and spine occur in some children with *diabetes*. Such limited joint mobility may indicate an increased risk for microvascular disease. Affected children may not be able to touch a flat surface with their entire palm or to oppose the palms of each hand tightly with the fingers fanned. The skin over the dorsum of the hand may be thick, tight and waxy.

Rosenbloom, A. L.: Skeletal and joint manifestations of childhood diabetes. Pediatr. Clin. North Am. 31:569, 1984.

Digital neurofibrosarcoma usually presents early in infancy as a nontender, firm, glistening, pea-sized tumor fixed to the overlying skin, most frequently the lateral or dorsal surface of the distal phalanx of a finger or toe. Multiple tumors may be present.

Juvenile aponeurotic fibromas occasionally occur as infiltrative or discrete tumors involving the palms or soles or both.

Acute, painful, warm, nonpitting swelling of the dorsa of the hands, fingers, feet and toes *(hand-foot syndrome)* accompanied by fever and leukocytosis may be the earliest clinical manifestation of sickle-cell disease in infants or young children. A purple-red discoloration and indurative edema of the hands and feet occur in *Kawasaki's disease*.

Damage to the digital epiphyses by *frostbite* may lead to deformity of the fingers.

LOWER EXTREMITIES

Shortening of the lower extremities may be documented by measuring the distance from the anterior superior spine to the lower end of the medial malleolus bilaterally. If muscle atrophy appears to be present, the circumference of each thigh or calf is measured at the same level above and below the patellas.

Shortening of an extremity may occur with a congenitally short femur or tibia, congenital dislocation of the hip, slipped femoral capital epiphysis, coxa plana, poliomyelitis, Ollier's disease and premature arrest of epiphyseal growth owing to infection or trauma. The involved extremity in infants with hemiplegia may be short and underdeveloped, with the changes usually greater in the upper than in the lower extremities.

Femoral hypoplasia, characterized by absence of one third to two thirds of the proximal femur, may occur in infants of diabetic mothers along with an unusual facies. Dimpling may occur over the thigh.

Enlargement of an extremity may be associated with hemangiomas, the Klippel-Trenaunay-Weber syndrome, hemihypertrophy, arteriovenous fistula, neurofibromatosis, lymphangiectasia and stimulation of epiphyseal growth following osteomyelitis or a fracture near an epiphysis.

Tibial Torsion

Internal or medial torsion of the tibia, present in most newborn and young infants, is the most common cause of a pigeon-toed or toeing-in gait. Tibial rotation decreases gradually over the first year after the onset of walking.

Bowing (Genu Varum). The tibias of infants appear to be bowed, and mild bowing is normal up to age two or three. Lateral bowing of the tibias may be caused by rickets or unilateral or bilateral osteochondrosis of the medial tibial condyle (Blount's disease). Early differentiation between marked physiologic bowing and Blount's disease may be difficult.

Congenital pseudarthrosis, characterized by anterior bowing of the lower tibia evident in the newborn period or not until later in infancy, is often associated with neurofibromatosis.

Bilateral or unilateral *anterior bowing of the tibia* may be caused by fetal positioning. Cutaneous dimpling may be present in the center of the curvature. Dimpling and anterior angulation of the leg may be associated with congenital absence of the fibula.

Knock-Knee (Genu Valgum). Just as mild bowing is normal in infants and children before two or three years of age, mild knock knee or genu valgum is common between two and one-half and four years of age. Genu valgum may occur with rickets, hypophosphatasia, Morquio's disease, Hurler's syndrome and pes valgus.

FEET

Congenital clubfoot or talipes equinovarus is characterized by adduction of the forefoot, inversion of the hindfoot and an equinus position (plantar flexion) of the heel. Muscular resistance and pain result when an attempt is made to correct this fixed deformity. Full dorsiflexion of the foot is possible with metatarsus varus but not with a true clubfoot. Many newborn infants hold their feet in a somewhat inverted position, but this position can be readily overcorrected. With a clubfoot, the space between the navicular tubercle and the medial malleolus is much diminished, and the two bony landmarks may be in complete apposition. Normally, the little finger may be placed in this space.

Clubfoot may be a manifestation of arthrogryposis, caudal regression syndrome, cerebral palsy, craniocarpotarsal dysplasia, diastrophic dwarfism, Larsen's syndrome, meningomyelocele, the peroneal type of progressive muscular atrophy or spinal cord tumor.

Metatarsus varus, characterized by adduction and inversion of the forefoot and often caused by an abnormal intrauterine position, differs from a clubfoot in the absence of an equinus deformity and in the ability to dorsiflex the foot fully. The position of the heel may be neutral, varus or valgus. If the hindfoot is held in a fixed position, the forefoot cannot be brought to the midline by manipulation. If inversion is absent, the term *metatarsus adductus* applies. Metatarsus adductus may be flexible or rigid.

Metatarsus varus is to be differentiated from the common medial tibial torsion that occurs in young children and accounts for a pigeon-toe or toeing-in gait. Children with marked toeing-in may stumble over their feet when walking rapidly or running. Differentiation can readily be made by placing the child supine so that the patellas point straight up. In patients with metatarsus varus, the forefoot is held in adduction, and the hindfoot is straight in line with the patella. With tibial rotation, both the forefoot and the hindfoot are held in the pigeon-toe position and not in line with the patella.

In-toeing may also be caused by increased femoral anteversion. Patients with anteversion turn their knees in when walking and tend to sit with their legs under them in a "W" rather than in a tailor, cross-legged or "M" position. Pronated feet are a common cause of toeing-in gait.

Internal rotation may be measured by having the child lie prone with his knees flexed and the pelvis held level. The legs are allowed to fall laterally into full internal rotation by gravity. Normally, the angle they assume from the vertical (the angle of internal rotation) will be less than 70 degrees. When the angle is greater than this, increased femoral anteversion is usually present to a mild degree (between 70 and 80 degrees) and severe (over 85 degrees). With the child in the supine position and the hips and knees extended, the femur can be rotated internally (the log roll test) up to 90 degrees but externally rotated less than the normal 40 to 50 degrees.

Staheli, L. T.: Torsional deformity. Pediatr. Clin. North Am. 24:799, 1977.

Infants and young children may walk with the forefoot in abduction or toeing out owing to femoral retroversion or external tibial torsion.

Talipes calcaneovalgus is characterized by eversion, abduction and dorsiflexion of the foot. The heel is the most dependent portion of the foot, and the dorsum may lie against the anterolateral aspect of the tibia. Usually the soft tissues on the lateral aspect of the foot are tight. This position is easily corrected by passive manipulation. A small depression may be present just anterior to the lateral malleolus. Equinovalgus also occurs in Larsen's syndrome.

The foot can be acutely dorsiflexed in many normal infants because of a congenitally long Achilles tendon.

An *equinus position* of the foot may develop with spastic cerebral palsy. Heel cord shortening is also a relatively early finding in pseudohypertrophic muscular dystrophy. Tightness of the Achilles tendon may be evaluated by slightly inverting the foot to lock the heel before the foot is dorsiflexed. If the foot cannot be flexed more than 30 degrees, the heel cord is tight.

Pes cavus, or high longitudinal arch, may be congenital or develop with Friedreich's ataxia, spina bifida, a cauda equina lesion, metatarsus varus, diastematomyelia, peroneal muscular atrophy and Hurler's syndrome.

Pes planus, or *flat feet,* are normal during infancy. Because of the fat pad present in the arch of the infant foot, the longitudinal arch does not become apparent until about the third year. Flat feet are often accompanied by pronation or eversion of the forefoot and, at times, by a hallux valgus. The medial malleolus is prominent with pronated feet, and an unusual amount of wear occurs on the medial surface of the heel. Flat or pronated feet are frequently hereditary or occur along with knock knees in children who have generalized ligamentous relaxation.

Congenital "rocker bottom" foot or *congenital vertical talus* causes a severe, rigid flat foot with a boat-shaped deformity of the sole. The talus and calcaneus are in equinus. The heel points downward and the forefoot is dorsiflexed on the hindfoot and abducted. Rocker bottom feet occur with trisomy 18.

Tarsal coalition with a bony bridge between two of the bones causes peroneal muscle spasm and a rigid, spastic foot that may become painful early in adolescence. Multiple sprains may occur with sports activities. On inversion of the foot, pain occurs in the region of the peroneal tendons on the lateral aspect, accounting for the synonym *peroneal spastic flatfoot.*

An *accessory navicular bone* may cause pain, swelling and a palpable protrusion on the medial aspect of the foot just dorsal to the arch.

Ehrlich, M. G.: Foot disorders in infants and children. Curr. Probl. Pediatr. 4:3, 1974.

Osteochondrosis of the tarsal navicular (Köhler's disease), most common between three and six years of age, may also appear later. Localized tenderness, redness, swelling and, occasionally, pain occur over the tarsal navicular bone on the medial side of the foot. Pain and limping may be accentuated by walking and jumping.

Osteochondrosis of the *head of the second metatarsal*, which usually appears during adolescence, is characterized by local pain and, at times, redness, swelling and a slight limp.

Achilles tendinitis, usually unilateral, is characterized by swelling, tenderness and, perhaps, pain over the insertion of the Achilles tendon, especially after running and jumping. Limping may occur. Achilles tendinitis and tenosynovitis, occurring in episodes of two or three days' duration, may be an early manifestation of familial Type II hyperlipoproteinemia. Achilles tendinitis or heel pain with plantar fasciitis may be a rheumatoid variant.

Shapiro, J. R., Fallat, R. W., Tsang, R. C., and Glueck, C. J.: Achilles tendinitis and tenosynovitis. Am. J. Dis. Child. 128:486, 1974.

Apophysitis of the os calcis (Sever's disease), which occurs in adolescents, is characterized by swelling and tenderness on pressure over the apophysis of the os calcis. The heel cord may also be tight. Involvement is usually bilateral.

Calluses or corns are produced by thickening of the skin in areas subjected to abnormal pressure as a result of improperly fitting shoes or foot abnormalities. Plantar warts also occur in children.

Staheli, L. T., and Griffin, L.: Corrective shoes for children: A survey of current practice. Pediatrics 65:13, 1980.

Morton's neuroma causes pain between the third and fourth toes when the metacarpal heads are squeezed together.

TOES

Polydactylism is characterized by accessory toes and fingers.

Syndactylism represents fusion or webbing of the toes or fingers.

Macrodactyly, or enlargement of a digit, is usually idiopathic.

Varus toe occurs when one of the toes lies above or below the adjoining medial toe. A *hammer toe,* one held in a position of flexion, may be congenital, occur with trisomy 18 or develop with acquired pes cavus. In patients with *Friedreich's ataxia*, the proximal phalanx of the large toe is dorsiflexed while the distal phalanx is plantar flexed.

Hallux varus, or medial deviation of the large toe, is common in infants. In *hallux valgus*, the large toe points laterally. The majority of children with *myositis ossificans progressiva* demonstrate hallux valgus with the large toes held underneath the second toes. Both the large toes and the thumbs may also be abnormally short.

In *Pfeiffer's syndrome*, the middle phalanges of all toes are absent.

In newborn infants, the large toenails may appear to be ingrown, and the ends of the toenails are often slightly elevated from the nail beds. In infants with Down's syndrome, the cleft between the first and second toes is wider than normal and may extend backward as a shallow crease.

Marked swelling, redness and edema of a distal portion of a toe or finger may be caused by constriction by a hair or a fine thread from a garment.

Narkewitz, R. M.: Distal digital occlusion. Pediatrics 61:922, 1978.

GAIT

Many variations occur in the gait of children who are beginning to walk. A change in gait, especially a report of ataxia, staggering, or walking into door frames requires careful evaluation. Gait is best evaluated by having the child walk up and down a well-lighted corridor for about 20 feet or so when he does not know he is being observed.

A *change in gait* may have serious implications. In a young child it may be an early manifestation of a cerebellar or a spinal cord tumor. In a dwarf, one needs to evaluate compression of the cord or of the base of the brain. Dislocation secondary to atlantoaxial stability in children with Down's syndrome and other disorders may cause deterioration of and fatigue in walking. With a young child who refuses to stand or walk, the possibility of discitis should be considered. For a discussion of discitis, see page 150.

An *atalgic gait,* owing to a painful extremity, is characterized by a short stance phase, the time that the extremity bears the body weight. An occult *stress fracture* is a common cause of a disturbed gait and refusal to walk in young children. A hairline fracture of the tibia in preschool children may require scintigraphy for early identification.

Singer, J., and Towbin, R.: Occult fractures in the production of gait disturbance in childhood. Pediatrics 64:192, 1979.

A *waddling gait* may be seen with:
Exstrophy of the bladder owing to separation of the pelvic bones
Bilateral dislocation of the hips
Pseudohypertrophic muscular dystrophy
Polymyositis
Bilateral slipped epiphysis
Bilateral coxa vara
Achondroplasia
Morquio's disease
Engelmann's disease (progressive diaphyseal dysplasia)
Myelodysplasia

Toe-walking or an *equinus gait* may occur with spastic cerebral palsy, pseudohypertrophic muscular dystrophy or other disorders characterized by shortening of the Achilles tendon. *"Toe walking,"* a normal phase in some children, is also observed with autism.

A *scissors gait* may occur with spastic cerebral palsy and in slipped femoral epiphysis.

The *hemiplegic gait* is characterized by abduction and internal rotation of the thigh, flexion of the hip and knee, and walking on the toes with the heel not touching the floor. In the upper extremity, the elbow is flexed and the shoulder abducted. The abnormality of the gait is accentuated when the child runs or walks fast.

The *steppage gait* seen in patients with foot drop is characterized by the involved foot being raised higher than the contralateral one so that the toes clear the floor.

Chronically ill children may have a *shuffling gait*. A similar gait may occur in dermatomyositis. Patients with tetralogy of Fallot characterisically *squat* to rest for a few minutes after they have walked a short distance. Unusual types of gait may be seen with *conversion disorder*.

Dubowitz, V., and Hersov, L.: Management of children with non-organic (hysterical) disorders of motor function. Dev. Med. Child Neurol. 18:358, 1976.

An *ataxic* gait is characterized by walking in a wide-based, staggering, unsteady fashion. The causes of ataxia are presented on page 119.

An in-toeing gait may be associated with metatarsus varus, tibial torsion, femoral neck anteversion or pronated feet.

Singer, J.: Evaluation of acute and insidious gait disturbance in children. Adv. Pediatr. 26:209, 1979.

THE ETIOLOGIC CLASSIFICATION OF LIMP

I. TRAUMA is the most frequent cause of limp in young children.

A. Sprains
B. Fractures, especially the greenstick variety, involving the lower extremities. Stress fractures and traumatic hairline fractures of the tibia (toddler's fracture) are often missed on radiographic examination until a callus or subperiosteal new bone forms; however, a bone scan is diagnostically helpful early.
C. Traumatic periostitis. Because the periosteum in young children is not firmly attached to the underlying bone, minor trauma to the tibia or femur may result in subperiosteal hemorrhage with local tenderness and, at times, fullness, along with limp or refusal to walk. Symptoms may persist for several days. When the child is first seen, roentgenograms are negative, but subperiosteal ossification is often evident a week or two later.
D. Contusions

E. Splinter or other foreign body in the foot, stone bruises, improperly fitted shoes
F. Fracture of long bones in patients with idiopathic juvenile osteoporosis or osteogenesis imperfecta tarda

II. OSTEOCHONDROSES. Along with local tenderness, pain and, perhaps, swelling, patients with an osteochondrosis may limp.

A. Osteochondrosis of the tarsal navicular (Köhler's disease)
B. Osteochondrosis of the head of the second metatarsal
C. Osteochondrosis of the patella
D. Osteochondrosis of the tibial tubercle
E. Osteochondrosis of the femoral capital epiphysis
F. Calcaneal apophysitis
G. Osteochondritis dissecans
H. Avascular necrosis of bone occurs in systemic lupus erythematosus.

Bergstein, J. M., Wiens, C., Fish, A. J., Vernier, R. L., and Michael, A.: Avascular necrosis of bone in systemic lupus erythematosus. J. Pediatr. 85:31, 1974.

III. JOINT DISEASES

A. Arthritis (See page 141.)
B. Diseases of the hip
1. Congenital dislocation of the hip
2. Osteochondrosis of the femoral capital epiphysis (coxa plana, Legg-Calvé-Perthes disease) occurs between four and ten years of age. The onset is insidious with an almost imperceptible limp. A bone scan may be diagnostically helpful.
3. Slipped femoral epiphysis. Pain in the knee or along the medial aspect of the thigh above the knee is the *earliest* sign of a slipped epiphysis. Limp does not develop until later.
4. Coxa vara. With a congenital coxa vara, a painless limp is noted shortly after the child has begun to walk. With an acquired coxa vara, the time of appearance of limp depends on the primary etiology.
5. Otto's pelvis, in which an abnormally deep acetabulum is present, becomes symptomatic during adolescence. Symptoms include limp and complaint of pain in the inguinal region or medial aspect of the knee. Motion of the hip joint, especially rotation and abduction, is limited.
6. Transient synovitis of the hip joint ("observation hip"). The presenting complaints in this common condition are mild or severe pain or limp or both. Patients are usually under ten years of age. The onset may be acute or insidious. Pain is present in the region of the hip or referred to the thigh or knee. Low-grade fever may occur. Motion at the hip is limited, and the lower extremity is held in flexion, external rotation and adduction. Internal rotation and abduction are restricted. Symptoms persist from a few days to several weeks. Differential diagnosis includes septic arthritis, Legg-Calvé-Perthes disease, osteomyelitis of the femur, tuberculosis, osteoid osteoma, slipped femoral capital epiphysis and rheumatoid arthritis.

Jacobs, B. W.: Synovitis of the hip in children and its significance. Pediatrics 47:558, 1971.

7. Hemarthrosis
C. Pyogenic arthritis of the sacroiliac joint

IV. TUMORS AND NEOPLASTIC DISEASE

A. Leukemia. A limp is often an early finding.
B. Metastases from neuroblastoma
C. Ewing's tumor
D. Osteogenic sarcoma

V. OTHER ORTHOPEDIC DISORDERS

A. Leg length discrepancies
B. Osteomyelitis, including pelvic osteomyelitis. Chronic, recurrent multicentric osteomyelitis affecting the distal metaphyses of long bones may present with a unilateral limp.
C. Progressive diaphyseal dysplasia
D. Calcaneal bursitis
E. Cerebral palsy
F. Vertebral disorders
G. Infections of the intervertebral disc; discitis
H. Herniated intervertebral disc
I. Osteoid osteoma. The neck of the femur is a common site.

VI. NEUROLOGIC DISORDERS

A. Tight filum terminale
B. Spinal cord tumor
C. Muscle weakness or paralysis

VII. MUSCLE

A. Muscular dystrophy
B. Polymyositis

VIII. Miscellaneous

A. An anal fissure may rarely cause a child to limp.
B. Iliac adenitis
C. Appendicitis with irritation of the psoas muscle
D. Conversion disorder

JOINTS

Term newborn infants lie with their elbows, hips and knees in partial flexion. Generally some resistance to passive movement of the joints is present, and full extension of the elbows, hips and knees may not be possible.

Joint disease may be manifested by swelling, redness, heat, pain and limitation of motion. For detection of excessive fluid in the knee joint, the fluid is expressed from the capsular reflections into the main joint space by placing the examiner's palms above and below the knee and pushing downward and upward respectively. With the joint so compressed, depression of the patella by one index finger followed by rebound indicates the presence of excessive fluid. The examiner may also place his index fingers opposite each other just beyond the edge of the patella. In the presence of joint effusion, downward pressure by one finger lifts the other as a result of transmitted pressure.

Brewer, E. J., Jr., and Gedalia, A.: The child with joint pain: An algorithmic approach. Cont. Pediatr. 2:18, 1985.

Etiologic Classification of Arthritis, Arthralgia and Joint Swelling

I. Infectious Arthritis

A. Pyogenic or septic arthritis may be caused by the *Staphylococcus aureus,* hemolytic *Streptococcus, Pneumococcus, Meningococcus, Haemophilus influenzae,* Brucella organisms, *Escherichia coli, Shigella* and *Salmonella.* All suspicious joints should be tapped and the synovial fluid cultured.

Pyogenic arthritis usually involves one of the larger joints. Systemic symptoms such as fever, chills, irritability and malaise may be prominent, or the complaints may be mainly confined to the joint. Pain and exquisite local tenderness are early findings followed by redness, swelling, protective muscle spasm and limitation of motion. Both active and passive motion of the joint is extremely painful. Inflammatory changes in peripheral joints are more apparent than with the shoulder and hip. Suppurative arthritis of the hip is frequently overlooked in infants, since early recognition is often difficult. Diagnostic needle puncture of the hip joint may be indicated in the presence of swelling of the upper part of the thigh in young infants. Flexion contracture and limitation of abduction of the hip are other suggestive signs. Pyogenic arthritis of the hip may be followed by dislocation. Osteomyelitis presents with many of the same signs and symptoms as does septic arthritis, but joint motion in the former is moderately good and less painful.

Pyogenic arthritis of the sacroiliac joint, an infection occurring in school-age children, is characterized by pain referred to the buttock and evoked by stressing the sacroiliac joint, marked tenderness over the joint and on rectal examination, and limp.

Nelson, J. D.: The bacterial etiology and antibiotic management of septic arthritis in infants and children. Pediatrics 50:437, 1972.
Rotbart, H. A., and Glode, M. P.: *Haemophilus influenzae* type b septic arthritis in children: Report of 23 cases. Pediatrics 75:254, 1985.
Schaad, U. B.: Pyogenic arthritis of the sacroiliac joint in pediatric patients. Pediatrics 66:375, 1980.

B. Transient synovitis of multiple joints may occur early in meningococcemia with pain and, perhaps, tenderness and redness. Monoarticular, usually sterile, arthritis may appear late in the first week of the illness. Brucellosis may cause arthralgia and, rarely, inflammatory changes, most commonly involving the hip joint.
C. Gonococcal arthritis may be characterized by migratory polyarthritis that may simulate acute rheumatic fever. An acute monoarticular arthritis, tenosynovitis of the flexor tendons of the hands and characteristic skin lesions may also occur.
D. Arthritis may be associated with mycoplasma and many viral infections such as rubella, hepatitis B, mumps, chickenpox, adenovirus, coxsackie B, Epstein-Barr and herpes.
E. Reactive arthritis may occur 10 to 14 days after an episode of salmonella diar-

rhea. The involvement is frequently migratory, polyarticular and distal, affecting the interphalangeal joints. Similar reactions may occur after *Yersinia* and *Shigella* intestinal infections.

Jacobs, J. C.: *Yersinia entercolitica* arthritis. Pediatrics 55:236, 1975.
Levine, J., Honig, P. J. and Boyle, T.: *Salmonella* reactive arthritis: Clues to diagnosis. J. Pediatr. 94:596, 1979.

F. Acute, painful, migratory polyarthritis may occur with rat-bite fever or Haverhill fever. Fever and a maculopapular or petechial rash may occur on the palms and soles.

Raffin, B. J., and Freemark, M.: Streptobacillary rat-bite fever: A pediatric problem. Pediatrics 64:214, 1979.

G. Toxic arthritis characterized by pain, redness and swelling, usually of a single joint, may occur with pharyngitis, scarlet fever and other acute infections, especially those caused by *Streptococcus.* Arthralgia of one or more joints occurs with toxic shock syndrome

H. Lyme arthritis occurs chiefly in the summer or early fall in patients who live in wooded areas. Joint swelling suddenly appears, usually involving the knee, elbow or wrist. Musculoskeletal pain is characterized by generalized achiness and stiffness of muscles and joints, severe back and leg cramps or migratory arthralgias. Myalgias and pain in tendons and bursae may also occur along with stiffness of the hands and digital joints. Fever, malaise, weakness and fatigue are other symptoms. Recurrences of the arthritis, each episode lasting a week to months, are followed by remissions, usually of several months duration. A characteristic rash, which progresses from a papular lesion to a large ring with a clearing center, may precede the onset of arthritis.

Doughty, R. A.: Lyme disease. Pediatr. Rev. 6:20, 1984.

I. Tuberculous arthritis is usually monarticular with swelling and a thickened, doughy consistency of the periarticular tissues. Effusion and inflammatory changes usually do not develop although some warmth and redness may be present early. Joint pain is not prominent at this time. Spasm of the adjacent muscles may be severe, and muscle atrophy rapidly develops. A negative tuberculin test almost completely excludes tuberculosis as an etiologic possibility.

J. Penetration of a joint, usually the knee, by a thorn (blackthorn, date palm, cactus, rosebush or sea urchin spine) may cause synovitis or pyogenic arthritis.

II. COLLAGEN-VASCULAR AND CONNECTIVE TISSUE DISEASES

A. Rheumatic fever may be characterized by an acute migratory arthralgia, usually of larger joints such as the ankles, knees, hips, wrists, elbows and shoulders. Involved joints may be swollen, tender, red, hot and painful. The joint is usually symptomatic for two or three days, and then the migratory arthritis moves on to other joints. The inflammatory arthropathy usually resolves within one week without residuae. Similar arthropathy may occur with leukemia, inflammatory bowel disease, gonorrhea and meningococcal infections.

B. Lupus erythematosus may be characterized by migratory, transient joint involvement with arthralgia; pain on motion; redness; swelling; and stiffness. These manifestations may simulate those of rheumatic fever or early rheumatoid arthritis.

C. Serum sickness may be characterized by joint redness, swelling, pain, stiffness and considerable effusion. Arthralgia may be part of a serum sickness–like syndrome caused by penicillin sensitivity.

D. Juvenile rheumatoid arthritis usually begins during the preschool years but may occur at any age. Juvenile rheumatoid arthritis has three chief modes of onset: (1) systemic with high, spiking fever, pericarditis, pleuritis, leukemoid reaction, evanescent rash, abdominal pain, hepatosplenomegaly and, possibly, marked generalized lymphadenopathy with concurrent or later appearance of arthritis; (2) polyarticular (rheumatoid factor seronegative or seropositive) with involvement of five or more joints; and (3) pauciarticular (early onset, ANA positive or late onset, HLA-B27) with four or fewer joints. The chronic arthritis of juvenile rheumatoid arthritis is characterized by swelling and restriction of motion which persists for at least six weeks, along with pain, warmth, erythema or tenderness. Some children with juvenile rheumatoid arthritis do not complain of pain. Arthralgia is defined as joint pain without objective physical findings.

The onset of juvenile rheumatoid arthritis is frequently insidious with the gradual onset of pain and swelling of the knee or ankle and a limp. The involved joints may be slightly warm, and passive motion is often painful and limited. Systemic symptoms such as easy fatigability, morning stiffness, anorexia and poor growth progress may be present, or the clinical manifestations may be confined to the joints. Fever, low-grade or spiking, persistent or intermittent, may be the earliest symptom. *Rheumatoid arthritis is to be considered a definite possibility in children with spiking fever of undetermined origin.* The fever, at times accompanied by chills, may be over 105°F (40.5°C) and persist for weeks. It is quotidian in type with wide swings from hyperpyrexia to a normal or subnormal temperature once or twice a day. In other patients the onset of joint involvement is acute with transient, migratory polyarthritis and fever. The differentiation between rheumatoid arthritis and rheumatic fever may be difficult in some instances.

In children, the knees, ankles or elbows are commonly first involved with other joints, including those of the hands and feet, affected later. The vertebral column usually remains normal, except for the cervical spine, in patients who develop ankylosing spondylitis.

Muscle atrophy, especially about the joints, may be severe. The combination of joint effusion and muscle atrophy causes the fusiform swelling often evident in spindle-shaped proximal and distal interphalangeal joints. The overlying skin may be red, shiny, smooth and atrophic.

Other manifestations of rheumatoid arthritis include a transient, usually nonpruritic, erythematous or salmon-pink, macular or maculopapular skin rash chiefly on the trunk, face, neck and inner aspects of the extremities, especially during febrile periods. Hepatomegaly and splenomegaly may occur in a few patients. Children with early childhood onset of pauciarticular arthritis have up to a 50 per cent chance of developing iridocyclitis whether or not the rheumatoid process is active. With school age or adolescent-onset pauciarticular arthritis, involvement of the sacroiliac joints, lumbar and thoracic vertebrae and pain in the lower back, hips or thighs occur. Initially, symptoms may be mild and intermittent. Acute iridocyclitis may be a complication.

Ansell, B. M.: Rheumatic Disorders of Childhood. London, Butterworth and Co., Ltd., 1980.
Schaller, J. G.: Juvenile rheumatoid arthritis. Pediatr. Rev. 2:163, 1980.

E. Patients with dermatomyositis may have joint involvement suggestive of rheumatoid arthritis. *Mixed connective tissue disease* has features of systemic lupus erythematosus, scleroderma and polymyositis. Polyarthritis and Raynaud's phenomenon are commonly present at the onset.

Singsen, B. H., Bernstein, B. H., Kornreich, H. K., King, K. K., Hanson, V., and Tan, E. M.: Mixed connective tissue disease in childhood. J. Pediatr. 90:893, 1977.

III. MISCELLANEOUS CAUSES OF ARTHRITIS AND ARTHRALGIA

A. Arthritis-like symptoms and signs may precede by months other manifestations of leukemia and neuroblastoma. Interphalangeal as well as larger joints may be exquisitely painful, warm and swollen. Migratory joint involvement may occur.

Fink, C. W., Windmiller, J., and Sartain, P.: Arthritis as the presenting feature of childhood leukemia. Arthritis Rheumatism. 15:347, 1972.
Schaller, J.: Arthritis as a presenting manifestation of malignancy in children. J. Pediatr. 81:793, 1972.

B. Some immunodeficient patients develop a polyarthritis that is indistinguishable from rheumatoid arthritis.

McLaughlin, J. F., Schaller, J., and Wedgewood, R. J.: Arthritis and immunodeficiency. J. Pediatr. 81:801, 1972.

C. Disseminated lipogranulomatosis, or Farber's disease, simulates rheumatoid arthritis to some extent. Painful joint enlargement in infants is followed by joint fixation. Subcutaneous and periarticular nodules are also present along with hepatomegaly, lymphadenopathy and hoarseness.

D. Acute, severe pain, swelling, and warmth of one or several large or small joints may occur with sickle cell disease.

Espinoza, L. R., Spilberg, I. and Osterland, C. K.: Joint manifestations of sickle cell disease. Medicine 53:295, 1974.

E. Reiter's syndrome is characterized by arthritis, conjunctivitis and urethritis.

Rosenberg, A. M., and Petty, R. E.: Reiter's disease in children. Am. J. Dis. Child. 133:394, 1979.

F. Gouty arthritis is rare in infants and children.

Yarom, A., Rennebohm, R. M., Strife, F. and Levinson, J. E.: Juvenile gouty arthritis. Am. J. Dis. Child. 138:955, 1984.

G. Psoriasis is a rare cause of arthritis in children with primary involvement of the distal interphalangeal joints. Symptoms may simulate those of seronegative juvenile rheumatoid arthritis.

Shore, A., and Ansell, B. M.: Juvenile psoriatic arthritis—an analysis of 60 cases. J. Pediatr. 100:529, 1982.

Sills, E. M.: Psoriatic arthritis in childhood. Johns Hopkins Med. J. 146:49, 1980.

H. Familial osteolysis of the carpal and tarsal bones begins at about five years of age with symptoms of an acute arthritis of the wrists and ankles. Slow, progressive and painless dissolution of the carpal and tarsal bones then occurs.

Gluck, J.: Familial osteolysis of the carpal and tarsal bones. J. Pediatr. 81:506, 1972.

I. Intermittent hydarthrosis or recurrent effusion of the knees occasionally occurs in adolescent girls.

J. Schönlein-Henoch purpura may be characterized, in part, by joint swelling, usually of the ankle or knee, with redness, tenderness, pain, swelling and heat. Multiple joints may be involved in a migratory fashion. The joint symptoms may be the initial manifestation.

K. Pigmented villonodular synovitis may cause intermittent pain and swelling, usually of the knee, in older children and young adults after minimal trauma or activity. Synovial fluid is dark brown or serosanguineous.

L. Arthritis may occur with periodic neutropenia and in familial Mediterranean fever. The involvement is usually initially monoarticular, but then other joints, including the sacroiliac, become involved.

Lehman, T. J. A., Hanson, V., Kornreich, H., Peters, R. S., and Schwabe, A. D.: HLA-B27-negative sacroiliitis: A manifestation of familial Mediterranean fever in childhood. Pediatrics 61:423, 1978.

M. Sarcoid arthritis is characterized by extensive joint swelling, effusion and boggy synovial thickening of joints and tendon sheaths. The fingers, wrists, ankles, knees, elbows and spine are involved. Little or no pain or limitation of motion occurs.

North, A. F., Jr., et al.: Sarcoid arthritis in children. Am. J. Med. 48:449, 1970.

N. Behçet's disease may be associated with synovitis, arthritis or arthralgia affecting the larger joints along with mouth ulcers and erythema nodosum.

O. Chronic active hepatitis may be accompanied by arthralgia or arthritis of a single or multiple large joints.

P. Inflammatory bowel disease may be preceded or accompanied by arthralgia and arthritis involving large joints or the spine in a manner that resembles ankylosing spondylitis.

Haslock, I., and Wright, V.: The musculoskeletal complications of Crohn's disease. Medicine 52:217, 1973.

Lindsley, C. B., and Schaller, J. G.: Arthritis associated with inflammatory bowel disease in children. J. Pediatr. 84:16, 1974.

Q. Stickler syndrome may be suspected at birth on the basis of bony enlargement of ankles, knees and wrists and hyperextensibility of the knees, elbows and fingers. Some infants have manifestations characteristic of the Pierre Robin syndrome or spondyloepiphyseal dysplasia. Progressive myopia may be followed by retinal detachment or cataracts.

R. The hypermobility syndrome may be characterized by pain, swelling of multiple joints and joint crepitus.

S. Episodic arthritis may occur with cystic fibrosis.

Newman, A. J., and Ansell, B. M.: Episodic arthritis in children with cystic fibrosis. J. Pediatr. 94:594, 1979.

T. Arthralgia is an occasional complaint in adolescents with hypothyroidism.

U. Arthralgia is a common psychogenic complaint.

V. Juvenile episodic arthritis/arthralgia is a benign disorder characterized by recurrent episodes in which the affected joint, abruptly extremely painful or tender, is held in flexion. Swelling may or may not be present. Laboratory and roentgen examinations are normal. The episodes last from a few hours to several weeks.

W. Arthralgia and arthritis occur late in the acute or subacute stage of Kawasaki syndrome.

X. Spondyloarthritis is a designation that may be applied to a number of syndromes that share common clinical manifestations. These disorders include ankylosing spondylitis, Reiter's syndrome, familial Mediterranean fever, reactive arthritis associated with *Salmonella, Shigella* or *Yersinia* dysentery, psoriasis and inflammatory bowel disease as well as rheumatoid arthritis.

Jacobs, J. C., Berdon, W. E., and Johnston, A. D.: HLA-B27-associated spondyloarthritis and enthesopathy in childhood: Clinical, pathologic, and radiographic observations in 58 patients. J. Pediatr. 100:521, 1982.

Y. Eosinophilic fasciitis presents with arthralgia, swelling and tenderness of the metacarpophalangeal joints, stiff hands, flexion contraction of the fingers and thickened skin over the extremities.

Brewer, E. J., Giannini, E. H., and Person, D. A.: Juvenile Rheumatoid Arthritis. 2nd ed. Philadelphia, W. B. Saunders Co., 1982, pp 81-82.
Patrone, N. A. and Kredick, D. W.: Eosinophilic fasciitis in a child. Am. J. Dis. Child. 138:363, 1984.

IV. TRAUMATIC ARTHRITIS

A. Sprain
B. Hemarthrosis is common with hemophilia, intra-articular fracture, patellar dislocation or tear of the arterior cruciate ligament.
C. Acute traumatic synovitis after an acute knee injury is characterized by distention of the joint capsule, discomfort and restriction of motion. The distention is usually delayed until six hours after the injury.
D. "Little League elbow" in young baseball pitchers may be characterized by pain, tenderness and swelling over the involved medial epicondyle.

Collins, H. R., and Evarts, C. M.: Injuries to the adolescent athlete. Postgrad. Med. 49:72, 1971.
Harvey, J.: Ankle injuries in children and adolescents. Pediatr. Rev. 2:217, 1981.
Schaller, J. G.: Arthritis and infections of bones and joints in children. Pediatr. Clin. N. Amer. 24:775, 1977.
Torg, J. S., Pollack, H. and Swelterlitsch, P.: The effect of competitive pitching on the shoulders and elbows of preadolescent baseball pitchers. Pediatrics 49:267, 1972.

HYPEREXTENSIBLE JOINTS

Hyperextensibility of joints may occur in the Ehlers-Danlos, Marfan's and Stickler syndromes, homocystinuria, hyperlysinemia, osteogenesis imperfecta, primary hyperparathyroidism, and a variety of neuromuscular disorders. Hypotonia and unusual mobility of the joints are often present in Down's syndrome and in infants with cerebral hypotonia. Hyperextensibility of the fingers and hands is marked in the cartilage-hair hypoplasia syndrome. Ligamentous laxity may also be part of a syndrome with cutis laxa, delayed growth and development, congenital dislocation of the hips and emphysema.

The *hypermobility syndrome,* which may be associated with joint pain or swelling or both, may be characterized by the patient's ability to extend the wrist so that the fingers are parallel to the dorsum of the forearm; appose the thumbs to the ventral aspect of the forearm; hyperextend the elbows and knees; and place the palms of the hands on the floor by bending over with the knees extended.

Biro, F., Gewanter, H. L., and Baum, J.: The hypermobility syndrome. Pediatrics 72:701, 1983.

The generalized relaxation and pliability of newborn infants during the first week of life permits them to be "folded" into a position which simulates their intrauterine posture.

Larsen's syndrome may be characterized by multiple joint dislocations involving the knee, elbow and, most commonly, the hip. Other anomalies include hypertelorism, frontal bossing, a low nasal bridge, cylindrical fingers, spatulate thumbs and short metacarpals.

Latta, R. J., Graham, C. B., Aase, J., Scham, S. M., and Smith, D. W.: Larsen's syndrome: A skeletal dysplasia with multiple joint dislocations and unusual facies. J. Pediatr. 78:291, 1971.

Patients with *diastrophic dysplasia* have a tendency to dislocate many joints, especially the hip.

LIMITATION OF JOINT MOTION

Limitation of joint motion occurs with arthralgia, arthritis, synovitis, osteomyelitis, diffuse fasciitis with eosinophilia and spastic cerebral palsy.

In *Morquio's disease,* extension of the thighs at the hip is limited so that the child walks in a crouched position with the hips and knees partially flexed.

Joint stiffness and limitation of extension, especially at the elbow, may occur in *Hurler's syndrome.* Stiffness may also be noted in the major joints in Sanfilippo's syndrome.

Patients who are paralyzed may develop joint contractures unless preventive measures are taken.

In its late stages, *dermatomyositis* is characterized by joint contractures.

Volkmann's ischemic contracture may complicate fractures about the elbow, especially the supracondylar type. Once the contracture has developed, the involved extremity is held in flexion at the elbow, wrist and interphalangeal joints, the forearm is pronated, and the metacarpophalangeal joints are hyperextended.

Contractures and joint dislocations may also occur in children with arthritis, particularly rheumatoid arthritis.

Joint motion is restricted in *diastrophic dysplasia* and in Cockayne's syndrome.

Arthrogryposis congenita multiplex is a congenital syndrome of diverse neuropathic, myopathic, connective tissue or mechanical etiology characterized by complete or moderate limitation of motion at one or many joints. Usually all four extremities are involved. Joint fixation may occur in either flexion or extension. Talipes equinovarus is frequently present. Dislocation of the hip and knees may occur. The periarticular tissues may appear thickened, and the extremities may taper from the hip to the ankle and from the shoulders to the wrists. Skin dimpling may be present over the patella, the styloid process of the ulna and other joints, and the usual skin creases are absent. Muscles of the extremities are often hypotonic or hypoplastic. The Pierre Robin syndrome may also occur in some patients.

Beckerman, R. C., and Buchino, J. J.: Arthrogryposis multiplex congenita as part of an inherited symptom complex: two case reports and a review of the literature. Pediatrics 61:417, 1978.

Symposium on arthrogryposis multiplex congenita. Clin. Orthop. Rel. Res. No. 194. April, 1985, pp. 2–125.

The infant with *myelodysplasia* may have joint contractures.

With *iliac adenitis* the child may keep the lower extremity on the affected side flexed at the hip because of spasm of the iliopsoas muscle.

Limited joint mobility, especially of the interphalangeal and metacarpophalangeal joints, is present in children with *diabetes mellitus* who are at increased risk for microvascular complications.

HIP JOINT

The diagnosis of *congenital dislocation of the hip* should be established early by screening examinations in the newborn period and repeated at three and six months of age. It is important that the infant be quiet and relaxed during these examinations.

In the newborn, the *Barlow test* may be used to diagnose an unstable or potentially dislocatable hip. This test is usually not useful after six weeks of age. With the infant supine, the hip flexed to 90 degrees and the knee fully flexed, the examiner places his palm over the infant's knee, his thumb in the femoral triangle opposite the lesser trochanter and his index or middle finger over the greater trochanter. The hip is then brought into mid-abduction with the thumb exerting gentle pressure laterally and posteriorly while the palm exerts posterior and medial pressure on the knee. In the presence of a dislocatable hip, the femoral head can be felt to click as it dislocates across the posterior lip of the acetabulum. When the thumb pressure is released, the femoral head returns to the acetabular socket.

In the *Ortolani test* for hip dislocation, the baby is placed supine on a hard surface, and the knee is fully flexed while the hip is flexed to 90 degrees and fully abducted. The thigh is held between the middle finger placed on the greater trochanter and the thumb placed over the medial thigh, with the pelvis stabilized by the examiner's other hand. As the femoral head moves across the posterior rim of the acetabulum into the socket, the examiner can hear a click or feel a jerk or a jolt. Likewise, redislocation can be detected with adduction of the hip.

In infants with unilateral dislocation of the hip, the inguinal and gluteal folds are higher on the involved side; however, an extra skin crease on the involved side below the gluteal fold is not of diagnostic help since such creases also occur normally, especially in obese infants. If the hips and knees are flexed so that the soles are placed flat on the table, the knee on the affected side is lower than the normal one.

Normally, when an infant is placed in the supine position with the thighs flexed to 90 degrees, the knees may be abducted 160 degrees or so. After the second or third month of life, limitation of abduction of the hip may be noted in congenital dislocation of the hip. Such limitation of abduction may not be present during the first weeks of life. A normal, crying infant may offer considerable resistance to abduction, as may the infant with spastic cerebral palsy. Limitation may also be caused by arthrogryposis multiplex or coxa plana. An acquired dislocation of the hip may occur in spastic cerebral palsy, myelodysplasia and rheumatoid arthritis.

If not detected early in infancy, dislocation of the hip may be overlooked until the child is observed to limp on beginning to walk. A waddling gait and lordosis are present with bilateral dislocation of the hip. A positive Trendelenburg sign may also be present in a child old enough to stand. When a child with a unilateral dislocation uses the involved extremity for weight bearing, a downward tilt or sinking of the pelvis occurs on the normal side. When the normal extremity is used for weight bearing, elevation of the pelvis occurs on the other side.

Legg-Calvé-Perthes disease, or osteochondrosis of the femoral capital epiphysis, occurs most commonly in boys between the ages of four and ten years. The onset is insidious with an almost imperceptible limp that is usually accompanied by pain in the groin, lateral hip or the medial aspect of the thigh and knee. The pain, which is usually relatively slight and simulates that of myalgia or muscle stiffness, may increase with activity. Initially, symptoms may be intermittent. Limitation of motion, particularly extension, abduction and internal rotation, is usually noted on examination. Muscle atrophy about the hip and shortening of the lower extremity may develop later.

Slipped capital femoral epiphysis occurs most commonly between the ages of 12 and 15 years. Although the incidence is greatest in obese children and in tall, thin adolescents who have recently experienced a rapid growth spurt, others may also be affected. Pain in the knee or along the medial aspect of the thigh above the knee, referred along the course of the obturator nerve, is usually the earliest symptom. Actual hip pain is a late complaint. Early pain may be accentuated by activity and alleviated by rest. A slight limp without pain may be the presenting complaint. When a limp develops, the patient walks with his foot in external rotation. Limitation of abduction may cause adduction of the lower extremities. As a result, the adolescent may have to cross his legs in order to sit, and he may walk with a scissors gait. Limitation of internal rotation of the hip, an early finding, is best demonstrated with the patient in the prone position and the knee flexed. The range of extension may, however, be greater than on the un-

involved side. In another characteristic finding elicited by asking the supine patient to flex his knee and hip, flexion of the hip in the neutral position blocks before a 90 degree angle is reached. Then, with further flexion, the hip externally rotates and abducts. A slipped capital femoral epiphysis should be considered whenever a patient complains of pain in the knee. *Anteroposterior and lateral roentgenograms of both hips are indicated in all patients with unexplained pain in the knee.*

Coxa vara represents a congenital or acquired decrease in the normal 135 degree angle between the shaft and the head and neck of the femur. Shortly after beginning to walk, the child may be noted to have a painless, lurching limp. Later, pain, perhaps referred to the knee, may also be present. Limitation of abduction and internal rotation are also found. Muscle atrophy, shortening and external rotation of the involved extremity may appear, and the greater trochanter may be elevated and more prominent than normal. A positive Trendelenburg sign is present on the involved side. Bilateral coxa vara causes a waddling gait and a lumbar lordosis.

Acquired coxa vara may follow or be associated with slipped femoral epiphysis, Legg-Calvé-Perthes disease, osteomyelitis, tuberculosis, pyogenic arthritis, rickets, chondrodystrophy, osteogenesis imperfecta, hypothyroidism, spastic cerebral palsy, trauma to the epiphysial plate and congenital dislocation of the hip and fractures.

SHOULDERS

In *Sprengel's deformity,* the scapula is elevated and rotated with its lower angle directed toward the spine. An omovertebral bone may extend as an osseous bridge between the medial aspect of the scapula and a cervical vertebra. Abduction of the arm on the involved side is limited to about 90 degrees. Scoliosis and torticollis with tilting of the head to the ipsilateral side may also be present.

CLAVICLE

Children with *cleidocranial dysostosis* can approximate their shoulders in the midline. In addition to drooping shoulders, delayed cranial ossification, large fontanels, open suture lines and fontanels, parietal and occipital bossing may also be present.

With fracture of the clavicle during birth, the arm on the involved side may not be used, or its motion may be limited; therefore, the Moro reflex causes a unilateral rather than a bilateral response. Crepitus, angulation and irregularity at the fracture site may be noted immediately and a lump palpated in a few weeks.

Pseudarthrosis of the clavicle is extremely rare.

PELVIS

Diastasis of the symphysis pubis occurs with extrophy of the bladder. Prominence of the anterior superior spine or horn-like projections from the iliac crests occur in the *nail-patella syndrome.*

KNEE

Genu recurvatum, hyperextension or "back" knee, not uncommon in newborn infants, is attributable to generalized ligamentous relaxation and to fetal posture. Occasionally, congenital dislocation of the knee causes the tibia to lie anterior and lateral to the femur and the knee to be hyperextended. Congenital lateral dislocation of the patella occurs rarely.

Hypoplasia of the patella occurs in the *nail-patella* syndrome.

A *popliteal hernia* (Baker's cyst) appears as a smooth, transilluminable cystic mass in the popliteal space accompanied, at times, by swelling of the knee joint. Rheumatoid arthritis may lead to cyst formation. Dissection downward or rupture of the cyst may simulate deep vein thrombophlebitis (pseudothrombophlebitis syndrome) because of a swollen and extremely painful calf.

Congenital discoid lateral cartilage may cause a palpable and audible clicking or snapping sound with movement of the knee joint, especially at the limits of flexion and extension. Localized tenderness may be present over the cartilage.

In adolescents, osteochondrosis of the tibial tubercle, or *Osgood-Schlatter disease,* is characterized by localized pain, tenderness on deep pressure and swelling of the tibial tubercle. The pain may be especially severe after physical activity such as kicking, prolonged kneeling, running or forceful extension of the knee against resistance. A slight limp may appear. The pain of jumper's knee is localized to the lower edge of the patella rather than the tibial tuberosity.

Patellofemoral pain syndrome (chondromalacia patella), a disorder that begins in adolescence, may cause knee pain, a retropatellar grinding sensation, clicking, popping, locking or buckling. The pain, which may be described as aching or restlessness behind, medial to or around the patella or in the popliteal fossa, is precipitated or exacerbated by activities that involve flexion of the patellofemoral joint; prolonged sitting with the knees flexed, standing after sitting, stair-climbing, running, squatting, kneeling or walking up inclines. Patellofemoral crepitus is palpated as the patient actively flexes and extends the knee. Tenderness is found medially and below the patella on the physical examination along with atrophy of the quadriceps, especially the vastus medialis, effusion and patellar hypermotility. A high-riding patella (patella alta) may appear to point upward. Patellar malalignment occurs in many patients with the patellofemoral pain syndrome owing to genu valgum, increased femoral anteversion, external tibial torsion and excessively pronated feet. The quadriceps or "Q" angle may be greater than the normal 10 to 15 degrees. The "Q" angle is that described between a line from the anterosuperior iliac spine to the center of the patella and another line from that point to the tibial tubercle. "Squinting" patellae with the patella pointing medially when the patient stands with the feet straight ahead suggests excessive femoral anteversion or femoral torsion.

Subluxation of the patella, with the patella slipping partially out of the intercondylar groove when the quadriceps contracts with the knee flexed and the foot placed on the ground in a position of external rotation, may cause patellofemoral pain. When the patient sits with his knees flexed to 90 degrees, the patella should face anteriorly and its anterior surface should be vertical; otherwise, the patella may be regarded as unstable. Such instability may be documented by the Fairbanks or apprehension sign in which the patella is pushed laterally while the knee is flexed 30 degrees, the foot supported, quadriceps relaxed and the patient reassured. Normally, the patella can be displaced laterally a centimeter or so. In the presence of excessive laxity, when a hypermobile patella is subluxated up on the lateral femoral condyle by a force applied to the medial patellar border, a reactive contraction of the quadriceps and extension of the knee occurs to move the patella medially in response to the patient's apprehension that the patella will dislocate.

Dislocation of the patella is more likely to occur in girls with genu valgum and in athletes after vigorous quadriceps contraction when the knees are flexed and in a valgus position as in a basketball jump shot. Patellofemoral pain may also be caused by a torn medial meniscus.

Carson, W. G., Jr., James, S. L., Larson, R. L., Singer, K. M., and Winternitz, W. W.: Patellofemoral disorders: Physical and radiographic evaluation. Part I: Physical examination. Clin. Orthop. No. 185, May 1984. p. 165.

Hemarthrosis of the knee associated with a rapid, tense and painful swelling always implies an intra-articular fracture or patellar dislocation in patients who do not have hemophilia. A less acute swelling suggests a tear of the anterior cruciate ligament.

The *popliteal pterygium syndrome* consists of a skin web or pterygium, usually bilateral, that extends from the heel to the ischial tuberosity; anomalies of the hand and feet; genitourinary defects; cleft lip and palate; and lip pits.

Garrick, J. G.: Knee problems in adolescents. Pediatr. Rev. 4:235, 1983.
Smith, J. B.: Knee problems in children. Pediatr. Clin. North Amer. 24:841, 1977.

Adolescents, especially boys, may have *osteochondritis dissecans* with limp, intermittent aching pain and joint stiffness. Either one or both knees may be involved. The patient may be aware of something moving within the joint, and the knee may intermittently click, "give way" or lock. Joint effusion, crepitus and periarticular muscular atrophy may develop. The medial femoral condyle is most commonly involved. Localized tenderness may be present at that site when the knee is flexed. Locking of the knee may also be caused by a torn fragment of a meniscus.

BACK

The newborn infant has a slight convexity of the spine in the thoracic and sacral regions. Cervical and lumbar curves do not appear until the end of the first year of life when the infant assumes a standing posture. With standing, infants and young children have a physiologic lumbar lordosis accentuated by a prominent abdomen. A slight lumbar kyphosis may be apparent in the sitting position .

Scoliosis is characterized by a lateral curvature of the spine associated usually with a rotary deformity. The initiating, primary curve is accompanied by a secondary or compensatory one.

Children between the ages of 8 and 15 years should be regularly screened for scoliosis in the following three positions:

1. From the back, with the child unclothed except for shorts and halter and standing erect with feet together, the examiner looks for unilateral elevation of a shoulder, prominence or elevation of a scapula, deeper crease on one side at the waist line, prominence of one hip, asymmetrical arm-flank distance, asymmetry of the hips or pelvis or curvature of the spine. The occiput should be aligned over the intergluteal cleft. Curves of under 30 degrees may be missed in this position.
2. The child is asked to bend 90 degrees forward at the hips with the knees straight and the arms dangling from the shoulders or pressed together in the prayer position. Inspection is made parallel to the back from either end for a thoracic or lumbar paravertebral prominence or hump.
3. Standing upright, the child is examined from the side for excessive thoracic kyphosis or lumbar lordosis.

Berwick, D. M.: Scoliosis screening. Pediatr. Rev.5:238, 1984.

Standing anteroposterior and lateral x-rays of the entire spine should be obtained when scoliosis or kyphosis is suspected on the screening examination. Functional scoliosis disappears when the patient lies down, sits or bends over; persistent or structural scoliosis does not.

Etiologic Classification of Scoliosis

I. Functional or Nonstructural Scoliosis may result from poor posture. A mild compensatory type of scoliosis, characterized by a long C curve, is present in patients who have a shortened lower extremity. The pelvis is tilted downward on the affected side.

II. Idiopathic Scoliosis occurs between 10 and 14 years of age, most commonly in girls, in the dorsal and dorsolumbar regions as an S-shaped curve with the primary curvature to the right in 85 per cent of cases. If the scoliosis progresses rapidly, a compensatory curvature does not develop, and the shoulders and pelvis are not parallel.

III. Acquired Scoliosis

A. *Neurofibromatosis* produces an acutely angulated, rapidly progressive but compensated scoliosis, usually in the thoracic area. The etiology may be suggested by the presence of *cafe-au-lait* lesions.

B. Muscle imbalance owing to paralysis of the muscles of the back may occur with spastic cerebral palsy, poliomyelitis, muscular dystrophy and other myopathies.
C. Syringomyelia
D. Hemihypertrophy
E. Marfan's syndrome
F. Friedreich's ataxia, Charcot-Marie-Tooth disease, Roussy-Lévy syndrome and other spinocerebellar degenerative disorders
G. Dystonia musculorum deformans
H. Tuberculosis
I. Diastematomyelia
J. Spinal cord tumor
K. Noonan's syndrome
L. Familial dysautonomia
M. Radiation of the spine
N. Conversion reaction
O. Prader-Willi syndrome

IV. Congenital Scoliosis

A. Hemivertebrae cause an acutely angulated scoliosis.
B. Persistent congenital torticollis may be followed by a compensatory scoliosis.
C. Pectus excavatum may be associated with a kyphoscoliosis.
D. Myelomeningocele
E. Chondrodysplasia punctata
F. Diastrophic dysplasia (kyphoscoliosis)
G. Spondyloepiphyseal dysplasia congenita
H. Metatropic dysplasia is characterized by the development of a rapidly progressing kyphoscoliosis when the child becomes older.
I. Pseudoachondroplasia
J. Congenital rib fusions

Jones, M. C.: Clinical approach to the child with scoliosis. Pediatr. Rev. 6:219, 1985.

Etiologic Classification of Kyphosis

I. A Mild Functional Kyphosis may be caused by poor posture. The normal rounding of the spine present in infants when they first begin to sit may be especially pronounced in those with muscular atony and ligamentous relaxation. Such functional kyphosis disappears in the prone position.

II. Hemihypertrophy

III. Generalized Skeletal Disorders

A. Kyphosis (gibbus) of the dorsolumbar spine may be an early physical sign in infants with Hurler's syndrome, Sandhoff's disease and spondyloepiphyseal dysplasia congenita.
B. The kyphosis in Morquio's disease usually does not appear until late infancy or the preschool years.
C. Hypophosphatasia.
D. A mild thoracolumbar kyphosis may appear with achondroplasia.

IV. Vertebral Epiphysitis (Scheuermann's disease) occurs during adolescence. Largely asymptomatic, involvement of the epiphyses of the vertebral bodies with consequent anterior wedging causes kyphosis of the thoracic or upper lumbar spine that may progress over several years.

V. Tuberculous Spondylitis (Pott's Disease) develops insidiously, usually during the first decade. Because of paravertebral muscle spasm, the child characteristically walks stiffly erect or on tiptoe and squats rather than bends over to pick up objects from the floor. Depending on the level of involvement, pain may be referred to the arms, the abdomen or the lower extremities.

VI. Kyphoscoliosis may occur with pectus excavatum.

VII. Tumors of the Spinal Cord

VIII. Noonan's Syndrome

IX. Kyphoscoliosis may be a sequela of irradiation of the spine.

Lordosis denotes an exaggeration of the normal anterior curvature of the lumbar spine. The abdomen may also be protuberant and the buttocks prominent. Some degree of lordosis is normal in older infants and young children and in children with poor posture. Thoracic kyphosis may lead to a compensatory lumbar lordosis. Lordosis may accompany congenital dislocation of the hips, pseudohypertrophic muscular dystrophy, spondylolisthesis, achondroplasia, spondyloepiphyseal dysplasia congenita, congenital deficiency of the abdominal musculature and hyperextensibility of joints.

Flattening of the normal curvatures of the spine or a mendicant, stooped posture may occur in patients with asthma, bronchiectasis, cystic fibrosis, other chronic and debilitating diseases and conversion reaction.

Stiffness of the back occurs with tetanus, poliomyelitis and tuberculous spondylitis, spinal cord tumors and discitis.

Infections of the intervertebral disk (dis-

citis) occur primarily in the lumbar region in young children. Symptoms include irritability; refusal to sit, stand or walk; limp; crying at night; stiffness of the back; loss of lumbar lordosis; vague back pain; abdominal pain; mild fever, and, occasionally, localized tenderness. Movement of the pelvis or thigh may cause pain. A positive Kernig's or Brudzinski's sign may be present. Roentgenographic changes may not occur for two to four weeks, but bone scans are diagnostic earlier.

Fischer, G. W., Popich, G. A., Sullivan, D. E., Mayfield, G., Mazat, B. A., and Patterson, P. H.: Diskitis: A prospective diagnostic analysis. Pediatrics 62:543, 1978.

Wenger, D. R., Bobechko, W. P., and Gilday, D. L.: The spectrum of intervertebral disc-space infection in children. J. Bone Joint Surg. 60-A:100, 1978.

Herniated intervertebral disc is a rare cause of low back pain in older children and adolescents. The most frequent physical findings are pain on deep pressure between the fifth lumbar and the first sacral vertebrae, limited ability to elevate the extended lower extremity unilaterally or bilaterally, restriction of back movement and flattening of the lumbar spine.

Calcification of the intervertebral discs, usually involving the cervical spine in children between five and ten years of age, may be accompanied by pain, spasm, tenderness and torticollis.

Swick, H. M.: Calcification of intervertebral discs in childhood. J. Pediatr. 86:364, 1975.

Vertebral osteomyelitis may be characterized by localized back pain and fever.

Spondylolisthesis, caused usually by L5 slipping forward on S1, and *spondylolysis* are rare causes of low back pain in adolescents. The pain, which may radiate into the buttocks, legs or groin, may be accompanied by tight hamstrings and limited ability for straight leg raising. Scoliosis may be present. Symptoms are decreased when the patient leans forward.

Winging of the scapulae may occur with juvenile muscular atrophy or facioscapulohumeral muscular dystrophy.

The *Klippel-Feil syndrome* is characterized by limitation of movement and shortening of the neck owing to a decrease in the number, abnormal width, fusion or irregular segmentation of the cervical vertebrae. Hemivertebrae may also be present.

Ankylosing spondylitis, which may be seen after the age of 15, is characterized by recurrent, transient stiffness and pain involving the lumbo-sacral spine, sacroiliac joints, buttocks, thighs and hips. Pain may radiate into the lower extremities. Tenderness may be present over the sacroiliac joints and lumbar spine. Anterior flexion of the lumbar spine may be limited. Peripheral arthritis may precede or accompany the spondylitis. Spondyloarthritis is discussed on page 145.

Pain, stiffness and limitation in motion of the neck may be an early manifestation of *juvenile rheumatoid arthritis.*

Tuberculous spondylitis may present with back pain, stiffness and limitation of motion.

Bone tumors of the spine such as aneurysmal bone cyst, osteoid osteoma, Ewing's sarcoma, osteogenic sarcoma, neuroblastoma, lymphomas and leukemia may cause back pain.

Spinal cord tumors may present with neck, back or extremity pain that is exacerbated by coughing, sneezing, straining or straight leg raising; motor weakness; muscle atrophy; paraspinal muscle spasm; positive Babinski reflex or a change in bladder and bowel habits.

Bunnell, W. P.: Back pain in children. Pediatr. Rev. 6:183, 1984.

Hoppenfeld, S.: Back pain. Pediatr. Clin. North Am. 24:881, 1977.

Back pain may be caused by vertebral collapse and compression with *leukemia, chronic corticosteroid therapy, eosinophilic granuloma* or *idiopathic osteoporosis.*

SACROCOCCYGEAL AREA

A *postanal dimple* is frequently present in the sacrococcygeal area. Nevi, hemangiomas, cystic lymphangiomas, lipomas and tufts of hair are other cutaneous lesions in the sacrococcygeal area that may be accompanied by neurologic and spinal cord defects.

A *pilonidal sinus* may also open in this area. Infection of an associated *pilonidal cyst* may be accompanied by inflammatory skin changes, perhaps with fluctuation and purulent drainage from the sinus tract.

Any mass that involves the sacrococcygeal area, the buttocks or the perineum in newborn infants is to be considered a *sacrococcygeal teratoma* until proved otherwise. The mass, which can be palpated rectally, may range in size from a few centimeters in diameter to almost half the size of the baby. The tumor may be hard or largely cystic in consistency. Dermoid cysts, anterior myelomeningoceles, lipomas, sarcomas and hemangiomas also occur in this region.

Differentiation of a completely cystic teratoma from a meningocele may be difficult except that a meningocele may be accompanied by neurologic abnormalities in the lower extremities and roentgenographic evidence of a spina bifida. The meningocele may also become tense when the infant cries or strains with a bowel movement. Pressure applied to a meningocele may be transmitted to the fontanel. Similar transmission of pressure may occur on palpation through the rectum.

Lemire, R. J., Graham, C. B., and Beckwith, J. B.: Skin-covered sacrococcygeal masses in infants and children. J. Pediatr. 79:948, 1971.

Agenesis of the sacrum, caudal dysplasia or the *caudal regression* syndrome, owing to congenital deformities of the lower lumbar, sacral and coccygeal vertebrae and related portions of the spinal cord may be characterized by neurologic impairment of the bladder and lower extremities and orthopedic deformities. Maternal diabetes may be present.

Thompson, I. M., Kirk, R. M., and Dale, M.: Sacral agenesis. Pediatrics 54:236, 1974.

BONE TUMORS

Clinical and roentgenographic differentiation between benign and malignant bone tumors is frequently not possible except by biopsy.

I. Ewing's Tumor is a common bone tumor in children and adolescents. Because systemic symptoms such as fever and malaise occur along with local pain, swelling and tenderness, the symptoms may simulate osteomyelitis.

II. Osteogenic Sarcoma, the most common bone tumor in children and adolescents, has its peak incidence in the decade from age 15 to 25. The distal femur or proximal tibia, the most frequently involved sites, may be characterized by pain, swelling, increased warmth and a limp. Chondrosarcoma is usually a low-grade malignancy.

Tebbi, C. K., and Freeman, A. I.: Osteogenic sarcoma. Pediatr. Rev. 6:55, 1984.

III. Osteochondroma, a benign tumor that most frequently involves the distal end of the femur or proximal end of the tibia and humerus, is generally discovered after trauma. Multiple osteochondromas occur in hereditary multiple exostoses.

IV. Osteoid Osteoma, a benign tumor, may cause chronic, boring or aching bone pain. Limp may be present if the tumor site is in the lower extremity. Muscle atrophy may also be noted. Pain episodes are usually intermittent, last an hour or two, and are worse at night, often awakening the child. Although long bones are the most common tumor site, any bone in the body may be involved. A fusiform swelling and inflammatory changes may be noted over the site. Pain may be localized or referred, (e.g., from the proximal or middle femur to the thigh or knee). Striking relief of pain follows aspirin therapy.

Orlowski, J. P. and Mercer, R. D.: Osteoid osteoma in children and young adults. Pediatrics 59:526, 1977.

GENERAL REFERENCES

Ferguson, A. B: Orthopedic Surgery in Infancy and Childhood. 4th ed. Baltimore, Williams & Wilkins, 1975.
Lovell, W. W., and Winter, R. B.: Pediatric Orthopaedics. Vols. I and II. Philadelphia, J. B. Lippincott Co., 1978.

17 / THE MUSCULAR SYSTEM

MUSCLE TONE

Muscle tone varies considerably, even among normal newborns and infants, depending upon the type of delivery, duration of labor, amount of anesthesia and central nervous system status.

MUSCLE HYPOTONIA AND WEAKNESS

Generalized ligamentous relaxation, accompanied by extreme hypotonia of the muscles, is present in many otherwise normal children. Characteristically, many of the joints are hyperextensible. Dorsiflexion of the feet, genu valgum and flat, everted feet are often present. Affected children may walk relatively late, fall frequently, and complain of leg pains after exercise.

Benign congenital myopathies are characterized by mild generalized or proximal, nonprogressive muscle weakness that appears in early infancy. Syndromes in this group include central core disease, nemaline myopathy, mitochondrial myopathy, congenital fiber-type disproportion, myotubular myopathy, multicore myopathy, reducing body myopathy, fingerprint body myopathy and familial myopathy with probable lysis of myofibrils in type I fibers.

Saper, J. R.: Benign congenital myopathy. Am. J. Med. 57:157, 1974.

Muscular hypotonia may occur in patients with Down's syndrome, Miller-Dieker syndrome, hypopotassemia, hypothyroidism, primary hypoparathyroidism, glycogenosis Type II (Pompe's disease, acid maltase deficiency), arthrogryposis, Werdnig-Hoffmann disease, Marfan's syndrome, the Zellweger cerebrohepatorenal syndrome, platybasia, gliomas of the hypothalamus and optic chiasm, medulloblastoma and astrocytoma. Muscle tone is absent in infants asphyxiated secondary to central respiratory depression or central nervous system injury. Muscle hypotonia associated with tumors of the cerebellar hemispheres may be generalized or present only on the ipsilateral side. Striking muscular hypotonia may occur in patients with idiopathic hypercalcemia. Generalized muscle weakness and hypotonia may occur in infantile botulism. Severe malnutrition is usually characterized by muscular hypotonia, although hypertonia may occur in marasmic infants. Wasting and decreased muscle tone and mass occur in kwashiorkor.

Muscle atony and hypotonia may be important indicators of cerebral palsy in infancy. These manifestations may later be replaced by those of spasticity or athetosis. Tay-Sachs disease is characterized by generalized hypotonia of muscles in the presence of hyperactive deep reflexes. Similar findings may occur in patients with brain stem tumors. Infants with congenital myotonic dystrophy may demonstrate marked floppiness. The Prader-Willi syndrome is characterized in the early months of life by generalized hypotonia so severe as to suggest flaccidity especially since the deep tendon reflexes are diminished or absent. In addition, the infant may demonstrate little motion.

In patients with hyperthyroidism, the presence of otherwise inapparent muscle weakness may be demonstrated by having the patient sit on an examining table or in a chair and extend his lower extremities straight out. Normally, such extension can be maintained for over two minutes. Easy fatigability and some atrophy may accompany the muscle weakness. Generalized muscle tenderness and weakness, especially involving the pelvic and shoulder girdles, often occur in hypothyroidism.

Rosman, N. P.: Neurological and muscular aspects of thyroid dysfunction in childhood. Pediatr. Clin. North Am. 23:575, 1976.

Muscle weakness may also be a manifestation of Addison's disease, Bartter's syndrome and Cushing's disease. Periodic, severe muscular weakness is a manifestation of primary aldosteronism. Hyperparathyroidism may cause proximal muscle weakness, wasting, hypotonia, muscle pain and cramps. Myopathy may be a complication of prolonged corticosteroid therapy. Muscle weakness occurs with carbon monoxide poisoning. Profound generalized weakness and pain may occur in patients with rhabdomyolysis and myoglobinuria.

Periodic paralysis and muscle weakness may be associated with either hypo- or hyperkalemia. With *primary hypokalemic periodic paralysis*, episodes of weakness and flaccid paralysis, predominantly proximal and mild, but in some instances extending to complete quadriplegia, usually begin early in the morning and last from 2 to 24 hours. The extent and duration of the paralysis varies. In *hyperkalemic periodic paralysis* (adynamia episodica hereditaria), a familial disorder, the episodes, which occur during the day, especially on resting after exercise, are briefer and less severe. Muscles of the trunk, pelvic girdle and extremities are predominantly involved.

MUSCLE HYPERTONIA

The so-called hypertonic infant demonstrates heightened muscle tone and tenseness and cries excessively and easily. Muscle tone is increased in infants with hypernatremia and the neonatal narcotic withdrawal syndrome. Hypertonus with decrease of or resistance to joint movement is a frequent finding in patients with cerebral palsy.

MUSCLE CRAMPS

Painful muscle cramps followed by transient myoglobinuria, weakness and stiffness may be precipitated by physical exertion in patients with *McArdle's syndrome* (phosphorylase deficiency) and in those with muscle phosphofructokinase or carnitine palmital transferase deficiency.

Fattah, S. M., Rubulis, A., and Faloon, W. W.: McArdle's disease. Am. J. Med. 48:693, 1970.
Layzer, R. B.: McArdle's disease in the 1980s. N. Engl. J. Med. 312:370, 1985.

In the exercise-induced type of *idiopathic rhabdomyolysis* and *myoglobinuria*, muscle pain, cramps, weakness, hypoactive deep tendon reflexes and myoglobinuria occur within a few hours after exercise.

Robotham, J. L., and Haddow, J. E.: Rhabdomyolysis and myoglobinuria in childhood. Pediatr. Clin. North Am. 23:279, 1976.
Roelofs, R. I., and Engel, W. K.: Myopathies associated with systemic diseases. Postgrad. Med. 50:95, 1971.

Muscle heat cramps may occur with exercise on hot, humid days. Muscle aches and cramps are characteristic of *diffuse fasciitis with eosinophilia*.

MYOSITIS

Dermatomyositis is characterized by muscle weakness that may range from mild to severe, stiffness, pain, tenderness, firmness and edema, all of which may develop early and insidiously, along with systemic symptoms such as easy fatigability, fever and malaise. Involvement may be extensive and symmetrical. Pharyngeal and esophageal muscles may be involved. Eventually, swallowing, speech and respiration are affected. Muscle weakness, although generalized, is predominantly proximal and involves the limb girdle and anterior neck flexors. The child may experience fatigue and difficulty in climbing stairs or turning door knobs. Muscle atrophy, fibrosis and woody induration develop later, along with joint contractures and periarticular swelling. The skin manifestations of dermatomyositis are reviewed on page 181. Skeletal muscle enzymes, especially creatine phosphokinase, are elevated.

Pachman, L. M., and Cooke, N.: Juvenile dermatomyositis: A clinical and immunologic study. J. Pediatr. 96:226, 1980.
Schaller, J. G.: Dermatomyositis. J. Pediatr. 83:699, 1973.
Spiro, A. J.: Childhood dermatomyositis and polymyositis. Pediatr. Rev. 6:163, 1984.

Polymyositis presents with clinical manifestations that simulate dermatomyositis, except for the skin involvement. Chronic polymyositis may closely resemble muscular dystrophy. The musculoskeletal findings in hypothyroidism and myopathic carnitine deficiency may occasionally simulate those in polymyositis. Occasionally, postinfectious polymyositis may be associated with myoglobinuria.

Bohan, A., and Peter, J. B.: Polymyositis and dermatomyositis. N. Engl. J. Med. 292:344, 403, 1975.
McGarry, J. D., and Foster, D. W.: Systemic carnitine deficiency. N. Engl. J. Med. 303:1413, 1980.

Chronic myositis may accompany other connective tissue or collagen-vascular diseases such as lupus erythematosus, polyarteritis nodosa and, occasionally, rheumatoid arthritis. Proximal muscle weakness may be present.

Clostridial myositis or gas gangrene is characterized by severe pain, crepitance, edema, discoloration and extreme toxicity.

Acute myositis, caused by influenza and other viruses, may be preceded by 2 to 4 days of fever, headache and symptoms of an upper respiratory illness. Severe muscle pain and tenderness begin suddenly in the gastrocnemius, soleus, and, occasionally, the thigh muscles, and the child has difficulty in walking. The feet are held in plantar flexion. The serum creatinine phosphokinase and glutamic oxaloacetic transaminase levels are elevated.

Farrell, M. K., Partin, J. C., and Bove, K. E.: Epidemic influenza myopathy in Cincinnati in 1977. Pediatrics 96:545, 1980.

Primary suppurative myositis, unusual in temperate climate zones, consists of abscess formation in one or more skeletal muscles. *Staphylococcus aureus* is the most common pathogen.

Sirinavin, S., and McCracken, G. H.: Primary suppurative myositis in children. Am. J. Dis. Child. 133:263, 1979.

Myositis fibrosa generalista, a rare disease in childhood, is characterized by painless muscle stiffness, induration, atrophy and contractures. Initially, the extent of involvement is usually slight, but the process gradually progresses until entire muscle groups are affected, most commonly those of the lower extremities. Except for the masseter muscles, the face is uninvolved.

Progressive myositis ossificans begins most commonly in the muscles of the neck and back as localized, tender, pliable or firm masses. Transient edema and erythema of the skin may appear over the involved area. Remissions occur, but over a period of months calcification develops in the connective tissue of the muscle, and the induration is replaced by a bony hardness. As the process gradually extends to involve most of the body's striated musculature, limitation of movement and ankylosis of joints appear. Shortening of the digits, particularly of the thumb and large toe, hallux valgus and other digital anomalies may also occur.

Localized myositis ossificans may be caused by trauma. Swelling, tenderness and pain on use of the involved muscle may occur. The brachialis anticus is the most frequently affected muscle. This complication may also appear in the quadriceps femoris after a thigh injury.

MYALGIA

Myalgia occurs with leptospirosis, Rocky Mountain spotted fever, bubonic plague and systemic lupus erythematosus. Profound, diffuse myalgia, predominantly affecting the proximal limb, trunk and neck muscles, occurs in the *toxic shock syndrome.* Muscle tenderness may be exquisite. Generalized musculoskeletal pain, at times with muscle cramps in the calves, thighs, and back, may be a prominent feature of *Lyme disease.* Muscle tenderness may be present along with weakness in *Guillain-Barré syndrome.*

Fibromyalgia in adolescents is characterized by musculoskeletal aches and pains, stiffness and multiple tender trigger points involving the back, the trapezius muscles and peripheral joints.

MUSCLE HYPERTROPHY

Congenital *muscular hypertrophy* occurs in association with mental retardation and cerebral palsy. Idiopathic benign congenital muscular hypertrophy may also occur. Rarely, generalized muscular hypertrophy may be observed in patients with hypothyroidism (the Kocher-Debré-Sémélaigne syndrome). Because of an absence of subcutaneous fat, the muscles of the extremities may appear prominent in patients with lipoatrophy.

Hopwood, N. J., Lockhart, L.H., and Bryan, G. T.: Acquired hypothyroidism with muscular hypertrophy and precocious testicular enlargement. J. Pediatr. 85:233, 1974.

MYOTONIA

Myotonia congenita is a familial disease that usually begins early in childhood with myotonia and hypertrophy of the muscles. The patient has difficulty in initiating muscular action, especially after a period of inactivity or quickly releasing his grip as in a handshake. Muscular relaxation occurs slowly. Local contraction and dimpling, occurring when a muscle such as the deltoid or the thenar eminence is struck with a reflex hammer, may persist for 30 to 60 seconds. Symptoms are exacerbated by cold, fatigue or excitement.

Paramyotonia congenita is characterized by myotonia after exposure to cold. Attacks of muscle weakness and stiffness may occur with or without such exposure. Elevation of the serum potassium is present in some instances.

Morning stiffness and *gelling* following a period of inactivity are common in active juvenile rheumatoid arthritis.

Muscular stiffness and twitching may occur in *tetany*. Rigidity may be an early finding in *malignant hyperthermia*.

The *Schwartz-Jampel syndrome* is characterized by myotonia, muscle stiffness, muscle hypertrophy, dwarfism, blepharospasm, micrognathia and pectus carinatum.

MUSCULAR DYSTROPHY

In addition to clinical evaluation of muscle involvement, other diagnostic procedures for *muscular dystrophy* include serum aldolase, creatinine phosphokinase, transaminasc (SGOT and SGPT), electromyography and muscle biopsy. Muscle testing and electromyography help select the appropriate muscle for biopsy. In the clinical differentiation between myopathy or neuropathy as causes for muscle weakness, muscle fasciculations suggest the latter. The deep tendon reflexes are never increased with a myopathy, although they may be when neurogenic weakness is associated with involvement of the corticospinal tracts.

Munsat, T. L., Baloh, R., Pearson, C. M., and Fowler, W., Jr.: Serum enzyme alterations in neuromuscular disease. JAMA 226:1536, 1973.

Pseudohypertrophic muscular dystrophy becomes clinically manifest during infancy or early childhood, predominantly in boys. The progression of the disease is variable, with many patients becoming wheelchair-bound in adolescence; however, in the more benign type, the patient remains ambulatory 25 to 30 years after onset of the disease. Symptoms, usually first noted when the child begins to walk, include toe walking, inability to run well, difficulty in climbing stairs, a waddling gait and a history of frequent falls. The gastrocnemius, soleus, gluteus, deltoid and triceps muscles are most commonly involved. Weakness and atrophy also occur in the muscles of the abdomen, pelvis, thighs and back, but usually not in those of the face. Early, many of the affected muscles, especially those of the calves, the triceps and the deltoid, are enlarged and have a firm, doughy or rubbery texture. As the disease progresses, muscular atrophy develops, initially at the musculotendinous

insertions, and the tendon reflexes gradually diminish until they are unobtainable. Atrophy is not preceded by pseudohypertrophy in the Leyden-Möbius type of progressive muscular dystrophy. The Achilles tendon becomes shortened, and flexural contractures develop at the hips, knees and elbows along with a lumbar lordosis. Because the Achilles tendon is short, the child walks on his toes. The gait is waddling, with the trunk swaying from side to side. The muscles of the shoulder girdle are extremely weak so that the patient seems to slip through the examiner's hands when an attempt is made to pick him up by the axillae. Winging of the scapulae also occurs.

Involvement of the flexors of the neck makes it difficult or impossible for the patient to elevate his head from the supine position. The loss of strength in the abdominal and other trunk musculature compromises the patient's ability to sit or stand from the supine position. *Gower's sign* refers to the manner in which the patient achieves the standing position by "climbing up himself." The child first turns on his side, flexes his hips and knees, and uses his extended arm as a pivot to assume a kneeling position. The feet are then brought forward and the lower extremities straightened by extension at the knee. Finally, the hands are lifted from the floor and placed sequentially over the tibias, the knees and the thighs until the child stands upright. Gower's sign, consistently present with progressive muscular dystrophy, may also occur in patients whose pelvic girdle weakness is caused by other disorders.

Emery-Dreifuss dystrophy, which has an insidious onset of weakness and muscle contractures, is characterized by toe-walking, flexion of the elbows and inability to fully flex the neck and spine. Atrial conduction disorders may occur in childhood or early adulthood.

The *facioscapulohumeral* type of muscular dystrophy begins between 12 and 20 years of age with weakness of the facial muscles and lack of facial expression (myopathic facies). The patient has difficulty closing his eyelids, elevating his eyebrows, frowning, raising the corners of his mouth on smiling and puckering his lips to whistle. Progression of the disease leads to weakness and atrophy of the muscles in the scapulohumeral and pectoral areas. Generalized involvement similar to that of the pseudohypertrophic type may eventually result. A form of neurogenic muscle atrophy that may simulate the facioscapulohumeral form of muscular dystrophy is discussed on page 124.

Limb-girdle dystrophy is intermediate between the Duchenne and facioscapulohumeral forms. Pseudohypertrophy of the calves and marked elevation of the serum enzymes usually do not occur. The pelvic girdle is principally involved, with the shoulder girdle less often affected. The onset is usually between 10 and 40 years of age.

Children with late onset *acid maltase deficiency* may demonstrate chronic progressive proximal muscle weakness that may simulate limb-girdle dystrophy. A neurogenic form of muscle atrophy may also simulate limb-girdle dystrophy. Dermatomyositis and polymyositis may have a similar distribution.

Tanaka, K., Shimazu, S., Oya, N., Tomisawa, M., Kusunoki, T., Soyama, K., and Ono, E.: Muscular form of glycogenosis Type II (Pompe's disease). Pediatrics 63:124, 1979.

Juvenile muscular atrophy, or Erb's type of muscular dystrophy, which begins at puberty or somewhat later, is characterized by weakness of the shoulder girdle. The facial muscles are uninvolved.

Congenital muscular dystrophy, a rare cause of the "floppy baby" syndrome, is present at birth and rapidly progressive.

Myotonic muscular dystrophy, a familial disorder, may be present at birth or first noted between 10 and 15 years of age. In newborn infants born to mothers with myotonic dystrophy, manifestations include facial diplegia, a tent-shaped mouth, difficulty in sucking, swallowing and breathing difficulties, muscle weakness, severe hypotonia with deep tendon reflexes preserved and retardation of motor development. Edema involving the head and extremities may be present. On chest x-ray, the ribs are abnormally slender. Myotonia usually appears later. Patients with early onset myotonic dystrophy also demonstrate lumbar lordosis and proximal muscle weakness. Arthrogryposis, talipes deformities or other joint immobility may be noted. In the older child and adolescent, the involvement begins distally in the hands and feet. When the onset is in early childhood, myotonia, characterized by slow relaxation of a muscle after contraction, may be the initial manifestation.

Carroll, J. E.: Diagnosis and management of Duchenne muscular dystrophy. Pediatr. Rev. 6:195, 1985.
Dyken, P. R., and Harper, P. S.: Congenital dystrophia myotonica. Neurology 23:465, 1973.
Pearse, R. G., and Howeler, C. J.: Neonatal form of dystrophia myotonica. Arch. Dis. Child. 54:331, 1979.
Sarnat, H. B., O'Connor, T., and Byrne, P. A.: Clinical effects of myotonic dystrophy on pregnancy and the neonate. Arch. Neurol. 33:459, 1976.
Zatz, M.: Diagnosis, carrier detection and genetic counseling in the muscular dystrophies. Pediatr. Clin. North Am. 25:557, 1978.

GENERAL REFERENCE

Dubowitz, V.: Muscle Disorders in Childhood. Philadelphia, W. B. Saunders Co., 1978.

18 / THE SKIN

SKIN OF THE NEWBORN INFANT

Easterly, N. B., and Solomon, L. M.: Neonatal dermatology. II. Blistering and scaling dermatoses. J. Pediatr. 77:1075, 1970.
Hodgman, J. E., Freedman, R. I., and Levan, N. E.: Neonatal dermatology. Pediatr. Clin. North Am.18:713, 1971.
Solomon, L. M., and Easterly, N. B.: Neonatal Dermatology. Philadelphia, W. B. Saunders Co., 1973.
Solomon L. M., and Easterly, N. B.: Neonatal dermatology. I. The newborn skin. J. Pediatr.77:888, 1970.

Premature infants have little subcutaneous tissue and their skin is delicate, with vessels visible through their almost transparent skin. The skin of the term infant is soft, smooth, and velvety, especially during the first few days of life. The skin over their hands and feet is often cold, bluish-red, and sometimes glossy. A few hours after birth, the skin becomes intensely red, and this color persists for several hours. The premature infant is highly vulnerable to severe zinc deficiency states.

Hambridge, K. M.: Zinc deficiency in the premature infant. Pediatr. Rev. 6:209, 1985.

In·the *postmature infant*, the vernix caseosa is minimal in amount or absent. The skin is dry, cracked and parchment- or collodion-like. Peeling is noted at birth. With a greater degree of postmaturity, the umbilical cord and skin are stained green or golden yellow.

The *vernix caseosa* is a soft, cheesy, clay-colored material that covers the skin of newborn infants. The amount varies considerably, being almost absent at times, especially in postmature infants. Meconium or yellow staining of the vernix caseosa, abnormal except in breech presentations, may occur in hemolytic disease of the newborn, postmature infants and fetal distress.

Branny or flaky *desquamation* of the skin, including that of the palms and soles, occurs to some extent in nearly all term infants during the first few days of life, but not until the second or third week in premature infants. In some, however, the desquamation is more extensive and sheetlike, especially over the trunk, with transverse creases or cracks. Babies subjected to acute intrauterine hypoxia show desquamation at birth.

The soles of premature infants are smooth, with only one or two creases present at 32 weeks. The creases appear distally and gradually extend toward the heels. Two thirds of the sole has creases at 37 weeks, while in term infants the entire sole, including the heels, is creased.The postmature infant has deeper sole creases.

Lanugo, a fine, downy kind of hair, is usually present over the face, ear lobes, back and shoulders of premature babies but is practically absent in term infants.

The skin of newborn infants reacts to pressure and irritation with erythema, tiny papules and nonspecific eruptions. The terms *flea bite dermatitis* and *toxic erythema of the newborn* describe one type of common nonspecific, transient, blotchy and erythematous lesion in the newborn. These lesions have tiny, central, yellow or white vesicles or wheals, most evident when the skin is stretched. The so-called pustular form of toxic erythema, characterized by yellow or white papular or pustular lesions, 1 to 3 mm in size and containing eosinophils, are usually found in skin creases.

Pustular melanosis, more common in black than in white newborn infants, is characterized by non-pruritic, vesicopustular lesions, without surrounding erythema, that on rupture leave a scaly fringe. The lesions are usually present on the chin, neck, lower back, pretibial region or palms and soles. Pigmented macules remain in black, but usually not in white, infants.

Ramamurthy, R. S., Reveri, M., Esterly, N. B., Fretzin, D.F., and Pildes, R. S.: Transient neonatal pustular melanosis. J. Pediatr. 88:831, 1976.

Newborn infants who are very active sometimes develop abrasions over their elbows, knees, ankles, heels, toes and other pressure areas. Scratch marks are not infrequently seen on the face.

Cutis marmorata, a purplish mottling of the skin, may occur in healthy infants and young children and is especially prominent in premature, hypothyroid, debilitated or dehydrated infants.

Shock or hypotension in the newborn infant is manifested by a pale, gray or cyanotic color; clammy skin;· respiratory distress; lethargy; and hypotonia.

"Harlequin" color change occurs in an occasional newborn infant, more commonly of low birth weight. Half of the body suddenly becomes pale or reddened with a sharp line of demarcation down the midline. These episodes last seconds to minutes and are without pathologic significance. Episodes of flushing, pallor or cyanosis may accompany *neonatal hypoglycemia.*

Erythema, vesiculation and depressed, hyperpigmented scars may be caused by the heated electrodes used in *transcutaneous oxygen monitoring* in the newborn.

Boyle, R. J., and Oh, W.: Erythema following transcutaneous pO$_2$ monitoring. Pediatrics 65:333, 1980.

Depressed, dimple-like scars may result from *fetal puncture* during third trimester amniocentesis or intrauterine transfusion.

Acne, with papules, pustules and comedones owing to maternal hormonal stimulation, may appear in newborn infants about the first week of life.

Milia are yellowish-white, somewhat shiny vesicles, pinpoint-sized or larger and usually grouped. They are caused by plugging and distention of sebaceous ducts. Milia may be noted during the first or second week of life on the forehead, nose, nasolabial folds, chin and cheeks.

Intertrigo, or chafing, refers to the moist, erythematous areas in creases of the skin. The folds of the neck, axillae, inguinal region and perineum are commonly involved. Seborrheic dermatitis and moniliasis may be etiologic agents.

Subcutaneous fat necrosis may occur during the neonatal period as single or multiple, indurated, button-like lesions, 1 to 2 cm in diameter or larger. Sites of predilection are the back, cheeks, buttocks and extremities. The overlying skin may be reddened or purple. Usually the lesions are not attached to the underlying subcutaneous tissue. Gradual disappearance over a period of weeks or months is the rule, but fluctuation and external drainage occasionally ensue. Subcutaneous calcification and hypercalcemia may develop as complications.

Sclerema neonatorum, an intense, non-pitting hardening of subcutaneous tissues, usually of the trunk and proximal portions of the extremities, occurs rarely in premature or debilitated newborn infants. This nonspecific finding usually accompanies life-threatening disorders such as septicemia, pneumonia, peritonitis and severe gastroenteritis. The process may begin on the buttocks, cheeks, thighs, calves or trunk and become generalized. The overlying skin is cold, hard, bound-down and mottled reddish-purple or waxy white in color.

Scleredema is an extremely rare, brawny, pitting edema that usually appears first on the lower extremities, then extends to involve the entire body. Premature or debilitated infants may be affected during the first or second week of life. Findings include feeble respiratory movements, a weak pulse, a subnormal temperature and listlessness.

Impetigo neonatorum is usually characterized by single vesicles or pustules surrounded by an erythematous areola. Rupture of the vesicle leaves a red, moist base with a wrinkled fringe. The lesions occur most commonly in skin folds and over the lower abdomen but may be more extensive. Bullae appear suddenly, coalesce and become widespread. Large areas of skin may become denuded. Initially, with *Ritter's disease*, a generalized erythema of the skin develops rapidly. The skin then becomes wrinkled and loose and exfoliates in sheets, leaving large, bright red, raw patches. Nikolsky's sign is positive (e.g., the skin separates in sheets as a result of friction by the examiner's finger).

Facial and mandibular cellulitis, at times associated with regional lymphadenitis, may be caused by group B streptococcus.

Baker, C. J.: Group B streptococcal cellulitis-adenitis in infants. Am. J. Dis. Child. 136:631, 1982.

Congenital cutaneous candidiasis is characterized by numerous vesiculopustular lesions that promptly desquamate with residual collarettes of scale. Coalescence of lesions leads to diffuse desquamation and erythroderma. The lesions appear principally on the trunk, neck, hands and flexural areas at birth.

Kam, L.A., and Giacoia, G. P.: Congenital cutaneous candidiasis. Am. J. Dis. Child. 129:1215, 1974.

A blueberry muffin rash, consisting of 2- to 8-mm dark blue or magenta-colored macules and papules, may be caused by *congenital viral infections* such as cytomegalovirus and rubella. Petechiae, or dark red, grey-purple or copper brown macular lesions, may also occur. Blueberry muffin—like skin lesions may also be a result of *cutaneous erythropoiesis* secondary to prolonged intrauterine anemia. Congenital leukemia or neuroblastoma may account for similar lesions. Skin biopsy of the lesion may be required for diagnosis.

Schwartz, J. L., Maniscalco, W. M., Lane, A. T., and Currado, W. J.: Twin transfusion syndrome causing cutaneous erythropoiesis. Pediatrics 74:527, 1984.

Transient neonatal pustular melanosis consists of 3- to 4-mm vesiculopustular lesions that are present at birth or shortly thereafter and appear most commonly on the palms, soles, neck and chin. The lesions transform in a few days to brown-pigmented macules that have a collarette of scales. Recurrent crops appear until three to four months of age.

Ramamurthy, R. S., Reveri, M., Esterly, N. B., Fretzin, D.F., and Pildes, R. S.: Transient neonatal pustular melanosis. J. Pediatr. 88:831, 1976.

Congenital herpes simplex infection produces a clustered, vesicular rash a few days after birth. Fulminant systemic symptoms and signs may follow.

Congenital syphilis is a diagnostic consideration whenever an eruption occurs on an infant's palms or soles. The lesions are thick, diffuse and either moist or covered by shiny, desquamating scales. Bullae may also occur on the palms and soles. The face and much of the body may be involved. Individual lesions are usually small, slightly elevated, annular, shiny, reddish-brown maculopapules. Moist, flat condylomata may appear in the perianal and genital regions. The moist fissures that occur about the mouth and nose heal with rhagades, or linear scars, that radiate from the corners of the mouth.

Flat, light red *capillary hemangiomas* occur commonly over the base of the nose, upper eyelids, upper lip and nape of the neck. These lesions, which blanch on pressure and are more prominent during crying, usually fade over a period of months. Unless they are intensely red, these lesions completely disappear. A prominent facial flame nevus over the center of the forehead and upper eyelids occurs in Beckwith's syndrome and in trisomy 13. Petechiae may appear on the head, along with cyanosis and edema, when a baby is born with the umbilical cord wrapped around his neck.

Mongolian blue spots are irregularly shaped, bluish or bluish-gray pigmented areas over the buttocks, sacrum, upper back and extremities. More common in black, Indian or Oriental infants, they are occasionally also noted in Caucasians. The pigmented area, which may be 10 cm or more in diameter, gradually disappears during infancy.

Localized defects of the hair, skin and subcutaneous tissue 1/2 to 1 inch in diameter may rarely be present at birth. Such defects most commonly involve the scalp, especially the vertex. Aplasia cutis, occurring in the midline over the lumbosacral spine, may be a marker of occult spinal dysraphism. The *focal dermal hypoplasia syndrome* is characterized by areas in which the skin or scalp is either absent or very thin, hyper- or hypopigmented and covered by telangiectasia. Reddish or brownish-yellow fatty tissue herniations occur through the dermis and multiple wart-like papillomas are present on the buccal mucous membrane, the skin of the genitalia or general body surface. Anomalies of the hands, eyes and teeth may occur.

Goltz, R. W., Henderson, R. R., Hitch, J. M., and Ott, J. E.: Focal dermal hypoplasia syndrome. Arch. Dermatol. 101:1, 1970.

Higginbottom, M. C., Jones, K. L., James, H. E., Bruce, D. A., and Schut, L.: Aplasia cutis congenita: A cutaneous marker of occult spinal dysraphism. J. Pediatr. 96:687, 1980.

Neonatal lupus erythematosus is characterized by the appearance, predominantly on the head and neck, of erythematous, oval-shaped, slightly atrophic macules with peripheral scaling. Associated findings may include congenital heart block, thrombocytopenia, anemia and leukopenia.

DERMATOGLYPHICS

The arches, loops and whorls of the fingers may be examined either from finger prints or with a magnifying lens. Unusual dermatoglyphic markings or patterns may be found in conditions such as the trisomy 21, trisomy 13, trisomy 18 and 5p syndromes, but they are not specific for an individual syndrome. Patients with Down's syndrome have a distal axial triradius of the palms, ulnar loops on all fingers, a simian line and a single flexion crease of the fifth finger along with clinodactyly.

Preus, M., and Fraser, F. C.: Dermatoglyphics and syndromes. Am. J. Dis. Child. 124:933, 1972.

PIGMENTATION

The symptom of *jaundice* is discussed in Chapter 28. Jaundice appears more readily in some patients and in some areas of the skin than in others. Clinically evident jaundice usually is present when the serum bilirubin level is between 5 to 7 mg per 100 ml. Jaundice may persist in tissues for some time after plasma levels have begun to fall. The affinity of elastic fibers for biliary pigments may explain the early appearance and persistence of pigmentation in the sclera and other areas of the body in which elastic tissue is plentiful. Jaundice is less evident in the presence of edema. Its clinical detection may also be difficult in the black patient except by inspection of the sclera. The greenish component sometimes noted in jaundiced patients is thought to be caused by biliverdin. Increased melanin pigmentation may occur in patients with chronic jaundice as a result of pruritus and scratching.

Bronze pigmentation may occur as a complication of phototherapy for neonatal hyperbilirubinemia.

Kopelman, A. E., Brown, R.S., and Odell, G. B.: The "bronze" baby syndrome: A complication of phototherapy. J. Pediatr. 81:466, 1972.

Cyanosis is discussed in Chapter 51. *Cold-induced acrocyanosis*, with cyanosis of the tongue, nose, lips and digits on exposure to cold, may occur with infectious mononucleosis. Acrocyanosis may appear in patients with anorexia nervosa, in infants who are dehydrated and in dyskeratosis congenita.

Carotenemia and *carotenoderma* in infants account for the lemon-yellow coloration of the skin frequently observed along the nasolabial folds, over the tip of the nose, chin and the forehead, on the palms and soles, around the nails, over the knuckles, around the eyes, along body folds and over pressure areas. The sclerae and mucous membranes are not pigmented. Carotenoderma may be especially prominent in infants who perspire profusely, since some of the pigment is excreted in the sweat and then deposited in the stratum corneum. Carotenemia may also occur in children with hypothyroidism.

A lemon-yellow, gray or tan skin tint may be present in patients with thalassemia; a dusky, brown or grayish pigmentation occurs in children who have received large numbers of transfusions because of chronic hemolytic or hypoplastic anemias. Dark yellow to brown coloration of the skin, more prominent over joints and exposed parts, especially the lower extremities, is sometimes noted in patients with Niemann-Pick disease. Quinacrine hydrochloride causes a diffuse yellow discoloration of the skin.

Addison's disease may be characterized by dirty brown, tan or bluish-black pigmentation, especially around the genitalia, breast areolae, umbilicus, in the skin folds and over the joints and exposed parts. The pigmentation may occasionally be more generally distributed over the body as freckle-like lesions. Depigmented areas within a zone of increased pigmentation have been described. Pigmented spots may also appear on the oral and buccal mucous membrane. A generalized brown pigmentation of the skin may be seen with *adrenoleukodystrophy*.

The *Rothmund-Thomson syndrome* is characterized in early infancy by redness and swelling of the cheeks and ears followed by pigmentation, depigmentation, atrophy and telangiectasia, along with hyperkeratoses over the joints, palms and soles. Bilateral cataracts develop.

Large, often unilateral, flat, brown *café au lait spots* are present in patients with *Albright's syndrome*, along with polyostotic fibrous dysplasia and sexual precocity. Present at birth or developing soon thereafter, these lesions have a more irregular edge than those of neurofibromatosis.

Under the age of five years, up to six *café au lait spots* over one-half inch in diameter are within normal limits. The lesions are light brown in white children and darker brown in black children. Café au lait spots, ranging in size from 1 to over 15 mm, are usually the first sign of *neurofibromatosis*. Numerous, freckle-like spots may occur in the axillae, in inguinal and cervical regions or over the entire body. Neuromas are small, soft, boggy, raised or pedunculated tumor masses in the skin and subcutaneous tissue. Café au lait spots also occur in Gaucher's disease, ataxia-telangiectasia, tuberous sclerosis, Fanconi's anemia and chronic myelogenous leukemia.

Riccardi, V. M.: Von Recklinghausen neurofibromatosis. N. Engl. J. Med. 305:1617, 1981.

Melanin spots occur on the lips, mouth and fingers in patients with generalized intestinal polyposis (Peutz-Jeghers syndrome). The macules range in size from 0.2 to 5 mm and are light brown to deep blue-black in color.

Acanthosis nigricans, which rarely appears at puberty, is characterized by thickened, reddish-brown or black, verrucous, scaling lesions with small papillomatous tumors in the axillary and inguinal folds, over the nape of the neck and about the nipples. Glucose intolerance and insulin resistence may also be present. Disorders associated with acanthosis nigricans include leprechaunism, lipotrophic diabetes and the type A insulin resistance with hyperandrogenism that has its onset about the time of puberty.

Kahn, C. R., Flier, J. S., Bar, R. S., Archer, J. A., Gorden, P., Martin, M. M., and Roth, J.: The syndromes of insulin resistance and acanthosis nigricans. N. Engl. J. Med. 294:739, 1976.

Dyskeratosis congenita, occurring in males on a familial basis, is usually first manifested by ridging and atrophy of the nails. Reticulated, gray-brown pigmentation of the skin occurs on the face, neck and chest with telangiectasia and atrophy. Hyperhidrosis and hyperkeratosis of the palms and soles, acrocyanosis, oral lesions, sparse hair and hypoplastic anemia are other characteristic features.

Incontinentia pigmenti is characterized in about 80 per cent of cases by the appearance at birth or early in infancy of bullous or vesicular lesions. These may be followed by a keratotic or warty stage and then by the appearance, chiefly over the trunk and extremities, of irregular, sharply outlined, non-elevated brownish or slate-colored areas that simulate the irregular veins present in marble or the splashing or spraying of brown paint on a light-colored surface. The bullous and keratotic stages do not occur in all patients. Other ectodermal anomalies and neurologic disorders may be present.

Hypomelanosis of Ito is characterized by the appearance during infancy of whorled, streaked, speckled and marbled areas of hypopigmentation, most evident with the Wood's light. Central nervous system impairments are frequently associated.

Schwartz, M. D., Esterly, N. B., Fretzin, D. F., Pergamente, E., and Rozenfeld, I. H.: Hypomelanosis of Ito (incontinentia pigmenti achromians): A neurocutaneous syndrome. J. Pediatr. 90:236, 1977.

In *albinism* the skin and hair are devoid of pigment. Partial albinism is characterized by patches of congenital hypopigmentation. A white forelock of depigmented hair may also occur. Partial albinism occurs in the Chédiak-Higashi syndrome.

Vitiligo refers to acquired, white, depigmented areas, encircled at times by a zone of increased pigmentation. The lesions tend to spread. The uveomeningoencephalitic syndrome (*Vogt-Koyanangi-Harada*) may be characterized by vitiligo and loss of hair pigment. Vitiligo also occurs in juvenile diabetes mellitus, sometimes preceding other clinical manifestations, in connective tissue disorders and in ataxia-telangiectasia. *Schmidt's syndrome* consists of vitiligo, thyroiditis, Addison's disease, diabetes and pernicious anemia.

Lerner, A. B., and Nordlund, J. J.: Vitiligo. What is it? Is it important? JAMA 239:1183, 1978.
Macaron, C., et al.: Vitiligo and juvenile diabetes mellitus. Arch. Derm. 113:1515, 1977.

Pityriasis alba, probably a form of atopic dermatitis, is characterized by round or oval patches of depigmentation with fine adherent scales 2 or 3 cm in diameter, present on the face, neck, trunk and extensor surfaces of the upper extremities.

Dull, white, ash leaf macules may be the initial manifestation of *tuberous sclerosis*. These 1- to 3-cm, well-demarcated lesions are round at one end and tapered at the other (lance-ovate). Present at birth or appearing in early infancy, predominantly on the trunk, the lesions may be few or over 100 in number. The Wood's light accentuates the hypopigmentation.

Hurwitz, S., and Braverman, I. M.: White spots in tuberous sclerosis. J. Pediatr. 77:587, 1970.

Areas of pigmentation and hypopigmentation, along with a macular-papular rash and peeling of the skin, occur in patients with *kwashiorkor*.

PIGMENTED NEVI

Junctional nevi, small brown or black lesions, occurring in about 3 per cent of newborn infants, are more commonly noted between three and five years of age. These lesions gradually increase in number until they reach a maximum of 20 to 40 in adolescence.

Giant hairy or bathing trunk nevus may involve 15 to 35 per cent of the skin surface, commonly the trunk, buttocks or an extremity. The nevus is light brown to deep black in color, may contain hairs and warty lesions and has a leathery texture. Malignant melanoma may occur as a complication.

Compound nevi are discrete, hairy, pigmented, usually raised, verrucous or dome-shaped lesions, 2 to several centimeters in diameter, evident at birth or somewhat later.

Spindle and epitheloid nevi generally appear before puberty, usually on the face but at times on the extremities or trunk as 1- to 3-cm dome-shaped lesions that are usually smooth, but occasionally rough, and pink or reddish in color.

Nevus unius lateris (linear nevus) may be present at birth, usually unilaterally, as dark brown papules in longitudinal streaks that tend to become verrucous over time. Mental retardation and seizures are accompanying manifestations.

Nevus linearis sebaceus are slightly raised, yellow-brown, warty lesions, present at birth, occurring partially in a linear distribution over the forehead or body and accompanied, at times, by yellow or dark brown skin plaques. Mental retardation and seizures may be associated findings. The *sebaceous nevus* present at birth or appearing in early infancy on the face or scalp is a waxy orange or orange-brown granular, hairless plaque up to 10 cm in diameter.

Ichthyosis hystrix are light brown or dark gray marbling or brush stroke hyperkeratoses.

Halo nevus refers to a depigmented halo around a nevus that develops in adolescence. Involution of the nevus occurs over time.

Blue nevus, an oval, raised, dome-shaped, usually single, gray or steel blue lesion may occur at birth or in early infancy on the face, hands or extremities.

Malignant melanoma rarely occurs in children.

Esterly, N. B., and Solomon, L. M.: Neonatal dermatology. III. Pigmentary lesions and hemangiomas. J. Pediatr. 81:1003, 1972.

Holden, K. R., and Dekaban, A. S.: Neurological involvement in nevus unius lateris and nevus linearis sebaceus. Neurology 22:879, 1972.

Jacobs, A. H.: Birthmarks: II. Melanocytic and epidermal nevi. Pediatr. Rev. l:47, 1979.

Trozak, D. J., Rowland, W. D., and Hu, F.: Metastatic malignant melanoma in prepubertal children. Pediatrics 55:191, 1975.

Walton, R. G.: Pigmented nevi. Pediatr. Clin. N. Am. 18:897, 1971.

Black heel refers to the benign, linear areas of punctate purple or black pigment that occur on both heels just above the plantar surface owing to capillary leakage of red cells in adolescents who have a history of frequent running on hard surfaces, as in basketball or other sports. The lesion, which at first glance may be mistaken for a melanoma, disappears within a few weeks after interruption of the physical activity.

The *multiple lentigenes (leopard) syndrome* is composed of several defects in addition to the *lentigenes*. These include electrocardiographic conduction defects, ocular hypertelorism, pulmonary stenosis, abnormalities of the genitalia, retardation of growth and deafness. The skin lesions are less than 5 mm in diameter, oval or round dark brown spots that occur anywhere except on the mucosal surfaces but are most concentrated on the neck and upper trunk. Although they may be present at birth, the lesions usually develop between two and five years of age.

Xeroderma pigmentosa may become evident late in infancy as numerous frecklelike lesions, especially prominent on the face, neck and extremities. The skin is abnormally sensitive to sunlight. Atrophic depigmented areas develop, along with scattered telangiectasia and flat verrucous lesions. Superficial ulcerations of the skin, which may appear during the course of the disease, most commonly about the facial orifices, heal with scarring and contractures. In time, malignant epitheliomas develop.

Striae sometimes appear in adolescent children who have gained weight rapidly. These children are usually, but not always obese. The striae may be light pink or white in color. Prominent red or purple striae, perhaps 1/2 inch in width and a few inches in length, may occur in infants and children with Cushing's syndrome, chiefly on the lower part of the abdomen, over the hips, the upper part of the chest and the extremities. Striae may also occur in children treated with corticosteroids.

EDEMA

The discussion here concerns localized edema. Edema as a symptom is discussed in Chapter 56.

In young infants minimal edema may be evident on the dorsum of the hands and feet. Nonpitting edema of the hands and feet may occur in infants with *Turner's syndrome* and occasionally in tetany of the newborn. Facial edema occurs in infants with hypothyroidism. In neonatal myotonic dystrophy, edema may be especially noted on the extremities and head.

Puffiness of the face occurs in patients who have frequent severe paroxysms of coughing owing to pertussis.

Angioedema is discussed on page 409.

With *Schönlein-Henoch purpura*, migratory massive areas of edema, which may involve an extremity, part of the abdominal wall, the face or scalp, may precede the appearance of purpura by one or more days. *Insect bites* on the face or ear often lead to localized edema in infants and children. *Serum sickness* may be characterized by facial or periorbital edema. The lips, tongue, buccal mucous membrane, larynx or external genitalia may also be involved. Edema may be a component of the serum sickness-like reaction that may complicate penicillin administration. Edema, especially of the face, may be a rare side effect of insulin treatment. Presternal edema may occur in patients with mumps, five to eight days after swelling of the salivary glands, especially when the submaxillary glands are involved. Edema of the hands and feet occurs in *Kawasaki disease*.

Doughy edema of the skin is a common manifestation of *dermatomyositis*. The swelling may be either generalized or localized to the lower eyelids and involved areas.

Periorbital edema is common in *acute glomerulonephritis*.

Massive edema of an extremity may occur in infants with osteomyelitis. Painful swelling of an extremity in infants may also be associated with cryofibrinogenemia.

Some patients with paralysis at the thoracic level develop dependent edema of the lower extremities because of impaired lymphatic and venous return. Obesity accentuates this tendency.

The physical findings caused by congenital or acquired *obstruction of the inferior vena cava* depend upon the site. When distal to the hepatic veins, a superficial collateral circulation develops over the lower part of the chest, abdomen and the inguinal regions. The lower extremities may or may not become edematous. Hepatomegaly and ascites develop with obstruction proximal to the hepatic veins. Thrombosis of the inferior vena cava may occur in children with cyanotic congenital heart disease. Patients with Chiari's syndrome or obliterative endophlebitis of the hepatic veins demonstrate hepatomegaly, ascites, abdominal pain and hepatic insufficiency. The superior vena caval syndrome, owing to obstruction of the superior vena cava, may be a complication of surgery for correction of a congenital heart lesion, a lymphoma or mediastinal fibrosis caused by histoplasmosis. Edema is localized to the arms, face and neck. Dyspnea and localized cyanosis or plethora may be evident. Minimal collateral circulation develops when the obstruction is distal to the azygos vein. Obstruction below the azygos vein is followed by a prominent superficial collateral circulation over the chest and abdomen with the blood returning through the inferior vena cava.

Issa, P.Y.: Superior vena caval syndrome in childhood: report of 10 cases and review of the literature. Pediatrics 71:337, 1983.

Edema of the face, including the eyes and lips, may occur in the *Melkersson-Rosenthal* syndrome along with a furrowed tongue and recurrent peripheral facial paralysis.

Myxedema usually is nonpitting. The skin is thickened and puffy.

LYMPHEDEMA

Milroy's disease is an autosomal dominant disorder evident at birth. The edema, which is usually confined to the lower extremities, does not pit except with firm pressure. *Meige's* disease, likewise an autosomal dominant disorder, becomes evident in the first or second decade of life. Lymphangiectatic edema of the hands and feet, pterygium colli and other congenital anomalies may accompany gonadal dysgenesis or Turner's syndrome in infants. Noonan's syndrome may be accompanied by lymphedema.

Lymphedema praecox or *late-onset lymphedema*, a primary disorder of lymphatic drainage of the lower extremities, may appear insidiously at adolescence, usually in girls. Initially the soft and pitting

edema involves the foot or ankle in a buffalo hump configuration, but spares the toes. The swelling at first may be intermittent and subside with rest; however, the edema eventually extends proximally and is nonpitting. The involved skin becomes thickened and has a "pig skin" appearance.

Lewis, J.M., and Wald, E.R.: Lymphedema praecox. J. Pediatr. 104:641, 1984.

One form of hereditary lymphedema in childhood is characterized by *recurrent streptococcal lymphangitis*. Another type is associated with *distichiasis* (extra eyelashes) and a widened spinal canal. In the lymphedema with yellow nails syndrome, the nail deformity may precede the lymphedema by a period of years. The Aagenaes syndrome is characterized by recurrent cholestasis and lymphedema of the lower extremities.

Fonkalsrud, E. W., and Coulson, W. F.: Management of congenital lymphedema in infants and children. Ann. Surg. 177:280, 1973.
Holmes, L. B., Fields, J. P., and Zabriskie, J. B.: Hereditary late-onset lymphedema. Pediatrics 61:575, 1978.
Kleiman, P. K.: Congenital lymphedema and yellow nails. J. Pediat 83:454, 1973.
Robinow, M., Johnson, G. F., and Verhagen, A. D.: Distichiasis lymphedema: A hereditary syndrome of multiple congenital defects. Am. J. Dis. Child. 119:343, 1970.

Most instances of acquired lymphedema are of postinfectious etiology.

Cat-scratch disease may cause secondary lymphedema in an extremity.

Acquired lymphedema involving one lower extremity may be secondary to a pelvic or retroperitoneal neoplasm, retroperitoneal fibrosis, deep calf vein thrombosis or thrombophlebitis.

Peterson, A. S., Besecker, J. A., and Hutchison, W.A.: Retroperitoneal fibrosis and gluteal pain in a child. J. Pediatr. 85:228, 1974.

PURPURA

Purpura refers to hemorrhage into the skin or mucous membranes. Pinpoint or pinhead-sized, scarlet or bluish-purple extravasations of blood are referred to as *petechiae*. Larger areas are usually termed *ecchymoses*. At first the lesions are bluish-purple, and the color does not fade on pressure. With local conversion of the extravasated hemoglobin to hemosiderin, the color gradually changes to brownish-green and then to yellow. Petechiae or larger purpuric spots may first occur about the ankles, wrists and neck folds. *Meningococcemia, Haemophilus influenzae type B bacteremia and meningitis must always be immediately ruled out in patients with unexplained petechiae and purpura, even in the absence of evidence of arthritis or meningitis.* Although the rash of meningococcemia is frequently petechial or purpuric, it may consist only of faint pink macules. Petechiae may also occur in scarlet fever, streptococcal pharyngitis, and echovirus and adenovirus infections. In the Waterhouse-Friderichsen syndrome, the skin may appear mottled, livid or cyanotic. Petechial embolic lesions may be present in patients with subacute bacterial endocarditis.

VanNguyen, Q. V., Nguyen, E. A., and Weiner, L. B.: Incidence of invasive bacterial disease in children with fever and petechiae. Pediatrics 74:77, 1984.

In addition to hemorrhage into the skin, *anaphylactoid or Henoch-Schonlein purpura* may be accompanied by a variety of cutaneous lesions symmetrically distributed over the extensor surfaces of the extremities, the buttocks and the lower back. The lesions may be pink or brownish-red macules or maculopapules, 0.25 to 2 cm in diameter, which may remain small and slightly nodular or coalesce. Hemorrhage commonly occurs into the center of the lesion. The erythema and elevation of the lesions may then disappear. Purpura disappears more slowly over a period of one to two weeks, the color changing gradually from purple to brown to yellow. Urticarial and vesicular lesions, either very small or large and bullous, may precede or accompany the eruption. Hemorrhage may also occur into those lesions that resemble erythema nodosum. The cutaneous lesions tend to occur in crops for several weeks or months. Swelling of the hands, feet and joints and localized angioneurotic edema, especially in the scalp, are often present. The initial findings in Wegener's granulomatosis may simulate Henoch-Schönlein purpura.

Hall, S. L., Miller, L. C., Duggan, E., Mauer, S. M., Beatty, E. C., and Hellerstein, S.: Wegener granulomatosis in pediatric patients. J. Pediatr. 106:739, 1985.

Purpura fulminans (purpura gangrenosa) is characterized by the sudden occurrence and rapid progression of extensive areas of ecchymosis and gangrene usually involving the extremities in a symmetrical fashion. It may be preceded by an infectious disease such as scarlet fever, chickenpox, measles or meningococcemia.

Purpura also occurs in patients with disseminated intravascular coagulation.

Purpuric and seborrheic skin lesions can be almost pathognomonic as manifestations of *histiocytosis X* (Letterer-Siwe disease). Crusted papular lesions occur, along with petechiae and a scaling eruption that resembles seborrheic dermatitis. The scalp, external auditory canals and trunk may be predominantly affected. Infants with *severe combined immunodeficiency* may present with a similar skin rash.

Ecchymotic lesions associated with *erythema multiforme* may simulate bruising owing to physical abuse.

Cryofibrinogenemia may cause localized areas of purpura or severely tender swelling and erythema of the extremities and digits on exposure to cold. These patients are otherwise asymptomatic or only mildly ill.

Ireland, T. A., Werner, D. A., Rietschel, R. L., Patterson, J. H., and Spraker, M. K.: Cutaneous lesions in cryofibrinogenemia. J. Pediatr. 105:67, 1984.

Hyperglobulinemic purpura, owing to sludging, thrombosis and compromise of the microcirculation, may occur with an autoimmune disorder or with chronic infection.

Psychogenic purpura (Gardner-Diamond syndrome) is characterized by the recurrent appearance of bruises in nontraumatized sites. The ecchymotic lesions, often preceded by stinging or burning sensations in the affected area, may be superimposed on an inflamed base or form a ring around a pink area. Bruises may range from 1 to 2 cm to several inches in diameter. Some patients report bleeding through the skin or from hair follicles. Headaches, syncope and abdominal pain may be other complaints. The differential diagnosis includes self-induced or factitial disease in which the patient induces the purpuric lesions.

Ratnoff, O. D.: The psychogenic purpuras: A review of autoerythrocyte sensitization, autosensitization to DNA, "hysterical" and factitial bleeding, and the religious stigmata. Semin. Hematol.. 17:192, 1980.

Tests of capillary fragility permit a crude evaluation of vascular integrity. In the *Rumpel-Leede test* a pressure midway between systolic and diastolic is maintained by a cuff wrapped around the upper arm for 5 to 10 minutes. Five minutes later, the skin distal to the cuff is examined for petechiae.

If none are found, the procedure is repeated on the other arm, using a pressure of 100 mm for 10 minutes. Normally, not more than 15 petechiae appear in a circular area 2 inches in diameter on the flexor surface of the forearm.

PRURITUS

Pruritus may be marked in patients with atopic eczema, the hyper-IgE (Job's) syndrome, contact dermatitis, fiberglass dermatitis, scabies, pediculosis, flea bites, hypervitaminosis A, fungal skin infections, urticaria, neurofibromatosis, Hodgkin's disease, lichen urticaria, dermatitis herpetiformis, photosensitivity, hydroa aestivale, infantile acropustulosis, hyperparathyroidism, chronic renal failure, chronic cholestasis and gypsy-moth-caterpillar dermatitis. *Circumscribed neurodermatitis*, probably produced by chronic pruritus and scratching, occasionally occurs in older children as a sharply defined, slightly raised, lichenified patch. *Skin picking* occurs in most children with the Prader-Willi syndrome.

In factitial dermatitis, scratching and picking at the skin may lead to deep, linear, crusted lesions, most common on the extremities and face, which may heal with scarring.

Spraker, M. K.: Cutaneous artifactual disease: An appeal for help. Pediatr. Clin. North Am. 30:659, 1983.

HEMANGIOMAS

Capillary hemangiomas, which occur commonly in young infants in the form of a *nevus flammeus*, are poorly defined, flat, diffuse, salmon pink to dark blue lesions over the root of the nose, upper eyelids, upper lip and nape of the neck. The lesion blanches upon pressure, is more evident during crying and fades out over time. A prominent nevus flammeus is present in the trisomy 13 and Beckwith syndromes. The *portwine nevus*, another type of capillary hemangioma, is flat and slate or reddish-blue in color. A vascular nevus present on the face over the distribution of the trigeminal nerve may also involve the underlying meninges. Such a facial nevus accompanied by convulsions and intracranial calcifications constitutes the *Sturge-Weber syndrome. Von Hippel-Lindau disease* is characterized by hemangiomas in the skin, retina and cerebellum.

Strawberry capillary hemangiomas are sharply outlined, raised, moderately soft, smooth or irregularly lobulated lesions, a few millimeters to several centimeters in diameter and bright strawberry or raspberry in color. Present at birth or appearing during infancy, the lesions increase in size over a period of 6 to 12 months. Gray patches appear on the hemangioma as the lesion begins to involute. At times, a deep cavernous hemangioma is palpable below and beyond the superficial strawberry nevus.

Cavernous hemangiomas, noted at birth or in early infancy, may be small and localized above or beneath the skin, or deep, diffuse and extensive. Localized hypertrophy of a part of the body may occur in the presence of very large cavernous hemangiomas. Cavernous hemangiomas are usually moderately soft, lobulated and compressible. The overlying skin may appear normal, purplish or cloudy blue in color. *Giant hemangiomas* involve much of an extremity and may be accompanied by thrombocytopenia (Kasabach-Merrit syndrome).

Jacobs, A. H.: Birthmarks: I. Vascular nevi. Pediatr. Rev. 1:21, 1979.

The *Bannavan syndrome* consists of hemangiomas, lipomas, subcutaneous hamartomas and macrocephaly.

Klippel-Trenaunay-Weber syndrome consists of a port-wine nevus with multiple hemangiomas, varicosities and, in some cases, arteriovenous fistulas, hemihypertrophy and localized overgrowth of an extremity, part of the trunk or face.

Angiokeratomas begin to appear between seven and ten years of age on the buttocks, genitalia, lower back, abdomen, umbilicus, and thighs in *Fabry's disease*. The lesions consist of 2- to 4-mm, round, purple or bluish-red and blood-filled macules or papules. Burning, lightening pain, warmth and perspiration occur in the hands and feet, especially the fingers and toes.

The *spider nevus* consists of dilated capillaries that radiate from a slightly raised, pinpoint center. Sites of predilection are the dorsum of the hands and the face. Although spider angiomas may occur in patients with chronic hepatitis, cirrhosis or Wilson's disease, they are without diagnostic significance in children who are otherwise healthy. Groups of dilated capillaries or telangiectasia are commonly present in infants and children, especially on the face, over the nose, below the eyes and over the upper back. These benign lesions, which have a familial predisposition, may simulate spider nevi.

Telangiectasia of the skin and conjunctiva, appearing between two and eight years of age, may be accompanied by ataxia, respiratory disease and other findings in the ataxia-telangiectasia syndrome. The dilated venules are noted initially on the bulbar conjunctiva, followed by telangiectasia on the ears, neck and flexure folds of the extremities.

Telangiectatic erythema of the cheeks, nose, eyelid margins, forehead, ears and extensor surfaces of the forearms and hands occurs in *Bloom's syndrome*, along with photosensitivity and understature. Telangiectasia is also present in the focal dermal hypoplasia syndrome, in moyamoya and in generalized or systemic sclerosis.

LYMPHANGIOMA

Cavernous lymphangiomas or cystic hygromas are soft, boggy, somewhat compressible, poorly demarcated, thin-walled tumors in the skin, subcutaneous or muscle tissue, most commonly occurring in the neck, but also in the tongue and mediastinum.

Lymphangioma circumscriptum consists of closely and irregularly grouped, glistening or crusted, flesh-colored, thick-walled and deep-seated vesicles that contain a colorless liquid. Scattered, raisin-sized, wartlike, brown shiny papules may also occur.

Lymphangiectasias, or enlarged lymph spaces in the subcutaneous tissue, may cause enlargement of an extremity. *Generalized lymphangiectasia* may involve the bone and be accompanied by chylothorax.

PERSPIRATION

Although newborn infants of 36 weeks or more gestation are able to sweat on the first day, visible perspiration usually begins on the face on the third day and on the palms somewhat later, especially in the premature infant. *Hyperhidrosis* persisting for hours or days occurs in both term and premature infants experiencing *narcotic withdrawal*. *Miliaria*, or *heat rash*, is produced by keratinous plugging of sweat glands. Perspiration that occurs about the head and causes moistening of the underlying sheet is not uncommon in normal infants. *Miliaria crystallina*, owing to sweat retention, consists of numerous, fine, pin-head-sized, clear vesicles unaccompanied by inflammatory changes in the skin. *Miliaria rubra* are discrete erythematous papular lesions owing to sweat retention in the dermis.

Excessive and inappropriate perspiration may occur in children who are chronically ill and in patients with cystic fibrosis, hyperthyroidism, pheochromocytoma, vasoactive intestinal peptide-secreting ganglioneuroma or ganglioneuroblastoma, hypoglycemia, familial dysautonomia, Russell-Silver dwarfism, dyskeratosis congenita and febrile illnesses. Night sweats may be reported in patients with Hodgkin's disease. Children with labile vasomotor control become flushed and perspire excessively with little provocation. Increased sweating may occur in infants and children with congestive heart disease or acute respiratory failure.

Excessive sweating of the palms, along with nailbiting and dilatation of the pupils, usually indicates anxiety. Warmth and perspiration of the hands and feet occur in *Fabry's disease*.

Hyperhidrosis of the hands and feet may be accompanied by *dyshidrotic dermatitis (pompholyx)* (see page 178).

"Sweaty sock" dermatitis is caused by hyperhidrosis and wearing socks made of synthetic fibers.

Ectodermal dysplasia of the anhidrotic type is a familial disease characterized by absence of visible perspiration. The skin in the flexural areas and around the base of the nose is dry, thin, white, glossy and eczematoid. Characteristic facies, anodontia, absence or dysplasia of the nails and atrophic rhinitis are other findings.

Absence of sweating below the site of the lesion may follow spinal cord injury.

Congenital sensory neuropathy with anhidrosis is characterized by the absence of sweating and pain.

Although anhidrosis is usually a major manifestation of heat stroke, active sweating may still occur in persons with exertional heat stroke.

SKIN TEXTURE

Tissue turgor and *skin elasticity* are helpful clinical signs in evaluating dehydration. Elasticity, measured by the way in which the pinched abdominal skin snaps back into place, is lost when a 10 per cent (100 mg/kg) volume loss occurs. In these instances, the pinched skin will remain standing in folds. Elasticity is similarly lost with malnutrition in the absence of dehydration. Turgor is determined by pinching the skin to squeeze out the blood and determining the speed at which the color returns. A slow return of color indicates a loss of turgor. In patients with *hypernatremia*, the skin may feel doughy or velvety. The earliest clinical signs of dehydration usually reflect an acute volume loss equivalent to 5 per cent of weight. Babies who have lost 10 per cent of their body weight show early circulatory impairment, while those with 15 per cent loss are in shock and near death.

Finberg, L.: Treatment of dehydration in infancy. Pediatr. Rev. 3:113, 1981.

The skin may be warm and moist in hyperthyroidism and dry, coarse and scaly in hypothyroidism. In dehydrated and malnourished patients the skin is dry.

Premature wrinkling of the skin about the eyes and mouth occurs in older adolescents with pituitary dwarfism.

Thickening and brawny texture of the skin occur in children with Hurler's syndrome. Patients with chronic idiopathic hypoparathyroidism may also have a thickened and roughened skin texture. *Shagreen patches*, may occur with tuberous sclerosis, especially on the face, trunk or lumbosacral area. These patches are raised, flat, light brown or skin-colored, leathery plaques, that simulate sharkskin or demonstrate horizontal wrinkling and range in diameter from a few millimeters to several centimeters.

A collodion-like skin covering may rarely be observed in the newborn. This brownish-yellow, shiny "varnished" appearance may be generalized or localized to the hands and feet. In those with *lamellar desquamation of the newborn*, the skin is normal after desquamation of large sheets is complete. On the other hand, in some infants, collodion skin represents the first manifestation of *sex-linked ichthyosis, bullous or nonbullous congenital ichthyosiform erythroderma* or *lamella ichthyosis*.

All of the ichthyoses are characterized by scaly, desquamating skin. *Ichthyosis vulgaris*, the most common form that is inherited in an autosomal dominant manner, is not usually present in the early months of life. The scales are fine, whitish or brown and occur primarily on the back and other extensor surfaces. Hyperkeratoses may be present on the elbows, knees and ankles. Keratosis pilaris and chapping of hands and feet may be noted. In the other ichthyosiform dermatoses, the scales are large, yellow or dark brown and periodically desquamate. Hyperkeratoses involve portions of the skin, palms and nails. In some of these disorders, redness of the underlying skin

occurs, or crops of large or small bullae that leave a raw surface on rupture develop. The term *harlequin fetus* describes infants with the most severe form of nonbullous congenital ichthyosiform erythroderma characterized by an "O" shaped mouth; diamond-shaped or triangular, hyperkeratotic plaques on the trunk and extremities; and deep fissures.

The *Sjögren-Larsson syndrome* is characterized by nonbullous congenital ichthyosis, spasticity and mental retardation. Ichthyosis also occurs in *Refsum's syndrome*.

Sandberg, N. O.: Lamellar ichthyosis. Pediatr. Rev. 2:213, 1981.

During the winter months, many children show mild dryness and follicular hyperplasia. Too frequent bathing and synthetic clothing finishes may be etiologic.

Vitamin A deficiency results in a dry, scaly, rough skin with "goose pimple" hyperkeratosis over the extensor surfaces of the arms, thighs, shoulders and buttocks and the flexor surfaces of the legs.

Keratosis pilaris, pinhead-sized keratotic papules on the sides of the arms and thighs, occurs, along with dry skin, in atopic dermatitis and ichthyosis. Follicular psoriasis with "horny spikes" may need to be considered in the differential diagnosis.

Keratosis palmaris et plantaris is a rare familial disorder characterized by a yellowish-brown, dry, fissured thickening of the palms and soles. Hyperkeratosis of the palms and soles may be associated with periodontoclasia, which causes premature loss of the deciduous and permanent teeth. Similar involvement of the palms and soles may occur with *pityriasis rubra pilaris, dyskeratosis congenita* and in the *Rothmund-Thomson syndrome*. Thickening of the skin of the palms, soles, elbows and knees may be accompanied by ringlike constrictions of the middle phalanx of the digits and congenital deafness. Hyperkeratosis of the palms and soles accompanied, at times, by bullae, occurs in *pachyonychia congenita*. Palmoplantar keratoderma may be a manifestation of hidrotic ectodermal dysplasia.

Keloid formation with excessive formation of scar tissue may complicate wounds and operative scars.

Seborrheic dermatitis is a moist, greasy, scaly, dirty yellow or yellowish-red crusting eruption ("potato chip" scales) that usually begins over the scalp, chiefly over the anterior fontanel ("cradle cap"), eyebrows, the sternal region, flexural areas and behind the ears. The diaper area and the skin folds are commonly involved. Fissuring or intertrigo in the skin creases is often present. Lesions may also appear on the trunk. Infants with histiocytosis X may have a seborrheic type of dermatitis over the scalp, face, neck and trunk. This brown, scaly, papular and vesicular rash may have both petechial and crusting components. Extensive involvement of the skin with seborrheic dermatitis occurs in *Leiner's disease*.

Leiner's disease, which occurs during the first few months of life, is characterized by severe seborrheic dermatitis, intractable diarrhea, recurrent infections, and failure to thrive. Affected infants have a functional deficiency of C5 or serum opsonic activity.

Jacobs, J. C., and Miller, M. E.: Fatal familial Leiner's disease: A deficiency of the opsonic activity of serum complement. Pediatrics 49:225, 1972.

Cutis laxa may appear at birth or later. The loose but not hyperelastic skin may form large folds of redundant skin that can be drawn out from the body. The neck may appear webbed. The drooping eyelids and cheeks give the patient a bloodhound appearance. Emphysema, which may develop in some patients, is lethal in infancy. Redundant skin occurs in the cartilage hair hypoplasia syndrome.

Sakati, N. O., Nyhan, W. L., Shear, C. S., Kattan, H., Akhtar, M., Bay, C., Jones, K. L., and Schackner, L.: Syndrome of cutis laxa, ligamentous laxity and delayed development. Pediatrics 72:850, 1983.

In *cutis hyperelastica*, a fold of skin may be grasped and stretched several inches. When released, the skin returns without folds. Hyperelasticity may be limited to localized parts of the skin. The mucous membrane of the mouth may also be involved. The thin and fragile skin tends to split with slight trauma. Healing of the resultant gaping wound occurs with shiny, white, wrinkled, thin and, perhaps, pigmented scars that may bulge or balloon out from the skin. Capillary hemorrhage occurs readily in these patients, and large hematomas may develop. These findings are present in the *Ehlers-Danlos syndrome*, along with joint hypermobility and subcutaneous lipomas.

Hollister, D. W.: Heritable disorders of connective tissue: Ehlers-Danlos syndrome. Pediatr. Clin. North Am. 25:575, 1978.
Prockop, D. J., and Kivirikko, K. I.: Heritable diseases of collagen. N. Engl. J. Med. 311:376, 1984.

Calcification may occur in the skin and underlying tissues in cavernous heman-giomas, neonatal subcutaneous fat necrosis, Ehlers-Danlos syndrome, dermatomyositis, other connective tissue disorders and progressive myositis ossificans. Calcinosis of unknown etiology may also appear in clusters, most commonly over the scrotum. Necrosis and ulceration of the skin may follow, with discharge of gritty, chalklike material. *Metastatic calcinosis cutis* may also occur with hyperparathyroidism, hypervitaminosis D and sarcoidosis. Calcinosis of the skin may be manifested by yellow or white specks that are extruded several months following multiple heel sticks in newborns.

Sell, E. J., Hansen, R. C., and Struck-Pierce, S.: Calcified nodules on the heel: A complication of neonatal intensive care. J. Pediatr. 96:473, 1980.

Calcinosis cutis may occur at the sites of EEG electrode placement.

Wiley, H. E. III, and Eaglstein, W.E.: Calcinosis cutis in children following electroencephalography. JAMA 242:455, 1979.

Scleredema adultorum, which usually follows a respiratory infection, is characterized by a hard, nonpitting, induration of the skin first present along the sides of the neck and then extending to the face, scalp, arms, neck and chest. The skin cannot be wrinkled or picked up in a fold. The facial expression may be masklike.

Findings in the Hurler, Hunter, Morquio and Scheie type of mucopolysaccharidoses include thickened, roughened skin and papular or nodular plaques on the trunk and upper extremities. These have an orange peel texture. In the *stiff skin syndrome*, stony-hard, localized lesions develop in the skin, especially over the buttocks and upper thighs, along with mild hirsutism and limitation of joint motion. The dermis contains an abnormal amount of mucopolysaccharide.

Esterly, N. B., and McKusick, V. A.: Stiff skin syndrome. Pediatrics 47:360, 1971.

ATOPIC AND CONTACT DERMATITIS; ECZEMA

Atopic dermatitis in infancy usually begins on the cheeks and forehead, with later involvement of the scalp and the extremities. Eczema rarely appears on the back or the diaper area. The lesions may be acute, exudative, subacute or chronic. These stages may occur sequentially or concurrently in different parts of the body. During the acute phase, a rough, orange-red, glossy erythema of the skin occurs, especially over the cheeks, along with fine scales. This is usually followed by an intensely pruritic, papulovesicular eruption. Itching is always present with atopic dermatitis, while it is often absent or minimal in seborrheic dermatitis. Rupture and coalescence of the minute vesicles produce raw, weeping and crusted lesions. In the subacute stage the weeping lesions begin to dry. Epithelization, thickening and scaling of the skin follow. Scattered symmetrical patches may appear on the trunk and extremities. In older infants and children, thickening, drying and lichenification of the skin occur, with involvement of the wrists, ankles, flexural areas and skin folds and with circumscribed scaly patches. The child scratches and rubs his skin relentlessly. Lighter and darker areas of pigmentation may develop and persist. The eyelids may appear wrinkled. *Keratosis pilaris*, a follicular hyperplasia that gives the skin a plucked-chicken appearance, is a common finding on the trunk, buttocks and extensor surfaces of the extremities in children with atopic dermatitis. Eczema also occurs, at times, in infants with phenylketonuria and in some children with ectodermal dysplasia of the anhidrotic type. Atopic dermatitis with papular and petechial lesions may involve the scalp and trunk in histiocytosis X. Atopic eczema may need to be differentiated from seborrheic dermatitis, and at times, the latter precedes the former. Weeping of the skin and severe or persistent pruritus is, however, more characteristic of atopic dermatitis.

Norins, A. L.: Atopic dermatitis. Pediatr. Clin. North Am. 18:801, 1971.

Kaposi's varicelliform eruption, a vesicular eruption caused by herpes or coxsackie A16 virus, may occur in infants with atopic eczema. The lesions appear in crops for several days and progress through vesiculation, umbilication, rupture and desiccation, with various stages present simultaneously.

The *Wiskott-Aldrich syndrome*, a sex-linked recessive disorder, is characterized by eczematoid dermatitis, draining ears, bloody diarrhea, petechiae and thrombocytopenia. Atopic dermatitis also occurs in patients with other disorders of neutrophil chemotaxis, e.g., the hyper-IgE (Job's) syndrome.

Contact dermatitis may be caused by innumerable substances, including scented or strongly alkaline soaps, skin lotions, cosmetics, wool clothing and plastic toys. Involvement occurs chiefly on the exposed areas of skin, although in reactive persons the eruption may become widespread. Acute involvement is characterized by erythema, edema and vesiculation. The lesion is usually sharply demarcated. Chronic involvement results in drying and lichenification.

Circumoral dermatitis may occur in infants who drool excessively.

Dermatitis venenata, owing to contact with poison ivy or similar agents, is characterized by erythema, edema and an intensely pruritic vesicular eruption over the exposed parts of the body, especially along scratch marks.

Infectious eczematoid dermatitis may result from the irritation produced by the purulent discharge associated with chronic rhinitis, suppurative otitis media and other draining lesions. Occasionally, the term "infectious eczematoid dermatitis" is applied to raised, infiltrated, sharply marginated patches covered with scales, tiny papules, vesicles or a purulent and crusting exudate.

Nummular eczema is characterized by round or oval, discrete plaques, 1/2 to 2 inches in diameter, covered by minute vesicles, exudate and crusts that occur chiefly on the extensor aspects of the extremities.

Gypsy-moth-caterpillar dermatitis, characterized by erythematous blotches, papules and vesiculopapules that appear in late April or May, especially on the extremities, may be caused by contact with airborne moth larvae.

ERUPTIONS IN THE DIAPER AREA

Primary irritant dermatitis is a bright erythematous, glazed or finely wrinkled, parchment-like or papulovesicular eruption with small superficial ulcers over the diaper area, occasionally severe enough to simulate a first-degree burn. Scaling may be noted on the upper thighs. The dermatitis may be limited to sites such as the abdomen and thighs where they are constricted by the diaper. The deep skin folds are usually spared. The eruption is most commonly caused by ammonia and the action of putrefactive bacterial enzymes on urinary amino acids with the production of irritant byproducts. In *noduloulcerative diaper dermatitis*, a few 1- to 3-cm nodules with central erosions occur on the genitalia or anterior thighs.

In *candidal diaper dermatitis*, the characteristic lesions on the glabrous skin begin in or involve the deep creases as small papules, transform into vesicles, and on rupture leave a denuded erythematous patch surrounded by a "white collar." Small patches may fuse into a larger beefy red one with pea- to dime-sized satellite lesions around the periphery. A psoriasiform *id* reaction (napkin psoriasis) may occur. Oral thrush is usually present.

Seborrheic diaper dermatitis usually begins at three or four weeks of age in the inguinal skin creases and then extends to adjacent areas with a beefy-red, sharply demarcated rash. Intertrigo with greasy scales may be noted in other skin folds, along with cradle cap. Small erythematous papules or pustules with peripheral scaling, owing to secondary infection with *Candida albicans*, may occur as satellite lesions. In addition to satellite lesions in the diaper area, other body areas may become affected, especially the flexural creases.

Psoriasis in infants may first present in the diaper region, including the skin folds. "Napkin" psoriasis may also be caused by infection with *Candida albicans*.

Acrodermatitis enteropathica appears in early infancy with erythematous, vesiculobullous, pustular and eczematoid skin lesions around the body orifices, scalp and the distal extremities, along with persistent diarrhea and alopecia. *Zinc deficiency* secondary to prolonged *parenteral* alimentation may cause similar findings.

Sturtevant, F. M.: Zinc deficiency, acrodermatitis enteropathica, optic atrophy, subacute myelooptic neuropathy and 5,7-dihalo-8-quinolinols. Pediatrics 65:610, 1980.

A red, pruritic rash in the perineal area followed by desquamation may be the chief and initial manifestation of *Kawasaki disease*.

Granuloma gluteal infantum appears on the buttocks in infants with diaper dermatitis as firm, reddish-blue oval or round, painless, cherry- or plumsize, slightly protruding nodules up to several centimeters in diameter. Spontaneous resolution occurs slowly.

Jacobs, A. H.: Eruptions in the diaper area. Pediatr. Clin. North Am. 25:209, 1978.
Rasmussen, J. E.: Diaper dermatitis. Pediatr. Rev. 6:77, 1984.

SKIN INFECTIONS

Impetigo contagiosa, usually caused by the *Staphylococcus* or Group A beta hemolytic *Streptococcus*, begins as purulent vesicles, bullae or pustules that rupture quickly

to be followed by the formation of a sticky, purulent honeycomb crust. The staphylococci are more likely to cause bullae, while the streptococci tend to cause crusting. Lesions are most frequent on the hands and lower extremities and around the nose and mouth. Some children have recurrent boils.

Periporitis staphylogenes may be a complication of miliaria owing to infection with the *staphylococcus*. A few or many small to pea-sized papules and pustules occur with a predilection for the scalp, forehead, neck and upper trunk.

Ecthyma is characterized by deep-seated, pustular lesions covered by a thick, sticky crust. The lesions, which may be primary or secondary to scratching in patients with scabies or insect bites, occur most frequently on the lower extremities, the buttocks and the forearms. Healing may be followed by brownish pigmentation or scarring.

Furunculosis, which results from suppuration involving the follicles and sebaceous glands of the skin, is characterized by large, elevated, exquisitely tender, erythematous patches.

Skin abscesses are most commonly caused by *Staphylococcus aureus* and group A *beta-hemolytic streptococci*.

Brook, I.: Aerobic and anerobic bacteriology of cutaneous abscesses in children. Pediatrics 67:891, 1981.

Pyoderma gangrenosum, which begins as a tender erythematous nodule and progresses to a pustule followed rapidly by ulceration and extension of the lesion, occurs in patients with leukemia and inflammatory bowel disease.

Lewis, S. J., Poh-Fitzpatrick, M. B., and Walther, R. R.: Atypical pyoderma gangrenosum with leukemia. JAMA 239:935, 1978.

The cutaneous manifestations of *gonococcemia* are initially maculopapules on an erythematous base. Later, these become painful and hemorrhagic, vesiculopustular or necrotic in the center. The lesions predominantly occur over the distal extremities.

Toxic epidermal necrolysis, or the scalded skin syndrome, owing to coagulase-positive staphylococci, occurs primarily in infants and young children and is characterized by the abrupt onset of diffuse erythema, perhaps with periorbital edema. Exquisite tenderness of the skin is prominent early, and the patient does not want to be touched. Involvement spreads rapidly, followed by loosening and separation of the epidermis and the formation of clear, fluid-containing bullae, which, at times, are very large. The skin is wrinkled and separates in large sheets with slight stroking or trauma (Nikolsky's sign), leaving extensive raw, red and oozing scalded-appearing areas, especially involving the skin folds. Cracks occur in the skin creases, particularly around the eyes and mouth. Healing begins in a week with disappearance of erythema and loss of irritability followed by scaling and desquamation.

A generalized scarlatiniform rash followed by desquamation may also be caused by staphylococci.

Toxic shock syndrome is characterized by fever, syncope, hypotension, myalgia, inflammation of the mucous membranes and a diffuse, evanescent erythema that involves the trunk and extremities. A full-thickness desquamation of the hands and fcct occurs within 7 to 14 days. Hair and nail loss may occur 2 to 3 months later.

Melish, M. E., and Glasgow, L. A.: Staphylococcal scalded skin syndrome: The expanded clinical syndrome. J. Pediatr. 78:958, 1971.
Tofte, R. W.: Toxic shock syndrome: Clinical and laboratory features in 15 patients. Ann. Intern. Med. 94:149, 1981.

Recurrent, severe staphylococcal infections of the skin and subcutaneous tissue, often without local inflammatory signs, occur in several neutrophil disorders, e.g., hyper-IgE (Job's) syndrome, Chédiak-Higashi syndrome and chronic granulomatous disease.

Infections of the skin caused by *pseudomonas* may cause clusters of vesicular lesions that have an inflammatory base and contain an opalescent fluid. These quickly become green, purulent and hemorrhagic blebs that rupture to leave round, indurated, ulcerated areas with necrotic, black centers and bright red areolae (ecthyma gangrenosa). The anogenital region is a common site of involvement. Areas of cellulitis with hemorrhage, necrosis and erythematous or violaceous nodules with or without fluctuation may also occur.

Reed, R. K., Larter, W. E., Sieber, O. F., Jr., and John, T. J.: Peripheral nodular lesions in *Pseudomonas* sepsis: The importance of incision and drainage. J. Pediatr. 88:977, 1976.
Thomas, P., Moore, M., Friedman, S., Decker, J., Shayegani, M., and Martin, K.: Pseudomonas dermatitis associated with a swimming pool. JAMA 253:1156, 1985.

Cellulitis of the face is discussed on page 183.

Herpes simplex infections are discussed on page 178.

The cutaneous manifestations of *tuberculosis* are extremely protean. Primary tuberculous infection of the skin is characterized by a papular, granulomatous or ulcerated lesion ranging in size from a few millimeters up to 2 cm. Scrofuloderma results from involvement of the skin overlying tuberculous lymph nodes or osseous tuberculosis. The cervical region is most frequently involved. Purplish discoloration, thinning and ulceration of the skin are followed by draining sinuses. Lupus vulgaris is a chronic, slowly growing, discrete, tuberculous skin lesion which appears most commonly on the face as a discrete, small, flat, red or brown plaque. The classic apple butter color is noted when pressure is applied with a glass slide. The lesion then becomes elevated and extends peripherally, up to several centimeters, with central clearing. The papulonecrotic type of tuberculid is a superficial, small, red papule that appears acutely in crops, persists for a few weeks and then either disappears or becomes crusted and heals with central umbilication.

Erysipelas occurs as a bright red, hot, slightly elevated lesion over the butterfly area of the face, the genitalia, about the umbilicus or on the hands and feet. The border is usually sharply circumscribed except in infants in whom it may be less well-demarcated. Central clearing and peripheral extension of the lesion occur. Erysipeloid lesions occasionally occur in patients with nephrosis.

Eosinophilic cellulitis, a disorder that may simulatc bacterial cellulitis, is characterized by acute cutaneous swelling without local warmth or tenderness. Eosinophilia occurs in the range of 30 to 50 per cent. Skin biopsy is required for diagnosis.

Blistering distal dactylitis is characterized by a superficial blister over the finger or thumb fat pad that contains thin, white pus.

Hays, G. C., and Mullard, J.E.: Blistering distal dactylitis: A clinically recognizable streptococcal infection. Pediatrics 56:129, 1975.

Human scabies is a diagnostic consideration in patients with chronic, marked pruritus. The lesions consist of tiny, 1- to 2-mm papulovesicles, slightly raised papules or burrows. The burrow is evident in only a minority of patients. Because of scratching and secondary infection, the primary lesions may be obscured by excoriations and pustular, crusted lesions that may be mistaken for infantile eczema. Areas most commonly involved are the flexor surfaces of the wrists, the interdigital spaces, nipples, axillae, groin, umbilicus, the waist, the genitalia in boys and the buttocks. In infants, the palms, soles and sometimes the face are sites of predilection. In many children, pruritic, reddish-brown nodules on the covered parts of the body may persist for months. The diagnosis may be confirmed by scraping the lesion gently with a No. 15 scalpel blade after a drop of mineral oil has been placed on a suspected lesion and examing the scrapings microscopically. *Animal scabies* are usually contracted by young children who have had skin contact with a puppy with mange.

Orkin, M., and Maibach, H. I.: Scabies in children. Pediatr. Clin. North Am. 25:371, 1978.

Myiasis, a tropical disease caused by fly larva that grow subcutaneously and then emerge through the skin, may simulate a boil or cellulitis.

FUNGAL INFECTIONS

Tinea capitis is discussed on page 16.
Tinea corporis begins as small red papules that undergo peripheral spread and central clearing to produce a ringlike effect. Small vesicles or scales may be present about the margin of these circular, pinkish, 1- to 2-cm lesions. Lesions suspected to be tinea should be examined by the Wood's lamp. The etiology may be confirmed by culture and KOH examination.

Tinea versicolor, caused by *Pityrosporum orbiculare,* is characterized by yellowish-brown (either slightly lighter or darker in pigmentation than the surrounding skin), nonpruritic, finely scaling, macular or irregular, sharply demarcated patches. Some large lesions occur over the face, neck, upper part of the back, chest and upper arms in older children and adolescents who perspire profusely. The Wood's light examination demonstrates a gold fluorescence over the involved skin. A KOH preparation demonstrates mycelia.

Tinea cruris is a brownish, erythematous, clearly demarcated lesion over the upper medial surfaces of the thighs usually first noted in adolescent males. Peripheral spreading may extend down the thigh. Central clearing and fine scaling along the border may be present. The scrotum is not affected.

Tinea pedis, or athlete's foot, which usually involves the interdigital spaces, especially between the fourth and fifth toes, may cause the skin to be erythematous, vesicular, scaling, macerated or fissured. Patches of vesicles or thickened, scaly, dry areas may occur on the soles and sides of the feet. Dermatitis involving the top of the toes have a contact or allergic etiology.

Dermatophytids or secondary fungus eruptions consist of pinkish maculopapules; tiny vesicles; or scaly, eczematoid patches on the sides of the fingers, palms, legs and trunk of children with inflammatory tinea infections. Slight pruritus may be present.

Intertriginous candidiasis occurs in the diaper area and skin folds as deeply red, confluent plaques of moist skin with sharply demarcated borders containing vesicopustules. Congenital cutaneous moniliasis may also occur.

Chronic cutaneous candidiasis may occasionally result in hyperkeratoses with hornlike lesions or verrucous plaques on the face and scalp. Chronic mucocutaneous candidiasis may accompany hypoparathyroidism, Addison's disease, multiple endocrinopathies, immunodeficiency disorders, disorders of neutrophil chemotaxis, Hodgkin's disease, sarcoidosis and leukemia.

Schlegel, R. J., et al.: Severe candidiasis associated with thymic dysplasia, IgA deficiency, and plasma antilymphocyte effects. Pediatrics 45:926, 1970.

Congenital cutaneous candidiasis is discussed on page 159.
In patients with *sporotrichosis,* subcutaneous nodules occur in linear distribution along the lymphatics from the primary indolent ulcer at the inoculation site to the enlarged regional lymph nodes. The primary lesion is a firm, painless, red papule that slowly enlarges to a 2- to 4-cm violaceous, ulcerated nodule with an undermined or raised border and crusting. The clinical picture associated with sporotrichosis may be simulated by nocardiosis. *Actinomycosis* may involve the face, neck, or abdomen with hard, nodular masses and sinus tracts that drain yellow granule-containing pus. *Blastomycosis* proceeds slowly from a papular stage to a chronically ulcerated, crusted lesion. Disseminated coccidioidomycosis may cause subcutaneous abscesses.

Easterly, N. B.: Fungal infections in children. Pediatr. Rev. 3:41, 1981.
Lynch, P. J., and Botero, F.: Sporotrichosis in children. Am. J. Dis. Child. 122:325, 1971.

VASCULAR MANIFESTATIONS

Capillary pulsation may be observed in the lips or fingernails of patients with increased pulse pressure.

Livedo reticularis is a reddish-blue mottling or reticular pattern of the skin, chiefly over the extremities and the trunk, most evident on exposure to cold. *Cutis marmorata*, the mildest form of this disorder, occurs transiently in young infants and in some older children. *Cutis marmorata telangiectatica congenita* is a benign condition characterized at birth by a reticular, bluish-red mottled appearance, phlebectasia, telangiectasia and ulceration with crust formation. Macrocephaly, limb asymmetry and delayed development may be associated symptoms. Episodic mottling of the skin may be the first manifestation of hereditary angioedema or of systemic lupus erythematosus. *Acrocyanosis* is a persistent cyanotic discoloration that involves the hands or feet, accompanied perhaps by livedo reticularis.

Kurczynski, T. W.: Hereditary cutis marmorata telangiectatica congenita. Pediatrics 70:52, 1982.

In *familial dysautonomia,* blotching of the skin occurs with crying, eating and excitement. *Blotching* may also occur in patients with congenital sensory neuropathy with anhidrosis and in those with congenital autonomic dysfunction with universal pain loss.

Gangrene, usually of part of an extremity, occurs rarely in infancy owing to severe dehydration, shock, sepsis or arterial needle puncture. The cause is often unknown. Gangrene of the skin may rarely occur with chickenpox, meningococcemia, *Pseudomonas* infection, Rocky Mountain spotted fever and other infectious diseases. Massive areas of gangrene occur in purpura fulminans. Gangrene of gluteal tissues may be a complication of calcium infused through an umbilical artery catheter. Gangrene may also follow peripheral arterial injuries.

Smith, E. W. P., Garson, A., Jr., Boyleston, J. A., Katz, S. L., and Wilfert, C. M.: Varicella gangrenosa due to Group A beta-hemolytic Streptococcus. Pediatrics 57:306, 1976.

Flushing of the skin may occur with psychomotor seizures, hypoglycemia, jimson weed poisoning, migraine and cluster headaches, phencyclidine toxicity and atropine poisoning. Flushing is rarely seen in patients with pheochromocytoma; facial pallor is more commonly encountered. Hot or cold flashes occur in panic attacks.

Acral blanching or *cyanosis* of part of an extremity owing to arterial spasm may be precipitated by arterial puncture or umbilical artery catheterization.

Vascular thrombosis may occur with homocystinuria, with paroxysmal nocturnal hemoglobinuria and in patients receiving corticosteroid therapy.

Pseudophlebitis of the calf may be caused by extension downward into the calf muscles and rupture of a Baker's cyst. Bleeding into the muscles of the calf in Henoch-Schönlein purpura may simulate a deep vein thrombosis. In children, thrombophlebitis is nearly always secondary to intravenous therapy. It may, however, occur with lupus erythematosus. With nonseptic, nonsuppurative thrombophlebitis, findings over the affected vein include pain, redness and tenderness. With infection of an intraluminal clot, a septic, nonsuppurative or a suppurative thrombophlebitis with purulent exudate, periphlebitic abscess and vein necrosis may occur.

Bernstein, M. L., Salusinsky-Sternbach, M., Bellefleur, M., and Esseltine, D. W.: Thrombotic and hemorrhagic complications in children with lupus anticoagulant. Am. J. Dis. Child. 138:1132, 1984.

Kitterman, J. A., Phibbs, R. H., and Tooley, W. H.: Catheterization of umbilical vessels in newborn infants. Pediatr. Clin. North Am. 17:895, 1970.

Sears, N., Grosfeld, J. L., Weber, T. R., and Kleiman, M. B.: Suppurative thrombophlebitis in children. Pediatrics 68:630, 1981.

Wise, R. C., and Todd, J. K.: Spontaneous, lower-extremity venous thrombosis in children. Am. J. Dis. Child. 126:766, 1973.

Disseminated intravascular coagulation, which may occur in a wide variety of disease states, including meningococcemia or Rocky Mountain spotted fever, may cause purpura of the extremities.

Vasculitis involving the skin may be characterized by purpuric papules, hemorrhagic bullae or cutaneous infarcts. Periungal, purpuric lesions owing to vasculitis may occur in patients with systemic lupus erythematosus. *Bacterial* embolization may also cause necrotic skin lesions.

Lakhanpal, S., Conn, D. L., and Lie, J. T.: Clinical and prognostic significance of vasculitis as an early manifestation of connective tissue disease syndromes. Ann. Intern. Med. 101:743, 1984.

Leg ulcers, often just above the medial malleolus, may occur in adolescents with sickle cell anemia.

Brown recluse spider (Loxosceles reclusa) bites produce little immediate reaction; however, in a few hours, intense pain and erythema, at times extensive, and vesiculation occur, along with fever, chills, nausea and vomiting. Acute hemolysis and thrombocytopenia may develop. Necrosis begins at about 24 hours and continues over 5 to 6 days.

Acute necrotizing fasciitis, a serious bacterial infection of subcutaneous tissue and fascial sheaths, may follow a surgical wound, trauma, a circumcision, bacteremia or an abscess. Swelling, edema, erythema, extreme pain and warmth occur over involved areas, usually the trunk or an extremity, followed by purple-black discoloration of the skin, bullae and necrosis. Approximately one-half of the reported cases have occurred in newborn infants.

Wilson, H. D., and Haltalin, K. C.: Acute necrotizing fasciitis in childhood. Am. J. Dis. Child. 125:591, 1973.

Gas gangrene is characterized by crepitance in the affected tissues.

Raynaud's phenomenon is manifested by intermittent, transient bilateral attacks of pallor, cyanosis and, often, erythema of the digits, most commonly the fingers, precipitated by cold or emotional stress. This disorder occurs in systemic lupus erythematosus, dermatomyositis, scleroderma, mixed connective tissue disease, polyarteritis and leukemia.

Redness of the fingers and toes and occasionally of the cheeks and nose may be seen in patients with arterial desaturation. Redness of the fingers and toes is also a nonspecific finding in some intellectually retarded children.

Decubitus ulcers may occur at pressure points in the absence of skin sensation.

Reflex neurovascular dystrophy is characterized by soft tissue swelling or vasomotor instability or both (e.g., mottled bluish or erythematous discoloration, decrease in skin temperature or alteration in perspiration, along with tenderness and pain in an extremity).

ERYTHEMA

Toxic erythema, characterized by blotchy, erythematous areas or a reddish, macular eruption, may occur in patients with pharyngitis, rheumatoid arthritis and other illnesses. A diffuse, erythematous eruption may appear in patients with rat-bite fever.

An evanescent rash is frequently noted in patients with *rheumatoid arthritis* during febrile periods. The lesions are erythematous blotches, salmon pink, discrete, 1 cm or less in diameter, maculopapules that often have a central area of clearing.

In patients with *pellagra,* a symmetrical, erythematous eruption, often accompanied by scaling, bleb formation and pigmentation, occurs over the exposed areas of the body. A pellagra-like rash on skin exposed to sunlight occurs in the Hartnup syndrome along with ataxia and mental retardation.

The lesions of *erythema multiforme* are polymorphous with erythema, macules, papules, vesicles, bullae and wheals. Usually one type of lesion predominates. The papular lesions may show peripheral spread and central clearing. In iris lesions, a purplish center is surrounded by a light red margin; in the cockade lesions, concentric colored rings (red, white and blue) are evident. At times the lesions coalesce, and the aggregate is surrounded by an annular or serpiginous border. Ecchymotic lesions may also occur with a blister in the center of the lesion. Erythema multiforme may be caused by drugs, viral infections (adenovirus 7 and herpes simplex virus 1), connective tissue diseases and malignancies.

Edmond, B. J., Huff, J. C., and Weston, W. L.: Erythema multiforme. Pediatr. Clin. North Am. 30:631, 1983.

In the *Stevens-Johnson syndrome,* or *erythema multiforme exudativum pluriorificialis,* the skin lesions of erythema multiforme are complicated by mucous membrane involvement. Stomatitis and pharyngitis may be accompanied by bullae, ulcers, pseudomembrane formation and hemorrhagic crusting. Mucopurulent conjunctivitis and uveitis may also be present. The anal, vaginal and urethral orifices are involved. Kawasaki disease may have a similar presentation.

Erythema chronicum migrans, a diagnostic feature of *Lyme arthritis,* begins on the proximal portion of an extremity or the trunk, especially the thighs, inguinal or axillary region, as a red macule or papule that enlarges after a few days or weeks to form a large, round ring-like area (5 to 60 cm). The rash often causes a burning sensation and is hot to touch. Its flat outer border is intensely red, and the center of the lesion is indurated and deep red in color. Clearing occurs between these two areas. Subsequent lesions are usually smaller. Fever, systemic symptoms and arthritis may occur concurrently with the rash or the joint manifestations may appear months later.

Berger, B. W.: Erythema chronicum migrans of Lyme disease. Arch. Dermatol. 120:1017, 1984.
Steere, A. C., et al.: The early clinical manifestations of Lyme disease. Ann. Intern. Med. 99:76, 1983.

Erythema nodosum is characterized by crops of painful, tender, firm, raised, yet deep-seated, round or oval subcutaneous nodules 2 to 4 cm in diameter. Most commonly, lesions occur over the anterior thighs and tibiae, but they may also appear on the extensor aspects of the arms, the lateral aspect of the thighs and elsewhere. The overlying skin is tense and, at first, bright red. In a few days these areas become lusterless and change first to a bluish-purple and then to a reddish-brown color. Erythema nodosum may occur in patients with a streptococcal infection; viral infection, including herpes simplex; tuberculosis; sarcoidosis; coccidioidomycosis; blastomycosis; lupus erythematosus; cat-scratch disease; cystic fibrosis; inflammatory bowel disease; histoplasmosis; chronic aggressive hepatitis; tinea capitis; Behçet's syndrome; *yersinia enterocolitica* infection; and, rarely, in rheumatic fever.

Kawasaki disease is characterized by fever of one to two weeks' duration, conjunctivitis, erythema of the lips and mouth, a "strawberry" tongue and cervical lymphadenopathy. An erythematous macular or maculopapular rash appears on the third to fifth day. In some patients the exanthem is pruritic and urticaria-like or consists of large, irregularly shaped plaques. Occasionally, the lesions have an erythema multiforme-like appearance. Intense purple-red discoloration of the palms and soles and firm, indurative swelling of the hands, feet, fingers and toes is followed in 10 to 14 days by desquamation in the form of a cast that begins at the juncture of the nails and skin at the tips of the toes and fingers.

Melish, M. E.: Kawasaki syndrome: An update (the mucocutaneous lymph node syndrome). Pediatr. Ann. 11:2, 1982.

Erythromelalgia is characterized by intermittent episodes of redness, increased skin temperature and burning pain involving the extremities, usually the fingers and toes or hands and feet.

Mandell, F., Folkman, J., and Matsumoto, S.: Erythromelalgia. Pediatrics 59:45, 1977.

Palmar erythema may occur with chronic liver disease.

Tache cérébrale, a dermatographic streak observed after drawing a fingernail or other sharp object across the skin, may be elicited in patients with encephalitis, meningitis and other acute central nervous system inflammatory diseases.

Photosensitivity on exposure to sun or ultraviolet light may be caused by systemic drugs, (e.g., phenothiazine), topical agents (e.g., perfumes and cosmetics), photoallergy (e.g., deodorant soaps) and biochemical disorders (e.g., porphyrias and genetic diseases

such as Bloom's syndrome). Symptoms include erythema, edema, blistering, burning, itching, vesiculation, weeping, eczema and crusting.

Ramsay, C. A.: Photosensitivity in children. Pediatr. Clin. North Am. 30:687, 1983.

Erythropoietic porphyria is characterized by severe photosensitivity. Erythema is followed by vesicles, bullae and weeping lesions on exposed areas with pigmented scars on healing. *Erythropoietic protoporphyria* is characterized by intense burning and itching on exposure to ultraviolet light. Severe erythema, edema, vesicles and bullae develop. Thickening, scaling and scarring occur over time. *Hepatic porphyria* may be accompanied by abdominal, neurologic and hematologic symptoms. *Porphyria cutanea tarda*, a hepatic porphyria, is characterized by increased fragility of the skin, bullae, hypertrichosis, hyperpigmentation and sclerodermoid changes.

DeLeo, V., Poh-Fitzpatrick, M., Mathews-Roth, M., and Harber, L.: Erythropoietic protoporphyria. Am. J. Med. 60:8, 1976.

Grossman, M. E., Bickers, D. R., Poh-Fitzpatrick, M., DeLeo, V. A., and Harber, L. C.: Porphyria cutanea tarda. Clinical features and laboratory findings in 40 patients. Am. J. Med. 67:277, 1979.

Ampicillin may cause a dull red, slightly pruritic, macular or maculopapular rash, especially in patients with infectious mononucleosis. The rash appears first on the trunk and then spreads peripherally to involve the face and the extremities.

Kraemer, M. J., and Smith, A. L.: Rashes with ampicillin. Pediatr. Rev. 1:197, 1980.

The *Cockayne syndrome* is characterized by microcephaly, large ears and nose, sunken eyes, mental retardation, dwarfism and photosensitivity. Sensitivity to sunlight also occurs in the Rothmund-Thomson and Bloom's syndromes.

Schmickel, R. D., Chu, E. H. Y., Trosko, J. E., and Chang, C. C.: Cockayne syndrome: A cellular sensitivity to ultraviolet light. Pediatrics 60:135, 1977.

Although *rheumatic erythemas* occur chiefly with rheumatic fever, they represent a "toxic" reaction rather than being pathognomonic for rheumatic activity. Erythematous papules are discrete, dull, red lesions, usually 2 to 4 mm in diameter, which appear transiently for a few hours or days in some patients with rheumatic fever. Most frequent about the joints and on extensor surfaces, the eruption may occur in crops. At times, it has an urticarial as well as a papular component. *Erythema marginatum* is characterized by transient, annular, erythematous patches with raised, dull red, discrete edges and brownish, flat centers. The lesions usually appear on the trunk but are occasionally also present on the extremities. Characteristically, the lesions vary widely in size, with some lesions many inches in diameter. Coalescence may occur with the formation of polycyclic forms. A brownish pigmentation of the skin may persist after the lesions fade. An erythema marginatum–like rash may occur in some patients with Kawasaki disease. *Erythema annulare* is similar to erythema marginatum except that the lesions are flat, undergo rapid change in form and recur frequently. When erythema annulare occurs in the newborn, *lupus erythematosus* should be suspected in the mother.

Watson, R. M., Lane, A. T., Barnett, N. K., Bias, W. B., Arnett, F. C., and Provost, T. T.: Neonatal lupus erythematosus. Medicine 63:362, 1984.

OTHER PAPULAR LESIONS

The lesions of *molluscum contagiosum* are shiny, pearly white, firm, rounded papules that range in size from 2 to 5 mm. They have a central umbilication from which a white, cheesy material can be extruded upon pressure.

Papular urticaria usually occurs during the spring and summer. The lesions are small, indurated, intensely pruritic, pale red papules, 3 to 10 mm in diameter, distributed chiefly over the extensor surface of the extremities, the buttocks, face and neck. Initially, the lesions have a vesicular component. Later, secondary infection, crusting and pigmentation may be noted. The lesions often persist for weeks, and recurrences are frequent. Papular urticaria may be caused by enteroviruses and insect bites.

The *Gianotti-Crosti syndrome*, or *papular acrodermatitis*, which occurs especially in young children, consists of crops of erythematous papules. The papules are usually large, nonpruritic and, at times, hemorrhagic and infiltrative, and they occur on the face, extremities, palms, soles, buttocks and back. The lesions, which persist for two to eight weeks, become confluent with the formation of plaques of flat-topped papules. Generalized lymphadenopathy and some hepatomegaly persist for up to three months. This disorder is often associated with the hepatitis B virus but papular acrodermatitis may have other etiologies.

Rubenstein, D., Esterly, N. B., and Fretzin, D.: The Gianotti-Crosti syndrome. Pediatrics 61:433, 1978.

Granuloma annulare is characterized by deep-seated waxy, whitish or pinkish, flat-topped papules arranged in a raised circle about 1 inch or more in diameter or in a crescent around a center that is clear, erythematous or atrophic. Sites of predilection include the sides of the fingers, the dorsum of the hands or feet, the knees and the buttocks.

Insect bites are common over exposed skin. Examination usually reveals a small punctum or elevation in the center of the lesion. Lesions are usually grouped, and localized edema may occur. Flea bites are especially likely to produce pruritic papules about the ankles. Insect stings may produce a localized reaction, extensive in some cases, consisting of pain, redness and swelling.

Fire ant bites are followed immediately by a wheal and flare ranging in size from 1 mm up to 10 cm. Several hours later, vesiculation develops at the site, surrounded by marked erythema and edema.

Ginsburg, C. M.: Fire ant envenomation in children. Pediatrics 73:689, 1984.

The lesions associated with *pityriasis rosea* are salmon-pink, irregular, maculopapular, oval patches usually distributed along lines of cleavage, especially over the covered part of the body, the trunk, proximal portions of the extremities, and the scalp. Individual lesions are 1/2 to 1 1/2 inches in diameter and characterized by a yellowish-brown central clearing ("crinkly cigarette paper center"). Thin, flaky scales are attached along the peripheral border of the lesions. The generalized eruption consists of about 100 lesions, with new patches continuing to appear over a five or six week period. The rash is usually preceded by a period of 10 days by one or more "herald" patches—annular or oval lesions, 1/2 to 2 inches in diameter with no raised border or central clearing. Rarely, the rash may be hemorrhagic.

Psoriasis is characterized by sharply defined, round or oval, elevated plaques in which the primary lesion is an erythematous papule covered by a shiny silvery or mica scale. Bleeding points may be noted on removal of the scale. The lesions coalesce to form plaques up to several centimeters in diameter with discrete borders. Although psoriasis may appear anywhere, the sites of predilection are the scalp, elbows, knees and the presacral and intergluteal regions. Acute *guttate psoriasis* may appear suddenly as 2-mm to 1-cm teardrop-shaped macules that occur principally over the trunk and proximal extremities but spare the face. A streptococcal pharyngitis precedes the eruption in many cases. Pitting of the fingernails may be noted. When it occurs in the diaper area, psoriasis has an eczematous appearance. Differentiation between seborrheic dermatitis, pityriasis rosea and psoriasis may be difficult.

Watson, W., and Farber, E. M.: Psoriasis in childhood. Pediatr. Clin. North Am. 18:875, 1971.

Pityriasis rubra pilaris, which may be mistaken for seborrheic dermatitis or psoriasis, is characterized by orange to deep red, very dry papular lesions that give a grater sensation on stroking the skin. Patches of yellowish scales occur on the face, knees, elbows, wrists and buttocks. Palmar and plantar hyperkeratosis also occurs.

Huntley, C. C.: Pityriasis rubra pilaris. Am. J. Dis. Child. 122:22, 1971.

VESICLES AND VESICOPUSTULES

Urticaria may occur either as white, pink or red macular wheals or as edematous, vesicular lesions that have pseudopodia and, in some cases, an erythematous flare. The lesions, which range from several millimeters to over an inch in diameter, may be present for only a few minutes or may persist for hours. Pruritus may be intense. Chronic urticaria may occur in systemic lupus erythematosus. Medications such as ampicillin, foods, salicylates, soaps, or detergents may be etiologic. Acute urticaria may be caused by viral infections (Epstein-Barr, enterovirus, mumps, hepatitis B) or streptococcal infections.

Schuller, D. E., and Elvey, S. M.: Acute urticaria associated with streptococcal infection. Pediatrics 65:592, 1980.

Cold urticaria, which occurs on exposure to cold, may be an inherited trait or a manifestation of a connective tissue disease, cold hemolysins, cryoglobulinemia, cryofibrinogenemia or a viral illness such as infectious mononucleosis.

Cholinergic urticaria occurs with exertion, fever, or a warm bath or shower.

Twarog, F. J.: Urticaria in childhood: Pathogenesis and management. Pediatr. Clin. North Am. 30:887, 1983.

Urticaria pigmentosa begins in infancy as red, urticarial, macular or papular lesions, 1/2 to 1 inch in diameter, which gradually change to a yellowish-red or deep brown color and become predominantly macular. Thirty or forty lesions may be present or they may involve the skin more generally. Wheals or bullae may appear when the macular lesions are stroked with a tongue blade. Vesicular and bullous lesions may also occur spontaneously. Dermatographia may be noted. The eruption tends to disappear at puberty. Urticaria pigmentosa may be associated with generalized mast cell infiltration.

Dyshidrotic dermatitis or pompholyx consists of tiny, deep, slightly pruritic vesicles that seem to be embedded in the palms and along the lateral aspects of the fingers and the feet. Excessive palmar perspiration is common.

Palmoplantar pustulosis may be associated with chronic, recurrent multifocal osteomyelitis.

Björksten, B., Gustavson, H-H, Erikson, B., Lindholm, A, and Nordström, S.: Chronic recurrent multifocal osteomyelitis and pustulosis palmoplantaris. J. Pediatr. 93:227, 1978.

Epidermolysis bullosa is characterized by bullae and large vesicles that appear spontaneously or secondary to slight trauma. In the simple form the lesions occur chiefly on the hands and feet, and healing proceeds without scarring. The dystrophic form is characterized by involvement of the mucous membranes and by large bullae. Epidermolysis bullosa hereditaria letalis is a progressive disorder that usually leads to early death. Rupture of the bullae, some of which are hemorrhagic, produces a raw surface that may be extensive. Healing occurs with scar formation. The nails may be lost, and secondary infection of the skin becomes a major problem. Epidermolysis bullosa in the newborn must be differentiated from bullous impetigo.

Herpes simplex occurs on the lips as single or grouped lesions, but may involve the skin elsewhere, either as a complication of eczema or as a primary skin infection. The herpes lesion usually begins as an erythematous macule, rapidly becomes papular and is capped by a minute, painful vesicle.

Crusting and secondary infection may follow rupture of the vesicle. In generalized skin infections, the lesions appear in crops for eight to nine days.

Herpes zoster begins as erythematous, papular and sometimes painful patches over the cutaneous distribution of cranial and spinal nerves. Vesicular lesions then develop to be followed by crusting.

Feldman, S., Hughes, W. T., and Kim, H. Y.: Herpes zoster in children with cancer. Am. J. Dis. Child. 126:178, 1973.

Rogers, R. S., III, and Tindall, J. P.: Herpes zoster in children. Arch. Dermatol. 106:204, 1972.

Hydroa aestivale is a rare eruption that begins in late infancy or early childhood. Photosensitivity of the skin to sunlight is present, and lesions recur throughout the summer. Remissions occur in winter and usually after puberty. Lesions, which are preceded by pruritus, begin as small reddish macules that become vesiculated, last for a few days and then become crusted. After separation of the crusts, a pigmented, pitlike scar remains. Involvement is confined to exposed surfaces such as the face and hands. Many of these patients have congenital porphyria.

Dermatitis herpetiformis is a rare skin disease in childhood characterized by frequent relapses and remissions. The eruption, which may be polymorphous but is usually bullous or papulovesicular, may persist for two or three months at a time. Lesions may be confined to the extensor surface or forearms and hands or be generally and symmetrically distributed over the extremities, trunk, buttocks and perineum. The bullous or vesicular lesions appear suddenly, usually on the trunk, pelvis and thighs. Clear and tense, and ranging in size from 0.5 to 2 to 4 cm or more, they may be confluent, grouped like herpetic lesions, or arranged in an annular fashion. Rupture of the lesions eventually occurs, leaving a raw surface that may become excoriated, crusted and secondarily infected. The papulovesicular lesions usually occur on the elbows, knees and thighs. The maculopapular lesions may demonstrate peripheral spreading with central clearing. Pruritus may be absent or mild in the bullous form and severe with a burning quality in the papulovesicular type. Healing may be followed by pigmentation of the skin. Gluten-induced enteropathy may be an associated finding.

Bean, S. F., Jordon, R. E., Winkelmann, R. K., and Good, R. A.: Chronic nonhereditary blistering disease in children. Am. J. Dis. Child. 122:137, 1971.

Hertz, K. C., Katz, S. I., and Aaronson, C.: Juvenile dermatitis herpetiformis. Pediatrics 59:945, 1977.

Acropustulosis, which occurs predominantly in black infants and begins usually between two and ten months of age, is characterized by intensely pruritic, erythematous, 1- to 4-mm papules that progress within 24 hours to vesiculopustules and crusted lesions predominantly on the hands, palms, feet, soles and trunk. The eruption has a duration of 7 to 10 days and recurs over a period of several months with remissions lasting two to three weeks.

Esterly, N. B.: Infantile acropustulosis and granuloma gluteal infantum. Pediatr. Rev. 5:59, 1983.

NODULES, PLAQUES AND TUMORS

Subcutaneous nodules (antigen cysts) may occur after routine immunization. Subcutaneous nodules also occur with *rheumatic fever* and *rheumatoid arthritis*. Those associated with rheumatic fever persist for a much shorter time. The oval, hard nodules are about 1/4 inch in diameter or smaller, with those in rheumatoid arthritis usually slightly larger than those of rheumatic fever. The nodules may appear in crops in the scalp, especially over the occiput; the scapulae; the spinous processes of the vertebral column; elbows; malleoli; patellae; and the dorsa of the hands and feet. Since they are deep in the subcutaneous tissue, the nodules may be more easily palpated than seen, but they become apparent if the overlying skin is made taut.

Benign rheumatic nodules in the subcutaneous tissues on the scalp, face, feet and elsewhere or over fascia or tendons may represent an unusual reaction to trauma.

Simons, F. E. R., and Schaller, J. G.: Benign rheumatoid nodules. Pediatrics 56:29, 1975.

Mucopolysaccharide infiltration may cause subcutaneous nodules in *Hunter's syndrome*.

Subcutaneous nodules are present in *disseminated lipogranulomatosis*.

Sporotrichosis may be characterized by nodules in a linear distribution along the lymphatics draining from the inoculation ulcer to the regional lymph nodes.

Extremely tender, indurated and erythematous subcutaneous nodules, occurring in crops, may present on the soles of the feet, calves and pretibial surfaces in patients with *periarteritis nodosa*. Fever and other systemic symptoms may be present.

Magilavy, D. B., Petty, R. E., Cassidy, J. T., and Sullivan, D. B.: A syndrome of childhood polyarteritis. J. Pediatr. 91:25, 1977.

Lymphosarcoma involving the skin and scalp may appear as pinkish or purplish plaques.

The lesions of *leukemia cutis*, appearing most commonly about the eyes or elsewhere on the face, may be small or moderate-sized, discrete or confluent, livid red or purple papules and plaques.

Acute febrile neutrophilic dermatosis (Sweet's syndrome) is characterized by painful, erythematous plaques, 0.5 to 4 cm in diameter, most common on the face and extremities. The lesions may have an annular appearance with a sharply defined papulovesicular border and central clearing or crusting. The disorder may persist for several months. Spiking fever and a neutrophilic leukocytosis also occur. Sweet's syndrome may precede or follow other manifestations of acute myelogenous leukemia.

Levin, D. L., Esterly, N. B., Herman, J. J., and Boxall, L. B. H.: The Sweet syndrome in children. J. Pediatr. 99:73, 1981.

Mucosal neuromas, white nodules that appear on the anterior tongue, palpebral conjunctiva or commissures of the lips along with a characteristic facies occur in the syndrome of *multiple mucosal neuromas and medullary thyroid carcinoma*.

Brown, R. S., Colle, E., and Tashsian, A. H.: The syndrome of multiple mucosal neuromas and medullary thyroid carcinoma in childhood. J. Pediatr. 86:77, 1975.

The *Gardner syndrome* consists of multiple soft tissue tumors, including cysts, lipomas, fibromas and bone tumors, usually involving the mandible. Intestinal polyps, if present, may undergo malignant change.

The nevoid basal cell carcinoma syndrome consists of cutaneous tumors, skeletal anomalies and cysts of the jaw. The nevoid basal cell cancers appear in the first years of life, usually in crops of flesh-colored or pigmented papules. The face is the most frequent site, especially around the eyes, the eyelids, the nose, the malar region and upper lid. The trunk and upper extremities may also be involved. Tiny pits, which are pathognomonic for this syndrome, appear on the hands and feet in young adults.

Juvenile fibromatosis is the general designation given to connective tissue tumors that may appear as localized soft tissue masses in or about the muscles, especially of the neck or extremities, or as more generalized involvement. In *juvenile aponeurotic fibroma*, small to moderate-sized, poorly marginated tumors may gradually develop on the hand, wrist, or sole of a young child. *Recurring digital fibrous tumors* are smooth, dome-shaped, nodules on the distal extensor surface of a digit.

Beckett, J. H., and Jacobs, A. H.: Recurring digital fibrous tumors of childhood: A review. Pediatrics 59:401, 1977.
Sprecht, E. E., and Konkin, L. A.: Juvenile aponeurotic fibroma. JAMA 234:626, 1975.

Porokeratosis, a heritable disease, causes keratotic lesions arranged in an interrupted linear fashion on an extremity. The eruption consists of hyperpigmented, scaling plaques with central clearing and a peripheral, fine keratinous ridge.

Cox, G. F., and Jarratt, M.: Linear porokeratosis and other linear cutaneous eruptions of childhood. Am. J. Dis. Child. 133:1258, 1979.

Nodular panniculitis, characterized by firm, usually pruritic and tender subcutaneous nodules, may develop after massive corticosteroid therapy.

Relapsing, nodular, febrile panniculitis (Weber-Christian disease) is characterized by a chronic febrile course with recurrent crops of elevated, sometimes tender, nodular subcutaneous lesions that range in diameter from 0.5 to 10 cm. The overlying skin may be either erythematous or normal. The lesions disappear slowly, followed by atrophy of the subcutaneous tissue and, at times, by pigmentation.

SARCOIDOSIS

The cutaneous manifestations of sarcoidosis include papules, nodules and plaques. The papules, which are the most common lesion, are usually small, firm but elastic, well-circumscribed and round or oval. They may be brown, bluish or yellowish-red. Lesions may range in number from few to many. Sites of predilection include the face, especially about the eyelids and nose, the neck, shoulders and back, and the extensor aspects of the arms. The surface of the lesions may be smooth and covered by delicate telangiectasia or by small scabs.

XANTHOMAS

Xanthomatous lesions may appear as yellow, orange or brownish-red papules, plaques, nodules, striae or pigmentation.

Xanthoma disseminatum (juvenile xanthogranuloma) occurs predominantly in infants, especially over the trunk, face, scalp, axillary and inguinal folds and the mucous membranes. Individual lesions, which may number over 100, are bright orange, reddish-yellow or golden brown discrete macules or papules that range in size from pinhead to several millimeters. The lesions are usually benign and spontaneously disappear.

Xanthoma tuberosum or planum is associated with hypercholesterolemia. Close relatives often have hypercholesterolemia, if not xanthomatous lesions. The lesions, which are usually large, brownish-yellow or golden papules, nodules, infiltrated plaques or yellow striae, are most frequently distributed over the extensor surfaces and about the large joints. Areas of predilection include elbows, knees, hip, heels, palms and knuckles. Tendons may also be involved.

Primary type I hyperlipoproteinemia is often characterized in infancy by crops of xanthomas. In the type II homozygote, xanthomas often occur at birth or a few years later.

Xanthomatous lesions may appear transiently in disease states characterized by prolonged hyperlipemia. The xanthomas are small, reddish-yellow or orange papules or plaques that occur especially on the extensor aspects of the extremities and on the palms and soles.

West, R. J., and Lloyd, J. K.: Hypercholesterolemia in childhood. Adv. Pediatr. 26:1, 1979.

COLLAGEN-VASCULAR AND CONNECTIVE TISSUE DISEASES

Lupus erythematosus most commonly involves the butterfly area of the face, over the cheeks and across the nose, with well-circumscribed, maculopapular, violaceous or reddish-brown patches ranging from 1/4 to 1/2 inch in diameter. Thin, whitish scales may adhere to the lesions. Erythema, edema and capillary telangiectases may occur over the involved areas. Lesions may also occur along the nails and on the palms and other exposed parts. Bullae may appear if inflammatory changes are severe. Although some lesions recede rapidly and without residua,

more persistent ones result in local atrophy and pigmentation. Photosensitivity or Raynaud's phenomenon may be reported. A few patients with systemic lupus erythematosus do not develop skin manifestations. *Discoid lupus erythematosus*, characterized by red, elevated, indurated lesions on the face and exposed areas often followed by scarring, is not accompanied by systemic manifestations. *Neonatal lupus erythematosus* is discussed on page 160.

Patients with *rheumatoid arthritis* often have widespread, blotchy erythematous lesions or a migratory, reddish macular eruption that may be pruritic. *Koebner's phenomenon* in these patients may be evoked by scratching the skin; maculopapules appear along the scratch mark several minutes later.

The skin eruption associated with *serum sickness* may be characterized by dermatographia, pruritus and urticarial wheals. Occasionally, the skin manifestations may be erythematous, morbilliform, scarlatiniform or purpuric. Angioedema may also occur.

Dermatomyositis may be accompanied by a variety of skin manifestations, including erythema and morbilliform, purpuric or urticarial lesions. Brawny induration or doughy edema is common. A dull red or deep crimson (heliotrope) color and scaling dermatitis may be present on the upper eyelids, along with periorbital edema. An erythematous, scaling dermatitis and telangiectasia over the knees, elbows, knuckles, interphalangeal joints (Gottron's sign) and malar prominences is virtually pathognomonic. Generalized edema may occur in some children. As the disease progresses, the tight, glossy and bound-down skin gives an indurated, thickened and leathery feel. The skin breaks down easily, and atrophy of the involved skin may occur with calcification of the subcutaneous tissue. Gritty calcium deposits may occasionally extrude through the skin. Joint contractures may occur over time.

In *periarteritis nodosa*, presenting symptoms may be subcutaneous nodules, calf pain and spiking fever.

Systemic sclerosis or scleroderma may be *systemic* or *localized*. In the former, rare before puberty, the involvement may affect the distal extremities especially the fingers or face (*acrosclerosis*), with loss of subcutaneous tissue; or, the involvement may be more diffuse with bound-down, tight, shiny and indurated skin that is not sharply demarcated from normal tissues. Raynaud's phenomenon may be the presenting complaint. Dysphagia may occur owing to esophageal involvement.

Focal scleroderma occurs, often unilaterally, as sharply demarcated, indurated, shiny plaques (*morphea*) or linear bands (linear scleroderma). The underlying subcutaneous tissue, muscle and bone may undergo atrophy. Arthralgia, stiffness and flexion contractures may occur. The lesions are usually white or flesh-colored, but they may also be yellow-brown and have a violaceous edge. The term *coup de sabre* is applied to lesions that involve the scalp or face.

Tuffanelli, D. L., and LaPerriere, R.: Connective tissue diseases. Pediatr. Clin. North Am. 18:925, 1971.

Eosinophilic fasciitis is characterized by an acute onset, often after strenuous physical exertion, of thickened, bound-down, scleroderma-like subepidermal tissue over the distal extremities, along with arthralgia and stiffness of the metacarpophalangeal joints with flexion contractures of the hands and fingers. Initially tender to touch, the skin later may have a puckered orange peel appearance. Laboratory examination demonstrates hypergammaglobulinemia and eosinophilia.

Britt, W. J., Duray, P. H., Dahl, M. V., and Goltz, R. W.: Diffuse fasciitis with eosinophilia: A steroid-responsive variant of scleroderma. J. Pediatr. 97:432, 1980.

SUBCUTANEOUS TISSUE

The thickness of the skin and subcutaneous tissue may serve as an index of nutrition. Except for premature infants, well-nourished infants have a firm layer of subcutaneous fat with bony landmarks such as the ribs, clavicles, scapulae and the interspaces of the chest that are not prominent on inspection.

Partial or progressive lipodystrophy is a disorder in which subcutaneous fat is gradually lost from the upper half of the body, especially from the cheeks, while the lower half of the body remains normal or becomes obese. Renal disease occurs commonly in these patients.

Total lipodystrophy or *lipoatrophy* is characterized by generalized loss of subcutaneous fat, present at birth or appearing later, hyperglycemia, hepatomegaly, hyperlipemia, hirsutism, hyperpigmentation or acanthosis nigricans, prominent muscles, increased stature, advanced bone age, en-

larged genitalia, renal and central nervous system disorders, and insulin-resistent hyperglycemia. In the congenital form, patients may have an acromegalic appearance with large hands and feet.

Huseman, C., Johanson, A., Varma, M., and Blizzard, R. M.: Congenital lipodystrophy: An endocrine study in three siblings. I. Disorders of carbohydrate metabolism. J. Pediatr. 93:221, 1978.

Insulin atrophy with loss of subcutaneous adipose tissue or local subcutaneous fat hypertrophy may occur at sites of insulin injection. Thickened, waxy, bound-down skin may be present over the dorsal aspect of the hands.

Lupus profundus, a nonsuppurative panniculitis, may cause induration of the subcutaneous tissue in patients with lupus erythematosus.

Cold panniculitis, characterized by tender, slightly reddened, disclike subcutaneous lesions, usually involving the cheeks or submental region, may occur on exposure to severely cold weather.

Patients with *progeria* have little subcutaneous fat.

Subcutaneous plaques and calcification of tendons may occur in *pseudohypoparathyroidism*.

Subcutaneous emphysema secondary to mediastinal emphysema or pneumothorax produces a crinkling, crepitant and crunching sensation on palpation of the skin. Involvement may include the neck, the upper thorax, the axillae and, at times, the trunk and genitalia.

Gas gangrene causes crepitation in the tissues.

SOME LESIONS FOUND ON THE FACE

Adenoma sebaceum consists of shiny, waxy, skin-colored, discrete or grouped papules, 2 to 6 mm in diameter, or red, seed-like lesions distributed over the butterfly area of the face and chin, sometimes accompanied by telangiectasia. This manifestation may not appear until late childhood. Adenoma sebaceum, mental retardation, sexual precocity and convulsions occur in *tuberous sclerosis*. A patch of dark, thickened, shark-like skin (shagreen patch) may be present over the lumbosacral area or elsewhere.

Acne is a common problem in adolescents. Preadolescent acne may occur with the adrenogenital syndrome. The openings of the

skin follicles may appear enlarged. Comedones or "blackheads" are frequently associated findings. Scarring and pitting of the
skin may occur with cystic acne.

Esterly, N. B., and Furey, N. L.: Acne: current
concepts. Pediatrics 62:1044, 1978.
Tunnessen, W. W., Jr.: Acne: An approach to
therapy for the pediatrician. Adv. Pediatr.
31:325, 1984.

Steroid rosacea, caused by the use of
topical fluorinated glucocorticosteroids, is
characterized by erythematous papules,
pustules and telangiectasia on the eyelids,
cheeks and chin.

Franco, H. L., and Weston, W. L.: Steroid rosacea
in children. Pediatrics 64:36, 1979.

Cellulitis of the face may be caused by
Haemophilus influenzae type b, *streptococcus pneumoniae* and group B streptococci.
Involvement of the cheek begins with little
in the nature of prodromata other than fever
and irritability for 24 to 36 hours. A central
indurated area develops, surrounded peripherally by a nonindurated edematous zone
without elevated or sharply demarcated borders. The involved area is tender, warm to
hot, and has a dusky or reddish-purple color
resembling a fading hematoma. The buccal
mucosa is slightly edematous on the involved side. Group B streptococcal cellulitis
of the face or submandibular areas may
occur in the first two months of life.

Rapkin, R. H., and Bautista, G.: Hemophilus influenzae cellulitis. Am. J. Dis. Child. 124:540, 1972.

Plexiform neurofibromas appearing in the
distribution of cutaneous nerves may give a
thickened sensation on palpation or feel like
a tangle of worms. The overlying skin may
be normal, thickened or pigmented. Neurofibromas commonly appear on the head or
neck, especially around the eyes.

A faint or prominent violaceous or erythematous discoloration of the upper eyelids
and, at times, periorbital tissues along with
periorbital edema, is an early manifestation
of *dermatomyositis*. These findings occasionally extend across the bridge of the nose
to involve the malar prominences. In some
cases the involvement is limited to the
cheeks, perhaps accompanied by periorbital
edema.

VERRUCAE

Verruca vulgaris occurs commonly as
single or multiple lesions over the hands
and fingers and occasionally under the

nails. The lesions, which have a diameter
of up to 1 cm, are firm, discrete, gray or
brownish-gray papules. The surface may be
flat and smooth early, but later it becomes
rough and fissured. Multiple flesh-colored or
yellow-brown, flat warts, millet-seed to pea
size, may occur on the face, lips, tongue and
neck as well as on the hands. These lesions
are slightly elevated, sharply circumscribed
and round or polygonal in shape. An explo-
sion of warts may occur in children who are
receiving chemotherapy or corticosteroids.

Plantar warts are thick, firm, plaquelike,
sometimes painful lesions on the soles and
occasionally on the palms. Tiny black dots
or seeds may be present on their surfaces.

*Verrucae acuminata (condylomata acu-
minata)* are filiform, papular, sometimes
coalescing, lesions in the perineal and genital areas usually associated with poor hygiene or possible sexual abuse.

NAILS

Postmature infants have long nails that
extend beyond the tips of the digits.

Fingernail biting in older children may
be correlated with other evidences of anxiety or tension.

Spoon-shaped nails (koilonychia), characterized by a concavity in the nail, may be
congenital, associated with iron deficiency
anemia in infants or rarely associated with
hypo- or hyperthyroidism. The significance
of longitudinal or transverse ridging is often
obscure except that this finding may occur
with hyperthyroidism, rheumatoid arthritis
or other severe or chronic illnesses. *Brittle-
ness* of the nails occurs with fungus infections, rheumatoid arthritis, hypoparathyroidism and chronic hypochromic anemia.
Deep, transverse grooves in the nails occur
during convalesence from Kawasaki disease.

Psoriasis may cause ridging and pitting
of the nails, subungal keratosis and loosening of the nail plate. *Pitting* of the nails
may also be noted in atopic dermatitis and
fungus infections along with thickening and
ridging.

The clinical diagnosis of *fungus infections* of the nails *(onychomycosis)* may be
difficult without studies of nail scrapings for
fungi. Involved nails may be pitted, friable
and scaly with hypertrophy in some and
atrophy in other areas. Ridging and fissuring may occur, as may separation of the
clouded, lusterless and dull yellow nail from
its bed.

White spots or lines in the nails *(leuko-*

nychia) may be caused by trauma, nutritional deficiency and illness. Congenital leukonychia may be accompanied by knuckle pads over the interphalangeal joints of the digits and hearing loss.

Hemorrhage beneath the nail secondary to trauma may cause nail loss. Such hemorrhage may also represent embolic phenomena in patients with bacterial endocarditis.

Firm, skin-colored or red subungual and periungual fibromas arising from the groove of the nail bed of the fingers and toes may occur in adolescents with *tuberous sclerosis*.

In patients with *hypoparathyroidism*, the nails may be deformed, atrophic, brittle, thickened, and covered by overgrowing skin. Monilial infections of the nails and skin may be a manifestation of hypoparathyroidism.

The *Coffin-Siris syndrome* is characterized by bilateral absence of the nails of the fifth fingers and toes, sparse scalp hair, coarse facial features, hypotonia, and mental retardation.

Feingold, M.: The Coffin-Siris syndrome. Am. J. Dis. Child. 132:660, 1978.

Paronychia is characterized by an inflammatory swelling around the edge of the nails.

A *herpetic whitlow*, caused by herpes simplex virus, is characterized by a painful swelling and erythema of a distal phalanx followed by local vesiculation. In contrast to a bacterial felon or paronychia, the lesion does not contain pus. A primary herpes simplex infection is usually present. A Tsanck test is diagnostically helpful.

Feder, H. M., and Long, S. S.: Herpetic whitlow. Am. J. Dis. Child. 137:861, 1983.

Nails may be congenitally absent in congenital ectodermal dysplasia.

In *pachyonychia congenita*, the nails are congenitally thickened, hard and discolored, have longitudinal striations and are elevated at their distal end. The undersurface of the nail contains a yellow-brown horny material. Other findings may include hyperhidrosis and hyperkeratosis of the palms and soles, follicular keratosis and leukokeratosis of the oral mucosa, especially the tongue.

Hyperpigmentation of the nails may occur with doxorubicin (Adriamycin) therapy.

Yellow nails may precede by many years the development of lymphedema.

Hidrotic ectodermal dysplasia is characterized by dystrophic nails, alopecia and palmoplantar keratoderma. Nail dystrophy may also occur with *alopecia areata*.

Patients with chondroectodermal dysplasia have abnormally small, friable and deformed nails. Dysplasia of the nails may be accompanied by absence or hypoplasia of the patella, elbow dysplasia and iliac horns in the *nail-patella* or *hereditary onycho-osteodysplasia (Hood) syndrome*.

The fingernails in *porphyria* may have a reddish-purple discoloration. Nail loss may occur. Loss of nails also occurs in the dystrophic form of *epidermolysis bullosa* and as a complication of tetracycline therapy.

Lasser, A. E., and Steiner, M. M.: Tetracycline photo-onycholysis. Pediatrics 61:98, 1978.

Nail dysplasia may occur in the *fetal alcohol* and *phenytoin syndromes*.

EXANTHEMS

Rubeola. Beginning behind the ears, along the hair line, over the forehead and the sides of the neck, the eruption of rubeola extends downward to the trunk on the second day and to the extremities by the third day. The rash, which lasts about five days, begins to fade from the face on the third day and continues to disappear in the order of its appearance. Individual lesions begin as discrete, brownish-red macules, which later become papular or morbilliform, blotchy and confluent. Unusually, the lesions may become hemorrhagic. Unless deeply colored, the rash fades on pressure. The skin between confluent areas is normal. With fading of the eruption a brownish, coppery pigmented color and a powdery desquamation may be noted for a few days. A prodromal transient rash may be blotchy and erythematous, urticarial or scarlatiniform.

The occurrence of the rash on the face in rubeola and its characteristic absence there in scarlet fever is a point of differentiation. The lesions of scarlet fever are also more macular, and the intervening skin is erythematous. The appearance of Koplik's spots just before and for 12 to 24 hours after the emergence of the rash of rubeola is also diagnostically helpful.

Atypical measles, occurring in adolescents and young adults previously immunized with inactivated measles vaccine, is characterized by a yellowish-red, maculopapular rash that begins on the ankles, wrists, palms and soles and spreads to the upper extremities and trunk. The lesions often become petechial or vesicular. Edema may occur over the shins and dorsa of the hands and feet.

Martin, D. B., Weiner, L. B., Nieburg, P. I., and Blair, D. C.: Atypical measles in adolescents and young adults. Ann. Intern. Med. 90:877, 1979.

Rubella. A rubelliform rash may be caused by many viruses, so a diagnosis on clinical grounds alone is usually unreliable. The rash of rubella usually begins on the face and extends over the body within a few hours. The eruption, which consists of fine, light pink, discrete macules, may change rapidly, perhaps resembling rubeola during the first 24 hours and becoming punctate or scarlatiniform during the second day. The lesions may become confluent to produce erythematous, flushed areas that fade on pressure. When the rash begins to fade after two to four days, a fine desquamation may occur. Transitory pigmentation of the skin is not present after the eruption disappears. The presence of the eruption about the mouth in patients with rubella as contrasted with the characteristic circumoral pallor in scarlet fever is a differential feature. Enlarged and tender suboccipital and postauricular and suboccipital nodes may precede and persist for a week or more after the appearance of the rash.

Scarlet Fever. The rash of scarlet fever, which usually begins in the axillae, inguinal areas, about the neck and over the chest or back, is frequently most evident along the skin folds. The exanthem extends over the body rapidly, reaching maximal intensity in one or two days, after which it begins to fade. Total duration of the eruption is four to seven days. Except for flushing of the cheeks and circumoral pallor, the face is usually not involved. The rash is characterized by a generalized, bright red erythema and a fine, pinpoint, papular, "goose-flesh" eruption that blanches on pressure. The skin is hot and dry. At times, the rash on the extremities is blotchy and morbilliform. In severe cases pinhead-sized blebs may be found over the chest. In black children the diagnosis may be difficult. The palms and soles may be brightly erythematous and covered by a pinpoint papular rash. A similar rash may be noted over the general skin surface.

Pastia's sign refers to the transverse hyperemic or petechial lines in the skin folds of the antecubital fossae, axillae and inguinal creases. These do not fade on pressure. Desquamation in the form of fine, branny or large flakes, which usually begins at the end of the first week over the neck and chest, around the nails and over the tips of the fingers and toes, may continue for weeks.

Differentiating the rash of scarlet fever from so-called toxic eruptions may be difficult. The latter are usually chiefly erythematous and without the fine, pinpoint papular or punctate characteristics of scarlet fever. Toxic eruptions are usually much briefer in their duration.

Roseola infantum or *exanthem subitum*, common in infants and young children, is preceded by a three day febrile course and appears as the temperature begins to fall. Beginning over the trunk, the rash extends chiefly to the neck and arms with slight involvement of the face and lower extremities. Individual lesions are rose-pink, discrete, small macules or maculopapules that fade on pressure. The eruption usually begins to fade shortly after its appearance but may persist for one or two days.

Other Viral Exanthems. Other viral exanthems may be macular, maculopapular, rubelliform, petechial, purpuric or vesicular. Papular, vesicular or ulcerated oral lesions may occur. A macular, erythematous rash may occur in infectious mononucleosis, especially with the administration of ampicillin. Enteroviruses may also cause an erythematous macular rash. Maculopapular exanthems are commonly associated with adenovirus infections. Coxsackie viruses A9 and B5 and echoviruses 4, 9 and 16 may cause a maculopapular rash. Echovirus 9 and other enteroviruses may cause a petechial rash. Because of the great variability of lesions, a specific etiologic clinical diagnosis is usually not possible. Differentiation of viral rashes from drug rashes may be difficult.

Cherry, J. D.: Viral exanthems. Cur. Probl. Pediatr. 13:5, 1983.

Chickenpox lesions begin in the scalp or on the trunk and spread centripetally to the face and, to a limited extent, to the extremities. The palms and soles may be minimally involved. As few as five or ten lesions or a large number of lesions may be present. Progression of the lesions is from macules to papules, vesicles, pustules and crusts. These occur in crops, with new lesions continuing to appear for four days. Consequently, various stages of progression may be present simultaneously. The papules appear as small, red, elevated lesions that continue to enlarge and rapidly develop into flat, unilocular vesicles that simulate a "tear drop" surrounded, usually, by a ring of erythema 1/4 to 1/2 inch in diameter. The vesicles are soft, do not have the central umbilication characteristic of smallpox lesions and rupture easily with subsequent crusting. Regressing lesions may appear slightly umbilicated. Pruritus is intense. Some papules do not progress to later stages, and vesicles may be noted in the absence of a preceding papule. The duration of the eruption is 8 to 14 days. Bullous lesions rarely occur.

Preblud, S. R., Orenstein, W. A., and Bart, K. J.: Varicella: Clinical manifestations, epidemiology and health impact in children. Pediatr. Infect. Dis. 3:505, 1984.

Rocky Mountain spotted fever begins with discrete pink or bright red macular lesions, a few millimeters in diameter, which initially blanch with pressure. In a few hours the rash becomes papular and later purpuric or petechial. The lesions appear first on the surface of the wrists and about the ankles, usually on the second to fourth febrile day, and spread centripetally over the next day or two to the rest of the body. The rash usually involves the palms and soles and is always most marked on the extremities. Nonpitting edema may develop around the eyes, on the face and over the extremities.

Riley, H. D., Jr.: Rickettsial diseases and Rocky Mountain spotted fever. Part I. Curr. Probl. Pediatr. 11:5, 1981.

Leptospirosis may be accompanied by a maculopapular, petechial or purpuric rash that is followed by peripheral desquamation. The clinical manifestations may resemble those in Kawasaki disease.

Wong, M. L., Kaplan, S., Dunkle, L. M., Stechenberg, B. W. and Feigin, R. D.: Leptospirosis: A childhood disease. J. Pediatr. 90:532, 1977.

Hand-foot-and-mouth disease, usually caused by coxsackie A16 and other Coxsackie strains, begins in the summer and fall with a sore mouth or throat followed by lesions on the hands and feet. The oral lesions, usually five to ten in number, begin as macules and progress rapidly to vesicles and then to ulcers with an erythematous halo. In some patients, 2- to 10-mm, tender, painful vesicles appear on the hands and feet preceded by a red macular stage. The papulovesicular lesion may be oval, angular or streaked. Occasionally, maculopapular lesions may develop elsewhere.

Tindall, J. P., and Callaway, J. L.: Hand-foot-and-mouth disease—It's more common than you think. Am. J. Dis. Child. 124:372, 1972.

In *rat-bite fever,* a diffuse erythematous eruption may occur in addition to induration and ulceration at the site of the bite.

Erythema infectiosum (fifth disease) usually begins with a bright red, confluent eruption over the cheeks, malar prominences and bridge of the nose in an otherwise asymptomatic patient. The involved area has a raised, sharply delimited edge. Lesions may then appear as macules over the lateral aspect of the extremities and the buttocks. These progress to papules that begin to fade on the sixth day with areas of central clearing, leaving a lace-like, reticular or geographic pattern. The eruption, which lasts seven to nine days, may disappear and recur for weeks. Constitutional symptoms are mild.

Balfour, H. H., Jr.: Fifth disease: Full fathom five. Am. J. Dis. Child. 130:239, 1976.

Infectious mononucleosis is occasionally accompanied by a morbilliform or scarlatiniform eruption.

Rose spots are small, reddish macules that blanch on pressure and last about three days. They appear on the abdomen in typhoid, other salmonella infections and shigellosis.

Goscienski, P. J., and Haltalin, K. C.: Rose spots associated with shigellosis. Am. J. Dis. Child. 119:152, 1970.

DRUG RASHES

Drug rashes may be produced by atropine, penicillin, ampicillin, barbiturates, salicylates, phenobarbital, hydantoin and many other drugs. The lesions may be polymorphous or chiefly erythematous, papular, vesicular, pustular or purpuric. Therapeutic or "overtreatment" dermatitis, occurring after the use of some remedial agent on the skin, may be characterized by pruritus and erythema over the site of application. Occasionally, a generalized and severe dermatitis may result. The following chemicals and substances are frequently involved: local anesthetics, penicillin, phenol, tar, menthol, camphor, iodine and salicylic acid. Almost any chemical substance may cause a contact dermatitis.

Knutsen, A. P., Anderson, J., Satayaviboon, S., and Slavin, R. G.: Immunologic aspects of phenobarbital hypersensitivity. J. Pediatr. 105:558, 1984.

BURNS

Burns may be characterized according to their depth and the extent of the surface area involved. A *first degree burn* is limited to the epidermis and characterized by erythema. The *second degree burn*, which represents a partial thickness injury, is manifested by erythema, blisters and marked pain if it is superficial and whitish skin and absence of pain if deeper. *Third degree burns*, which are full thickness thermal injuries, are not painful. If less than 10 per cent of the skin surface area is involved by a second degree burn or less than 1 per cent by a third degree burn, the lesion is characterized as minor. A severe burn is characterized by involvement of greater than 20 per cent of the surface area by a second degree and 10 per cent by a third degree burn.

Electrical burns of the mouth may be misleading because the initial minimal edema and white mucosal coagulum may be followed 7 to 10 days later by extensive loss of tissue and hemorrhage.

Burns characteristic of *child abuse* include cigarette or match tip burns, which are round, uniform and well-demarcated; circumferential, forced scalding burns of the perineum, buttocks, posterior legs, thighs, feet, stocking level on the legs or glovelike burns of the hands; and heating grate or radiator burns. In the case of forced immersion burns, a donut hole–like area of sparing may occur if that part of the body has been compressed against the side of a container and thus has no contact with the hot liquid. Similarly, if the child is held in extreme flexion during the burn, the flexural area will be spared. Splash burns, in which hot liquid is poured or thrown on a child, have an arrow-head appearance owing to the hot fluid running off the main part of the burn.

Lenoski, E. F., and Hunter, K. A.: Specific patterns of inflicted burn injuries. J. Trauma 17:842, 1977.

CHILD ABUSE

In addition to the burns described above, other cutaneous indications of child abuse include multiple bruises in areas not usually traumatized, bite marks, multiple scars or bruises with the imprint of a hand, loop marks from a cord or rope or the multiple linear bruises on the back or buttock caused by a belt. Bruises inflicted by physical

trauma undergo a series of color changes, but an exact estimation of the duration of a contusion is difficult. During the first day, a reddish-blue or purple color is present. A blue or blue-brown color appears from the first to the third day, a greenish hue from the fifth to seventh day, a yellow color by the tenth day and then a brown color with fading over two or four additional days.

Bittner, S., and Newberger, E. H.: Pediatric understanding of child abuse and neglect. Pediatr. Rev. 2:197, 1981.
Ellerstein, N. S.: The cutaneous manifestations of child abuse and neglect. Am. J. Dis. Child. 133:906, 1979.
Kempe, H. C., and Helfer, R. E. (eds.): The Battered Child. 3rd ed. Chicago, University of Chicago Press, 1980.

HAIR

Scalp hair is discussed on page 15.

The fine, unpigmented *lanugo hair* present during the last trimester of fetal life gradually disappears within weeks after birth. Lanugo hair is observed most commonly in the premature but occasionally is noted over the shoulders and upper arms in the term infant. *Vellus* or *down hair*, which begins to appear shortly before birth and is similar to lanugo hair, is the predominant type seen during childhood. Eventually, gradual and partial replacement of vellus hair by the coarser, longer and more pigmented *terminal hair* occurs. During the preschool and school-age periods, vellus and then terminal hair appears on the extensor surfaces of the extremities, along the spine, in the interscapular region, across the shoulders and sometimes in the pilonidal or sacral area. The prominence of body hair is variable, being extensive in some children but minimal in most. Silken, blond hair may also appear on the sides of the face and over the upper lip in early childhood. The hair in children with albinism is nonpigmented, fine and silky. Fine lanugo-like hair may be noted in patients with anorexia nervosa.

Hypertrichosis, the excessive growth of body hair not attributable to an endocrine disorder and most evident on nonsexual areas of the body, may be a familial characteristic. Excessive hair may also be seen in chronically ill patients and in those suffering from starvation. Patients with porphyria cutanea tarda may have excessive hair growth over exposed areas. Hairiness may rarely occur as a side-effect of hydantoin therapy. Hypertrichosis occurs in the Coffin-Siris and de Lange syndromes. Hair on the side of the face may occur with the Treacher Collins syndrome. Hair growth may be noticeably slowed in hypothyroidism and chronic illness.

Adrenal cortical androgens are responsible for the growth of axillary, pubic and facial hair. This growth is conditioned by the level of circulating androgen and the responsiveness of the hair follicles. The latter may show considerable normal variation.

In the Tanner maturational scale, *stage 1* is preadolescence, in which vellus hair is present over the pubic area in prepubescent boys and over the labia in prepubescent girls. In the adolescent male, pubic hair appears after the growth of the testes and penis has begun. In Tanner *stage* 2, a sparse growth of long, slightly pigmented, downy hair on the pubis, chiefly at the base of the penis, occurs. In *stage* 3, the hair is darker, coarser and more curled. In *stage* 4 the hair is more adult in type but covers a smaller area than in the mature adult. With *stage* 5, the adult quantity and type are achieved with extension of the hair growth to the adjacent medial surface of the thighs and upward to and around the umbilicus.

In the adolescent girl, the beginning of breast development usually antedates the appearance of pubic hair. Unpigmented down or *stage 1* usually appears between the ages of 10 1/2 and 12 1/2 years with long, sparse, slightly pigmented down hair present in *stage* 2. In *stage* 3, a few more pigmented, semi-terminal darker and coarser hairs appear. In *stage* 4, full length, pigmented, wiry, sparse, terminal hairs appear, but the area covered is less than in adults. In *stage* 5, dense, fully mature terminal hairs appear.

In most adolescents, the pubic hair usually has a characteristic male or female distribution. In the male, the distribution is in the form of a diamond, the superior apex of which extends upward toward the umbilicus. In the female, the pubic hair appears in the form of an inverted triangle.

Axillary hair usually does not appear until the second stage of pubic hair development has been attained. In general, its development is some six months behind that of pubic hair. In some adolescents, however, axillary hair may appear concomitantly with or even precede pubic hair. A small amount of axillary hair may be present in girls at the menarche.

In adolescent boys, facial hair appears shortly after axillary hair. Its distribution and other characteristics may reflect a familial pattern. Body hair becomes prominent in the male during adolescence and continues to develop throughout the post-adolescent period.

A greater amount of pubic and occasionally of axillary hair, at times coarse and curled, may sometimes be noted in young children, especially in girls, in the absence of other signs of sexual precocity or virilism (*precocious adrenarche*). Continued observation is important because of the possibility of an adrenocortical neoplasm, adrenocortical hyperplasia or isosexual precocity in the male. In the latter, however, other secondary sex characteristics or evidence of excessive androgen secretion are present or appear shortly.

Korth-Schutz, S., Levine, L.S., and New, M. I.: Serum androgens in normal prepubertal and pubertal children and in children with precocious adrenarche. J. Clin. Endocrinol. Metab. 42:117, 1976.

Sexual hair is decreased or absent in patients with hypopituitarism, in hypothyroidism and in adolescent girls with Addison's disease. It is decreased and may be delayed in Turner's syndrome.

Hirsutism, the appearance in a female of hair on the face, chest, breasts and abdomen with a male distribution of pubic hair with or without other virilizing signs, is usually caused by a subtle excess of androgen. It may be a manifestation of Cushing's disease, a virilizing adrenal neoplasm, very mild congenital adrenal hyperplasia or polycystic ovary (Stein-Leventhal) syndrome. A morning plasma testosterone level should be obtained to determine if hyperandrogenemia is present. In most instances a specific cause cannot be determined.

Leng, J-J., and Greenblatt, R. B.: Hirsutism in adolescent girls. Pediatr. Clin. North Am. 19:681, 1972.

Alopecia totalis, along with short stature, occurs in some patients with vitamin D–dependent rickets, type II.

GENERAL REFERENCES

Hurwitz, S.: Clinical Pediatric Dermatology. Philadelphia, W. B. Saunders Co., 1981.

Korting, G. W., Curth, W., and Curth, H. O.: Diseases of the Skin in Children and Adolescents. Philadelphia, W. B. Saunders Co., 1978.

Solomon, L. M., Esterly, N. B., and Loeffel, E.D. (eds.): Adolescent Dermatology. Philadelphia, W. B. Saunders Co., 1978.

Solomon, L. M., and Esterly, N. B.: Neonatal Dermatology. Philadelphia, W. B. Saunders Co. 1973.

Weinberg, S., Leider, M., and Shapiro, L.: Color Atlas of Pediatric Dermatology. New York, McGraw Hill Book Co., 1975.

Part Two

SIGNS AND SYMPTOMS

19 / THE PEDIATRIC INTERVIEW AND HISTORY

Discussion of the pediatric history in this chapter differs from the traditional presentation (chief complaints, present illness, past medical history, developmental and feeding history, family history and review of systems) in that it deals principally with the process of interviewing. This approach is taken not to devalue the customary practice—indeed, the entire volume is concerned with the presenting complaint, development and other traditional content—but to emphasize the value of the interview as the basic tool for history taking.

The importance of detail (e.g., an exact description of the symptoms or signs reported, their chronology and the circumstances surrounding their occurrence) cannot be over-emphasized. Pediatric diagnosis is a matter of having in mind the various possible explanations for presenting signs and symptoms, then utilizing the history, physical examination, laboratory procedures and other tools to clarify the specific cause or causes. For many symptoms, the interview is the quickest and often the only key to diagnosis, whether the etiology is biomedical, psychosocial or a combination of the two. Both biomedical and psychosocial diagnostic possibilities need to be integrated into the initial history. The interview provides not only an opportunity for obtaining data but also a way to help the patient* psychologically. Flexible and imaginative history taking develops when the physician modifies the conventional procedure, thereby enabling himself to acquire better understanding of the patient within a limited time while simultaneously establishing rapport and engaging in a therapeutic relationship. Certainly, the doctor's demonstration of diagnostic thoroughness and skill in eliciting a comprehensive history is, in itself, supportive.

The length and direction of the history depend upon the circumstances surrounding each case. In emergency situations, history-taking is, of course, limited to obtaining the data essential for immediate diagnosis and therapy. When seeing children who are acutely ill, exploring beyond the immediately pertinent facts is often inappropriate.

The pediatric history involves a triangular relationship among physician, child and parents. Pediatric diagnosis and management generally require a family focus. Whether the physician interviews parents and child or adolescent together or separately depends upon the presenting complaints. In many instances the physician may initially interview the parents and child together, then later interview them separately. Interviewing the family as a unit, including children above the age of eight years, has a place in pediatric diagnosis.

The following discussion relating to the technique of interviewing includes some general principles and recognizes that the process is highly dependent upon the personality and experience of the doctor. The interview is unique for every patient and for every clinician—no two people can be interviewed in exactly the same way; no two patients with the same disorder present the same history; and no two physicians who interview skillfully do it the same way. The extensive list of interviewing principles that follows reflects the central importance of the interview in pediatric diagnosis.

SOME GENERALIZATIONS

The interview is a powerful tool in that it offers both an effective method of collecting diagnostic data and a fruitful means of establishing a therapeutic relationship.

Biomedical and psychosocial diagnostic and etiologic possibilities should be considered currently.

The interview is a progressive, cumulative process.

The deft interviewer has a cultivated perceptiveness; a scientific curiosity about people; and a highly developed ability to

---

*The term *patient* will be used to refer to the child, to the parents or to both as appropriate in the text.

191

see, hear, feel, empathize with and read the patient.

The goal is verbal, nonverbal and affective *communication.*

The interview is an *active* process, an experience, a relationship. It should be flexible, spontaneous and, in part, intuitive.

The patient will scrutinize the doctor's face for evidence of interest, concern, indifference, censure, agreement, acceptance, anger, disapproval, shock, friendliness, surprise, reassurance and responsiveness.

The physician's facial expression and body language may facilitate the effectiveness of an interview. For example, an appearance of quiet attention demonstrates the physician's personal interest in what the patient is saying, while a concerned expression may underline his reaction to a child's prolonged absence from school due to school avoidance.

When a patient has many problems, the physician should focus on one at a time.

Open-ended questions that permit meaningful answers are preferred to those that can be answered simply by "Yes" or "No."

Determine what the patient wants and his readiness to accept help.

If the physician surmises at the start that a seeming interest on his part in psychosocial and family interactions would be sensed as irrelevant or intrusive, he should reserve those considerations until later. The initial concern should, in that event, be limited to biomedical factors, with any exploration of feelings pursued at a more propitious time.

Do not interrogate, prod or probe.

Minimal movement by the interviewer is usually facilitative and helps the patient concentrate on what he has to say.

The patient's initial questions and expectations must be answered at some level before the end of the visit.

Even though not always the real or primary problem, the chief complaint should remain as a focus of the interview. Other areas may be profitably explored, but the physician should return to that topic by the end of the session.

Interviews should be scheduled for a defined period and end within that time limit.

The success of an interview is likely to be compromised if the physician or patient feels pressured by lack of time.

Both parents should be asked to be present. Unless it is a one-parent family, upsetting findings (e.g., mental retardation), should, if possible, be conveyed to both parents together.

BEGINNING THE INTERVIEW

The interview begins with introductions and a few transitional social remarks. When seeing a child or adolescent alone, this introductory period may continue for a few minutes.

The experienced clinician has in mind one or several diagnostic hypotheses based on the presenting symptoms and signs. These may change in response to additional information and observation.

"Would you tell me what has been concerning you about Cynthia?" "What else? . . ." "Now, you've mentioned two concerns, one, _____, and two, _____." "What else?"

Overly vigorous note taking may suppress significant parts of the history, especially if the problem is psychologic; on the other hand, if parents appear wary of psychologic implications, initial meticulous note taking may allay their concerns until the tone of the interview changes.

Writing notes and observing the patient simultaneously is difficult. Observation may be as important as or may illuminate what is said.

LISTENING AND WHAT TO LISTEN FOR

The interviewer needs to *hear* and *receive* the patient's message.

Note the order in which the problems are mentioned, recurrent references and significant omissions.

Be attentive as to how words and phrases are used to conceal, reveal or imply the patient's thoughts, feelings or experiences.

The patient's spontaneous association of statements and events is of interest.

Listen carefully to the patient's first statement and his last one on leaving.

The patient's spontaneously disclosed opinion of and attitude toward previous clinicians is of interest.

If litigation may be in process (e.g., child custody, accidents involving presumed injury to the child, school avoidance or probation hearings in relation to antisocial behavior), be circumspect.

Note significant pause by the patient before answering a question.

Note quick, unsolicited and defensive protestations such as : "We have a wonderful marriage." "There couldn't possibly be anything emotionally wrong." "One thing I'm certain about, it's not his nerves!" "That doesn't bother me now." "That's all over now." "Everything is fine." "The other children are doing well." "I'm very happy."

When a patient says, "I don't see what that has to do with my problem," it's probably relevant.

Unexpected use of medical terminology by someone who is not a health professional may suggest Munchausen's syndrome by proxy.

Note an impersonal, clinical quality to the history.

Note whether one person speaks for another who is present (e.g., "He thinks . . .") or repeatedly answers questions directed to another family member.

Note whether the patient avoids a question by subtly changing the subject or appears to misunderstand while feigning eagerness to answer.

If the interviewer believes the patient's answer to a question is not a candid one, he should rephrase the question (e.g., "How do you *really* feel?") or return to the question later.

Sometimes a question to which a patient initially chooses not to respond may be answered later or in a subsequent interview.

Nonstop talking may be a cover for the patient's anxiety, perhaps serving as a defensive screen so as to preclude the opportunity for the interviewer to ask potentially troublesome questions.

ASSUMPTIONS

Although most patients come with the wish and the expectation to be helped, they may have reservations about both. They have their own agenda of concerns and ideas of what would be helpful. These considerations may condition the success of the visit.

Patients often present a facade. They may dissemble.

Seek to identify the *primary* patient and the *central* problem.

Regard the initial history as tentative and incomplete. The most important material may not be disclosed by the patient until later.

The patient may initially be unable to describe his problem comfortably or adequately. He may not be sure what it is.

The patient may not disclose the primary or real reason for coming until convinced that the interviewer will be empathetic.

The patient who feels the physician understands him will usually, if given a chance, share his real concerns and problems in addition to those mentioned in the chief complaint. The physician needs to listen for and *hear* those interjections.

The patient may be totally unaware of what may seem self-evident to the clinician.

The way patients perceive events may be very different from how the interviewer or another family member sees them.

A different or contradictory account of the history may be given by each parent and by the child or adolescent.

Symptoms may persist owing to secondary or conscious gains for the child, such as special solicitude, concern or privileges.

Some patients simply do not understand or are unable to accept that an etiologic relationship may exist between psychosocial factors and somatic complaints.

Some families do not have a language of affects. The parents' attention may be evoked by somatic complaints but not by feelings.

The psychosocial morbidity in many families is hidden, even to the family members themselves.

Parents of infants who fail to thrive or who are retarded, psychotic or handicapped are likely to have feelings of anger, shame, inadequacy, anxiety, despair and guilt.

When a patient says, "Let me ask you about a hypothetical situation," or asks a question about someone else, the question is probably related to the patient's own problem.

THE SETTING

Courtesy and cordiality of the appointment secretary, receptionist or other first-contact personnel are essential.

The physician's punctuality contributes to a positive impression.

Greeting of each patient by name should be accompanied by eye contact, a smile and, if it seems appropriate, a handshake. The greeting should not be perfunctory.

Assurance of privacy and a quiet setting are facilitative. The office door should be closed. A hospitable ambience promotes openness.

Comfortable chairs of the same height

should be arranged to permit eye contact between the physician and the patient without straining.

Soft lighting is helpful, and the patient should not face sunglare.

Depending upon the comfort of the patient, the doctor should not sit too close or too distant. A distance of five or more feet between physician and patient fosters an impersonal ambience. Sitting next to the patient is usually more facilitative.

Sitting behind a desk when interviewing children or adolescents may introduce a barrier to openness.

Unless unavoidable, the interview should not be interrupted by phone calls or by someone opening the door.

Patients may talk more freely during or after the intimacy and reassurance of the physical examination or if given a chance to talk about their strengths, successes and hopes. Listen carefully at these times or at the conclusion of the examination. Ask if they wish to ask or tell you about anything else.

See the parents and the child or adolescent together and separately. The order in which this is done will vary with the family and the physician.

If the parent is hesitant about talking, excuse the child from the room by saying, for example: "Why don't we have Johnny play (color, read) in the waiting room while we talk?" Then proceed to interview the parent.

If the parents appear comfortable when discussing sensitive matters in the child's presence, the child has probably heard it all before.

THE FACILITATIVE INTERVIEWER

The ideal physician is perceived as mature, unhurried, accepting, nonjudgmental, courteous, gracious, genuine, responsive, and trustworthy.

The doctor's expertise should be viewed by the patient as reassuring and comforting rather than as intimidating or patronizing.

The facilitative doctor's interest is shown by his alertness to what the patient is saying, by his facial expression and by his tone of voice.

Some patients respond best to an assertive interviewer, others to one who is gregarious, and still others to a physician who is perceived as quiet and thoughtful.

The patient's name and that of the parents and siblings should be used at appropriate points during the interview as a way of personalizing or individualizing the process.

The empathetic doctor senses in the patient such feelings as anxiety, depression, anger or fear. For example, he may comment: "You seem kind of sad today."

He respects the patient's dignity.

He is not too smoothly articulate.

He allows patients to talk and follows ensuing leads that he believes will be productive.

He is not prematurely reassuring.

INTERVIEWING CHILDREN

Unless they are already familiar with the physician, children may be initially apprehensive and fearful about the interview: "I'll bet you were a little nervous about coming here."

Introduce yourself. Explain what you do. Be yourself—an adult who is interested in helping children and adolescents.

Give the child a few moments to get acquainted with you and with the setting.

The doctor's comfortable friendliness will place most children at ease.

Whereas children will usually talk readily, an occasional child, especially one who is shy or anxious, may respond only to direct questions and even then circumspectly.

The doctor may play with very young children for a few minutes as a means of getting acquainted. Blocks, a ball, crayons, a pad of paper, picture books or a doll and bottle are useful facilitators, similar to "conversation pieces."

Since very young children can easily imagine that a stuffed animal or a hand puppet can talk and listen, part of the interview can be conducted through that medium if it seems developmentally appropriate.

Topics to talk about with children include
Family members
School experiences: "How are the teachers (the subjects, the other students)?" "What goes best for you at school?"
Friends
Sports and recreation
Possible career plans
Favorite television programs
Admired athletes, singers, actors or other performers
Pets

Provide the opportunity for the child to talk about some of his or her strengths, especially at the beginning of the interview: "Tell me about some of the things you're best at . . ." If the child protests that he has none, say: "Well, I think you're being modest. What comes the easiest for you?"

Other approaches

"Many girls your age are concerned about _____. I imagine that you may be also. Tell me about it."

Role playing: "Let's imagine that you're the doctor . . . Dr. Susan . . . and a girl your age . . . let's call her Marcia . . . tells you she has _____ (patient's symptom). What would you think might be causing her trouble?" Then later, "What do you think would help her?"

Important questions

"If your teachers asked you to write a story about your life . . . family, what would you write?"

"How are things going?"

"What kind of things do you do for fun—your favorite activities?"

"What kind of activities do you not enjoy?"

"Tell me how you spend a typical school day . . . say yesterday. A typical Saturday and Sunday?"

"What do you *and* your mother (father) do for fun?"

"Do you have a special friend?"

"To whom do you talk about things?" "How about things that trouble or worry you?" "Do you find that helpful?"

"How are the other children in your school, neighborhood?"

"Tell me about your mother (father, brother)."

"Tell me about your relationship with _____."

"How do you get along with your _____ (siblings, parents, peers)?"

"What would you like to do when you're finished with school?"

"What kind of discipline do your parents use?" "For what?" "Do you think that's fair?" "Is it effective?" "Do mother and father have the same ideas about this?" "What do you think the rules ought to be?"

"It's natural for everyone to get angry sometime. What are some of the things that make *you* angry?"

"What do you do when you get angry?"

"How could I tell if you were angry?"

"So what keeps you from letting people know when you're angry?"

"If a fairy godmother were here and granted you three wishes, what would you wish for?"

"How are you different from (like) your sister (brother)?"

"What makes you sad (worried, happy)?"

"Many children worry about their parents—their parents' health—something happening to them . . . or they may worry about themselves. Which member of your family do *you* worry about the most?"

"Who has been sick in your family?"

"Has anyone in your family died?"

"Draw me a picture." "Tell me a story about your picture."

INTERVIEWING ADOLESCENTS

The ground rules should be clarified at the start. The child should know he is free to discuss the interview with his parents if he wishes, but the doctor will not unless the patient concurs or if, in the doctor's judgment, the parents need to know to protect the patient's health or safety. The physician would then share with the patient what he plans to tell his or her parents.

After the introductory amenities, which give the patient time to look around, the doctor may simply ask, "John, I wonder if you would tell me why you came to see me (or why your parents brought you to see me)."

If the patient denies knowing why, ask what he thinks the reason might be—his best guess.

If he still says he does not know, respond with a statement such as, "I understand that you're having a problem at school . . ."

Adolescents will usually discuss their thoughts and feelings readily, especially when their parents are not present and confidentiality is assured.

If angry or offended about coming to see the physician, the adolescent may deny he has a problem.

If the patient has been brought by subterfuge, dissociate yourself from that tactic: "I'm sorry. That wasn't appropriate. Tell me why you think this happened."

If the doctor believes the child may be depressed or angry, the following statement that fronts for a question may be facilitative: "I would guess that things aren't going so well for you . . ."

If that is the case, the child will usually give his answer nonverbally by glancing quickly at the physician. This cue can be followed by the statement: "Tell me about it . . ."

The doctor should not feel challenged to make an adolescent talk, nor press him about subjects that the teen-ager obviously does not want to acknowledge, at least not at that time. The traditional review of symptoms may be used as a neutral introduction to enhance the initial communication. Or the physician can try these approaches:

"Your life is none of my business unless you would want to talk with me about how things are going."

"I can appreciate that you weren't wild

about coming here . . . that you don't feel it makes sense . . . but since we have this time, I'd be interested in hearing about how you think things are going . . ."

If the patient does not respond, it is generally fruitless to continue at length. Close the visit graciously, give the child your phone number and tell him you'd be pleased to see him again if he would like to come back.

Today, questions about sexuality, drugs and alcohol are not unexpected by the adolescent. However, if the patient appears embarrassed or uneasy, say: "If that's too personal we won't talk about it now."

Some questions for adolescents
"How have you felt lately?"
"How would you describe yourself . . . your usual mood . . . your feelings?"
"Tell me about some of the things you're really good at."
"Do you have a job?" "What do you do?"
"How do others—your family, your friends—feel about you?"
"What are your responsibilities or chores at home?"
"What sort of privileges do you have at home?"
"What rules do your parents have for you?"
"What happens if you bend or break them?"
"I don't know your mother (father, sibling) well. Could you describe them for me?"
"How do your parents feel about this problem?"
"What do your parents think of your friends?"
"Have you had a recent date?" "What did you do?"
"How would you change your life if you could?" "How about in relation to your mother (father) (boyfriend)?"
"What does (name of disease or symptom) mean to you? I know you came to find out, but I'm interested in knowing what *you* think might be causing this problem."
"Do you think the problem is serious?" "What have you been told about it?" "Tell me what that means to you."
"What are some of the changes that have occurred in your life lately?"
"What do you do for physical activity?"
"What makes you feel really stressed?" "What helps you cope with that?"
"Typically, adolescents have concerns, you know, about their body, their size, their growth, their development, and I would suppose that you have too. What thoughts have you had about your health?"
"I don't know" or "I forgot" are generally evasive statements. If the adolescent remains guarded, be patient. There is a reason for such reticence (e.g., parental

admonition not to talk, uncertainty about confidentiality, lack of trust in the doctor, shame, anxiety or being forced to come).
"What do the other teenagers at school think about drugs (drinking, sex)?" "What's your attitude about that?"
"Are you sexually active?" In the female adolescent, this question may be linked to those about menstruation. "Do you smoke?"

OBSERVE ACTIVELY

Visual clues are highly important since much is communicated nonverbally.

Note the patient's attitude on meeting the interviewer: Is he smiling? Pleased? Cool? Suspicious? Overly friendly? Unfriendly? Reserved? Indifferent? Depressed?

The physician needs to be aware of feelings engendered in himself during the interview—anger, anxiety, dislike, admiration, frustration or impatience.

Does what you see and feel match up with what the patient is saying?

Other clues to watch for

Perspiration, blushing or paling; controlled, uneven, or blocked speech; the plaintive voice; talking in a whisper; the patient's gait on entering the room; mendicant posture; tics

Frequent swallowing; tenseness, fidgetiness; a preoccupied air and avoidance of eye contact

Sudden glance at the interviewer or someone else in the family following a statement or question

Clenching, rubbing, wringing hands, scratching or nail-biting

The kind of clothing worn. Dark clothes may be a sign of depression in an adolescent.

Sudden request by parent or adolescent for permission to smoke

Reddening of eyes or crying

Frowns, smiles

Apparent concern or unconcern about symptom

Double messages, e.g., mother laughing while telling child to behave or smiling when talking about his bad behavior

The light that seems to go on in a patient's mind when he has made a significant association or achieved a new insight

Interactions between parents and child, parent and parent, and between child and physician during the visit

Developmentally inappropriate behavior, e.g., older child on parent's lap, difficulty in separating child from parent, or the mother laying a young infant on the examination table and then walking away

The way in which the infant or young child is held or helped during the interview and physical examination

The mother's "parenting presence"

The child's response to his parent's requests

The child's play and activity

ITEMS DIFFICULT FOR PATIENTS AND PARENTS TO VERBALIZE

The possibility of a serious disorder in their child, e.g., mental retardation or malignancy

Parental emotional problems, including alcoholism and depression

Their own physical health problems

Sexual problems

Marital discord or problems

Financial stresses

Child abuse

Sexual abuse

Anger, especially at other members of the family

NOTE: If the patient's concerns are thought to be conscious and relevant, it may be appropriate for the interviewer to provide an opening such as: "Many parents (children) in this situation have this sort of question (worry) . . . and it would be only natural if you did also."

QUESTIONS FOR PARENTS

When reviewing the prenatal period or early infancy, ask: "Was that a convenient time for you to be pregnant?" "How did your pregnancy go?" "What was your labor with _____ like?" "Your delivery?" "Did you have anyone to help you during this time?"

Questions about feeding, sleeping, toilet training and discipline may elicit helpful information.

Questions about the relationships parents experienced as children with their own parents and siblings and how they were reared may be highly relevant. Such questions might include: "How were things for you when you were growing up?" "Did you intend to raise your children pretty much as you were reared or somewhat differently?" "How do you think that has worked out?"

A review of the parent's life history may be helpful. If pertinent, ask what the health status of each parent was at earlier stages of the child's development.

Other important questions

"Often our children remind us of someone in our family or ourselves. Whom does _____ remind you of?"

"How does _____ get along with other children?"

"Why do you think that is?"

"What sort of temperament does _____ have?"

"Was _____ ever very sick?" "Were you or the doctors worried that he might not live?"

"What do you think would be helpful?"

"How do you think all this has affected _____?"

"How do you think _____ feels about that?"

"Tell me how _____ spends his day."

"Have you and (son, daughter) been separated for any length of time?"

"Does _____ become upset when you leave?"

"What changes would you like to see in (child, spouse, yourself)?"

"This has been going on for some time, and I was just wondering why you came in now?"

"Whose idea was it to come?"

"I'd be interested in what you think may be causing the problem."

"It would be helpful for me to know what you have been doing about this." "What have you been told about it?"

"Does this behavior also occur when he is with others? At school? At the day care center? With the grandparents?"

"Would you tell me what has been really worrying you the most about _____?"

"What were you expecting of this visit?"

"Do you ever have a chance to go out without the children?" "How often?" "Why not?"

"How have things been going between the two of you (parents)?"

"What are the arrangements for privacy (bathroom, bedroom) in your home?"

"What have you told _____ (the child) about your illness (his illness, the divorce, the stillbirth, the adoption, etc.)?"

CLARIFICATION

The clarifying function of the interview helps the patient gain a realistic view of his situation.

One way to encourage elaboration on a topic is for the interviewer to shift his posture and appear puzzled: "You know, I'm a little uncertain about what you consider your main concern to be. What would you say is the major difficulty?" or "I guess that I don't understand that. Would you please clarify it for me?"

If the patient disclaims an opinion on what the cause of his problem is ("I don't know." "I have no idea."), the physician may reply, "Well, I recognize that you don't know, but when a problem has been going on for some time, parents naturally develop some notions about it or ask around. It would be helpful to have your ideas."

Understand what the patient means by the words he uses. Verify that he understands the ones the physician chooses.

When the patient uses qualifying terms such as "reasonably well," "a little," "somewhat," "really," "fair," "in most respects," "average," "so-so," "OK . . . I guess," or "like everybody else," ask him to be more specific: "What do you mean 'somewhat'?"

Seek specificity about content and feelings rather than let vague references pass.

In a facilitative physician-patient relationship, clarifying information will generally be volunteered unless not consciously known to the patient.

When he surmises that the patient has not disclosed the pertinent facts, the physician may sidestep answering the question, "What do you think is wrong?" by a statement such as, "I'm not sure yet." or "This is obviously a complex matter, and it will take time for me to understand it."

If a specific diagnosis would seem blunt or premature, share it at a more appropriate time.

Significant differences of opinion in the family can be noted with a comment such as, "Both of you seem to have a little different view of this matter."

To obtain further elaboration of a statement, repeat the patient's preceding word or phrase.

The use of one or two syllable sounds—uh huh, yes, hum, ah—may encourage the patient to elaborate.

Other clarification techniques
"Why do you say *that*?"
"Why do you ask?"
"How do *you* feel about it?"
"And so . . ."
"Such as"
"So . . ."
"Well . . ."
"Give me an example."
"Tell me more about that."
"For instance . . ."
"Therefore . . ."
"Why is that?"
"You feel . . . "
"You mentioned _____?"
"As I get it, _____."
If the patient seems angry about something that he has not verbalized, say: "You seem to be angry about something. I don't know why, so can you tell me?"

If the patient brings up material that does not forward the purpose of the interview, show no interest in it.

If the patient is tearful or cries during the interview, the doctor may wait a moment and then comment: "This is difficult to think about." or "This seems to be upsetting you. Would you tell me about it?" Offering the patient facial tissues too quickly may prematurely shut off a useful elaboration of what is upsetting.

HELPING THE PATIENT TO FEEL BETTER

By the end of the interview, each patient should feel better about himself or believe that the session was worthwhile.

Commendation of the patient in some way during the interview contributes to his self-esteem: "What a beautiful child!" "That's quite an achievement!"

Patients who feel positively evaluated by their doctor are more likely to comply with his recommendations.

In addition to the problems and failures that patients disclose in the interview, the practice of encouraging them to talk about their successes and strengths places them in a less dependent and defensive posture and may help them to be more forthcoming with information.

The patient with multiple hypochondriacal symptoms needs to be encouraged to carry on in spite of his symptoms.

The clinician's interest and understanding are especially appreciated by the parents of retarded children. Such interest may be shown in many sensitive ways, including holding or cuddling a baby or by talking and playing with a child.

THE DIFFICULT PATIENT

Understanding the reason for a child's difficult or inappropriate behavior helps the physician work productively with the patient who otherwise would be even more disturbing, frustrating and anger-provoking.

The physician will, at times, feel calm and relaxed, whereas at other times and with different patients he may feel tense, impatient and angry.

The patient's anger may be a manifestation of anxiety; his cockiness a compensation for insecurity; and his "sweetness and light" a cover for hostility.

The patient's difficult behavior usually derives from previous unsatisfactory or nongratifying relationships with authority figures, including other physicians.

The patient's over- or underevaluation of the physician is usually unrelated to what the doctor says or does.

With patients who are angry, uncooperative, belittling, sarcastic, provocative, suspicious, disrespectful, attacking, irritating, resentful, blustering or challenging, the doctor should attempt to maintain his equanimity, avoid defensiveness, and bridle the natural tendency to flare with anger. At the same time, the physician should not accept abuse.

When a parent's anger is a cover for anxiety, his behavior may change dramatically in response to the physician's calm, empathetic remark: "I'm sure that you must be very worried about _____'s illness." "Tell me about it." Or, "You're obviously very angry about something. What happened?" Then listen without becoming defensive.

If one senses at the beginning of the interview that the patient is angry, try to disarm him by conveying your understanding of how he feels, by being careful not to be perceived as critical, by proceeding slowly, by avoiding premature interpretations that suggest the patient's emotional problems may be contributory. Instead, make a positive remark, initially confine questions to the presenting complaint, spend a moment or two at the start in talking about neutral matters and show your seriousness and concern.

Compulsive or highly narcissistic patients are difficult to help. They see no merit in changing their behavior or in accepting the suggestions of others.

Some patients are unable to form a trusting relationship with a physician.

A patient's needs and expectations may be so great or unrealistic that no physician can satisfy them.

Some patients display no overt emotion and respond with parsimonious, almost telegraphic answers that tend to conceal more than they reveal; other patients talk incessantly but assiduously avoid revealing their real feelings.

EXPRESSIONS OF EMPATHY

"How did you manage?"

"That must have made you angry (sad, happy)."

"That must have been a trying time for you."

"You must have been hurt (upset)."

"It's hard to talk about this."

"People don't seem to understand how you feel."

"You seem to be receiving a lot of unwanted advice."

"You seem to be kind of hard on yourself."

"I'd guess you find it difficult to trust anyone."

"The death of someone so close is hard to deal with."

"I suppose you were scared that you might lose (son, daughter)."

"This has been kind of a secret fear, I take it."

In addition, an understanding nod may convey that you're with them.

CAUTION

A history of failure by the patient to follow previous regimens generally foretells future noncompliance.

If a patient reports dissatisfaction with or anger at previous doctors, be prepared to experience a similar fate.

Rather than agree, disagree or ignore such pejorative remarks, the physician might quietly observe: "Well, you seem to have been unhappy with that experience."

It may be difficult to establish a constructive, continuing relationship with a nomadic patient who has consulted a succession of doctors in an effort to seek agreement with his own perception rather than receive an objective opinion.

The patient who is too friendly, overly interested in the doctor's personal life, too courteous, too agreeable or too flattering may be trying to control or vitiate the physician or to make the relationship a nonprofessional one. If unsuccessful in this, his or her behavior may change abruptly.

The pace of the interview should not exceed the patient's tolerance.

Respect the patient's defenses. Pushing him to reveal more than he is currently prepared to disclose is unwise.

Do not try to hurry the process. A certain amount of time is required. It is better to schedule additional sessions than to attempt to do too much too soon.

Discuss with the patient only those feelings that he has verbally expressed, even though you sense others of which he is unaware or does not currently wish to disclose. Premature verbalization by the physician of the patient's undisclosed feelings or gratuitous interpretation of behavior may cause resentment and defensiveness.

Take care when exploring matters not closely relevant to the patient's present expressed concerns or complaints, especially in the initial interview.

Avoid any approach that is or may be perceived as manipulative or devious.

Provide help at the level the patient is prepared to receive it. Do not give advice the patient cannot follow.

A very anxious patient has difficulty in concentrating; therefore, it is prudent to address only one item at a time. Explanations should also be brief; otherwise, the anxious patient may have an information overload.

It is generally wise to avoid judgmental terms such as "good," "bad," "right," "wrong," and "fault." It is wise not to express criticism of anyone.

In situations such as a divorce or a parent-child conflict, remember that the story has two sides that are often contradictory.

Let sleeping dogs lie. Know when not to intrude. Otherwise, one may arouse great anxiety and resistance. The patient's resultant failure to return may foreclose an opportunity to be helpful.

Avoid teasing, facetiousness, jocularity, sarcasm, or comments that make the patient believe he or his complaint is being made light of or is not being considered in a professional manner. Although helpful on occasion, humor should be used sparingly and with great discretion.

Avoid familiarity. Keep the relationship professional, not social. Avoid interjecting or discussing one's personal life, experiences or opinions.

Do not discuss other patients in any way, even if asked about someone specifically: "As you know, I cannot make any comments." The physician's ability to keep confidences is being tested.

Try to be prospectively aware of your own emotional blind spots, prejudices and situations that tend to make you anxious or angry. When the physician finds himself changing the subject or talking too much, it may be in order to steer the interview away from a topic or problem about which he feels anxious or uninformed.

In general, avoid the use of the personal pronoun "I," e.g., "I think," "If I were you."

Set a reasonable limit on the length of the interview. Spending an unlimited amount of time is wasteful to both physician and patient as well as expensive and, perhaps, antitherapeutic.

If the parents obviously have little insight into their problems, proceed with caution.

Do not comment on slips of the tongue or inconsistencies in the patient's story.

Have reasonable goals and expectations for what you can do to help each patient. Do not ask questions about matters if you do not know what to do with the answers.

The physician should not exceed the boundaries of his competency in either the biomedical or psychosocial arenas.

The pediatrician is not a marriage counselor.

Do not deny the reality of the patient's subjective somatic complaints, e.g., "pain," "weakness," "dizziness." And never announce that "There is nothing wrong with _____" or imply that "It's all in the patient's head."

Avoid giving quick, superficial advice or reassurance. The patient may have knowingly withheld the information necessary for a meaningful response.

Confronting parents with a direct interpretation of psychosocial etiologies, even when obvious to the doctor, is usually undesirable.

Patients tend to be defensive about gratuitous interpretations. They feel antagonistic if they are not ready to understand or accept the doctor's observations.

Give advice sparingly about psychosocial issues; however, authoritative advice may be given if the patient understands exactly what the doctor is saying, is not seriously emotionally disturbed, has been openly communicative, would welcome such counsel and can, in the physician's judgment, follow it.

Do not take at face value all the statements a patient makes.

Unless adequately explored, a patient's anxieties are not lessened by random reassurance.

Be alert to the manipulative patient who seeks, perhaps through slanted, inaccurate or incomplete data, to have the doctor do what the patient wants (e.g., delay hospitalization for the patient with anorexia nervosa, perform procedures and tests in the Munchausen syndrome by proxy, approve of a homebound teacher for a child who has school avoidance, offer an opinion as to child custody). When thwarted, even gently, these patients may become very angry, which is in itself a manipulative tactic.

Be cautious about listening to "secrets" from one of the parents transmitted privately in an attempt to control the doctor's actions. Although exceptions occur, it may be appropriate to suggest that the patient mention the material to other members of the family during the interview.

The patient who asks your opinion about someone else's behavior or problem is likely talking about himself.

The patient who requests or demands to be told exactly what to do may have no intention of following that advice. The physician might respond with: "Well, do you think you would follow those suggestions?" or "It's not quite that easy. It's going to take time to understand the problem and to see just what would be helpful."

If a mother indicates that the father will not agree to come in for the next visit, she may be expressing her ambivalence about his presence. Convey your belief that she can get him to come or offer to call him directly. "I'd like to have his ideas about _____'s situation."

If psychiatric referral is indicated, are the patient and his family ready for referral? Do they believe they need psychiatric help? Are they knowledgeable about potential benefits, limitations, costs and time? Do they have misconceptions?

Parents are extraordinarily sensitive to any implication that they have caused their child's emotional problem.

Although psychiatric referral may be declined, the pediatrician has the responsibility, at the appropriate time, to convey his recommendation clearly.

If psychiatric help is either unavailable or declined, the pediatrician may continue to be helpful.

Be cautious about initiating a discussion about placing of a retarded child outside the home unless the parents indicate their readiness for such discussion.

FACILITATING DISCUSSION OF POSSIBLE PSYCHOLOGIC ETIOLOGIC FACTORS

If a parent states that her child is "nervous," the physician may interject questions such as: "Who else in the family would you say is nervous?" "Who's the *nervous* one in your family?" "Does nervousness run in your family?" "Who does the *worrying* in your family?"

If the parent raises the possibility of an emotional cause, do not pounce on that suggestion. Be a little tentative: "Well, I guess that's possible. Would you explain a little more why you suggest that?"

Words such as "sensitive," or "blue" or "down" may be less charged than "anxious" or "depressed." "Tension" and "stress" usually do not create defensiveness. Say: "You seem kind of tense (worried)."

If the patient repeatedly denies the presence of problems when the physician believes they exist say: "OK—everything may not be as great as you say, but you seem to think that everything is fine." Ask permission to inquire about a sensitive matter. For example, "Could I ask you kind of a personal question? If it's too personal, you need not answer . . . but it would be helpful for me to know."

"Well, those are natural feelings."

FAMILY INVENTORY

Ask about symptoms or illnesses, parent's emotional and social adjustments, siblings, grandparents and other significant persons. "How is your health, Mr. _____ ?" "What kind of symptoms do you have?" "Are you seeing a doctor?" "What medicine are you taking?" "How do *you* feel?" "How are things going with you?"

If a parent seems sad or anxious, verbalize that observation and invite him to talk about it.

Important areas to explore

Time and cause of death of significant persons

Separations and losses the child has experienced

Parent's work, including hours and arrangements for substitute child care

How the parents have been getting along

Who lives in the house, including persons not in the family and recent additions to or departures from the household

Family crises

Sleeping arrangements

Privacy practices (bedroom, bathroom)

The father's participation in the family

Thoughts about discipline

The mother's time for herself away from the children

The parents' joint or individual social interests

Social support network. Helpful? Not helpful?

Community ties—church, clubs, and other organizations

Other important questions

"You've been telling me about what you regard as _____'s troublesome traits. Tell me about his good points—things you really like about him."

"What do you believe your (husband, wife, son, daughter) thinks about that?"

"Mr. _____, you're a key person in _____'s life—someone he admires a lot. I would find it most helpful to hear your thoughts about how he is getting along."

"What would you change, if you could, about your family?"

In the interviewer's judgment, does the family's equilibrium depend on the continuing presence of the patient's symptoms or illness?

BEING PSYCHOLOGICALLY HELPFUL

The physician's personal warmth, empathy, integrity, sincerity and acceptance of the patient and his problem are important ingredients of a therapeutic physician-patient relationship.

In being identified by the patient as reliable and trustworthy, the physician has developed a potentially helping relationship.

The physician's ability to promote confidence and facilitate communication of facts and feelings enhances his effectiveness.

The physician's understanding of people permits him to avoid being moralistic, judgmental or authoritarian.

The opportunity in the interview for the patient to sort out thoughts, communicate fears and worries and discharge feelings with an interested and facilitative physician, a person who has a special status in society, may be therapeutic.

The patient experiences the supportive interest of the physician in being valued as a person.

The physician offers a special therapeutic relationship through his ability to get a child to like, trust and admire him; to be comfortable and friendly; to relate in a strongly positive fashion and to identify with and assume, at least to some extent, his ideas and attitudes toward health and his view of the child's symptoms and life situation. In this way he also enables the patient to share important aspects of his or her personality and experiences.

Continuity of care and the appropriate investment of time and interest facilitate a constructive relationship.

The doctor's supportive interest in carefully identifying the patient's successes, strengths, resiliency and potentialities, in addition to his weaknesses, worries, feelings, puzzlements and vulnerabilities, helps establish a health-promoting bond among physician, parent and child. It also contributes to a patient's self-esteem, fosters his ability to assume an active role in the resolution or amelioration of his problem and promotes the development of new capabilities.

The interview offers an opportunity for self reflection, discovery and clarification. It helps the child be more open with his feelings.

The doctor need not understand all the psychodynamics in the evolution of a problem to be therapeutically effective.

The patient's spontaneous insight is more important than the physician's verbal interpretation.

Be aware of the patient's feelings and your own.

The right word or phrase at the right time may be extremely helpful.

The physician may at times be directive, giving members of the family assignments to be done before the next session, e.g., greater participation of the father, increased social experiences for the parents, enhanced communication within the family, efforts to alter behavior that is troublesome, and more open discussion of issues about which a conflict has arisen in the family.

IF THE INTERVIEW IS NOT GOING WELL

Is the patient uneasy because the doctor's interest in psychosocial matters was unanticipated or misunderstood?

Is the patient sufficiently psychologically or developmentally minded to understand the relevance of those factors?

Is the patient comfortable?

Did the interviewer do anything verbally or nonverbally to interfere with rapport?

Did the patient come against his own wishes? If one suspects this, ask the patient to clarify his feelings about coming.

Is the patient angry? Depressed? Psychotic? Retarded? Very shy?

Is the patient reluctant to talk in the presence of another family member?

Is the patient in the process of evaluating the physician's interest, competence and ability to keep confidences?

Are the doctor and patient incompatible?

Is the patient intimidated?

Does the patient really want help at this time?

Is the patient hesitant or unable to express feelings?

Some patients erect a barrier of rationalization and intellectualization.

The psychologically disturbed patient may omit significant details, alter others and resist the efforts of the interviewer to learn additional facts.

Because of the patient's anxiety, the history may be extremely diffuse.

The patient who does not volunteer information or elaborate may have been forced to come against his wish.

The patient may be afraid that such exploration and clarification may precipitate a divorce, lead to disclosure of personal or family secrets, or elicit the doctor's disapproval.

PERIODS OF SILENCE

If parent and child are hesitant about starting the interview, look at one of the parents or the child and say: "_____, why don't you start off?"

Pauses in the interview should not be too quickly interrupted.

If such a pause is prolonged, the physician may use an encouraging gesture, nod, smile or interject a word or phrase such as the following:

"Now, you've been telling me about _____. Could you tell me something about _____?"

"You said _____?"

"You mentioned _____?"

"Won't you go on?"

"You were about to say something."

"These things are hard to talk about."

"Well . . .?"

"So?"

An adolescent who is shy, embarrassed, unaccustomed to talking with an adult, depressed or anxious may tend to be silent.

Cultural or language barriers may be present.

ENDING THE INTERVIEW

The physician's ability to see the time without obviously "clock-watching" allows him to bring the discussion to an end within the scheduled period and prevents the termination from seeming abrupt and the interview from seeming incomplete.

"Well, I see that our time is up." The doctor should then stand and move to open the office door.

It may be helpful to offer, just before the time is up, a brief summary of the interview to illuminate important points made, to indicate the doctor's satisfaction with it and to commend the patient: "You've been very helpful."

"There are some other matters that we ought to discuss, so I believe that further sessions would be helpful."

"Think some more about all this, and we'll discuss it next time. Some other ideas will probably come to mind."

Both the doctor and the patient—the parents and the child—should have a clear understanding of what they are to do next or between visits, e.g., "We've decided on some assignments, so let's work on them between now and next _____."

If return office visits would be inconvenient or unnecessary, arrange follow-up by phone: "Call me Thursday at 4:00 to let me know how things are going."

If the patient raises a new problem at the end of the interview (e.g., "Oh, by the way . . .") do not attempt to deal with it then. Rather, suggest that she bring it up in the next session or make an appointment for another visit. Recognize that this belated complaint may be the most important issue for the patient.

The usual interval for supportive interviews is one week. Less frequent visits make continuity more tenuous.

Time between sessions is often an important diagnostic and therapeutic ally.

If both parents were present for the first interview, return visits may permit the interviewer to see each parent alone if that is desired: "Why don't each of you take turns in bringing _____ to see me."

The end of the interview *is* the end of the interview. The temptation to have a social chat is present during the let-down period after the intensity of the interview; however, such practice tends to undermine the interviewer's effectiveness.

GENERAL REFERENCES

Bernstein, L., Bernstein, R. S., and Dana, R. H.: Interviewing: A Guide for Health Professionals. 2nd ed. New York, Appleton-Century-Crofts, 1974.

Browne, K., and Freeling, P.: The Doctor-Patient Relationship. 2nd ed. New York, Churchill-Livingstone, 1976.

Byrne, P. S., and Long, B. E. L.: Doctors Talking to Patients. London, Her Majesty's Stationery Office, 1978.

Enelow, A. J., and Swisher, S. N.: Interviewing and Patient Care. 2nd ed. London, Oxford University Press, 1979.

Engel, G. L., and Morgan, W. L., Jr.: Interviewing the Patient. Philadelphia, W. B. Saunders Co., 1973.

Korsch, B. M., and Alvey, E. F.: Pediatric interviewing techniques. Curr. Probl. Pediatr. 3:3, 1973.

Senn, M. J. E.: The contribution of psychiatry to child health services. Am. J. Orthopsychiatry 21:138, 1951.

Senn, M. J. E.: Emotions and symptoms in pediatric practice. Adv. Pediatr. 3:69, 1948.

Senn, M. J. E.: The psychotherapeutic role of the pediatrician. Pediatrics 2:147, 1948.

Simmons, J. E.: Psychiatric Examination of Children. 3rd ed. Philadelphia, Lea & Febiger, 1981.

Walton, J. N., Duncan, A. S., Fletcher, C. M., et al.: Talking with Patients: A Teaching Approach. London, Nuffield Provincial Hospitals Trust, 1979.

20 / FEVER

CLINICAL CONSIDERATIONS

Fever in children is, in most instances, attributable to a readily identifiable infection, usually a respiratory one. Not infrequently, however, the cause of fever is not immediately apparent, and further observation or laboratory examinations are required. Fever may be accompanied by delirium, seizures and chills.

The mechanisms for heat loss are limited in the presence of a high environmental temperature and high humidity and in patients with congenital ectodermal dysplasia of the anhidrotic type in whom sweating does not occur.

Usually, during the first two years of life, no significant diurnal variation in body temperature occurs. Between the ages of six months and two years, some fluctuation may be noted, perhaps as much as 0.6° C (1° F). In children between the ages of two and six years, the diurnal variation may be as much as 0.9° C (1.6° F). In children above this age, the variation may be as much as 1.1° C (2° F). Usually, the highest body temperature is recorded in the late afternoon or early evening.

No one temperature reading can be given as *normal* for all children at all times. There is, instead, a *range* of normality. In the newborn period, fever has been defined as a rectal temperature greater than 37.4 to 37.8° C (99° to 100° F), whereas in infants, a temperature of 38.33° C (101° F) is considered fever. In older children, a rectal temperature of 38.5° C (101.3° F) or an oral temperature of 37.8° C (100° F) is usually regarded as abnormal. The child should be at bed rest or physically inactive for 30 minutes before the temperature is taken so that a basal determination may be obtained. Exercise may cause as much as a 1.1° C (2° F) rise in body temperature. The temperature should also not be taken within one hour after a meal, since a slight physiologic rise in body temperature follows eating. Oral temperatures are also affected by prior intake of cold or hot foods. In children under the age of six years, the temperature may be taken rectally or by placing the thermometer in the axilla for three minutes. The oral recording of the temperature is usually satisfactory in children above six years of age.

When the temperature is taken rectally, the thermometer should be inserted about 5 cm into the rectum of an infant, or up to 7 cm in an older child. Since the thermometer may perforate the colon, axillary temperature may appropriately be substituted, with the normal range being from 36.5° C (97.7° F) to 37.2° C (99° F). The rectal temperature is often considered to be as much as a degree higher (F) than the oral temperature and the axillary reading correspondingly lower.

The premature infant not only has difficulty in balancing heat production with heat loss but also is easily overheated. Skin temperature on the anterior abdominal wall should be between 36 and 36.5° C (96.8 to 97.7° F). The very premature infant requires an ambient temperature of 37° C during the first days of life. Imperfect thermoregulatory mechanisms are also present in the term newborn infant, but to a lesser extent than in the premature infant. Little concern need be shown over rectal temperatures in the range from 36.1 to 37.8° C (97 to 100° F) in term infants who appear healthy.

Sauer, P. J. J., and Visser, H. K. A.: The neutral temperature of very low-birth-weight infants. Pediatrics 74:288, 1984.

Since fever is such a common manifestation of disease, a comprehensive etiologic classification of fever would be impractically long. The classification given below is of disease states in which fever may be the presenting or prominent complaint. In many instances, the febrile course is acute and self-limited; in others, it is intermittent, recurrent or chronic. Patients with unexplained fever should be re-examined daily, since new physical findings may have become evident.

ETIOLOGIC CLASSIFICATION OF FEVER

I. INFECTIONS, especially those of the upper respiratory tract, are by far the most common cause of fever in childhood.

A. Respiratory infections
   1. Common cold
   2. Acute sinusitis may cause acute fever in children. Sinusitis may be a

cause of chronic fever, but such an etiology is uncommon.

3. Pharyngitis is probably the most frequent cause of fever in childhood. Fever occasionally precedes by some hours other symptoms and signs.
4. Otitis media, mastoiditis
5. Pneumonia. The etiologic classification of pneumonia is included on page 375.
6. Pulmonary tuberculosis is an important diagnostic consideration in infants and children with unexplained fever.

B. Urinary tract infections. *The importance of including the possibility of a urinary tract infection in the differential diagnosis of fever cannot be overstressed.* Repeated urine cultures are an essential part of the work-up in children with acute or chronic fever, even though urinary symptoms such as frequency are not present.

C. Exanthems. Fever is a prominent symptom in the prodromal phase of the exanthematous diseases, especially in the presence of a community outbreak or a history of recent exposure. Exanthem subitum, or roseola infantum, is a diagnostic consideration in children with acute, unexplained fever, especially in infants between the ages of six months and two years. Although the child usually does not appear ill, roseola may be ushered in by hyperpyrexia, convulsions and a bulging fontanel. A leukopenia and a relative lymphocytosis may be present. The fever continues for three to four days and is followed by an evanescent rash.

D. Enteric infections. Although other symptoms may be more prominent, fever may be an important complaint in patients with an enteric infection. Cultures and serologic tests are often helpful in arriving at a specific diagnosis.
1. Salmonellosis
2. *Campylobacter* enteritis
3. Ascariasis
4. Amebiasis

E. Infections of the central nervous system
1. Meningitis. In the presence of fever and such physical findings as a bulging fontanel, nuchal rigidity, convulsions, altered sensorium and positive Kernig's sign, meningitis is, of course, a likely diagnostic possibility. *The possibility of meningitis exists in every infant with unexplained fever*, even though the fever has been present for several days. Irritability, unusual drowsiness or failure to feed well may also occur. Unusual irritability is, at times, the only indication that meningitis has developed in a young infant. Fever may not be present when the patient is first seen. Meningitis caused by *Haemophilus influenzae* is especially likely to have an insidious onset, with fever the most prominent early symptom. Tuberculous meningitis is *always* a diagnostic consideration when irritability or unexplained fever occurs in a child with a positive tuberculin skin test or a known tuberculous infection. Examination of the cerebrospinal fluid is frequently indicated as a diagnostic measure in infants and children with an unexplained serious illness and in patients with unexplained fever. Persistence of fever 72 hours after initiation of adequate therapy in a patient with meningitis may be caused by a complicating subdural effusion. Other complications include brain abscess, arthritis, ophthalmitis, phlebitis and drug fever. Because persistent meningeal infection is a possibility, repeated cerebrospinal fluid examinations are indicated.

Balagtas, R. C., Levin, S., Nelson, K. E., and Gotoff, S. P.: Secondary and prolonged fevers in bacterial meningitis. J. Pediatr. 77:957, 1970.

Lin, T-Y., Nelson, J. D., and McCraken, G. H., Jr.: Fever during treatment for bacterial meningitis. Pediatr. Infect. Dis. 3:319, 1984.

2. Encephalitis. The possibility of postinfectious encephalitis is to be considered whenever fever recurs during convalescence from measles, chickenpox or other exanthems. Primary encephalitis is another cause of fever.
3. Poliomyelitis. Unexplained fever of a few days' duration may precede the appearance of paralysis in patients with poliomyelitis.

F. Infections of the liver and biliary tract
1. Infectious hepatitis
2. Chronic aggressive hepatitis
3. Cholangitis in a partially obstructed biliary tree may account for septic fever in patients with cystic fibrosis and may complicate Caroli's disease or congenital dilatation of the intrahepatic bile ducts.

Wyllie, R., and Fitzgerald, J. F.: Bacterial cholangitis in a 10 week old infant with fever of undetermined origin. Pediatrics 65:164, 1980.

4. Liver abscess
5. Granulomatous hepatitis due to sarcoidosis, tuberculosis, histoplasmosis or brucellosis

Simon, H. B., and Wolff, S. M.: Granulomatous hepatitis and prolonged fever of unknown origin: A study of 13 patients. Medicine 52:1, 1973.

G. Infections involving the heart
   1. Rheumatic fever
   2. Infective endocarditis
   3. Myocarditis. An electrocardiogram should be obtained in patients with unexplained fever when the tachycardia is greater than that ordinarily attributable to fever. The quality of the heart sounds in these patients may also be abnormal.
H. Systemic infections
   1. Bacteremia. *The practice of including bacteremia as a diagnostic consideration in infants and children with unexplained fever is essential, especially in the newborn, young infants and toddlers.* Blood cultures are of great diagnostic help in arriving at a specific etiologic diagnosis, not only in the patient with spiking fever or chronic fever of undetermined etiology, but also in patients with infectious diseases such as meningitis, pneumonia and diarrhea. In patients with spiking fever, blood cultures should be drawn, if possible, an hour or two before the spike. If this cannot be done, several blood cultures may be obtained during 24 hours. The clinical picture of sepsis in young infants is particularly deceptive, since fever may not be present. Bone marrow cultures may be diagnostic for fever due to bacterial, fungal or mycobacterial etiologies.
      Pneumococcal or *H. influenzae* type B bacteremia or meningitis is especially a possibility in children under the age of two years with acute fever over 38.9° C (102° F) of unknown origin; a WBC count of 15,000/cu mm or higher; an erythrocyte sedimentation rate of 30 mm or greater; evidence of pneumonia or upper respiratory tract infection; or absence of a localized focus of infection. Infants under three months of age with a fever of 38° C (100.4° F) or higher should usually be hospitalized and given a septic work-up of blood culture, urine culture, chest x-ray and lumbar puncture. Therapy with antibiotics may

be promptly undertaken in these instances, especially in infants under six weeks of age.
   Children with a history of leukemia or other malignancy, nephrosis, sickle cell anemia, immunodeficiency disorder or absence of the spleen are also at special risk of a bacteremia. Blood cultures should be obtained in such children. For those with a fever greater than 38° C and a WBC count of 15,000/cu mm or higher, presumptive treatment with agents effective against *Streptococcus pneumoniae* and *H. influenzae* type B would appear indicated. If the blood culture is positive, the child should be admitted for repeat blood cultures, lumbar puncture if clinically indicated, e.g., in the presence of irritability, and intravenous antibiotic therapy. Continued observation on an ambulatory basis is justifiable only if the child is afebrile, is playful and alert, does not appear ill and will be under close and adequate surveillance.

Klein, J. O.: Current concepts of infectious diseases in the newborn infant. Adv. Pediatr. 31:405, 1984.
Klein, J. O., Schlesinger, P. C., and Karasic, R. B.: Management of the febrile infant three months of age or younger. Pediatr. Infect. Dis. 3:75, 1984.
Klein, J. O.: Bacteremia in ambulatory children. Pediatr. Infect. Dis. 3:S5 (Suppl), 1984.
Liu, C-H., Lehan, C., Speer, M. E., Smith, E-O., Gutgesell, M. E., Fernbach, D. J., and Rudolph, A. J.: Early detection of bacteremia in an outpatient clinic. Pediatrics 75:827, 1985.
Long, S. S.: Approach to the febrile patient with no obvious focus of infection. Pediatr. Rev. 5:305, 1984.

   2. Infective endocarditis. An adequate number of blood cultures should be obtained whenever bacterial endocarditis is suspected. Because a small number of these patients consistently demonstrate negative blood cultures, six blood cultures for both aerobic and anaerobic organisms should be obtained over a period of several days. In the postoperative cardiac patient with bacterial endocarditis, fever may be the only presenting finding. Bacterial endocarditis may occur in the absence of a murmur.

Newburger, J. W., and Nadas, A. S.: Infective endocarditis. Pediatr. Rev. 3:226, 1982.

3. Infectious mononucleosis

Andiman, W. A.: The Epstein-Barr virus and EB virus infections in childhood. J. Pediatr. 95:177, 1979.

4. Acute infectious lymphocytosis
5. Epidemic influenza
6. Enterovirus infections in the newborn may cause fever, viral meningitis, diarrhea, hepatosplenomegaly, poor feeding, lethargy, irritability and rash. In the older child, fever may persist for 5 to 12 days or up to three weeks. Severe headache, abdominal pain, myalgia, a rubelliform rash and stiff neck may be associated symptoms.

Lake, A. M., Lauer, B. A., Clark, J. C., Wesenberg, R. L., and McIntosh, K.: Enterovirus infections in neonates. J. Pediatr. 89:787, 1976.

7. Colorado tick fever caused by *Dermacentor andersoni*
8. Tick-borne relapsing fever, caused by the blood spirochetes *Borrelia* and characterized by recurrent episodes of fever and influenza-like symptoms, may occur one to three weeks after an overnight stay in a log cabin at over 5000 feet elevation in the Western United States.

Le, C. T.: Tick-borne relapsing fever in children. Pediatrics 66:963, 1980.

9. Rat bite fever: Spirillary (Sodokin); streptobacillary (Haverhill fever)
10. Cytomegalovirus infection (CMV). Acquired cytomegalovirus infection may resemble infectious mononucleosis with atypical lymphocytes, low-grade fever that persists for several weeks, malaise and fatigue. The heterophil test is negative. Paired serum samples for CMV titers should be obtained from children with unexplained fever of more than two weeks' duration.
11. Leptospirosis may present as a febrile illness or as fever of undetermined etiology.
12. Q fever may present as a purely febrile syndrome.
13. Rocky Mountain spotted fever
14. Psittacosis may be considered when a history of exposure to psittacine birds is obtained in the presence of a pulmonary infiltration.
15. Epidemic myalgia
16. Tularemia
17. Histoplasmosis
18. Blastomycosis (nonpulmonary)

19. Visceral larva migrans
20. Malaria
21. Cat-scratch disease
22. Toxoplasmosis
23. Tuberculosis in nonpulmonary forms; e.g., disseminated tuberculosis or involvement of the peritoneum, pericardium, genitourinary tract or liver may be a cause of fever.
24. Toxic shock syndrome is characterized by the sudden onset of high fever followed by vomiting, diarrhea, myalgia, hypotension, shock and an erythematous rash.
25. Bubonic plague
26. Brucellosis

Street, L., Jr., Grant, W. W., and Alva, J. D.: Brucellosis in childhood. Pediatrics 55:416, 1975.

27. Trichinosis
I. Abscesses, localized infections
1. Osteomyelitis. In patients considered to have acute osteomyelitis, a number of blood cultures and a bone scan should be promptly obtained. The length of time during which therapy is withheld in an attempt to secure the etiologic organism depends upon the severity of the illness in each patient. It seems reasonable that even in the most toxic patients a minimum of two blood cultures may be obtained and that probably in no patient should therapy be withheld for more than 24 hours.
2. Intracranial abscess; cerebritis

Liston, T. E., Tomasouic, J. J., and Stevens, E. A.: Early diagnosis and management of cerebritis in a child. Pediatrics 65:484, 1979.

3. Lung abscess
4. Retropharyngeal abscess
5. Alveolar abscess
6. Perinephritic abscess. Both the urinalysis and the intravenous pyelogram are usually normal.
7. Appendiceal abscess
8. A pelvic abscess is to be considered with fever of unknown cause.
9. Mediastinitis
10. Liver abscess

Harrison, H. R., Crowe, C. P., and Fulginiti, V. A.: Amebic liver abscess in children: Clinical and epidemiologic features. Pediatrics 64:923, 1979.

11. Subphrenic abscess
12. Spinal epidural infection
13. Purulent pericarditis

14. Empyema
15. Bronchiectasis
16. Immunodeficiency diseases
17. Thrombophlebitis secondary to infected intravenous needle or catheter. The needle tip of the catheter should be cultured.
18. Intervertebral discitis is characterized by low-grade fever, irritability and refusal to walk or sit up.

II. COLLAGEN-VASCULAR OR CONNECTIVE TISSUE DISEASE

A. Rheumatic fever. A low-grade fever is occasionally the earliest manifestation of rheumatic fever, with the major and minor manifestations appearing later.
B. Serum sickness
C. Dermatomyositis
D. Periarteritis nodosa
E. Polyarteritis nodosa of infancy is characterized by a prolonged febrile illness, skin rash, conjunctivitis, convulsions, anemia and congestive heart failure.

Tang, P. H. L., and Segal, A. J.: Polyarteritis nodosa of infancy. JAMA 217:1666, 1971.

F. Lupus erythematosus. Initially, some of these patients may demonstrate intermittent fever.

Fish, A. J., Blak, E. B., Westberg, N. G., Burke, B. A., Vernier, R. L., and Michael, A.F.: Systemic lupus erythematosus within the first two decades of life. Am. J. Med. 62:99, 1977.

G. Juvenile rheumatoid arthritis is an important diagnostic possibility in children with fever of undetermined origin. Low or spiking, persistent or intermittent fever may be the earliest manifestation of this disease, appearing before the onset of arthritis. One or two spikes of 39° C (103° F) or higher may occur daily, most often in the late afternoon or evening, with the temperature usually returning to normal or subnormal between rises. Occasional hyperpyrexia with temperatures above 40.6° C (105° F) may occur. The onset of febrile episodes may be accompanied by shaking chills. Fever may persist for weeks or months before arthritis becomes evident. An evanescent rheumatoid rash may accompany the febrile episodes.
H. Mixed connective tissue disease

III. NEOPLASTIC DISEASES

A. Leukemia frequently presents with fever as the initial symptom. Peripheral blood examination may show only slight anemia and leukopenia at that time, with few or no blast cells. Fever in patients with leukemia as well as other malignancies is usually caused by infection, especially in the presence of granulocytopenia.
B. Hodgkin's disease is usually also manifested by lymphadenopathy by the time the patient becomes febrile.
C. Ewing's tumor
D. Neuroblastoma with bone metastases

IV. DEHYDRATION

A. Dehydration, especially in newborn and young infants, may cause fever and irritability.
B. Hypertonic dehydration (hyperosmolarity) may also be accompanied by fever.
C. Diabetes insipidus in infants may also cause fever.

V. DRUGS, IMMUNIZATION

A. Most drugs can cause fever, occasionally persistent fever of unknown origin. Drug fever rapidly disappears within 48 hours after the drug is stopped.
B. Atropine poisoning may be accompanied by hyperpyrexia.
C. Immunization reactions
D. Salicylate intoxication is frequently accompanied by fever, at times over 40.6° C (105° F). Young infants appear especially prone to hyperpyrexia due to salicylism.

VI. NEUROLOGIC DISORDERS

A. A number of central nervous system disorders may cause irregularities in control of body temperature that result either in hyper- or hypothermia. Such disorders include intracranial hemorrhage, brain tumors, infections, and surgical operations that involve the hypothalamus, the region of the third ventricle or the medulla. Because the anterior hypothalamus acts to prevent an abnormal elevation of the body temperature, injury to this structure may result in hyperthermia. The regulatory center for the prevention of excessive heat loss is thought to be in the posterior hypothalamus. Infants with intracranial hemorrhage due to birth trauma are especially prone to hyperpyrexia or hypothermia. Neurogenic hyperthermia may also occur in patients with bulbar poliomyelitis and in those with encephalitis. Febrile episodes due to autonomic dysfunction may occur in Guillain-Barré syndrome.

B. The association of febrile states and infectious diseases with seizures in young children is well known. Fever may not only result from the muscular contractions that occur during a convulsion, but may also, in rare instances, be the sole clinical manifestation of a paroxysmal seizure discharge from the hypothalamic region. Fever may also develop in patients in status epilepticus.

C. Infections of the central nervous system are discussed on page 337.

D. Children with familial dysautonomia often have episodes of unexplained fever.

E. Infants with congenital familial nonhemolytic jaundice with kernicterus have frequent febrile episodes, probably central in origin.

F. Neurogenic fever may occur in Krabbe's disease.

G. Fever may occur with a cervical spinal cord tumor.

H. Cerebral spinal fluid shunt infection

Odio, C., McCracken, G. H., and Nelson, J. D.: CSF shunt infections in pediatrics. Am. J. Dis. Child. 138:1103, 1984.

VII. Blood Diseases

A. Fever may be one of the primary manifestations of a hemolytic anemia, especially during a crisis.

B. Fever may also be a manifestation of a transfusion reaction.

C. Fever is a common manifestation of leukemia.

D. The occurrence of high fever (39.5 to 40.5° C) in children with sickle cell anemia raises the possibility of overwhelming bacterial infection due to *S. pneumoniae* or *H. influenzae*.

VIII. Hemorrhage

A. Hemorrhagic disorders may be characterized by fever if bleeding occurs into a viscus or other body tissue.

B. Intracranial hemorrhage in the newborn infant may cause fever.

C. Adrenal hemorrhage in the newborn infant is often accompanied by fever.

D. Hemorrhage into a tumor may be accompanied by fever.

IX. High Environmental Temperature

A. Premature and newborn infants readily develop elevation of body temperature owing to environmental overheating.

B. Sustained elevation of the environmental temperature, as occurs in very hot weather, may also cause an elevation of body temperature in term infants. This response is more likely in very young infants, but may also be noted in those who are older. Heat stroke may develop in otherwise normal infants if the environmental temperature is high enough to overtax the ability of the infant to dissipate heat. Infants left in closed automobiles in the summertime may die of heat stress.

King, K., Negus, K., and Vance, J. C.: Heat stress in motor vehicles: A problem in infancy. Pediatrics 68:579, 1981.

C. Infants with brain damage often tolerate high environmental temperatures poorly and, as a result, may manifest hyperpyrexia and heat stroke.

D. Patients with cystic fibrosis are also prone to severe electrolyte depletion heat prostration when subjected to a persistent high environmental temperature.

E. An infant wrapped or clothed too warmly may develop a fever.

X. Miscellaneous Causes for Fever

A. Kawasaki disease is characterized by the abrupt onset, without prodromal signs, of fever that spikes several times a day up to 40° C (104° F). Hyperpyrexia may also occur. The fever does not respond to aspirin or acetaminophen.

B. Periodic disease may be characterized by the episodic occurrence of fever, sometimes accompanied by abdominal pain or arthralgia. Cyclic neutropenia is manifested by neutropenia occurring at approximately 21- to 27-day intervals, along with fever, malaise, mouth ulcers, sore throat, arthritis and headache.

C. Familial Mediterranean fever or periodic polyserositis, an autosomal recessive disorder occurring primarily in Sephardic Jews and persons of Armenian descent, is characterized chiefly by recurrent fever and abdominal pain, but also by pleural, pericardial, meningeal and articular symptoms.

Cone, T. E., Jr.: Periodic diseases in children. Postgrad. Med. 50:242, 1971.

D. Takayasu's arteritis is characterized by fever, fatigue, dyspnea, arthralgia, carotid artery tenderness, hypertension and decreased pulse.

E. Virilizing adrenal hyperplasia. Episodes of periodic fever, headaches, abdominal pain, chills, cutaneous flushing and prostration have been described in a variant of virilizing adrenal hyperplasia.

F. Ectodermal dysplasia of the anhidrotic type may be responsible for episodes of unexplained fever in infants.

G. Infantile cortical hyperostosis may be characterized, in part, by fever that may range from 38.3 to 39.4° C (101 to 103° F). At times, fever is the initial symptom, followed shortly by irritability and swelling over involved bones.

H. Inflammatory bowel disease may be accompanied by fever. Crohn's disease may initially present as fever of undetermined origin.

I. Paroxysmal atrial tachycardia

J. Congestive cardiac failure. Although fever is known to be associated with congestive cardiac failure, the temperature usually does not exceed 37.8° C (100° F). Fever higher than this level should be ascribed to some other cause.

K. Hyperthyroidism during toxic crises

L. Sarcoidosis. The chest film is abnormal in 95 per cent of children with sarcoidosis.

M. The postpericardiotomy syndrome, which may occasionally follow pericardiotomy by two or three weeks, is characterized by persistent fever and precordial pain. A pericardial friction rub may be heard transiently.

Engle, M. A., Zabriskie, J. B., Senterfit, L. B., and Ebert, P. A.: Postpericardiotomy syndrome. Mod. Concepts Cardiovasc. Dis. 44:59, 1975.

N. A benign postperfusion syndrome, due to the cytomegalovirus and characterized by fever, splenomegaly and atypical lymphocytes, occurs occasionally after open heart surgery. The fever, which occurs six to seven weeks after operation, may persist from 7 to 21 days.

O. About one third of children may develop a transient elevation of body temperature up to 39° C (102° F) within 12 hours of cardiac catheterization and angiography.

P. Low-grade fever may occur with narcotic withdrawal in newborns.

Q. Fabry's disease may be characterized by bouts of fever.

R. Fever of undetermined origin. The criteria used to characterize fever of undetermined origin generally include fever of 38.3° C (101° F) or higher that persists for two or more weeks, an absence of localizing findings and inability to make an etiologic diagnosis by the use of usual laboratory means.

Many of the disorders listed above in this chapter are to be considered diagnostic possibilities in patients with fever of unknown origin. In many instances, fever of undetermined etiology spontaneously resolves before a cause can be established. In addition, what is reported by the parent as persistent fever may, on careful review of the history, represent a series of self-limited, usually viral illnesses rather than a persistent fever of undetermined origin. In other instances, the parent has a misunderstanding of what constitutes "fever" (a rectal temperature of 38.5° C or its equivalent), the normal diurnal variation of body temperature or the effect of activity and exercise on core temperature. The term *pseudo-fever of unknown origin* (pseudo-FUO) has been applied to characterize this frequent cause of consultation. In many instances, the parent is overly concerned about complaints such as fatigue. The temperature is taken frequently and the child is kept home from school. At times, this pattern represents masked school phobia, especially when coupled with complaints of "sore throat," tiredness or recurrent abdominal pain. Although the child's absence from school, often for weeks, is usually not mentioned by the parents as a presenting complaint or in the history, it should be explored by a question such as, "How much school has this illness caused Johnny to miss?"

Often these parents fear the presence of an occult malignant disorder. Children with pseudo-FUO do not appear ill. Useful screening examinations when a biomedical disease is considered as a diagnostic possibility in these children include a complete blood count, Westergren erythrocyte sedimentation rate, platelet count, urinalysis, urine culture, tuberculin skin test, perhaps a chest radiograph and, in endemic areas, histoplasmosis antibody titers.

Factitious fever may occur in older adolescents who report spiking fever. When the patient is asked to record his pulse rate at times of fever, the patient will not report it to be elevated.

Kleiman, M. B.: The complaint of persistent fever. Recognition and management of pseudo fever of unknown origin. Pediatr. Clin. North Am. 29:201, 1982.

Long, S. S.: Approach to the febrile patient with no obvious focus of infection. Pediatr. Rev. 5:305, 1984.

Murray, H. W.: Factitious fever updated. Ann. Intern. Med. 139:739, 1979.

HYPERPYREXIA

I. Hyperpyrexia with Elevation of the Body Temperature to 41.1° C (106° F) or above may occur in patients with neurologic disorders; Duchenne type muscular dystrophy; Reye's syndrome; central nervous system infections such as bacterial or aseptic meningitis; rickettsial diseases, including Rocky Mountain spotted fever; atropine poisoning; salicylate poisoning; bulbar poliomyelitis; and, terminally, in tetanus. In the newborn, hyperthermia may be a manifestation of adrenal hemorrhage, intraventricular hemorrhage or toxoplasmosis. Hyperpyrexia also is a late manifestation in patients with metachromatic leukodystrophy or subacute sclerosing panencephalitis. Hyperpyrexia may also occur in patients severely ill with fulminant infections, especially when accompanied by peripheral circulatory failure. Heat stroke, characterized by hyperthermia and hypohidrosis, may be preceded by fatigue, nausea, disorientation, incoherent speech and a staggering gait.

American Academy of Pediatrics Committee on Sports Medicine: Climatic heat stress and the exercising child. Pediatrics 69:808, 1982.

Pomerance, J. J., and Richardson, C. J.: Hyperpyrexia as a sign of intraventricular hemorrhage in the neonate. Am. J. Dis. Child. 126:854, 1973.

II. Malignant Hyperpyrexia, a syndrome precipitated by halogenated inhalational anesthetic agents or succinylcholine, may have either an insidious or fulminant course. The first sign may be intense muscle contraction and rigidity. Tachypnea, tachycardia, arrhythmias, and severe metabolic acidosis are frequently present. Hyperpyrexia may occur during anesthesia or several hours later. Susceptible patients have an underlying clinical or subclinical myopathic or neuropathic disorder, such as myotonia congenita, central core disease and elevation of serum creatinine phosphokinase. Malignant hyperthermia may be a complication associated with a progressive congenital myopathy in an understatured male with cryptorchidism, pectus carinatum, spinal defects, hypoplasia of the mandible, antimongoloid palpebral fissures, ptosis, low-set ears, webbed neck and weak serrati muscles. Malignant hyperpyrexia also occurs in the Schwartz-Jampel syndrome, which consists of dwarfism, skeletal anomalies and muscular stiffness.

Kaplan, A. M., Bergeson, P. S., Gregg, S. A., and Curless, R. G.: Malignant hyperthermia associated with myopathy and normal muscle enzymes. J. Pediatr. 91:431, 1977.

King, J. O., and Denborough, M. A.: Anesthetic-induced hyperpyrexia in children. J. Pediatr. 83:37, 1973.

Seay, A. R., and Ziter, F. A.: Malignant hyperpyrexia in a patient with Schwartz-Jampel syndrome. J. Pediatr. 93:83, 1978.

HYPOTHERMIA

Hypothermia, a body temperature under 35° C (95° F), may occur in premature infants and in infants with intracranial birth injury. If heat loss is not prevented, the body temperature of normal newborn infants may fall as much as 1.1 to 2.8° C (2 to 5° F) within the first hour after birth. In the newborn infant hypothermia may cause tachypnea, apnea, acidosis, hypoglycemia and disseminated intravascular coagulation.

An abnormally low body temperature may also occur in patients with shock, critical illness or heavy sedation. Encephalitis may also be accompanied by hypothermia. Hypothermia and instability of temperature is a persistent problem in patients with Menkes' kinky-hair syndrome. A rectal temperature of less than 35.5° C (96° F) may be recorded during the first two days of life in a newborn with hypothyroidism. Hyponatremia and water intoxication in infants may cause hypothermia and seizures.

Accidental hypothermia may be caused by wind chill, especially when the individual is wet, or by immersion in cold water.

Accidental hypothermia. Committee on Pediatric Aspects of Physical Fitness, Recreation and Sports, American Academy of Pediatrics. Pediatrics 63:926, 1979.

Although they do not usually demonstrate hypothermia, patients with anorexia nervosa or hypothyroidism may complain of feeling cold.

GENERAL REFERENCES

Feigin, R. D., and Shearer, W. T.: Fever of unknown origin in children. Curr. Probl. Pediatr. 6:3, 1976.

Jacoby, G. A., and Swartz, M. N.: Fever of undetermined origin. N. Engl. J. Med. 289:1407, 1973.

Pizzo, P. A., Lovejoy, F. H., Jr., and Smith, D. H.: Prolonged fever in children: Review of 100 cases. Pediatrics 55:468, 1975.

ETIOLOGIC CLASSIFICATION OF FEVER

21 / REGURGITATION AND VOMITING

REGURGITATION

Regurgitation, which refers to nonforceful expulsion of food and secretions from the esophagus or stomach through the mouth, is usually not accompanied by nausea or forceful contractions of the abdominal muscles.

ETIOLOGIC CLASSIFICATION OF REGURGITATION

I. "PHYSIOLOGIC" REGURGITATION. In the early weeks of life many normal babies regurgitate one or more times a day, bringing up a mouthful or two of food a short time after feeding. Mothers often refer to this as "spitting up." Frequently its cause cannot be determined. As long as normal weight gain continues, there is no cause for concern. Ordinarily the frequency of regurgitation tends to diminish as the baby becomes older and it ceases, usually, by seven to eight months of age.

II. FAULTY FEEDING TECHNIQUES. Frequently the cause of regurgitation may be found in the feeding technique. Observation of the mother feeding the baby may be informative. Babies who nurse either vigorously or slowly may require burping more than once during a meal. If the baby is put down without being burped, eructation of air may cause regurgitation.

Nipple holes that are too small unduly prolong the feeding time and increase the amount of air swallowed, leading to overdistention of the stomach and regurgitation. Retracted nipples may result in excessive air swallowing in the breast-fed infant. Bottle propping often leads to swallowing of air. If a baby's formula is inadequate calorically or if he is not fed frequently enough, an excessive amount of air swallowing may be a result of increased non-nutritive sucking; on the other hand, overfeeding may also cause regurgitation. Excessive handling of an infant immediately after feeding also facilitates regurgitation.

III. GASTROESOPHAGEAL REFLUX. Although vomiting occurs in most children with gastroesophageal reflux, effortless regurgitation may also be present. At times this food loss may be severe enough to cause an abnormally slow weight gain or a weight loss. Symptoms usually begin between the third and tenth days of life. Regurgitation, which usually does not appear until the infant is put down, may not occur if the baby is held or is set in an upright position for approximately 30 minutes after feeding. Gastroesophageal reflux may continue for weeks or a few months with gradual disappearance of symptoms; however, in other instances, the persistence of symptoms and failure to thrive may require surgery for their correction. Gastroesophageal reflux occurs in otherwise normal children, but it is also common in those with Down's syndrome, developmental delay and cystic fibrosis.

Bendig, D. W., Seilheimer, D. K., Wagner, M. L., Ferry, G. D., and Harrison, G. M.: Complications of gastroesophageal reflux in patients with cystic fibrosis. J. Pediatr. 100:536, 1982.

Herbst, J. J.: Diagnosis and treatment of gastroesophageal reflux in children. Pediatr. Rev. 5:75, 1983.

IV. CONGENITAL ESOPHAGEAL OBSTRUCTIONS

A. Esophageal atresia with or without tracheoesophageal fistula. Symptoms begin shortly after birth, and a history of maternal hydramnios may be noted. *The presence of an excessive amount of mucus in a baby's mouth and throat is always suggestive of this diagnosis.* Prompt regurgitation, choking and, perhaps, cyanosis occur with the first and subsequent feedings attempted. The diagnosis may be supported by failure in the attempt to pass a number 8 or 10 French soft rubber radiopaque catheter into the stomach. Radiopaque material instilled through this catheter at fluoroscopy pools in the proximal esophageal pouch. Esophageal atresia may be a component of the VATER association, which includes vertebral defects, anal atresia, radial dysplasia, renal defects and, at times, ventricular septal defect and a single umbilical artery.

B. Stenosis of the esophagus. A stenotic segment may be present in the midportion of the esophagus, causing regurgitation to begin after the first week of life. If the stenosis is minimal, difficulty is not experienced until solid foods are introduced into the diet. The infant may then be considered a "slow" or "fussy" eater. Less frequently, the diagnosis is not suspected until a foreign body lodges in the mid-esophagus.

C. Congenitally short esophagus may cause dysphagia, regurgitation and hematemesis due to esophageal ulceration. Symptoms may occur in infants but are usually not present until the late childhood or early adult years. These children are also "slow" eaters and present feeding problems. Gastric rugae can be visualized above the diaphragm on roentgenographic study. Rather than a congenital defect, this disorder is usually the result of cicatricial contraction associated with a chronic esophagitis caused by gastroesophageal reflux. A true congenital short esophagus is rare.

D. Esophageal hiatus hernia may cause "spitting up" or occasional projectile vomiting. Complications include tracheal aspiration with resultant pulmonary infiltration or peptic esophagitis. If esophagitis is present, the vomitus may be coffee-ground or blood-flecked. Contortions of the neck, including torticollis, opisthotonus and posturing of the trunk, may occur with esophageal reflux and hiatus hernia (Sandifer's syndrome). Rarely, laryngospasm following reflux and aspiration may cause apneic episodes, cyanosis and muscle stiffening.

E. Webbing of the esophagus

F. Cardiospasm

G. Congenital vascular ring. In addition to respiratory symptoms, infants with this anomaly demonstrate hesitancy in swallowing, choking and regurgitation. Dysphagia may first occur or become more notable after the introduction of solid foods.

H. Duplication of the esophagus occurring in the posterior mediastinum may cause dysphagia, regurgitation, respiratory obstruction, cough and, occasionally, hematemesis. Symptoms often occur during the first two years of life.

V. ACQUIRED ESOPHAGEAL LESIONS

A. Esophagitis usually represents a transient inflammation. Occasionally, however, ulceration occurs, followed by stricture formation and obstruction. Esophagitis may occur in the following situations:
1. Infectious diseases: pneumonia, candidiasis, scarlet fever, diphtheria, syphilis, typhoid fever and poliomyelitis
2. Ingestion of corrosive agents
3. Cardiac disease with chronic elevation of venous pressure
4. Chronic pulmonary infections
5. Gastroesophageal reflux

B. Strictures
1. Secondary to infectious diseases
2. Scleroderma
3. Corrosive agents, including lye, bleaches and ammonia
4. The reflux of gastric contents may cause peptic esophagitis, mucosal ulceration and, eventually, a stricture.
5. Ulceration or inflammation due to a foreign body may be followed by scarring.

C. Esophageal diverticulum. Rarely, a tracheobronchial lymph node, adherent to the esophagus after an inflammatory process, may cause a traction diverticulum.

D. Traumatic pseudodiverticulum of the pharynx in newborn infants may follow injury to the posterior pharyngeal wall and be mistaken for esophageal atresia. Because of the resultant cricopharyngeal spasm and functionally high esophageal obstruction, nasogastric tubes cannot be passed or the pharyngeal wall may be perforated in the attempt.

E. Foreign bodies may cause esophageal obstruction either because of their size or the inflammatory reaction they initiate. Esophageal stenosis should be suspected whenever a foreign body stops at some level other than one of the three anatomically narrow points of the esophagus.

F. Retroesophageal abscess
1. Extension of retropharyngeal abscess
2. Esophageal perforation
3. Foreign bodies
4. Vertebral tuberculosis
5. Ulceration from a tracheotomy tube
6. Suppurating mediastinal lymph nodes

VI. RUMINATION usually begins between the third and eighth months of age as the regurgitation of previously swallowed food with rechewing and reswallowing. The baby protrudes his tongue and lower jaw, slightly extends his head, and then makes rhythmical chewing and swallowing motions until regurgitation occurs. Part of the food then dribbles out of the baby's mouth and some is reswallowed. Rather than being distressed, the infant appears almost to enjoy the process.

Occasionally the baby initiates regurgitation by inserting his fingers or a toy into his mouth. Babies who ruminate are often markedly visually alert—"radar-like." Rumination occurs primarily when the infant is left to himself. Weight loss may be severe. The term "spitting up" is rarely used in the presenting complaint; rather, the parent reports vomiting or failure to gain. Rumination results from a parenting disability with the mother usually depressed, uninvolved or fearful of the infant's vulnerability to illness. Recovery is usually prompt when increased mothering and developmentally appropriate nurturing care are temporarily provided by nurses or a mother substitute. Persistent rumination may also occur in older infants and children who are severely mentally retarded or psychotic. Propionic acidemia may present with the symptom of rumination.

Sauvage, D., Leddet, I., Hameury, L., and Barthelemy, C.: Infantile rumination. J. Child Psychiatry 24:197, 1985.

VII. REGURGITATION may be the initial manifestation of pyloric stenosis, but vomiting soon supervenes.

VIII. MISCELLANEOUS CAUSES

A. Dyspnea may lead to air swallowing and gastric overdistention.
B. Ascites, abdominal cysts, organ enlargements and neoplasms may cause regurgitation as a result of increased intra-abdominal pressure.
C. Eventration of the diaphragm can cause frequent regurgitation, probably as a result of angulation of the lower esophagus or stomach.
D. Narcotic withdrawal in the newborn
E. A hemangioma at the cardia may interfere with gastroesophageal closure.

VOMITING

CLINICAL CONSIDERATIONS

Vomiting refers to the forceful expulsion of gastric contents through the mouth, usually accompanied by vigorous contractions of the abdominal muscles. The vomiting center is influenced by both excitatory and inhibitory neurologic and metabolic influences. In infants and young children, vomitus often comes through the nose as well as the mouth. Because of the danger of aspiration, vomiting is exceedingly hazardous in prematures and in infants with neuromotor disability.

The threshold of the vomiting center can be exceeded by emetic impulses from any sensory nerve. Stimuli come primarily from the labyrinth; pharynx; gastrointestinal, biliary and genitourinary tracts; heart; pelvic organs; and peritoneum. Unpleasant sights, odors or tastes may cause vomiting, as may any sufficiently painful stimulus. The threshold of the vomiting center can also be lowered, so that the subthreshold stimuli that continually enter the center may cause vomiting. This may be the mechanism through which psychogenic causes and increased intracranial pressure operate. Drugs that evoke emesis may have a direct action on the vomiting center or on a central chemoreceptor trigger zone separate from, but anatomically near, the vomiting center. Abnormal body metabolites in patients with diabetic ketoacidosis, liver disease, uremia and other disease states may act similarly.

Since nausea is a subjective sensation, its presence cannot be determined precisely in infants. Grimacing, restlessness, yawning, pallor, salivation, sweating, failure to suck their fist, and refusal to refeed after vomiting suggest the presence of nausea in this age group. Older children may complain that their "tummy" or their "throat" hurts.

Appearance of Vomitus

The appearance of the vomitus or stomach aspirate may be of diagnostic help. *In the newborn, gastric aspirate* greater than 20 ml or containing bile, especially in the presence of a history of maternal polyhydramnios, may suggest intestinal obstruction.

Undigested Food. Regurgitation of uncurdled milk in a newborn infant suggests esophageal atresia. In older children, regurgitation of undigested food suggests a stricture of the esophagus or other obstructive lesion at or above the cardia.

Absence of Bile. Absence of bile in the vomitus suggests an obstruction proximal to the ampulla of Vater. Bile may not be clinically apparent in freshly passed vomitus because its yellow color is often diluted with food and gastric juice. Shortly after exposure to air, however, oxidation of the bile pigments causes the pathognomonic green color.

Bilious Vomiting. In the term newborn infant, bilious vomitus should always be considered a sign of intestinal obstruction. It may also occasionally occur in the premature infant with an immature pyloric sphincter and in infants with sepsis as a result of adynamic ileus.

Fecal Vomiting. When the vomitus has a fecal odor, peritonitis or an obstruction of the lower bowel or colon is suggested.

HEMATEMESIS

Bright red blood in the vomitus indicates that the blood has had little or no contact with gastric juice and that active bleeding is present at or above the cardia or in the stomach. Rapid or massive duodenal bleeding may also be manifested by the vomiting of bright red blood. "Coffee-ground" emesis indicates that blood has been altered by gastric digestion and suggests slow bleeding from the esophagus, cardia, stomach or duodenum. Epistaxis is occasionally followed by the vomiting of fresh or altered swallowed blood. If blood is returned through a nasogastric tube introduced into the stomach, gastrointestinal bleeding may be assumed to be proximal to the ligament of Treitz; if no blood is present in the stomach, the bleeding is most likely distal to this point. The ability to diagnose causes of hematemesis has been greatly augmented by fiberoptic endoscopy and selective abdominal angiography.

Hematemesis may be associated with the following disease states:

1. Peptic ulcer
2. Esophageal or other enteric duplication
3. Esophageal varices are the most common cause of massive hematemesis.
4. Esophagitis in patients with a hiatus hernia or gastroesophageal reflux
5. Hematemesis may follow repeated vomiting due to any cause, including pyloric stenosis.
6. Acute gastritis during the course of a severe infectious disease such as pneumonia

7. Poisoning due to ingestion of iron sulfate
8. Theophylline toxicity may cause a hemorrhagic gastritis.
9. Hemangioma in the esophagus
10. Hematobilia
11. Thrombocytopenia
12. Vasculitis

ETIOLOGIC CLASSIFICATION OF VOMITING

I. MECHANICAL VOMITING is frequently secondary to an obstructive lesion of the stomach or intestinal tract, usually a congenital anomaly. Intestinal obstruction should be suspected in any newborn infant who (1) has over 20 ml of fluid in the gastric aspirate, especially if it is bile-stained; (2) vomits and has abdominal distention in the first 24 to 36 hours of life; or (3) does not pass stools. A history of maternal polyhydramnios raises the possibility of a high intestinal obstruction. Plain films of the abdomen in the upright and supine positions are important diagnostic aids.

A. Obstruction
1. Intestinal atresia. Symptoms due to obstruction begin in the first 24 hours of life. If the atretic area is proximal to the ampulla of Vater, the stools contain bile, but the vomitus does not. Distention is confined to the epigastrium or left upper quadrant, and gastric peristaltic waves may be seen. X-ray films show air in the stomach and duodenum but none in the small bowel. Duodenal atresia occurs with an increased frequency in babies with Down's syndrome. If the atretic area is distal to the ampulla of Vater, the vomitus contains bile but the stools do not. Abdominal distention is generalized when the atresia is within or distal to the jejunum. The ileum is the most common site of atresia.

Talbert, J. L., Felman, A. H., and DeBusk, F. L.: Gastrointestinal surgical emergencies in the newborn infant. J. Pediatr. 76:783, 1970.

2. Imperforate anus. Abdominal distention and vomiting begin within 24 to 36 hours after birth. Meconium is not passed. Most commonly the anus is imperforate, and the proximal rectal pouch ends blindly somewhere above. The site of the anus is revealed by dimpling or in-

creased pigmentation of the skin. Stroking of the area causes visible puckering. In other infants, a normal anus is present, but the rectal pouch is blind. A digital rectal examination reveals the site of obstruction. In a third type, a thin membrane separates the anus from the rectum. Dark meconium may be seen through the membrane, and the area may bulge when the baby cries. Anoperineal, rectovesical, rectourethral, rectovaginal and rectoperineal fistulas commonly accompany an imperforate anus. As a result, meconium may be present in the urine of boys and the vagina of girls.

3. Meconium ileus. Symptoms of obstruction beginning within the first 24 to 36 hours represent the earliest manifestation of cystic fibrosis. If passed, the meconium is thick, tenacious and tarry. Palpation may reveal firm, rubbery loops of bowel, giving the impression of a sausage-filled abdomen. A plain film of the abdomen reveals small bubbles throughout the meconium.

O'Neill, J. A., Jr., Grosfeld, J. L., Boles, E. T., Jr., and Clatworthy, H. W., Jr.: Surgical treatment of meconium ileus. Am. J. Surg. 119:99, 1970.

4. Meconium plug. Inspissated meconium in the distal colon may cause abdominal distention, bile-stained vomiting and failure to pass meconium. The obstruction may be relieved by enemas or digital rectal examination. The meconium plug syndrome may be a manifestation of cystic fibrosis or Hirschsprung's disease.

5. Intestinal stenosis
   a. Duodenal. Symptoms of partial obstruction may begin in the first week of life, and the obstruction may rapidly become complete. Differentiation from duodenal atresia is often difficult. If complete obstruction is not present, the baby may feed poorly, have frequent emeses and demonstrate poor weight gain.
   b. Jejunal or ileal. Complete obstruction may simulate atresia.
   c. Rectal. Symptoms of obstipation and megacolon present from birth may simulate aganglionic megacolon. Fecal impaction may cause intestinal obstruction.

6. Neonatal small left colon syndrome may be asymptomatic or associated with low intestinal obstruction. Uniform narrowing of the colon from the splenic flexure to the anus is demonstrable by barium enema. Incidence of maternal diabetes is high.

Davis, W. S., and Campbell, J. B.: Neonatal small left colon syndrome. Am. J. Dis. Child. 129:1024, 1975.

7. Malrotation of the bowel. In infants with malrotation of the bowel, the descending duodenum often becomes obstructed within the first three weeks of life. Obstruction may be caused by peritoneal bands that cross the duodenum and bind the cecum to the posterior abdominal wall or to direct pressure from the malrotated cecum itself. The vomitus usually contains bile, but rare exceptions occur. Because duodenal obstruction may be accompanied by midgut volvulus, immediate surgery is indicated. Infants with the syndrome of asplenia and congenital heart disease may also have malrotation.

8. Midgut volvulus. Incomplete fixation of the malrotated bowel may lead to volvulus of the midgut (duodenum to midtransverse colon). Delay in diagnosis is dangerous because of the threat of bowel infarction. Obstructive symptoms with bilious vomiting sometimes begin as early as three to four days after birth but may occur at any age. Gastric peristaltic waves may be noted. Distention may be epigastric or generalized but is often absent. Recurrent episodes of volvulus with spontaneous resolution occasionally cause cyclic vomiting in older children. Volvulus occurs at times around the atrophied cord of the omphalomesenteric duct. When intestinal obstruction occurs in an infant with the asplenic syndrome (cyanotic congenital heart disease and nucleated red blood cells in the peripheral blood), a midgut volvulus may be present.

Berdon, W. E., Baker, D. H., Bull, S., and Santulli, T. V.: Midgut malrotation and volvulus. Radiology 96:375, 1970.

9. Pyloric stenosis. Regurgitation in the first week of life is frequently the initial symptom in this disorder.

Usually, vomiting gradually becomes evident in the second and third weeks. As mucosal edema is superimposed on the muscular narrowing of the pyloric canal, vomiting becomes increasingly projectile. If the baby is given a small amount of fluid by mouth and examined in adequate light, vigorous gastric peristalsis is usually visible. The diagnosis depends upon an absence of bile in the vomitus and the presence of a palpable pyloric tumor.

10. Torsion of the stomach may cause vomiting in infants, beginning soon after birth and, at times, projectile in character. The diagnosis is established by roentgenologic examination.

11. Annular pancreas is a rare cause of complete or partial and recurrent intestinal obstruction.

12. Diaphragmatic hernia. Dyspnea, cyanosis or vomiting may occur in newborn babies with a massive herniation of the abdominal viscera through a congenital diaphragmatic defect.

13. Hiatus hernia may become symptomatic at any age. Recurrent episodes of colicky lower thoracic or epigastric pain, ulceration of the herniated stomach with hematemesis, discomfort after eating and vomiting may occur.

14. Duplications of the alimentary tract may cause partial intestinal obstruction with colicky pain and vomiting.

Grosfeld, J. L., O'Neill, J. A., and Clatworthy, H. W., Jr.: Enteric duplications in infancy and childhood: An 18-year review. Ann. Surg. 172:83, 1970.

15. Incarcerated or strangulated hernias

16. Intussusception usually causes vomiting early. In the older child intussusception may be a complication of cystic fibrosis.

Holsclaw, D. S., Rocmans, C., and Shwachman, H.: Intussusception in patients with cystic fibrosis. Pediatrics 48.51, 1971.

17. Adhesive bands

18. Foreign bodies in the gastrointestinal tract
   a. Trichobezoar
   b. Lactobezoar. Intestinal obstruction may occur 5 to 14 days after birth owing to inspissated milk curds. This disorder occurs primarily in premature infants who receive a high-calorie powdered milk formula. Abdominal x-rays reveal dense, round or elongated masses in the bowel surrounded by air halos.

Schreiner, R. L., Brady, M. S., Franken, E. A., Stevens, D. C., Lemons, J. A., and Gresham, E. L.: Increased incidence of lactobezoars in low birth weight infants. Am. J. Dis. Child. 133:936, 1979.

19. Paralytic ileus
   a. Peritonitis
   b. Postsurgical complication
   c. Acute infectious diseases such as pneumonia
   d. Severe hypokalemia

20. Intramural hematoma of the intestine secondary to even slight blunt abdominal trauma may cause nausea, bilious vomiting, abdominal pain, tenderness, ileus and, at times, fever. Symptoms and signs may follow immediately or be delayed several days. An abdominal mass may be palpable. A "coil spring" deformity on an upper gastrointestinal series is diagnostic.

Stewart, D. R., Byrd, C. L., and Schuster, S. R.: Intramural hematomas of the alimentary tract in children. Surgery 68:550, 1970.

21. Aganglionic megacolon may cause neonatal vomiting.

22. Sigmoid volvulus, which may occur in patients with a large redundant sigmoid loop attached to a narrow mesenteric base, is usually a fulminant process with early necrosis of the bowel. Chronic constipation may be a contributing factor. A barium enema is required for diagnosis.

Hunter, J. G., Jr., and Keats, T. E.: Sigmoid volvulus in children. Am. J. Roentgenol. 58:621, 1970.

23. The chronic idiopathic pseudo-obstruction syndrome in infants and children is characterized by intermittent vomiting, distention, abdominal pain, diarrhea, constipation and failure to thrive. The upper gastrointestinal series reveals abnormal motility and dilated small bowel loops.

Byrne, W. J., Cipel, L., Euler, A. R., Hapin, T. C., and Ament, M. E.: Chronic idiopathic pseudo-obstruction syndrome in children—clinical characteristics and prognosis. J. Pediatr. 90:585, 1977.

24. Ascariasis may cause vomiting owing to mechanical obstruction by masses of parasites.

B. Gastroesophageal reflux may become symptomatic in the first week of life with projectile vomiting or regurgitation. The vomitus may be blood stained. Associated symptoms include apnea; wheezing; a chronic, barking cough; dysphagia; weight loss; and cyanosis due to laryngospasm. Older children may complain of heartburn. Recurrent aspiration pneumonia may occur. Sandifer's syndrome, characterized by torticollis and a peculiar head-cocking position, may occur in patients with severe esophagitis secondary to gastroesophageal reflux. Barium esophagogram, esophageal monometry, pH monitoring (Tuttle test), gastroesophageal scintiscan and endoscopy are frequently used diagnostic procedures.

C. Mechanical vomiting due to severe cough. The vigorous contractions of the abdominal muscles and diaphragm that occur during severe coughing may result in vomiting.

II. REFLEX CAUSES

A. Reflex vomiting due to stimuli from the gastrointestinal tract
1. Swallowing of amniotic fluid. Often no definitive cause can be found for retching and vomiting in the first two to three days of life. Excessive swallowing of amniotic fluid has been suggested as an explanation.
2. Postnasal drip and pharyngeal mucus may stimulate the gag reflex and lead to vomiting, especially on arising.
3. Edematous uvula. Rarely, a long uvula that has become inflamed during a respiratory infection may stimulate gagging and retching.
4. Respiratory infections. Many babies and young children vomit in association with respiratory infections. Whether this is caused by simultaneous infection of the gastrointestinal and respiratory tracts or by the irritant effect of swallowed secretions is not known.
5. Viral gastroenteritis (See page 225.)
6. Bacterial gastroenteritis
7. Gastritis
   a. Candidiasis
   b. Scarlet fever
   c. Diphtheritic pseudomembranous gastritis
   d. Corrosive gastritis: lye, bleaches, ammonia

8. Spontaneous gastric perforation may occur during the first week of life in the newborn infant. Findings include bilious vomiting, rapid abdominal distention, lethargy and shock.
9. Gastrointestinal allergy; milk and soy-induced enterocolitis.
10. Peptic, gastric or duodenal ulcer. The presenting symptom in premature, debilitated or acutely ill infants may be vomiting, which may simulate that of pyloric stenosis. In other infants, colic, loose stools and, occasionally, melena occur. Early in childhood, anorexia and abdominal pain are the predominant complaints, and vomiting is infrequent. Occasionally, vomiting occurs without abdominal pain.
11. Necrotizing enterocolitis is characterized by abdominal distention, poor feeding, bilious vomiting, respiratory distress, abdominal distention, jaundice, diarrhea, apnea, lethargy, hypothermia and blood in the stools. The infant appears septic and in shock. X-rays reveal free peritoneal air, pneumatosis intestinalis or hepatic portal venous gas. Necrotizing enterocolitis occurs most frequently in premature infants on the third to fifth day of life, especially in those who have experienced perinatal stress. It may also occur in the term infant in the second and third weeks of life. Signs of peritonitis, e.g., resistance to palpation, induration, discoloration and edema of the abdominal wall may be present.

Santulli, T. V., Schullinger, J. N., Heird, W. C., Gongaware, R. D., Wigger, J., Barlow, B., Blanc, W. A., and Berdon, W. E.: Acute necrotizing enterocolitis in infancy: A review of 64 cases. Pediatrics 55:376, 1975.

12. Vomiting may be the initial manifestation in patients with celiac disease.
13. Appendicitis. Vomiting, usually preceded by pain, is the rule in acute appendicitis. A history of pain may not be elicited in infants and young children, and vomiting may be the only early symptom. An appendiceal abscess may cause bowel obstruction or persistent fever.
14. Acute peritonitis. Fecal vomiting often occurs owing to ileus.
15. Hemorrhagic diseases with upper gastrointestinal tract bleeding

16. Superior mesenteric artery syndrome is characterized by intermittent duodenal dilatation and stasis without evidence of mechanical obstruction. Symptoms include frequent vomiting, abdominal cramps, poor weight gain or weight loss. Severe vomiting occurs after the application of a body cast (cast syndrome).

Burrington, J. D.: Superior mesenteric artery syndrome in children. Am. J. Dis. Child. 130:1367, 1976.

17. Mesenteric vascular occlusion leads to vomiting, abdominal distention, intermittent abdominal pain, blood in the stools and diarrhea or constipation.

B. Reflex vomiting due to stimuli from the genitourinary tract. Vomiting may be the only symptom of genitourinary tract disease in infants and young children.
1. Acute pyelonephritis. Vomiting, often projectile and perhaps accompanied by visible peristaltic waves, may be the outstanding symptom.
2. Obstructive anomalies and hydronephrosis. Vomiting frequently occurs in the presence of anomalies of the urinary tract, especially those that cause intermittent obstruction.
3. Acute glomerulonephritis. Vomiting occasionally occurs as a prodrome.
4. Urinary calculi may cause vomiting.
5. Pregnancy may be a cause of persistent vomiting in adolescent girls.

C. Reflex vomiting due to labyrinthine disturbances
1. Otitis media with labyrinthitis
2. Motion sickness: car sickness; sea sickness; air sickness

D. Reflex vomiting due to drugs and poisons. The mucosa of the gastrointestinal tract is directly irritated in most instances, although some drugs also act centrally.
1. Salicylates
2. Mustard, ipecac
3. Digitalis
4. Vomiting may be an early symptom in children with lead poisoning.
5. Vomiting is an almost constant symptom of theophylline toxicity. The vomiting may be intractable with bloody or coffee-ground vomitus.
6. Withdrawal symptoms in fetal alcohol syndrome; narcotic withdrawal

E. Heat prostration
F. Hypoadrenalism in young infants with congenital virilizing adrenal hyperplasia may be accompanied by persistent or recurrent vomiting as well as by diarrhea. Visible peristaltic waves may occur. Dehydration may be more severe than would be anticipated from the amount of vomiting or diarrhea. Nausea and vomiting may be early manifestations of Addison's disease in older children.

G. Hypercalcemia. Vomiting, occasionally severe and projectile, may be the initial manifestation in infants with idiopathic hypercalcemia.

H. Neonatal tetany may be accompanied by vomiting along with convulsive seizures and edema of the hands and feet.

I. Renal insufficiency; uremia

J. Pancreatitis may account for vomiting and abdominal pain.

K. Infectious hepatitis. Vomiting may be an early symptom.

L. Reye's syndrome may be characterized early by an upper respiratory infection, chickenpox or influenza followed by repetitive vomiting, irritability, changes in sensorium (delirium, lethargy and stupor) and combativeness. In infants, seizures, apnea, hyperventilation and diarrhea may occur. Vomiting is a constant feature.

Trauner, D. A.: Reye's syndrome. Curr. Probl. Pediatr. 12:5, 1982.

M. Acidosis. Vomiting may occur in patients in diabetic ketoacidosis or with other causes of metabolic acidosis.

N. An inborn error of metabolism, especially a disorder characterized by protein intolerance and metabolic acidosis, is to be suspected as a cause of persistent vomiting that begins after the institution of milk feedings in newborn infants. This group includes:
1. Urea cycle defects characterized by hyperammonemia, lethargy and coma. In addition to these disorders, hyperammonemia in newborn infants may be associated with severe perinatal asphyxia, hepatic failure due to sepsis and transient hyperammonemia of prematurity. Symptoms attributable to neonatal hyperammonemia include severe vomiting, lethargy, seizures, stupor and coma. Citrullinemia and argininosuccinic aciduria may occur in a subacute form characterized by anorexia, poor feeding, vomiting and neurologic symptoms.
2. Disorders of organic acid metabolism. These patients demonstrate profound lethargy and projectile

vomiting accompanied by metabolic acidosis, ketosis, neutropenia and thrombocytopenia.
  a. Methylmalonic acidemia. Other clinical features include hepatomegaly and failure to thrive.

Barness, L. A.: Methylmalonic acid. Pediatrics 51:1012, 1973.

  b. Propionic acidemia. These infants fail to thrive.

Wolf, B., Hsia, Y. E., Sweetman, L., Gravel, R., Harris, D. J., and Nyhan, W. L.: Propionic acidemia: A clinical update. J. Pediatr. 99:835, 1981.

  c. Isovaleric acidemia
  d. Lactic acidosis

Keating, J. P., Feigin, R. D., Tenenbaum, S. M., and Hillman, R. E.: Hyperglycinemia with ketosis due to a defect in isoleucine metabolism: A preliminary report. Pediatrics 50:890, 1972.
Snyderman, S. E., Sansaricq, C., Chen, W. J., Norton, P. M., and Phansalkar, S. V.: Argininemia. J. Pediatr. 90:563, 1977.

  3. Phenylketonuria may cause vomiting in the newborn.
  4. Fructose intolerance (fructosemia) and fructose-1,6-diphosphatase deficiency may be manifested by recurrent nausea, vomiting, abdominal pain, diarrhea, failure to thrive, hepatomegaly, malaise and hypoglycemia after ingestion of fructose-containing foods.

Rennert, O. M., and Greer, M.: Hereditary fructosemia. Neurology 20:421, 1970.

  5. Hereditary tyrosinemia
  6. Galactosemia

III. CENTRAL VOMITING

A. Central nervous system disorders
  1. Intracranial neoplasms. Chronic or pernicious vomiting, especially when associated with recurrent headaches, is a common symptom of an intracranial neoplasm in children. Although accompanied at times by other evidences of increased intracranial pressure, vomiting may occur initially in the absence of such pressure owing to direct involvement of the medullary vomiting center, as in patients who have a midline tumor of the cerebellum, a tumor involving the fourth ventricle, a pontine or a medullary tumor. *Vomiting in the absence of signs of increased intracranial pressure can be caused by an intracranial neoplasm.* Initially, the vomiting often occurs in the morning, a short time after awakening, and before breakfast. It may be projectile but commonly is not. Nausea may precede the vomiting. Remissions due to spontaneous decompression may occur after the child has been vomiting for several days. Vomiting recurs, however, within a short time unless surgical intervention occurs. *The presence of an intracranial neoplasm is a serious diagnostic consideration in every child with unexplained vomiting.*
  2. Cerebral edema
    a. Cerebral edema in the newborn infant may be accompanied by vomiting and convulsive seizures during the first two or three days of life.
    b. Traumatic cerebral edema: acute focal edema; acute general edema. Repeated vomiting after a head injury need not cause undue concern unless accompanied by alteration in consciousness or neurologic abnormalities.
  3. Intracranial hemorrhage
  4. Subdural hematoma. Vomiting, convulsions and irritability are the cardinal symptoms of this disorder in infants. Unexplained vomiting may be the only symptom. Usually, however, a subdural hematoma is accompanied by delay in neuromuscular development, convulsions, macrocephaly, widening of the biparietal diameter, fever and failure to thrive.
  5. Child abuse in the form of vigorous shaking of infants (whiplash) may cause projectile vomiting, irritability, seizures and a bulging fontanel.
  6. Hydrocephalus. Signs and symptoms of increased intracranial pressure owing to acute obstruction of cerebrospinal fluid shunts include vomiting, irritability, lethargy, headache, bulging of the fontanel or rapid increase in head size.
  7. Pseudotumor cerebri is characterized by headache, vomiting, blurred vision and diplopia.

Freeman, J. M., and D'Souza, B.: Obstruction of CSF shunts. Pediatrics 64:111, 1979.

  8. Meningitis and meningoencephalitis

9. Subdural effusions complicating bacterial meningitis
10. Intracranial abscess
11. Epilepsy. Rarely, abdominal pain and vomiting may, in themselves, constitute a form of epilepsy. These symptoms may also represent an aura in patients with major seizures.
12. Central nervous system leukemia may cause projectile vomiting, headache and meningismus.
13. Leigh's disease may be characterized by recurrent vomiting, lethargy and brainstem dysfunction with dysphagia, facial weakness, respiratory irregularity, extraocular palsies and ataxia.
14. Lead poisoning is accompanied by encephalopathy and increased intracranial pressure. Vomiting, often persistent and projectile, is a frequent and, at times, initial symptom.
15. Hypoglycemia
16. Migraine is frequently accompanied by vomiting.
17. Salicylism. Vomiting may be the initial manifestation.
18. Hypertensive encephalopathy
B. Central vomiting not caused by primary central nervous system disease
   1. Abnormal body metabolites
      a. Uremia
      b. Diabetic ketoacidosis
      c. Hepatic cirrhosis
      d. Chronic renal acidosis may be characterized by recurrent episodes of vomiting.
   2. Acute infections; sepsis or other infections, especially in young infants
   3. Acute mountain sickness may cause severe nausea and vomiting along with intense headache and malaise.
   4. Psychogenic vomiting. Vomiting occurs in some children when they are unduly stimulated or excited. Anorexia and vomiting are frequently present in infants and children living in a persistently stressful environment. Some children may gag and

vomit if an attempt is made to force them to eat a particular food or foods. Self-induced, recurrent vomiting is sometimes seen in moderately or severely retarded children. Occasionally, vomiting may be related to school avoidance. In this event, vomiting usually occurs before or shortly after breakfast while the child is still at home, or it may occur at school.

Dolgin, M. J., Katz, E. R., McGinty, K., and Siegel, S. E.: Anticipatory nausea and vomiting in pediatric cancer patients. Pediatrics 75:547, 1985.

5. Cyclic vomiting is characterized by episodes of vomiting that tend to recur two, three or more times a year. The episode may last for three to four days. Severe ketosis and, sometimes, acidosis and fever develop. The cause for this syndrome is unknown. These children, who are usually under six years of age, are often emotionally labile, and an episode of cyclic vomiting may be precipitated by some emotional upset or viral illness. Cyclic vomiting may occur in patients with a diverticulum of the small bowel or recurrent volvulus. Cyclic vomiting has also been described in children with familial dysautonomia and in those who later experience migraine headaches. Cyclic vomiting has also been considered an autonomic type of epilepsy.

Reinhart, J. B., Evans, S. L., and McFadden, D. L.: Cyclic vomiting in children: Seen through the psychiatrist's eye. Pediatrics 59:371, 1977.

6. Anorexia nervosa and bulimia may be accompanied by secret, self-induced vomiting. Both disorders may coexist or occur separately. Whereas patients with anorexia and bulimia may demonstrate serious weight loss, patients with bulimia do not. Bulimia also occurs in the Kleine-Levin syndrome.

Rich, C. L.: Self-induced vomiting. Psychiatric considerations. JAMA 239:2688, 1978.

ETIOLOGIC CLASSIFICATION OF REGURGITATION

ETIOLOGIC CLASSIFICATION OF VOMITING

Table continued on following page

ETIOLOGIC CLASSIFICATION OF VOMITING *Continued*

G. Hypercalcemia, 220
H. Neonatal tetany, 220
I. Renal insufficiency; uremia, 220
J. Pancreatitis, 220
K. Infectious hepatitis, 220
L. Reye's syndrome, 220
M. Acidosis, 220
N. Metabolic errors, 220
    1. Urea cycle defects
    2. Disorders of organic acid metabolism
    3. Phenylketonuria
    4. Fructosemia, fructose-1,6-diphosphatase deficiency
    5. Hereditary tyrosinemia
    6. Galactosemia
III. CENTRAL VOMITING, 221
  A. Central nervous system disorders, 221
    1. Intracranial neoplasms
    2. Cerebral edema
    3. Intracranial hemorrhage
    4. Subdural hematoma

    5. Whiplash due to child abuse
    6. Hydrocephalus; obstructed cerebrospinal fluid shunt
    7. Pseudotumor cerebri
    8. Meningitis and meningoencephalitis
    9. Subdural effusions
    10. Intracranial abscess
    11. Epilepsy
    12. Central nervous system leukemia
    13. Leigh's disease
    14. Lead poisoning
    15. Hypoglycemia
    16. Migraine
    17. Salicylism
  B. Other causes, 222
    1. Abnormal body metabolites
    2. Acute infections
    3. Acute mountain sickness
    4. Psychogenic vomiting
    5. Cyclic vomiting
    6. Anorexia nervosa, bulimia

22 / DIARRHEA

Diarrhea refers to an increased frequency and water content of the stools owing either to solute malabsorption, fluid secretion or motility disturbance.

ETIOLOGIC CLASSIFICATION OF DIARRHEA BY AGE PERIODS

I. THE NEWBORN INFANT

Diarrhea may begin insidiously with restlessness, irritability, lethargy, refusal of food, vomiting, and weight loss preceding a change in the frequency or consistency of the stools; on the other hand, the sudden passage of a large, watery stool may be the initial symptom.

A. Overfeeding may cause loose stools in the premature infant.
B. Viral diarrhea of the newborn may occur in epidemic form. Stools are yellow, liquid and explosive. Etiologic agents in viral diarrhea of the newborn include rotavirus, Norwalk virus, astro virus, calicivirus, ECHO virus types 11, 14 and 18, Coxsackie virus B-3 and sporadic adenovirus infections.

Lake, A. M., Lauer, B. A., Clark, J. C., Wesenberg, R. L., and McIntosh, K.: Enterovirus infections in neonates. J. Pediatr. 89:787, 1976.

C. Necrotizing enterocolitis, which occurs primarily in low birth weight infants who have experienced stressors such as hypoxia, polycythemia or respiratory distress, is characterized early by abdominal distention and grossly bloody stools. Other findings include lethargy, toxicity, apnea, poor feeding, diarrhea, bilious vomiting, abdominal distention, lethargy and signs of peritonitis such as abdominal tenderness or erythema. Roentgen examination reveals pneumatosis or pneumoperitoneum. The onset is usually in the first five days of life but may be delayed until three weeks of age.

Santulli, T. V., et. al.: Acute necrotizing enterocolitis in infancy: A review of 64 cases. Pediatrics 55:376, 1975.

D. Bacterial diarrhea of the newborn
1. Enteropathogenic, enterotoxigenic and enteroinvasive *Escherichia coli.* Certain serogroups of *E. coli* cause sporadic and epidemic outbreaks of diarrheal disease in newborn and older infants. The infection may be subclinical, mild, severe or fulminant. The enterotoxigenic form, the most frequent in infants, causes green, foul-smelling stools with mucus.
2. Salmonella. The stools are green, mucoid and may contain blood. Abdominal distention, vomiting, dehydration, rapid weight loss, fever, stupor and convulsions may occur. Splenomegaly and jaundice may also be noted. Bacteremia, meningitis, peritonitis, pyogenic arthritis, osteomyelitis and pleurisy are possible complications. The course may be mild, severe with sepsis, or prolonged and typhoidal. Salmonella enteritis in the mother may cause infection of the newborn infant during delivery.
3. Campylobacter enteritis may occur in newborn infants.
E. Parenteral diarrhea refers to the occurrence of loose stools in the presence of extraintestinal infections (e.g., respiratory or urinary tract infections).
F. Dietary factors. Few episodes of diarrhea are caused by the usual formulas used in the feeding of newborn infants. Cow's milk allergy may become symptomatic in the first weeks of life with colic, loose stools and, perhaps, bright red blood in the stools.
G. Congenital enterokinase deficiency, an extremely rare defect in the intestinal mucosa, causes diarrhea and hypoproteinemia.

Haworth, J. C., Gourley, B., Hadorn, B., and Sumida, C.: Malabsorption and growth failure due to intestinal enterokinase deficiency. J. Pediatr. 78:481, 1971.

H. Congenital alkalosis with diarrhea (congenital chloridorrhea), a rare familial disease, is characterized by intractable, watery diarrhea beginning shortly after birth. Extreme alkalosis results from excessive loss of chloride ion in the stools. Congenital Na^+ diarrhea has also been reported.

Holmberg, C., and Perheentupa, J.: Congenital Na+ diarrhea: A new type of secretory diarrhea. J. Pediatr. 106:56, 1985.
McReynolds, E. W., Roy, S., III, and Etteldorf, J. N.: Congenital chloride diarrhea. Am. J. Dis. Child. 127:566, 1974.

I. Diarrhea may be a symptom of neonatal drug withdrawal.

II. OLDER INFANTS AND CHILDREN
A. Infections
1. Parenteral diarrhea. Children may have loose stools at the onset of or during an acute respiratory or urinary tract infection.
2. Acute viral gastroenteritis syndrome (epidemic nausea and vomiting, viral diarrhea). Next to respiratory disease, acute gastroenteritis is the most common illness in children. About 20 to 30 per cent of episodes of acute infectious diarrhea have a bacterial etiology. Another 20 to 30 per cent are of undetermined etiology. The remaining 50 per cent have a viral etiology, most commonly the rotavirus. Rotavirus infections occur predominantly in infants between the ages of 6 and 24 months, especially during the winter months. The illness is characterized by the abrupt onset of vomiting, diarrhea, fever, lethargy, irritability and moderate dehydration. The fever and vomiting last only 24 to 48 hours, but the diarrhea may persist for a week. Other family members may become ill.
    The Norwalk virus causes endemic outbreaks of a 24- to 48-hour illness characterized by the explosive onset of vomiting, diarrhea, nausea, crampy abdominal pain, fever, anorexia and myalgia. Schoolage children and adults are primarily affected. Diarrhea, with 2 to 20 watery bowel movements a day, usually follows nausea and vomiting by a few hours.

Blacklow, N. R., and Cukor, G.: Viral gastroenteritis. N. Engl. J. Med. 304:397, 1981.
Hodes, H. L.: Gastroenteritis with special reference to rotavirus. Adv. Pediatr. 27:195, 1980.
Rodriguez, W. J., et al.: Clinical features of acute gastroenteritis associated with human reovirus-like agent in infants and young children. J. Pediatr. 91:188, 1977.
Steinhoff, M. C.: Rotavirus: The first five years. J. Pediatr. 96:611, 1980.
Tallett, S., MacKenzie, C., Middleton, P., Kerzner, B., and Hamilton, R.: Clinical, laboratory, and epidemiologic features of a viral gastroenteritis in infants and children. Pediatrics 60:217, 1977.

3. Infectious hepatitis. Mild diarrhea may occur during the preicteric phase.
4. Bacterial diarrhea.
    a. Staphylococcal food poisoning. Severe vomiting, retching, ab-

dominal pain and diarrhea occur within one to six hours after ingestion of food contaminated with staphylococcal exotoxin. Several members of a family may simultaneously become ill. Stools are watery and may contain blood. Shock and cyanosis may occur in severe cases.

b. Salmonella (excluding typhoid fever). Vomiting, abdominal pain, fever and diarrhea with watery, mucoid and sometimes bloody stools may be caused by a salmonella enteric infection. Bacteremia with localization in joints, bones, meninges or soft tissues may occur as complications. Splenomegaly, jaundice, meningismus, convulsions and stupor may appear.

c. Typhoid fever. Frequent watery or mucoid stools occur in approximately half of the patients with typhoid fever. Very young infants are often asymptomatic except for mild gastroenteritis.

d. Shigella (bacillary dysentery) usually occurs between one and five years of age with about 25 per cent of infections affecting infants under one year of age. The onset is abrupt with vomiting, abdominal cramps, high fever, prostration and explosive, odorless, greenish-yellow and watery stools. Within a few hours the stools may contain mucus, pus and streaks of bright red blood. Meningismus, disorientation, coma and convulsions may suggest the presence of encephalitis. Bacteremia is relatively infrequent. Bronchitis or pneumonitis may also occur. Diarrhea may continue intermittently for weeks or months. Other members of the family are usually carriers or have active disease. Amebae and other intestinal parasites are frequently present.

e. *Pseudomonas aeruginosa* may also cause severe diarrhea. Colonization or overgrowth of the intestinal tract by *Klebsiella pneumoniae* or staphylococci, pneumococci or streptococci may cause diarrhea.

f. Enteropathic *E. coli* may be etiologic in diarrhea in children with foul, green, loose and slimy stools. Enteroinvasive *E. coli* may produce symptoms that simu-

late shigella dysentery with fever, chills, vomiting, abdominal cramps and tenesmus as well as profuse diarrhea. Enterotoxigenic *E. coli* is the major cause of traveler's diarrhea.

g. Tularemia may be accompanied by diarrhea, vomiting and abdominal pain.

h. Brucellosis. Diarrhea or bloody stools may occur during the acute phases of this disease.

i. Tuberculous enteritis may have a protracted course with intermittent diarrhea and tenesmus. Blood in the stools is usually microscopic in amount.

j. Non-cholera vibrio infections

Hughes, J. M., Hollis, D. G., Gangarosa, E. J., and Weaver, R. E.: Non-cholera vibrio infections in the United States. Ann. Intern. Med. 88:602, 1978.

k. *Yersinia enterocolitica* may cause diarrhea in infants and young children. Usually mild and self-limited, the diarrhea may, however, be severe with blood in the stools, fever, crampy abdominal pain and vomiting. Symptoms may simulate acute appendicitis.

Marks, M. I., Pai, C. H., Lafleur, L., Lackman, L., and Hammerberg, O.: *Yersinia enterocolitica* gastroenteritis: A prospective study of clinical bacteriologic and epidemiologic features. J. Pediatr. 96:26, 1980.
Rodriquez, W. J., Controni, G., Cohen, G. J., Florence, B., Khan, W. N., and Ross, S.: *Yersinia enterocolitica* enteritis in children. JAMA 242:1978, 1979.

l. Campylobacter enteritis, a frequent cause of enteritis, may be characterized by bloody diarrhea, headache, fever, malaise, myalgia, abdominal tenderness, abdominal pain and fever. In the acute phase, the symptoms may suggest appendicitis, mesenteric adenitis or intussusception. The stools are watery, profuse, foul-smelling and may be grossly bloody. Although the symptoms may spontaneously resolve in one to seven days, relapsing manifestations may suggest inflammatory bowel disease.

Rettig, P. J.: Campylobacter infections in human beings. J. Pediatr. 94:855, 1979.
Torphy, D. E., and Bond, W. W.: Campylobacter fetus infections in children. Pediatrics 64:898, 1979.

m. The toxic shock syndrome is characterized by vomiting and diarrhea as well as myalgia, high fever, hypotension and dermatitis.

n. *Vibrio cholerae*

Drachman, R. H.: Acute infectious gastroenteritis. Pediatr. Clin. N. Am. 21:711, 1974.

Nelson, J. D., and Haltalin, K. C.: Accuracy of diagnosis of bacterial diarrheal disease by clinical features. J. Pediatr. 78:519, 1971.

Pickering, L. K.: Evaluation of patients with acute infectious diarrhea. Pediatr. Inf. Dis. 4:13 (May/June suppl.), 1985.

5. Protozoan diarrhea
   a. *Amebiasis* may be characterized by intermittent episodes of diarrhea with four to six liquid stools a day. The stools may contain only microscopic amounts of blood, mucus and pus. Constipation is often present between episodes of diarrhea. In the severe dysenteric form the stools initially are watery, green and slimy. Nausea, abdominal cramps, tenesmus and fever are also present. Blood-flecked stools and mucus appear within a short time, and as many as 15 to 20 stools may be passed in 24 hours. Chronic amebiasis may simulate ulcerative colitis with blood, mucus and pus intermittently present in the stools. Stool cultures for salmonella or shigella organisms are indicated.

Dykes, A. C., Ruebush, T. K., II, Gorelkin, L., Lushbaugh, W. B., Upshur, J. K., and Cherry, J. D.: Extraintestinal amebiasis in infancy: Report of three patients and epidemiologic investigations of their families. Pediatrics 65:799, 1980.

   b. *Giardia lamblia.* Giardiasis may cause explosive, watery, foul stools with abdominal distention, borborygmi, and flatulence. The celiac syndrome may be produced by extensive coating of the mucosal surfaces of the duodenum and jejunum by this protozoan. The cysts may be demonstrable by stool examination in 30 per cent of cases. Duodenal aspiration, biopsy with Giemsa-stained smears of the mucus or the string test may be diagnostic. Giardiasis is one of the causes of malabsorption in patients with immunodeficiency syndromes.

Ament, M. E.: Diagnosis and treatment of giardiasis. J. Pediatr. 80:633, 1972.

Burke, J. A.: Giardiasis in childhood. Am. J. Dis. Child. 129:1304, 1975.

Pickering, L. K.: Problems in diagnosing and managing giardiasis. Pediatr. Inf. Dis. 4:6 (May/June suppl.), 1985.

   c. Cryptosporidiosis

Wolfson, J. S., et al.: Cryptosporidiosis in immunocompetent patients. N. Engl. J. Med. 312:1278, 1985.

6. Diarrhea caused by other parasites
   a. Nematodes (roundworms)
      1. Trichuriasis (whipworm disease). Rarely, bloody, mucoid diarrhea may occur.
      2. Hookworm disease. Unformed, tarry stools may be present in patients with heavy hookworm infestation.
      3. Strongyloidiasis (threadworm disease). Mucoid diarrhea, at times severe, may persist or alternate with constipation. Patients may develop a malabsorption syndrome and a protein-losing enteropathy.
      4. Ascariasis may cause chronic diarrhea and colicky abdominal pain.
   b. Platyhelminthes (flatworms). During the early stages mucoid diarrhea is frequent with taeniasis (tapeworm) infestation.

Katz, M.: Parasitic infections. J. Pediatr. 87:165, 1975.

7. Fungal diarrhea
   a. Histoplasmosis. Diarrhea is frequent in the disseminated form of this disease. Blood may appear in the stools with ulceration of Peyer's patches.
   b. Candidiasis
B. Malabsorption syndromes
   1. Celiac disease is caused by an intolerance to wheat gluten (gluten-induced enteropathy). Vomiting may be the initial manifestation, and intermittent diarrhea may begin at any time from birth to the end of the second year. In an occasional child, symptoms begin later or are limited to understature. The stools are often fluid or mushy and vary in color from pale cream to greenish-yellow. Mucus may cause the stools to have a metallic sheen. Occasionally, oily or greasy droplets appear on the surface of a fluid stool. The volume is usually larger than normal and eventually the stools have an offensive odor. One to ten stools a day

may be passed during diarrheal episodes, which may last days, weeks or months. Irritability may be notable during these periods. Remissions are frequent at first, and the stools may be normal or constipated between episodes.

In addition to an increase in fecal fat, the laboratory findings most consistently present include a low concentration of serum proteins, serum folate and serum carotene. Serum carotene levels less than 20 μg/100 ml are seen almost exclusively in malabsorption states. The Sudan III stain for fecal fat may confirm a clinical impression that the stool contains excessive fat but may be falsely negative. Normal stools do not contain Sudan III staining material or only small particles. The one-hour xylose test may be useful as a screening examination. Biopsy specimens of the small intestinal mucous membrane demonstrate characteristic changes. The disorder should respond promptly to a gluten-free diet.

Dermatitis herpetiformis, discussed on page 179, may accompany celiac disease. Tropical sprue may also occur in children, causing a gluten-sensitive enteropathy or chronic malabsorptive-type stools.

Ament, M. E: Malabsorption syndromes in infancy and childhood. Parts I and II. J. Pediatr. 81:685, 867, 1972.
Santiago-Borrero, P. J., Maldonado, N., and Horta, E.: Tropical sprue in children. *J. Pediatr.* 76:470, 1970.

2. Cystic fibrosis. Early, the clinical manifestations may be chiefly those of a persistent respiratory infection. When solid foods are introduced, the stools may become foamy, bulky and foul-smelling. Often the stools remain formed or soft, although rarely they may be watery. Increased frequency occurs occasionally, but constipation is present in some cases. In infants up to one year of age who present with evidence of malabsorption but no history of respiratory infections, a sweat chloride determination should be obtained. At times, steatorrhea is the only presenting symptom.
3. Pancreatic enzyme deficiency may occur independent of cystic fibrosis in the Schwachman-Diamond syndrome characterized by steatorrhea,

failure to thrive, metaphyseal dysostosis, dwarfism, neutropenia and susceptibility to infections. Complete absence of trypsinogen or of lipase may also occur.
4. Short bowel syndrome owing to massive resection of the small bowel may be associated with malabsorption secondary to inactivation of the pancreatic enzymes and inability to reabsorb conjugated bile salts.
5. Other causes of steatorrhea include gastrointestinal allergy, absence of bile in the stools, bile salt deficiency, administration of broad-spectrum antibiotics, intestinal stenosis and intestinal malrotation. Steatorrhea may be associated with hypoparathyroidism and with Wolman's disease. Whipple's disease is characterized by chronic diarrhea, fever, arthritis and edema.
6. Parasites. Giardiasis is the parasite most commonly associated with malabsorption. Other etiologic agents are *Strongyloides stercoralis, Capillaria philippinensis* and coccidia.
7. Abetalipoproteinemia is characterized by steatorrhea, thorny projections on the erythrocytes (acanthocytosis), atypical retinitis pigmentosa, progressive ataxia and virtual absence of beta-lipoprotein (Bassen-Kornzweig syndrome). Diarrhea occurring in the first two years of life is usually the initial symptom. Neurologic symptoms occur many years later. A low serum cholesterol level in a young child with the celiac syndrome suggests this disorder. The diagnosis may be established by lipoprotein immunoelectrophoresis.
8. Primary immunodeficiency syndromes may be accompanied by gastrointestinal symptoms such as vomiting, diarrhea, steatorrhea, weight loss and protein-losing enteropathy. Giardiasis may be present in patients with primary B cell deficiency. Chronic watery diarrhea in patients with T cell defects is probably secondary to mucosal structural changes. Chronic diarrhea occurs in infants with the acquired immune deficiency syndrome.

Ament, M. E., Ochs, H. D., and Davis, S. D.: Structure and function of the gastrointestinal tract in primary immunodeficiency syndromes. A study of 39 patients. Medicine 52:227, 1973.
Gryboski, J. D., Self, T. W., Clemett, A., and Herskovic, T.: Selective immunoglobulin A defi-

ciency and intestinal nodular lymphoid hyperplasia: Correction of diarrhea with antibiotics and plasma. Pediatrics 42:833, 1968.

Horowitz, S., Lorenzsonn, M. S., Olsen, W. A., Albrecht, R., and Hong, R.: Small intestinal disease in T cell deficiency. J. Pediatr. 85:457, 1974.

9. Intestinal lymphangiectasis. In addition to chylous ascites and edema, diarrhea may be secondary to malabsorption of fat.

10. Carbohydrate malabsorption. The diarrhea of carbohydrate malabsorption results from the osmotic effects of nonhydrolysed, unabsorbed sugar in the small bowel and from the acid metabolites formed by bacterial fermentation of the sugars in the colon. Stools are watery, frothy, often profuse, acid and frequently accompanied by flatus and excoriation of the perianal skin.

Carbohydrate malabsorption states may be congenital or acquired and related to disaccharides or monosaccharides. The exceedingly rare congenital disorders may cause diarrhea, vomiting and failure to thrive from the first day of life (lactase deficiency and glucose-galactose malabsorption) or after the first month (sucrase-isomaltase deficiency) unless carbohydrates are removed from the diet. Secondary types of carbohydrate malabsorption include lactase deficiency, lactase deficiency with deficiency of other disaccharides and temporary monosaccharide malabsorption.

Secondary lactase deficiency, by far the most common, follows any disorder that damages the epithelium, especially the brush border of the intestinal mucosa. Acute gastroenteritis is the most frequent cause of secondary lactase deficiency, a disorder that lasts from a few days to several weeks. If the carbohydrate intolerance persists over three weeks, the infant usually becomes intolerant to all monosaccharides. Other disorders that lead to secondary deficiencies include celiac disease, giardiasis, cow's milk or soy protein isolate sensitivity, leukemia treated with antimetabolites, protein-calorie malnutrition and gastrointestinal tract surgery in the newborn. Secondary lactase deficiency is especially common following diarrhea in newborn infants. Disaccharidase deficiency also occurs in many children with immunologic disorders.

Carbohydrate malabsorption may be suspected on the basis of the history and examination of the stool. Screening stool examinations (1) determine the stool pH and (2) test the stool for reducing substances. In the screening tests, only the liquid portion of the stool uncontaminated by urine should be used. Stools should be collected on a piece of plastic inserted in the diaper and tested promptly. The pH may be determined by a Combistic or pH paper. Normally, the fecal pH is between 7 and 8. In carbohydrate malabsorption the pH is less than 5.5 to 6, an abnormally low value.

The screening test for sugar in the stool employs the Clinitest reagent. A Clinitest tablet is added to 15 drops of a mixture of one part fluid stool to two parts water. The resulting color is then compared to a color chart. Values above 0.5 per cent are abnormal. If sucrose is thought to be the offending sugar, the stool should be hydrolyzed using 1N HCl instead of water for dilution and boiling for 30 seconds to convert the sucrose to glucose and fructose.

In the presence of a suggestive history and positive screening tests, removal of the sugar from the diet should promptly relieve the diarrhea. If more sophisticated diagnostic tests are needed, specific carbohydrate tolerance tests may be used.

Dubois, R. S., Roy, C. C., Fulginiti, V. A., Merrill, D. A., and Murray, R. L.: Disaccharidase deficiency in children with immunologic deficits. J. Pediatr. 76:377, 1970.

Gracey, M., and Burke, V.: Sugar induced diarrhoea in children. Arch. Dis. Child. 48:331, 1973.

Lifshitz, F., Coello-Ramirez, P., and Gutierrez-Topete: Monosaccharide intolerance and hypoglycemia in infants with diarrhea. I. Clinical course of 23 infants. J. Pediatr. 77:595, 1970.

Lactose intolerance differs from congenital lactase deficiency in that the patients as young children usually do not have symptoms but demonstrate milk-induced abdominal cramps and diarrhea as adolescents or adults.

C. Gastrointestinal allergy. In the newborn period, gastrointestinal allergy to cow's milk may cause clinical manifestations that range from severe diarrhea and shock to chronic diarrhea with mucus, gross or occult blood in the stools and steatorrhea. Diagnostic criteria include cessation of symptoms with elimination of milk and their recurrence within 48 hours of a rechallenge on three occasions. Most patients develop symptoms during the first six weeks of life. Tolerance to milk is gradually acquired by 2 to 5 years of age. Some infants are also extremely sensitive to soy protein and develop vomiting, diarrhea and blood in the stools after its ingestion. Elimination diets may be helpful diagnostically when gastrointestinal allergy is suspected.

Bahna, S. L., and Heiner, D. C.: Cow's milk allergy: Pathogenesis, manifestations, diagnosis and management. Adv. Pediatr. 25:1, 1978.

Mendoza, J., Meyers, J., and Snyder, R.: Soybean sensitivity. Pediatrics 46:774, 1970.

Powell, G. K.: Milk- and soy-induced enterocolitis of infancy. J. Pediatr. 93:553, 1978.

D. Antibiotic diarrhea owing to alteration of the intestinal flora
E. Endocrine and metabolic diarrhea
1. Hyperthyroidism
2. Uremia
3. Nephrosis may be characterized by episodes of nonspecific diarrhea.
4. Cystinosis
5. Hereditary tyrosinemia
6. Wolman's disease
7. Chronic diarrhea with abdominal distention and wasting is the presenting symptom in some patients with a cervical, thoracic or abdominal ganglioneuroma or ganglioneuroblastoma. Bowel movements are foul-smelling, frequent, frothy and loose, watery or greasy. The patient may have a history of weight loss or failure to gain. Lethargy, irritability, flushing, excessive perspiration and hypertension may also be noted. Measurement of catecholamine and vasoactive intestinal peptides should be obtained if this disorder is considered. Complete reversal of symptoms follows removal of the tumor.

Kaplan, S. J., Holbrook, C. T., McDaniel, H. G., Buntain, W.L., and Crist, W. M.: Vasoactive intestinal peptide secreting tumors of children. Am. J. Dis. Child. 134:21, 1980.

Vorhess, M. L.: Functioning tumors. Am. J. Dis. Child. 134:14, 1980.

8. The Zollinger-Ellison syndrome is manifested by severe diarrhea with or without peptic ulcer and marked hyperchlorhydria.
9. Nonbeta islet cell hyperplasia may be associated with chronic diarrhea.

These patients have refractory watery diarrhea, elevated levels of vasoactive intestinal peptide (VIP) and pancreatic islet nonbeta cell hyperplasia.

Grishan, F. K., Soper, R. T., Nassif, E. G., and Younoszai, M. K.: Chronic diarrhea of infancy: Nonbeta islet cell hyperplasia. Pediatrics 64:46, 1979.

10. Zinc deficiency may cause diarrhea, acrodermatitis and alopecia in patients with acrodermatitis enteropathica or those receiving parenteral alimentation with zinc-deficient solutions.
F. Miscellaneous causes of diarrhea
1. Gastrointestinal hemorrhage (See page 258.)
2. Acute appendicitis with pelvic position of the appendix
3. Acute peritonitis. Diarrhea may occur early.
4. Laxatives, cathartics or high sulfate content of well water (over 400 mg of sulfate per liter) given to infants. Surreptitious administration of cathartics to children may occur in Munchausen's syndrome by proxy. If the agent contains phenolphthalein, red or pink staining of the diarrheal stools may occur.
5. Diffuse familial polyposis of the colon. Loose stools with or without mucus and blood are present in the majority of these patients.
6. Protein-losing enteropathy may be characterized by diarrhea as well as marked hypoproteinemia and edema. Serum protein electrophoresis may be indicated as part of the work-up of patients with chronic diarrhea.
7. Dietetic candies containing sorbitol may cause diarrhea when eaten in large quantities because of the osmotic effect of the sugar.
8. Foreign body in the intestine or rectum.
9. Aganglionic megacolon. Enterocolitis with the acute onset of diarrhea, vomiting, abdominal distention, lethargy, fever and dehydration at two or three weeks of age is a life-threatening complication. Massive dilatation of the colon may occur.
10. Rectal stenosis. Fluid stools may occur around a fecal impaction.
11. Starvation stools may be watery, greenish and mucoid.
12. Ulcerative colitis. Unexplained, intermittent, mucoid diarrhea may

precede by weeks or months the appearance of mucus, pus and blood in the stools. The onset may be sudden or insidious. In the latter event, the first symptom is an increased number of bowel movements. At times, rectal bleeding is the initial symptom. When involvement is localized chiefly to the rectum and rectosigmoid, blood, pus and mucus may be noted in the stools. In such cases the bowel movements may be of normal consistency or the patient may even be constipated. Blood in the stools in the absence of diarrhea may be the first symptom of ulcerative colitis. In severe ulcerative colitis, the patient has more than six diarrheal stools a day, and toxic dilatation of the colon may be a life-threatening complication. Fever and weight loss are common. Extra-intestinal complications include arthritis, erythema nodosum, pyoderma gangrenosum, aphthous ulcers in the mouth, growth retardation, anemia and delayed puberty. Crohn's disease involving the colon is a differential consideration. Abdominal cramps and tenderness may also be present. The sense of urgency and tenesmus may be severe, and the patient may be awakened several times a night to have a bowel movement. Bloody diarrhea, crampy abdominal pain and toxic megacolon may occur with antibiotic-associated pseudomembranous colitis.

Ament, M. E.: Inflammatory disease of the colon: Ulcerative colitis and Crohn's colitis. J. Pediatr. 86:322, 1975.

Hamilton, J. R., Bruce, G. A., Abdourhaman, M., and Gall, D. G.: Inflammatory bowel disease in children and adolescents. Adv. Pediatr. 26:311, 1979.

Kelts, D. G., and Grand, R. J.: Inflammatory bowel disease in children and adolescents. Curr. Probl. Pediatr. 10:5, 1980.

13. Crohn's disease (regional enteritis) may be characterized by chronic, persistent diarrhea. Cramping abdominal pain, loss of weight and fever may also be present. Initial symptoms, appearing before diarrhea, may include growth failure, delayed puberty and fever of undetermined origin. An abdominal mass consisting of matted loops of involved bowel or, more rarely, an abscess may be palpable on abdominal examination. Perianal disease with anal fissures and fistulae may also be a presenting finding.

14. Constipation with fecal retention may be accompanied by so-called paradoxical diarrhea with involuntary passage of liquid stool around a hard fecal mass in the rectum.

15. Antibiotic-associated pseudomembranous colitis is a serious disorder associated with the administration of oral or parenteral antimicrobial agents. Symptoms and findings include fever, vomiting, profuse, watery and, at times, bloody diarrhea, distended abdomen, abdominal tenderness, dehydration, toxic megacolon and, possibly, peritonitis, sepsis and shock. Severe colitis and a pseudomembrane are noted on endoscopic examination. The diarrhea is caused by a cytotoxin elaborated by *Clostridium difficile*.

Feigin, R. D.: Antimicrobial agent-induced pseudomembranous colitis. Pediatr. Rev. 3:147, 1981.

Viscidi, R. P., and Bartlett, J. C.: Antibiotic-associated pseudomembranous colitis in children. Pediatrics 67:381, 1981.

16. Reye's syndrome in infants is often accompanied by diarrhea.

17. Necrotizing cellulitis of the cecum (typhilitis), which may occur acutely in patients with acute leukemia, causes right lower quadrant pain and bloody diarrhea. Pseudomonas or other gram-negative bacilli are etiologic.

18. Kawasaki disease may be accompanied by frequent watery stools.

19. The hemolytic-uremic syndrome may begin with bloody diarrhea.

20. Severe combined immunodeficiency may be accompanied by intractable diarrhea.

G. Psychogenic diarrhea
   1. Fear or anxiety
   2. Encopresis (See page 239.)

H. Chronic nonspecific diarrhea (irritable bowel syndrome, psychogenic factors) is characterized by persistent or recurrent diarrhea in children between the ages of six months and three years. Three to ten stools are passed each day, with the early morning stool formed and the others small and containing mucus and vegetable fibers. These patients usually do not have a history of a significant weight loss. The cause is unknown. Excessive fluid intake has been suggested as one cause of the syndrome. Chronic diarrhea in young children may be etiologically related to emotional turmoil and conflict in the family. In such instances the periods of diarrhea parallel times of increased emotional tension and discord in the family. On hospital admission, the diarrhea dramatically ceases.

III. CHRONIC DIARRHEA

The etiologic possibilities in chronic diarrhea or diarrhea persisting more than three weeks include many of the causes listed above in this chapter. The most frequent causative disorders are:
A. Infections owing to bacterial or parasitic pathogens
B. Carbohydrate malabsorption secondary to infectious gastroenteritis
C. Malabsorption syndrome, especially cystic fibrosis and celiac disease
D. Inflammatory bowel disease
E. Neural crest tumors
F. Gastrointestinal allergy
G. Irritable bowel syndrome (psychogenic factors)
H. Immunodeficiency syndromes
I. Antibiotic-associated diarrhea
J. Excessive fluid intake

Fitzgerald, J. F., and Clark, J. H.: Chronic diarrhea. Pediatr. Clin. North Am. 29:221, 1982.
Fitzgerald, J. J.: Management of the infant with persistent diarrhea. Pediatr. Inf. Dis. 4:6, 1985.
Green, H. L., and Grishan, F. K.: Excessive fluid intake as a cause of chronic diarrhea in young children. J. Pediatr. 102:836, 1983.
Gryboski, J. D.: Chronic diarrhea. Curr. Probl. Pediatr. 9:5, 1979.
Rossi, T. M., and Lebenthal, E.: Pathogenic mechanisms of protracted diarrhea. Adv. Pediatr. 30:595, 1983.
Walker, W. A.: Benign chronic diarrhea of infancy. Pediatr. Rev. 3:153, 1981.

COMPLICATIONS OF ACUTE DIARRHEA

I. DEHYDRATION MANIFESTED BY:

A. Tachycardia
B. Visible dryness of the tongue and mucous membranes; stringy oral secretions
C. Sunken anterior fontanel
D. Reduced tissue elasticity and turgor (See also page 167.)
E. Weight loss. In acute illnesses weight loss is chiefly caused by dehydration.
F. Fever
G. Reduced frequency of urination
H. Dark urine

Finberg, L.: Treatment of dehydration in infancy. Pediatr. Rev. 3:113, 1981.

II. SHOCK

III. HYPOKALEMIA

IV. HYPERNATREMIA.
The infant with hypernatremia has a velvety or doughy feel to the skin. High fever may be present. Signs of central nervous system dysfunction include unusual irritability or lethargy, hypertonicity, meningismus, convulsions, stupor and coma.

Finberg, L.: Hypernatremic (hypertonic) dehydration in infants. N. Engl. J. Med. 289:196, 1973.

V. INTRACTABLE DIARRHEA SYNDROME AND FAILURE TO THRIVE
may occur secondary to mucosal atrophy, continued nutrient loss and inadequate protein-caloric intake owing to therapeutic fasting.

VI. BACTEREMIA.
The younger the patient, the greater the hazard of bacteremia.

VII. PYOGENIC ARTHRITIS

VIII. PERITONITIS

IX. PNEUMONIA

X. PYELONEPHRITIS

XI. MENINGITIS

XII. ENCEPHALOPATHY OWING TO THROMBOSIS OF CORTICAL VEINS OR HYPERNATREMIA

XIII. PHLEBOTHROMBOSIS

A. Thrombosis of the large cortical veins or dural sinuses in severely dehydrated infants and children may cause convulsive seizures, coma and paresis.
B. Thrombosis of the renal veins may be followed by sudden enlargement of one or both kidneys, shock, hematuria and azotemia. Symptoms may be minimal, however, and the urinary findings mistakenly attributed to the primary dehydration. Bilateral renal vein thrombosis may result in the nephrotic syndrome.
C. Renal artery thrombosis followed by oliguria, anuria, hematuria, albuminuria, casts and azotemia.

XIV. PERIANAL EXCORIATION
results from maceration and tryptic digestion of the per-

ianal skin. This complication is especially noted in disaccharidase deficiency.

XV. ANAL PROLAPSE

XVI. INTUSSUSCEPTION may occur during the course of severe diarrhea. The diagnosis may be overlooked if the abdominal pain and blood in the stools are attributed to dysentery.

GENERAL REFERENCES

Gall, D. G., and Hamilton, J. R.: Chronic diarrhea in childhood. Pediatr. Clin. North Am. 21:1001, 1974.

Gryboski, J. (ed.): Gastrointestinal Problems in the Infant. Philadelphia, W. B. Saunders Co., 1975.

Poley, J. R.: Chronic diarrhea in infants and children. Parts I and II. South. Med. J. 66:1035, 1133, 1973.

Roy, C. C., Silverman, A., and Cozzetto, F. J.: Pediatric Clinical Gastroenterology. 2nd ed. St. Louis, C. V. Mosby Co., 1975.

ETIOLOGIC CLASSIFICATION OF DIARRHEA BY AGE PERIODS

23 / CONSTIPATION

Constipation refers to difficulty in defecating. The stools may be normal cylindrical masses or hard, dry pellets. The bowel movements are characteristically infrequent; however, a few pellets may be passed several times a day. In the presence of a fecal impaction the stools may become fluid (paradoxical diarrhea). The symptoms of constipation include mild anorexia, tenesmus, straining and abdominal pain. Pain on defecating is frequent. The stools may be streaked with bright red blood as a result of anal fissures. Anal or rectal prolapse may occur in debilitated patients. Fecal material is often palpable in the lower abdomen as firm, irregular, cylindrical masses.

NORMAL STOOLS

Meconium stools are greenish-black, odorless, thick and sticky. Four or five are passed each day during the first three to four days of life. Delay in passage of meconium stools in the first day of life may be attributable to aganglionic megacolon, intestinal obstruction, a meconium plug, hypothyroidism, sepsis with adynamic ileus or maternal narcotic addiction.

Transitional stools are mixed, greenish-brown, thin and slimy, and may contain milk curds. Four to eight stools are passed per day between the fourth and seventh days of life.

The number of stools passed by normal infants during the first week of life gradually increases to reach a peak, usually on the fifth day. A relation exists between the number of stools and the infant's total food intake. During any one day a small number of normal newborns have no bowel movements; on the other hand, a few babies pass as many as 12 to 14 stools. The diagnosis of constipation or diarrhea in this age period, therefore, is not based on the frequency of stools alone, but also on their nature and other clinical findings. Since mothers are frequently concerned about the number of stools their babies pass, it is usually well to inform them of what to expect in the first week of life.

Milk stools are passed after the first week of life. *Breast-fed* babies have homogeneous, pasty, mushy (like cream soup), slightly sour-smelling, light yellow stools that cling to or sink into the diaper. One to eight are passed each day with an average of two to four a day. Many babies have a stool after each feeding. Faintly green stools containing a small amount of mucus are seen occasionally. An infant is rarely, if ever, constipated while exclusively on a breast milk diet. Babies fed on *cow's milk* have one to four putty-like, firm, pale yellow stools which do not cling to the diaper. The presence of tough curds may give the stool a scrambled-egg appearance. Milk stools turn green or brown on exposure to air.

The frequency of stools usually decreases between one and three months of age in both breast- and bottle-fed infants. A few normal babies may then have stools as infrequently as every second or third day. By one year of age the majority of infants have only one stool a day, but individual infants may have more or fewer.

When chopped foods are first added to a baby's diet, they may appear in the stool almost unchanged. Mucus is often present in the stools of babies during respiratory infections. A light-colored, seemingly acholic stool may occasionally be passed in normal infants and children, usually in relation to a respiratory infection. In some children seen because of constipation, the parents report that the stools are large enough to plug up the toilet.

PHYSIOLOGY OF DEFECATION

In the first year of life defecation is primarily a reflex act. Mass peristaltic movements initiated by fecal bulk traverse the entire colon (unless the myenteric plexus is not intact). These movements are influenced by parasympathetic (excitatory) and sympathetic (inhibitory) impulses. When the rectum becomes distended with feces, afferent fibers conduct impulses to the "defecation center" in the second, third and fourth sacral segments of the spinal cord. Motor impulses from this area then cause relaxation of the internal anal sphincter.

This sphincter is also subject to parasympathetic inhibition and sympathetic excitation. The afferent impulses that ascend the spinal cord also cause contraction of the voluntary muscles of defecation. Closure of the glottis and contraction of the diaphragmatic and abdominal muscles lead to an increase in the intra-abdominal and intra-rectal pressures. Dilatation of the external anal sphincter occurs reflexly. The levator ani muscles contract and lift the anus over the fecal mass.

During the first year of life, each mass peristaltic movement is followed by the passage of a stool, since defecation is not voluntarily inhibited. The defecation reflex normally prevents an excessive accumulation or desiccation of feces. In the second year of life and thereafter, voluntary cortical control of defecation is possible through the willful contraction or relaxation of the external anal sphincter (striated muscle). In older children the number of stools normally passed a day varies with the child. Most children have one bowel movement a day; some have two a day; and still others have a stool every other day or even less frequently without symptoms.

Bowel Training. A cultural concern accompanies gastrointestinal function. Many parents are still conditioned to believe that one bowel movement a day is essential, and they often place a premium on early cleanliness. These attitudes ignore individual differences in the natural frequency of the stools and the level of neuromuscular development as indications for initiating training. Since the passage of bowel movements often becomes a point of coercion and conflict between parent and child, constipation frequently arises during the training period, especially if upsetting events such as a divorce, a move or a mother's return to work outside the home occur concurrently.

1. "CATCHING" THE STOOL. After the first few months of life the majority of babies have stools at fairly predictable times, but a few infants remain totally irregular. If the baby is regular, has an adequate sense of balance, and can sit well alone, mothers sometimes attempt "catching" of the stool. Catching does not constitute training, and defecation continues to be a reflex activity without a voluntary component. When the baby begins to walk, however, the stools are often passed more irregularly and, therefore, become difficult to catch. Mothers who had prided themselves on early training may then find that all semblance of it has disappeared.

2. CHOICE OF A POTTY. The potty seat should facilitate defecation. This is possible if the following requirements are met: a seat small enough to support the ischial tuberosities, an adequate back and arm rest and a firm foot rest. Although a potty seat that can be placed on the floor would seem the most desirable type, the psychologic advantage of identification by the child with other members of the family has made the use of a potty seat attached to the adult seat seem more advantageous. Because of the fear of falling, the parent should remain with the child if the adult toilet is used. As the child grows older, small stairs to the adult toilet should be available so that he can go to the toilet as he desires.

The potty also should permit an optimal position for defecation. The infant must be able to lean forward with the thighs partially flexed on the abdomen, the feet firmly planted on the floor or a foot rest, and the ischial tuberosities adequately supported. This position permits a fulcrum action of the levator ani muscles and places the accessory muscles of defecation at a mechanical advantage.

3. TRAINING TECHNIQUES. The use of the toilet is a habit that need not be "trained into" a child. Bowel control is a complicated function that requires a relatively advanced degree of neuromuscular, social and emotional development. The baby must wish to please his mother by controlling bowel function. He must be aware that a movement is coming, be able to withhold it through cortical inhibition, be able to verbalize his need to defecate in some manner and understand what is expected of him when he is placed on the potty. These capacities are seldom present before the second year of life, develop slowly and cannot be accelerated by external pressure. Parents often have the erroneous idea, however, that bowel training requires an all-out effort on their part. Actually, little training is necessary. Children in other societies learn bowel control by imitation and are often spontaneously trained by the age of two years.

Training can be advantageously delayed until the infant is proficient at walking because until that time bowel movements are apt to be irregular as the new skill is being integrated. Usually walking has been mastered by 14 to 15 months of age, and training can be started then. If the baby has regular movements, he can be placed on the potty at the expected time. If he is irregular, the parent should wait until he grunts or strains or otherwise indicates the coming of the stool. He should not be placed on the potty at a predetermined time and given a suppository to induce a stool. The mother should use the same word for defecation each time. Ten minutes is usually sufficient for a sitting, and a baby may be removed from the potty sooner if he is resistant. Attempts at training may be stopped temporarily if resistance develops and when the baby is tired or ill. Lapses in training are frequent throughout the second year and are especially apt to occur during periods of integration of new skills or emotional stress.

4. RESISTANCE TO TRAINING. Resistance usually has an emotional basis and may be managed by a reduced emphasis on the training process. Early in the course of training, an infant may not use his word for defecation until after a movement has occurred. This indicates that he is learning to connect the word with the act, an essential feature of training. It does not represent resistance or cause for discouragement. A baby in the second year may have a bowel movement after he has been removed from the potty and dressed. This sometimes indicates resistance and often correlates with other aspects of personal-social behavior; on the other hand, it may be interpreted to the mother as an encouraging sign, e.g., that the child has just about mastered this complicated business and will likely soon be successful. This pattern is usually transient and should not become a matter of undue concern. If all goes well, the child usually manages his clothes and goes to the toilet alone by two or three years of age. Lapses, however, may still occur in the third year. The causes for true resistance to training include the following:

a. *Fear.* The baby may be afraid of the potty because he has had painful stools there or he may have a fear of falling from the adult toilet. Occasionally he is scared by the flushing of the toilet after defecation. Because the baby cannot verbalize these fears, his behavior is seen as resistance.

b. *Maternal Disgust.* A baby frequently has pride in his stool. He may admire it and even call his mother from another room to see it. Sometimes he may play with it. In contrast to this, his mother may disgustedly flush the stool down the toilet and react with revulsion when she discovers a stool in his pants or finds him playing with it.

c. *Disturbed Parent-Child Relations.* During training the infant learns that the passage of his stool on the potty pleases his parent. He also learns that he can withhold or pass it at will. From this time on he can either give up his stools for the approval of his parent or he can withhold them. Punishment, unpleasantness and coercion in bowel training may elicit reactive withholding of the stool and resistance to training.

ETIOLOGIC CLASSIFICATION OF CONSTIPATION AND INFREQUENT STOOLS

I. INTERFERENCE WITH MASS PERISTALTIC MOVEMENTS OF THE COLON

A. Reflex mechanisms of mass peristalsis anatomically intact
  1. Lack of fecal bulk causes an inadequate stimulus to mass peristaltic movements.
    a. Anorexia, underfeeding, vomiting and starvation. Constipation is a common complaint in patients with anorexia nervosa.
    b. Lack of roughage in the diet
      1) Continued use of pureed foods after 10 to 12 months of age
      2) Preponderance of highly refined starches in the diet
      3) High protein diet. Protein is almost completely digested and absorbed, leaving little residue.
    c. Enemas, laxatives and suppositories empty the colon and remove the stimulus to peristalsis for two to three days. Diarrhea is usually followed by infrequent stools for several days.
  2. Hard stools interfere with the effectiveness of mass peristaltic movements.
    a. Cow's milk stools
      1) Substitution of a supplemental bottle of cow's milk for one of the breast feedings may cause firmness of the stools and a decrease in frequency.
      2) Excessive cow's milk intake. Occasionally infants refuse solid foods in the latter half of the first year of life and satisfy their caloric needs by an excessive intake of cow's milk—as much as two quarts a day. The high calcium content of this diet leads to the formation of calcium caseinate and soaps in the stools, substances that supply bulk but do not stimulate peristalsis.
    b. Desiccated stools
      1) Dehydration and fever cause desiccation of the stools by diminishing intestinal secretions and increasing water absorption from the colon. A transient period of constipation is common during acute febrile illnesses. In hot

weather, babies may be constipated if not offered sufficient water. The stools may be desiccated in patients with infantile renal acidosis, diabetes insipidus or idiopathic hypercalcemia.

2) Withholding the stool. The longer a stool is withheld, the more water is reabsorbed in the rectum.

3. Mechanical obstruction blocks the fecal stream and interferes with the progress of a mass peristaltic movement. Obstipation or intractable constipation may result.

a. Intestinal atresia

b. Imperforate anus. Constipation may be the presenting complaint in infants with an imperforate anus and rectoperineal fistula.

c. Meconium ileus

d. Meconium ileus equivalent (kiotileus) refers to the intestinal obstruction that occasionally occurs in older children with cystic fibrosis. Firm, rubbery masses of stool are palpable on abdominal examination.

e. An inspissated meconium plug in the lower colon in the newborn infant may cause intestinal obstruction and failure to pass meconium. The signs and symptoms include those of intestinal obstruction with abdominal distention, vomiting that may be bilious and intestinal patterning. Roentgen examination results, other than being compatible with low intestinal obstruction, do not differentiate meconium ileus, small intestinal atresia or Hirschsprung's disease from the meconium plug syndrome. The barium enema, which reveals a normal caliber colon, is diagnostic and often therapeutic. Cystic fibrosis and aganglionic megacolon are among disorders associated with the meconium plug syndrome.

f. Intestinal stenosis, especially in the rectosigmoidal and anal regions.

g. Malrotation of the bowel

h. Volvulus

i. Duplication of the alimentary tract, especially of the rectum

j. Incarcerated hernia

k. Intussusception

l. Congenital or acquired adhesive peritoneal bands

m. Cholestyramine therapy prescribed for the pruritus in intrahepatic cholestasis syndromes may produce severe constipation and fecal impaction.

4. Paralytic ileus

a. Peritonitis

b. Postoperative ileus

c. Reflex ileus associated with pneumonitis or other acute illness

d. Severe hypokalemia

B. Anatomically defective reflex mechanisms of mass peristalsis

Aganglionic megacolon or Hirschsprung's disease is caused by a segmental absence of parasympathetic ganglion cells in the myenteric plexus. The affected segment usually begins at or near the anus and extends proximally some 5 to 20 cm. Occasionally, the defect may involve the entire colon and part of the ileum.

Symptoms may begin at birth or on the first day of life with delayed passage of meconium and abdominal distention. Most normal infants pass meconium in the first 24 hours. In other instances, evidence of intestinal obstruction does not appear until a few days later. Some newborn infants demonstrate severe obstipation, while others have intermittent episodes of constipation, abdominal distention and vomiting.

Rectal examination reveals a normal anal sphincter, well-formed anal canal and a small, empty rectal ampulla. That the baby evacuates the colon on rectal examination does not rule out aganglionic megacolon. Roentgenographic examination with a lateral view demonstrates a low intestinal obstruction and a small, air-containing rectum. The diagnosis may be confirmed by barium examination without prior preparation of the colon. With the patient in the oblique or lateral position, a small amount of barium is allowed to run slowly into the rectum. In patients with aganglionic megacolon, a narrowed, irregular segment of the rectum is visualized. Turbulent and purposeless peristalsis may also appear. The bowel proximal to the narrowed segment, usually at the junction of the rectum and sigmoid, may be dilated and redundant.

Accurate diagnosis of aganglionic megacolon may be difficult in newborn infants and during the first several months of life. The barium enema does not always demonstrate the classic findings as seen in older patients, since dilatation and hypertrophy of the proximal colon may not yet have developed. Such infants will have a normal-sized colon but may demonstrate delayed evacuation of the barium. X-rays, especially lateral views, should, therefore, be repeated at 24 and 48 hours. Normal infants usually pass the barium in 24 hours, but with aganglionic megacolon, the barium is retained and mixed with fecal material. Rectal biopsy is diagnostic in equivocal cases. Not infrequently these patients have associated anomalies in the urinary tract, (e.g., a large, atonic bladder with or without megaloureters). If surgical correction is not performed early, chronic abdominal enlargement gradually develops. Enterocolitis is a major complication, with massive dilatation of the colon, diarrhea, vomiting, fever, dehydration and lethargy.

Anatomic megacolon occurs secondary to a congenital anorectal stenosis or to stricture of the rectum that develops after surgical correction of an imperforate anus. Anterior displacement of the anus is a common cause of constipation. Rarely, intrinsic or extrinsic tumors may cause a megacolon. Anatomic megacolon can be diagnosed by history and by digital examination of the rectum. The onset of symptoms is usually gradual, and the time of onset depends upon the degree of obstruction.

Reisner, S. H., Sivan, Y., Nitzan, M., and Merlob, P.: Determination of anterior displacement of the anus in normal infants and children. *Pediatrics* 73:216, 1984.

II. INTERFERENCE WITH THE SPINAL ARC

A. Voluntary inhibition of defecation may cause the defecation stimulus to disappear. The stool may then become desiccated and its passage accompanied by pain. This, in turn, may cause further inhibition of defecation. Reasons for voluntary inhibition are:
   1. Children may be too busy to take time from their play.
   2. The child may be afraid of being late for school if he stops to defecate. At school he may be embarrassed to ask permission to leave the room or to use the toilet if the stall has no door.
   3. Hospitalized infants or young children may not be able to make their need to defecate known to the staff.
   4. After the age of four years or so a child may desire privacy when he uses the toilet.
   5. Traveling disrupts routines. The child may feel anxious or insecure when away from familiar surroundings, or a toilet may be inaccessible to him. Some children experience difficulty in using a toilet away from home.

B. Excessive use of suppositories, laxatives and enemas. These agents empty the colon so that stools are infrequent for two to three days. This may create the false impression that constipation has recurred or is still present. In patients who receive laxatives over a prolonged period of time, the bowel becomes insensitive to its own physiologic reflexes and dependent on artifical agents.

C. Spinal cord lesions. Interruption of the spinal cord above the defecation center in the second, third and fourth sacral segments causes a loss of voluntary control. Defecation then reverts to a reflex act so that the rectum empties automatically with each mass peristaltic movement of the colon. Destruction of the cord at the defecation center causes the loss of all rectal sensation and relaxation of the external anal sphincter with incontinence rather than automaticity. Fecal impaction frequently occurs in patients with either type of spinal cord lesion. It is rare for a neurologic lesion to produce fecal incontinence without a disturbance in bladder control.

Rectal continence is sustained through the actions of the internal sphincter, which is under reflex control, and of the striated muscle external sphincter, which is under both reflex and voluntary control. Rectal incontinence occurs only when the somatic innervation of the external sphincter has been impaired. In such instances, a full rectum produces reflex relaxation of the internal sphincter. Without adequate voluntary and reflex action of the external sphincter, incontinence results.

White, J. J., Suzuki, H., El Shafie, M., Kumar, A. P. M., Haller, J. A., and Schnaufer, L.: A physiologic rationale for the management of neurologic rectal incontinence in children. Pediatrics 49:888, 1972.

   1. Transection of the spinal cord
   2. Meningomyelocele
   3. Spina bifida occulta associated with myelodysplasia
   4. Diastematomyelia is characterized by difficulty in walking. Dribbling of urine and fecal incontinence occur frequently. Fecal impaction may develop.
   5. Spinal cord tumors

III. INTERFERENCE WITH THE RELAXATION OF THE ANAL SPHINCTERS

A. Anal fissures are a frequent cause of constipation in early infancy. A bowel movement may not occur for several days, and the stools are apt to be hard and streaked with bright red blood. The infant may be irritable and cry excessively, especially before and after a bowel movement. The majority of fissures can be visualized with the infant in a knee-chest position and the buttocks spread to reveal the mucocutaneous junction of the anus. Early lesions have the appearance of superficial erosions. More advanced fissures are seen as linear or elliptical breaks in the skin. Long-standing fissures are deep and indurated. In the presence of a suggestive history, rectal examination may be performed when a fissure is not visualized. Internal fissures are often visible through the relaxed anal sphincter as the examining finger is withdrawn.

Fissures involuntarily inhibit defecation by producing spasm of the external anal sphincter. This results in desiccation of the stools. The cycle becomes self-perpetuating because the passage of hard stools traumatizes the mucosa and prevents healing of the fissure. Anal fissures occasionally occur in patients with anal stenosis; in older children with pinworms, they may result from perianal scratching.

B. Anal stenosis
   1. Congenital anal stenosis is a common cause of constipation in young infants. Anal fissures are often also present.
   2. Acquired stricture may be a complication of surgery for imperforate anus.

IV. INTERFERENCE WITH CONTRACTION OF THE VOLUNTARY MUSCLES OF DEFECATION

A. Congenital deficiency or complete absence of the abdominal musculature is characterized by a protuberant and often asymmetrically shaped abdomen. Constipation is always a problem. The bladder may be enlarged, and hydroureter and hydronephrosis are usually present.
B. Floppy infant syndrome
C. Cerebral palsy
D. Poliomyelitis
E. Guillain-Barré syndrome
F. Infantile botulism may initially cause constipation. Subsequent findings include poor cry, lethargy, expressionless facies, weak suck, generalized weakness, dysphagia, loss of head control and absence of deep tendon reflexes.

Johnson, R. O., Clay, S. A., and Andarnon, S. S.: Diagnosis and management of infant botulism. Am. J. Dis. Child. 133:586, 1979.

G. Rickets may be accompanied by flabby, weak abdominal musculature.
H. Anemia may be associated with flabby, weak, hypotonic musculature.
I. Constipation in infants and children with hypothyroidism occurs secondary to hypotonia of the abdominal and intestinal musculature. Constipation may be an early symptom of congenital hypothyroidism.

V. INTERFERENCE WITH AUTONOMIC AND CORTICAL CONTROL OF DEFECATION

A. Irritable colon
B. Encopresis with functional megacolon secondary to chronic constipation in the absence of neurologic or other anatomic factors is characterized by repeated fecal soiling owing to the involuntary passage of small amounts of feces into the underpants of a child over four years of age. Fecal soiling of the underclothing with soft fluid stool is an almost constant finding. The child with encopresis often seems unaware of his odor. Periodically, voluminous stools are passed spontaneously. Rectal examination reveals a large rectal vault packed with feces that may be surprisingly soft in many cases but often firm or hard. Constipation is usually longstanding, so that enormous amounts of stool may be found on physical examination or a plain x-ray of the abdomen. Some children are found to have only rectal retention with a megarectum rather than a megacolon.

The child who has encopresis without constipation usually has major psychopathology. The severe constipation in children with encopresis may be secondary to painful defecation owing to an anal fissure, coercive bowel training, fear of the toilet, or reactive voluntary withholding of bowel movements. The accumulated fecal mass causes distention of the rectum. Sensory receptors in the rectal wall and puborectalis muscle then lead reflexly to relaxation of the internal sphincter. With subsequent relaxation of the levator ani and shortening of the anal canal, the external sphincter opens and encopresis occurs.

Colicky abdominal pain is frequent. Abdominal distention is less prominent than with aganglionic megacolon and is usually minimal, even after several years. When emotional factors are prominent, children with encopresis may refuse to use the toilet. Rather, they hold their lower extremities tightly together and strain in an apparent attempt to withhold the stool.

An intravenous pyelogram may be indicated in patients with chronic fecal impaction because secondary hydronephrosis and vesicoureteral reflux are often present.

Levine, M. D.: The school child with encopresis. Pediatr. Rev. 2:285, 1981.

C. Premenstrual syndrome

ETIOLOGIC CLASSIFICATION OF CONSTIPATION AND INFREQUENT STOOLS

I. INTERFERENCE WITH MASS PERISTALTIC MOVEMENTS OF THE COLON, 236
   A. Intact reflex mechanism of mass peristalsis, 236
      1. Lack of fecal bulk
      2. Hard stools
      3. Mechanical obstruction
      4. Paralytic ileus
   B. Defective reflex mechanism of mass peristalsis, 237
II. INTERFERENCE WITH SPINAL ARC, 238
   A. Voluntary inhibition of defecation, 238
   B. Overuse of suppositories, laxatives and enemas, 238
   C. Spinal cord lesions, 238
III. INTERFERENCE WITH RELAXATION OF ANAL SPHINCTERS, 239
   A. Anal fissures, 239
   B. Anal stenosis, 239

   1. Congenital anal stenosis
   2. Acquired stricture
IV. INTERFERENCE WITH CONTRACTION OF VOLUNTARY MUSCLES, 239
   A. Congenital deficiency or absence of abdominal musculature, 239
   B. Floppy infant syndrome, 239
   C. Cerebral palsy, 239
   D. Poliomyelitis, 239
   E. Guillain-Barré syndrome, 239
   F. Infantile botulism, 239
   G. Rickets, 239
   H. Anemia, 239
   I. Muscular hypotonia in hypothyroidism, 239
V. INTERFERENCE WITH AUTOMOMIC AND CORTICAL CONTROL OF DEFECATION, 239
   A. Irritable colon, 239
   B. Encopresis, 239
   C. Premenstrual syndrome, 240

---

24 / DYSPHAGIA

Dysphagia may be defined as difficulty in swallowing, characterized variously by choking, return of fluids and food through the nose, hesitation in swallowing, and pain or retrosternal discomfort or both during deglutition.

ETIOLOGIC CLASSIFICATION OF DYSPHAGIA

I. ANATOMIC

A. Congenital malformations
   1. Cleft palate
   2. Macroglossia

   3. Micrognathia
   4. Intrinsic esophageal lesions, e.g., atresia, stenosis, webs. With an H-type tracheoesophageal fistula, severe choking and coughing may follow feeding.
B. Acquired malformations
   1. Esophageal stenosis may occur postoperatively in infants with esophageal atresia and tracheoesophageal fistula.
   2. Esophagitis secondary to gastroesophageal reflux or hiatus hernia may cause marked dysphagia. Esophageal spasm may occur.
   3. Pseudodiverticulum of the esophagus may result from a perforation of

the mucosa or submucosa during suctioning, intubation or passage of a nasogastric tube. Findings include increased salivation, respiratory distress, vomiting and choking.

4. Esophageal involvement may occur with scleroderma, lupus erythematosus or dermatomyositis. Dysphagia may be the initial symptom in dermatomyositis.

5. Alkali burns of the esophagus may cause dysphagia and excessive salivation.

6. Esophagitis owing to *Candida albicans* may occur in chronic mucocutaneous candidiasis or in immunodeficient or immunosuppressed patients.

Kobayashi, R. H., Rosenblatt, H. M., Carney, J. M., Byrne, J., Ament, M. E., Mendoza, G. R., Dudley, J. P., and Stiehm, E. R.: *Candida* esophagitis and laryngitis in chronic mucocutaneous candidiasis. Pediatrics 66:380, 1980.

C. Encroachment; compression; displacement
   1. Enlarged tonsils
   2. Cardiac enlargement
   3. Vascular ring
   4. Mediastinal tumor
   5. Retropharyngeal abscess
   6. Goiter; chronic lymphocytic thyroiditis (Hashimoto's thyroiditis)
   7. Pneumomediastinum
D. Inflammatory lesions
   1. Herpetic gingivostomatitis
   2. Thrush
   3. Peritonsillar abscess
   4. Pharyngitis
   5. Epiglottitis

II. NEUROMUSCULAR

A. Cerebral damage. Difficulty in sucking and swallowing may be the first indication of maldevelopment of or damage to the central nervous system. The mother may report that the baby requires more than an hour to take one ounce of milk or that he does not seem to know how to suck or use his tongue. Saliva may accumulate in the infant's mouth, and constant drooling occurs.
B. Infants with hypothyroidism may feed poorly and have difficulty in sucking and swallowing.
C. "Floppy baby" syndrome. Infants with generalized hypotonia may have difficulty in feeding.
D. Pharyngeal paralysis
   1. Evidence of difficulty in swallowing is an early sign of bulbar poliomyelitis.
   2. Postdiphtheritic paralysis; tick paralysis; Guillain-Barré syndrome.

3. Isolated palatal paralysis may become manifest soon after birth with regurgitation of liquids through the nose while feeding.
4. Botulism produces dysphagia along with constipation, diplopia, photophobia, blurring of vision and generalized weakness occurring 18 to 36 hours after ingestion of the toxin.
5. Pseudobulbar or suprabulbar paresis may occur owing to involvement of nerve tracts from the cortical motor areas for the lips, palate and tongue to the medullary motor nuclei. Clinical manifestations result from weakness or spasticity of the lips, tongue, palate and pharyngeal muscles. A jaw jerk is present.
6. Congenital absence of cranial nerve nuclei
7. Möbius' syndrome may cause dysphagia in infants.

E. Pharyngeal or cricopharyngeal incoordination
F. Congenital myotonic dystrophy may be characterized by difficulties in sucking and swallowing along with facial diplegia, hypotonia and absence of spontaneous respiration.
G. Pontine glioma
H. The infantile form of Gaucher's disease may be characterized by dysphagia and laryngospasm.
I. Children with familial dysautonomia often have difficulty in swallowing and, as a result, may aspirate food.
J. Rabies
K. Phenothiazine toxicity
L. Lesch-Nyhan syndrome may cause athetoid dysphagia.
M. Myasthenia gravis may be characterized by dysphagia and by difficulty in chewing owing to weakness of the jaw muscles. Regurgitation may occur through the nose.
N. Subacute necrotizing encephalomyelopathy (Leigh's syndrome), which has its onset in infancy, may be characterized by dysphagia as well as other signs of brain stem dysfunction.
O. Kearns-Sayre syndrome is characterized by ptosis, ophthalmoplegia, retinal degeneration and cerebellar signs, in addition to dysphagia and dysphonia.
P. Narcotic withdrawal in the newborn may be accompanied by poor feeding and regurgitation.
Q. Wilson's disease

III. PSYCHOLOGIC AND FUNCTIONAL DISTURBANCES

A. Conversion reaction. Globus hystericus associated with spasm of the upper pharyngeal constrictors is characterized by a "lump" in the throat, difficulty in swallowing and, at times, by retrosternal discomfort.

B. A type of pseudodysphagia may occur in which a child refuses to chew foods that are chopped and restricts his diet to those that are pureed. Other children hold food in their mouths creating a "chipmunk" appearance with their distended cheeks. If the child is not retarded, this usually reflects problems in the mother-child relationship.

C. Achalasia (cardiospasm) occasionally occurs in older children and adolescents. Early, dysphagia for both liquid and solid foods is recurrent and transient. Only a brief delay may occur in swallowing, but the patients are described as slow eaters. Later, dysphagia is constant, with a feeling that food is caught in the lower esophagus, and undigested food is regurgitated or vomited. The patient may complain of chest pain, vague discomfort or pressure in the lower substernal region. Nocturnal cough and recurrent pneumonias may occur.

Berquist, W. E., Byrne, W. J., Ament, M. E., Fonkalsrud, E. W., and Eulher, A. R.: Achalasia: Diagnosis, management and clinical course in 16 children. Pediatrics 71:798, 1983.

D. Infants who have been maintained on prolonged total parenteral nutrition or gastrostomy feedings may refuse oral feedings, including the bottle.

IV. FOREIGN BODY LODGED IN THE ESOPHAGUS may cause dysphagia, total inability to swallow or pain on swallowing.

V. RESPIRATORY AND CARDIAC DISORDERS. Infants with dyspnea may have dysphagia because the act of swallowing accentuates their respiratory difficulty. Infants with hypoxia or shortness of breath may appear to have dysphagia, since they require a long time to take even small feedings.

A. Larynx
   1. Congenital laryngeal disorders such as inspiratory laryngeal collapse
   2. Epiglottitis, acute laryngotracheobronchitis
B. Pulmonary disease
C. Cardiac disease

ETIOLOGIC CLASSIFICATION OF DYSPHAGIA

25 / ABDOMINAL AND PELVIC PAIN

Abdominal pain is one of the most common and yet, at times, one of the most difficult symptoms to evaluate. In infants, abdominal pain may be suspected in the presence of screaming or persistent crying, restlessness, irritability, squirming, grunting respiration, flexion of the thighs on the abdomen and refusal to eat.

ETIOLOGIC CLASSIFICATION OF ABDOMINAL PAIN

I. Intra-abdominal Causes

A. Gastrointestinal tract and mesentery

  1. Colic is a nonspecific symptom occurring during the early months of life and characterized by vigorous and prolonged crying, presumably owing to intermittent abdominal pain. The episodes are sudden in onset and, in many cases, begin about the same time each day. The infant appears to be in great pain and is often inconsolable. His face becomes flushed, his abdomen distended, and he draws his extremities against his body. Often, his crying does not diminish, even though he is picked up and rocked. The incidence and frequency of colic appear to vary in different social groups and families, with the baby's temperament, and with his manner of relieving tension. In some, colic is rarely seen or occurs only occasionally, while other infants experience the discomfort almost every evening for two or three months. Many factors may be etiologic. Errors in feeding technique such as excessive air swallowing, improperly sized nipple holes, bottle-propping, failure to "burp" the infant and the ingestion of an excessive amount of a too dilute formula are considerations. Underfeeding, as well as overfeeding, should be investigated. Gastrointestinal allergy may play a role at times. In other instances, colic may reflect tenseness in the mother and the household.

  2. Peptic ulcer in children, usually duodenal rather than gastric and a relatively rare cause of abdominal pain, may be periumbilical, epigastric or poorly localized. Although the pain may be severe enough to cause the child to cry, it is usually described as more of a persistent stomach ache. Episodes of pain last from a few minutes to hours and are more frequent at night than during the daytime. Pain may occur in the morning before breakfast and before other meals, but it usually has no relation to meals. Pain may be relieved by milk or other food, but it also may become worse for a time after eating. Relief may occur after vomiting. Peptic ulcer occurs with a high frequency among adolescent heroin users.

  In premature and very young infants, vomiting is a more prominent clinical manifestation than abdominal pain. In young children, recurrent or cyclic vomiting, with or without nausea, may be the chief symptom. The occurrence of peptic ulcers in children with burns, head injuries, intracranial tumors, infections of the central nervous system, severe stress and steroid therapy is well known. Since hematemesis and melena may occur in children with a peptic ulcer, examination of stools for occult blood is indicated. Demonstration of an actual ulcer crater by x-ray or endoscopy is necessary for diagnosis.

Deckelbaum, R. J., Roy, C. C., Lussier-Lazaroff, J., and Morin, C. L.: Peptic ulcer disease: A clinical study in 73 children. Can. Med. Assoc. J. 111:225, 1974.

Rosenlund, M. L., and Koop, C. E.: Duodenal ulcer in childhood. Pediatrics 45:283, 1970.

  3. The Zollinger-Ellison syndrome, which consists of peptic ulceration, hypertrophy of gastric mucosa, gas-

tric hypersecretion with increased acidity and non–beta islet cell tumor of the pancreas, has been reported in children over seven years of age. Presenting complaints include abdominal pain, vomiting, hematemesis and melena. The ulcer is usually duodenal but may occur also in the stomach or jejunum.

Buchta, R. M., and Kaplan, J. M.: Zollinger-Ellison syndrome in a nine-year-old child: A case report and review of this entity in childhood. Pediatrics 47:594, 1971.

4. Dietary indiscretion, either overindulgence or the ingestion of foods not easily digested, is a common cause of acute abdominal pain in young children.

5. The diagnosis of appendicitis is often not difficult, but it may be most challenging. The classic history begins with abdominal pain followed by nausea, vomiting and fever. In the presence of these symptoms, appendicitis is always a diagnostic consideration. Initially, the pain may be periumbilical or epigastric. After a time, perhaps a few hours, the pain may become localized in the right lower quadrant or in the region of the umbilicus. Young children do not localize abdominal pain well. The pain, rarely severe, is usually constant, but may be colicky or intermittent. If the appendix ruptures, the child may complain less of pain for an hour or two; however, the pain soon returns with increased intensity. The symptoms associated with abdominal pain and appendicitis in infants and very young children—irritability, restlessness, unexplained crying, refusal of feedings and vomiting—are often overlooked.

   Vomiting, with or without nausea, may occur once, twice or repeatedly. Almost a constant feature in children with appendicitis, the diagnosis is less likely in the absence of vomiting. Younger children seem to vomit more often than those who are older. Fever is usually low grade and, unless a complication occurs, rarely exceeds 38.9° C (102° F). Bowel movements are usually normal, or constipation may be present. Diarrhea may occur if the inflamed appendix lies next to the terminal ileum or sigmoid. Diarrhea may also appear in children with early peritonitis. Appendicitis may occur as a complication of measles and in children who have an upper respiratory tract infection, enteritis or rheumatic fever.

   The physical findings, discussed on pages 91 and 106, are of great importance in deciding whether or not acute appendicitis is present. If these findings have not developed when the child is first seen, repeated examinations are indicated over a period of a few hours. A white blood cell count, urinalysis and a chest roentgenogram are indicated in the diagnostic work-up. A plain film of the abdomen may demonstrate the presence of a fecalith.

   Mesenteric lymphadenopathy owing to *Yersinia enterocolitica* or other causes may cause abdominal pain that closely resembles acute appendicitis. When a normal appendix is found in the presence of mesenteric adenitis, a node should be biopsied for culture.

   Typhlitis, a necrotizing lesion of the cecum usually caused by *Pseudomonas* or other gram negative bacteria, may cause severe, acute right lower quadrant pain.

6. Intussusception is an especially important diagnostic consideration in infants with abdominal pain. Immediate diagnosis and treatment are imperative if mortality is to be prevented. Brennemann's description of the pain is classic: "The onset is dramatic. Awake or asleep the baby suddenly cries out with a pain that is obviously extreme. He screams, claws, and clambers up on his mother, twists and squirms, and nothing gives any relief until, almost as suddenly, there is a lull with absence of pain, only to be followed by a similar painful episode. This sudden onset is of great diagnostic value. As in almost no other condition the mother usually states the exact hour at which the pain began. In the course of some hours the pains become less severe, as a rule not enough to cause the child to cry out as before. With each recurrence he merely squirms, throws himself to one side, doubles up, whimpers, moans or sighs. He appears calm, too calm, paying little attention to his surroundings and yet seems preoccupied and apprehensive."

   The history of abdominal pain, sudden in onset, lasting several seconds, and recurring every 5 to 15 minutes always means intussusception until that diagnosis is ruled out. In some instances, pain may not be a prominent feature or may be persistent rather than intermittent. Between the paroxysms of pain, the child may appear completely normal. Vomiting occurs early in many of these patients. Blood in the stools is usually a relatively late finding. The physical findings in patients with intussusception have been described on page 90. Although the diagnosis can usually be made readily on the basis of the history and physical examination, a barium enema is diagnostic and usually therapeutic. Since diarrhea may occur in patients with intussusception, this possibility should be considered in infants seen with an atypical picture of dysentery. At times, infants with intussusception present with limpness, lethargy, listlessness, obtundation or stupor. Intussusception should be considered a diagnostic possibility when these early signs appear.

Intussusception in children above the age of six years raises the possibility of an intestinal lymphoma. Adolescents with the Peutz-Jeghers syndrome may develop intussusception as a complication.

Chronic intussusception is a rare cause of recurrent pain in childhood. Intermittent vomiting and the passage of small amounts of blood in the stool may occur.

7. Intestinal malrotation may at times be responsible for recurrent abdominal pain. Nausea and vomiting may also be present.
8. Volvulus
9. Intra-abdominal hernia
10. Meckel's diverticulum. Blood in the stools, usually sudden and large in amount, suggests a Meckel's diverticulum. On the other hand, Meckel's diverticulitis may be characterized by abdominal pain, tenderness, vomiting and fever—symptoms indistinguishable from those of appendicitis. The findings, however, usually do not become localized in the right lower quadrant. Meckel's diverticulum may also cause recurrent, somewhat diffuse, periumbilical discomfort.
11. A mesenteric cyst may be responsible for recurrent abdominal pain or abdominal distention. Bleeding into the cyst may cause acute, severe pain that may suggest acute appendicitis.
12. Duplications of the intestinal tract may be characterized by intermittent, colicky abdominal pain and vomiting.
13. Intestinal polyps are a rare cause of intermittent abdominal pain and discomfort.
14. With an incarcerated hernia, the infant is irritable, fretful and in severe pain. The respiratory rate is increased. Refusal of feedings and vomiting may occur.
15. Intestinal obstruction is characterized by intermittent, colicky pain. The intensity of the pain varies with the degree of obstruction.
16. Constipation is a common cause of vague, chronic abdominal pain and discomfort in children.
17. Sigmoid volvulus may simulate some of the symptoms of intussusception, including anorexia, abdominal cramps, tenderness, a palpable mass and rectal bleeding.

Campbell, J. R., and Blank, E.: Sigmoid volvulus in children. Pediatrics 53:702, 1974.

18. The diagnostic work-up of children with abdominal pain should include examination of the stools for ova and parasites. Pinworms may rarely cause appendicitis.
19. The onset of diarrhea in patients with dysentery or other infectious gastroenteritis may be preceded by abdominal pain, tenderness, vomiting and fever. Usually the abdominal pain is not severe, and localization does not occur. Abdominal pain and diarrhea with watery, mucoid and sometimes bloody stools may occur in patients with *Salmonella* enteritis. *Campylobacter* enteritis may begin with periumbilical, intermittent and colicky abdominal pain relieved by the passage of a stool or flatus. The presence of fever, generalized abdominal tenderness, diarrhea and frank blood in the stools may simulate inflammatory bowel disease.
20. Aerophagia may cause abdominal pain.
21. An increase in the frequency of stools, abdominal discomfort and abdominal cramps may be the earliest clinical manifestations of ulcerative colitis. The abdominal cramps, tenesmus and urgency may be re-

lieved by passage of a stool. Abdominal pain is not present in all patients. See page 230.

22. Children with regional enteritis or Crohn's disease may have recurrent episodes of vague or crampy abdominal pain, usually periumbilical or in the right lower quadrant, anorexia, vomiting, diarrhea, fever and weight loss. Pain may be relieved by defecation. The symptoms of acute regional enteritis may closely simulate those of acute appendicitis.

Dubois, R.S., Rothschild, J., and Silverman, A.: The pediatric corner: The varied manifestations of Crohn's disease in children and adolescents. Am. J. Gastroenterol. 69:203, 1978.

Gryboski, J. D.: Crohn's disease in children. Pediatr. Rev. 2:239, 1981.

Hamilton, J. R., Bruce, G. A., Abdourhaman, M., and Gall, D. G.: Inflammatory bowel disease in children and adolescents. Adv. Pediatr. 36:311, 1979.

Kelts, D. G., and Grand, R. J.: Inflammatory bowel disease in children and adolescents. Curr. Probl. Pediatr. 10:5, 1980.

23. Rarely, colicky abdominal pain may be caused by an allergic response to specific foods. Diarrhea, nausea and vomiting may also occur.

24. Lactose intolerance, a genetic trait with increased prevalence among black, native American and Hispanic children and adolescents is characterized by bloating, flatulence, recurrent abdominal pain, diarrhea and cramps.

Barr, R. G., Levine, M. D., and Watkins, J. B.: Recurrent abdominal pain of childhood due to lactose intolerance. N. Engl. J. Med. 300:1449, 1979.

Committee on Nutrition, American Academy of Pediatrics: The practical significance of lactose intolerance in children. Pediatrics 62:240, 1978.

25. Abdominal pain, at times severe, may occur in patients with cystic fibrosis owing to such factors as steatorrhea with excessive fermentation of intestinal contents, irritability of the descending loop of the duodenum or pancreatitis. Epigastric pain may be caused by esophagitis secondary to gastroesophageal reflux.

26. Hereditary angioedema may cause recurrent episodes of severe abdominal pain owing to edema of the bowel wall. Concurrent cutaneous angioedema may not occur.

27. Retractile mesenteritis or mesenteric panniculitis, a subtype of systemic idiopathic fibrosis, may cause recurrent abdominal pain, fever and an elevated erythrocyte sedimentation rate.

Binder, S. C., Deterling, R. A., Jr., Mahoney, S. A., Patterson, J. F., and Wolfe, H. J.: Systemic idiopathic fibrosis: Report of a case of the concomitant occurrence of retractile mesenteritis and retroperitoneal fibrosis. Am. J. Surg. 124:422, 1972.

B. Urinary tract
   1. Abdominal pain, especially chronic or recurrent, is often attributable to urinary tract disease. Obstruction with or without superimposed infection is the most important renal disease associated with abdominal pain. Urologic abdominal pain may be localized to the back, the flank or the lower abdomen. Fever, nausea and vomiting may also be present.
   2. Patients with Henoch-Schönlein purpura, hemophilia or other systemic hemorrhagic disease may have colicky renal pain owing to the passage of blood clots down the ureter.
   3. A renal calculus may cause recurrent, persistent, or generalized abdominal pain, at times without hematuria. Nausea, vomiting and fever may be the presenting complaints, along with poorly localized abdominal pain. Classic renal colic with radiation of pain along the ureter to the genitalia is uncommon. Immobilization is an important etiologic factor in renal stone formation.

Walther, P. C., Lamm, D., and Kaplan, G. W.: Pediatric urolithiases: A ten-year review. Pediatrics 65:1068, 1980.

   4. Hypercalciuria may be associated with abdominal or suprapubic pain with or without calculi.
   5. Abdominal pain occasionally occurs as an early manifestation of acute glomerulonephritis.
C. Liver and gallbladder
   1. Infectious hepatitis may be characterized by abdominal discomfort and pain in the right upper quadrant. The possibility of nonicteric hepatitis is to be considered in patients with right upper quadrant or epigastric pain.
   2. Cholecystitis, although rare, does occur in childhood. It is characterized by severe abdominal pain, chiefly in the right upper quadrant,

and by nausea, vomiting and fever. Tenderness, guarding and a mass may be noted on physical examination. Jaundice may also occur.

Andrassy, R. T., et al.: Gallbladder disease in children and adolescents. Am. J. Surg. 132:19, 1976.

Pieretti, R., Auldist, A. W., and Stephens, C. A.: Acute cholecystitis in children. Surg. Gynecol. Obstet. 140:16, 1975.

Takiff, H., and Fonkalsrud, E. W.: Gallbladder disease in childhood. Am. J. Dis. Child. 138:565, 1984.

3. Patients with cholelithiasis may have repeated episodes of nausea, vomiting, colicky abdominal pain, chiefly in the right upper quadrant, tenderness and muscle guarding. Jaundice is an occasional symptom. Cholelithiasis is usually associated with a systemic disorder such as sickle cell anemia, chronic hemolytic anemia, Wilson's disease, cystic fibrosis or metachromatic leukodystrophy. Children receiving long-term total parenteral alimentation may develop cholelithiasis.

Ariyan, S., Shessel, F. S., and Pickett, L. K.: Cholecystitis and cholelithiasis masking as abdominal crises in sickle cell disease. Pediatrics 58:252, 1976.

Rosenfield, N., Grand, R. J., Watkins, J. B., Ballantine, T. V. N., and Levey, R. H.: Cholelithiasis and Wilson's disease. J. Pediatr. 92:210, 1978.

4. Passive congestion of the liver
5. Intrahepatic sinusoidal plugging during a sickle cell crisis may cause fever, jaundice, hepatomegaly, leukocytosis, elevated alkaline phosphatase and acholic stools.
6. Choledochal cyst or cystic dilatation of the gall bladder may cause abdominal pain. Jaundice of the obstructive type and a palpable mass in the right upper quadrant are also frequently present. The discomfort is usually localized in the right upper abdomen.
7. Hydrops or acute distention of the gallbladder may cause a right upper quadrant mass, severe pain and rigidity of the rectus muscle. Acute hydrops of the gallbladder occurs as a complication of Kawasaki disease.
8. Hepatic tumors may cause abdominal discomfort.
9. Chiari's syndrome or thrombosis of the hepatic veins is characterized, in part, by upper abdominal pain.

D. Spleen
1. Traumatic rupture of the spleen may cause tenderness and muscle spasm in the left upper quadrant.
2. Splenomegaly produces abdominal discomfort.
3. Congestive splenomegaly may be associated with left upper quadrant pain during episodes of hematemesis.

E. Pancreas
1. Acute pancreatitis is characterized by the abrupt onset of midepigastric or generalized, constant abdominal pain; nausea, protracted vomiting; jaundice; fever; and abdominal tenderness, most prominent in the epigastrium or around the umbilicus. The patient usually appears acutely ill and may be in shock. Physical examination reveals maximal tenderness in the midepigastric area with muscle guarding and rigidity. The abdomen is distended and has a firm, doughy feel. The child may assume the knee-chest position for pain relief. Bluish discoloration of the umbilicus or flanks may occur in the presence of intra-abdominal hemorrhage. Pleural effusion may develop in some patients. Daily determination of the serum amylase is indicated when pancreatitis is suspected. Pancreatic ultrasonography may be diagnostically helpful in children with acute or chronic abdominal pain of unknown etiology. Hyperglycemia and hypocalcemia may also occur.

Pancreatitis may be associated with mumps, mycoplasma infection, systemic lupus erythematosus, azotemia, increased intracranial pressure, congenital duodenal duplication in the head of the pancreas, sepsis, blunt or penetrating trauma or mechanical obstruction of the pancreatic ducts by *Ascaris*. Acute pancreatitis may also be induced by drugs such as azathioprine, isoniazid, valproic acid, 6-mercaptopurine, L-asparaginase and steroids. Obstruction of the pancreatic or distal common bile duct, usually owing to a congenital anomaly of the ducts, may be etiologic. Chronic relapsing pancreatitis is characterized by recurrences of pain and upper abdominal discomfort. Pancreatic calcifications, diabetes mellitus and steatorrhea may occur. Recurrent pancreatitis may be hereditary, including familial hyperlipoproteinemia, hyperlipemia, or a manifestation of hyperparathyroidism or cystic fibrosis. Fat necrosis associated with pancreatitis may cause fever, tender subcutaneous nodules, polyarthritis and bone pain.

Jordan, S. C., and Ament, M. E.: Pancreatitis in children and adolescents. J. Pediatr. 91:211, 1977.

Shwachman, H., Lebenthal, E., and Khaw, K.-T.: Recurrent acute pancreatitis in patients with cystic fibrosis with normal pancreatic enzymes. Pediatrics 55:86, 1975.

   2. Congenital fibrosis of the sphincter of Oddi may be associated with abdominal pain.

   3. Pseudocyst of the pancreas is characterized by abdominal pain, anorexia, nausea, vomiting, distention and an abdominal mass, usually tender and firm, in the upper abdomen. Ascites, weight loss or fever may also be noted.

F. Ovaries, uterus, fallopian tubes

   1. Torsion of an ovarian pedicle, cyst or tumor on the right may be accompanied by symptoms indistinguishable from those of acute appendicitis. Torsion of the adnexa is a diagnostic consideration with a history of a sudden onset of lower abdominal pain and vomiting, especially with a history of similar episodes. A pelvic mass can be palpated on rectal examination. Intermittent torsion may cause recurrent symptoms. Rupture of an ovarian follicle at ovulation (*mittelschmerz*), usually in adolescents over 16 years of age, may cause dull but, at times, sharp lower abdominal quadrant pain two weeks before a menstrual period. Abdominal and unilateral adnexal tenderness and some muscle guarding may be noted. Pelvic discomfort and cramps may also accompany menstruation.

Ein, S. H., Darte, J. M. M., and Stephens, C. A.: Cystic and solid ovarian tumors in children: a 44-year review. J. Pediatr. Surg. 5:148, 1970.

   2. Hematocolpos in adolescent girls may be accompanied by constant or intermittent abdominal pain.

   3. Dysmenorrhea is characterized by crampy lower abdominal pain that may radiate to the back and thighs, peripheral edema, bloating, headache, nausea, vomiting and diarrhea. Primary dysmenorrhea refers to painful menstruation in the absence of pelvic pathology, while secondary dysmenorrhea is associated with pelvic disorders such as endometriosis or pelvic inflammatory disease. The premenstrual syndrome may be associated with irritability, fatigue, depression, breast swelling and tenderness.

   4. Acute salpingitis caused by *Neisseria gonorrhoeae* is accompanied by fever, shaking chills, lower abdominal pain, nausea, vomiting, abdominal and adnexal tenderness, a purulent urethral and vaginal discharge and tenderness on movement of the cervix. Leukocytosis and an elevated sedimentation rate are present. Direct laparoscopy is the only definitive way to establish the diagnosis. Gonococcal perihepatitis may accompany acute salpingitis. Subacute pelvic inflammatory disease is characterized by lower abdominal and pelvic pain, fever, dysmenorrhea, menstrual irregularity and an elevated sedimentation rate.

Litt, I. F., Edberg, S. C., and Finberg, L.: Gonorrhea in children and adolescents: a current review. J. Pediatr. 85:595, 1974.

   5. Endometriosis in adolescent girls may cause cyclic pelvic pain, irregular menses, dysmenorrhea, bladder symptoms and vaginal discharge. Pelvic tenderness and nodularity are noted on pelvic examination.

Goldstein, D. P., deCholnoky, C., and Emans, S. J.: Adolescent endometriosis. J. Adolesc. Health Care 1:37, 1980.

Huffman, J. W.: Endometriosis in young teen-age girls. Pediatr. Ann. 10:12, 1981.

   6. Hematocolpos may cause cyclic abdominal pain in adolescents.

   7. Ectopic pregnancy may be characterized by amenorrhea, menorrhagia or irregular bleeding, lower abdominal pain and a tender adnexal mass unaccompanied by fever or a cervical discharge.

G. Lymph nodes

   1. Mesenteric lymphadenitis is a diagnosis made by exclusion. With a history of abdominal pain, vomiting and fever, the suspicion of acute appendicitis is always warranted. A period of observation may be required to eliminate or affirm this possibility. If the symptoms do not progress and significant tenderness is absent, appendicitis can eventually be excluded. When it cannot, laparotomy is indicated.

2. Iliac adenitis may cause lower abdominal pain, tenderness, fever and leukocytosis.
3. Leukemia and other lymphomas may cause abdominal pain through involvement of mesenteric or retroperitoneal lymph nodes.
4. Tuberculosis of the mesenteric lymph nodes may cause chronic abdominal pain.

H. Primary streptococcal or pneumococcal peritonitis is a rare occurrence in children. Generalized abdominal pain is present. Tuberculous peritonitis is characterized more by abdominal discomfort than actual pain, although at times the pain may be severe. After rupture of an appendix, the child may complain less of pain for an hour or two. The pain then becomes generalized, and the child lies very still in an effort to minimize the discomfort. Peritonitis in children undergoing continuous ambulatory peritoneal dialysis is characterized by cloudy peritoneal fluid, fever and abdominal pain.

Warady, B. A., Campoy, S. F., Gross, S. P., Sedman, A. B., and Lum, G. M.: Peritonitis with continuous ambulatory peritoneal dialysis and continuous cycling peritoneal dialysis. J. Pediatr. 105:726, 1984.

I. Mesenteric vein thrombosis
J. Pelvic osteomyelitis may cause right-sided abdominal pain without rebound tenderness.
K. Superior mesenteric artery syndrome is produced by duodenal obstruction proximal to the ligament of Treitz. Symptoms, which are intermittent or constant, include postprandial fullness, abdominal pain and cramps, nausea and vomiting, and failure to gain weight. Weight loss and a hyperextension body cast are among precipitating causes.

II. EXTRA-ABDOMINAL CAUSES

A. Right lower lobe pneumonia with diaphragmatic pleurisy may cause abdominal pain, vomiting and, perhaps, muscle guarding on the right, suggestive of appendicitis. A chest roentgenogram may be required for differentiation.
B. Heart
   1. Rheumatic fever. Diffuse or epigastric abdominal pain may be one of the initial symptoms. It may precede other manifestations or occur later. Fever, vomiting and leukocytosis may be present. Although abdominal tenderness and rigidity may be present, localizing findings may occur in the right lower quadrant so that differentiation from appendicitis is difficult or impossible.
   2. Pericarditis may be accompanied by epigastric complaints.
   3. Infants with congenital endocardial fibroelastosis may appear to have intermittent episodes of colicky abdominal pain.
C. Central nervous system, spinal cord and spine
   1. Abdominal epilepsy. Abdominal pain is a common aura of epileptic seizures. Unusually, paroxysmal episodes of abdominal pain may be ascribed to abnormal cerebral discharges. The abdominal pain is severe and colicky, sudden in onset and periumbilical or epigastric in location. Pain lasts only a few minutes and may be followed by postictal sleep. The occurrence of some clouding of consciousness, disorientation or confusion during the episode is an important diagnostic point. The electroencephalograph is abnormal. These patients may or may not have a history of convulsive seizures.

Babb, R. R., and Eckman, P. B.: Abdominal epilepsy. JAMA 222:65, 1972.

   2. Brain tumors and other intracranial lesions may rarely be accompanied by abdominal pain.
   3. Herpes zoster
   4. Tuberculous spondylitis
   5. Spinal cord tumors in the dorsolumbar region may cause recurrent abdominal pain.

Buck, E. D., and Bodensteiner, J.: Thoracic cord tumor appearing as recurrent abdominal pain. Am. J. Dis. Child. 135:574, 1981.

   6. Intervertebral discitis or vertebral collapse may cause abdominal pain radiating from under the ribs downward to the umbilicus or symphysis pubis.
D. Blood
   1. Abdominal pain may occur in patients with acute hemolytic anemia and during crises with chronic hemolytic anemia.
   2. The symptoms and signs of an abdominal crisis in patients with sickle cell anemia may simulate those of an acute surgical abdomen, acute hepatitis or cholecystitis with pain, jaundice, leukocytosis and elevation of liver enzymes. Usually the pain remains generalized. Splenic throm-

boses may be accompanied by pain in the left upper quadrant.

3. Abdominal pain may occur in patients with leukemia. A necrotizing typhlitis or inflàmmation of the cecum occurring as a complication during the treatment of acute leukemia may cause severe right lower quadrant abdominal pain and bloody diarrhea.

4. Abdominal pain in patients with anaphylactoid or Schönlein-Henoch purpura may occur either before or after the appearance of the purpura. The pain is often colicky and may be severe. Nausea, vomiting, hematemesis and melena may occur. Gastrointestinal hemorrhage in patients with other types of purpura may also cause abdominal pain.

Byrn, J. R., Fitzgerald, J. F., Northway, J. D., Anand, S. K., and Scott, J. R.: Unusual manifestations of Henoch-Schönlein syndrome. Am. J. Dis. Child. 130:1335, 1976.

5. Hemophilia may cause abdominal pain as a result of retroperitoneal hemorrhage.

6. Acute infectious lymphocytosis may be characterized by abdominal pain.

E. Metabolic

1. Lead poisoning may cause colicky abdominal pain and vomiting.

2. Hyperparathyroidism owing to a functioning parathyroid adenoma may be characterized by severe abdominal pain, nausea, vomiting, fever, azotemia, stupor and coma.

3. Addison's disease may be characterized by severe abdominal pain, vomiting and diarrhea.

4. Diabetic ketoacidosis may be accompanied by abdominal pain.

5. Hypoglycemia

6. Hyperlipoproteinemia may be characterized by attacks of colicky abdominal pain of one to four days duration along with abdominal tenderness, boardlike rigidity, anorexia, fever and, at times, physical collapse. Hepatosplenomegaly or lipemia retinalis may be present.

7. Acute intermittent porphyria may cause colicky abdominal pain.

8. Hereditary angioedema may be characterized by recurrent abdominal pain.

9. Familial paroxysmal polyserositis (Mediterranean fever) may be manifest as paroxysmal peritonitis with exquisite abdominal tenderness, muscle guarding, vomiting, fever

and leukocytosis. In some patients, paroxysmal pleuritis may occur independent of, precede or follow the abdominal episode.

F. Miscellaneous

1. Periarteritis nodosa. Abdominal pain, frequently in the right upper quadrant, may be a nonspecific symptom.

2. Arachnidism or black widow spider poisoning is characterized by severe abdominal pain and rigidity of the abdominal wall without localized tenderness.

3. Epidemic myalgia may be characterized by spasmodic abdominal pain, tenderness and muscle spasm.

4. Rheumatoid arthritis may cause abdominal pain, presumably owing to mesenteric adenitis or peritoneal inflammation.

5. Pain (stitch) in the upper or lower abdominal quadrants, usually on the right, or under the costal margins is frequently reported in older children and adolescents after running.

6. Mesenteric arteritis, a complication occurring three to six days following surgical correction of coarctation of the aorta, is characterized by hypertension, abdominal pain, tenderness, distention, vomiting, intestinal bleeding, fever and, if untreated, gangrene of the bowel.

III. PSYCHOGENIC ABDOMINAL PAIN

Psychogenic pain disorders are best approached developmentally through an understanding of the challenges and environmental stresses that a child is confronting at a given time. These are best determined in the pediatric interview, a process that allows both the collection of data and the development of a therapeutic relationship between the doctor and the child and family. The physician may open the interview with a statement such as: "In seeing many children with abdominal (or other) pain, I've found that it's sometimes due to physical causes, sometimes to stresses at this age and sometimes to both. But *pain is pain* no matter what the cause, so it's my practice to examine all possibilities thoroughly . . . physical . . . psychologic . . . whatever."

This preface precludes the possible conclusion on the part of the parents or child that the doctor, in a snap decision, has concluded that the pain is "in the child's head" or that the child is "making it up." It also conveys the message that psychosocial considerations are a legitimate part of the diagnostic process and recognizes that such possibilities are more easily accepted at the onset than after a fruitless work-up for organic disease. Ruling out an organic etiology *before* considering those of a psychological or developmental nature may be antidiagnostic and antitherapeutic.

As his most effective psychotherapeutic tool, the interview helps the physician understand the patient and the parents' past and current life situations, along with their feelings, beliefs, and anxieties. At the same time, the patient and his family sense the physician's expertise and interest. Sharing personal facts, feelings and problems with a physician often results in a dramatic lessening of anxiety and pain. In addition to illuminating linkages between the child's pain and the environmental or developmental stresses being experienced, the interview provides parents, who may be unaware of their child's feelings because of a preoccupation with their own difficulties, the opportunity to concentrate on their child, themselves and on their interactions in a clarifying fashion. The physician's personal warmth, empathy and capacity to understand how the patient feels helps him foster the child's identification with his knowledge of what is healthy.

The following kinds of personal, developmental or family stressors and problems are of interest in the interview:

A. Separation experiences that represent for the child a major life change and stressor.
　1. The death or the anticipated death of a significant person—a parent, sibling, grandparent, friend or pet.
　2. Divorce or anticipated divorce or desertion
　3. Social or vocational commitments that make the parents unavailable to the child. Such parents are little involved with their child psychologically and are frequently absent from the home.
　4. The fear of premature death in a child who has recovered from a critical illness or who has a long-term, life-threatening disease—the vulnerable child syndrome
　5. Lack of communication within the family
　6. Recent move of the family or a close friend
　7. Entrance to middle or junior high school
　8. The child placed outside his family
　9. Addition of a step-parent, other adult or adopted sibling to the family
　10. An older sibling's marriage, entrance to college or departure for military service
　11. Major change in parental career or lifestyle
　12. Social isolation of the family
B. Family illness
　1. Vulnerable parents or siblings
　　a. Medically vulnerable owing to a physical illness (e.g., cancer or myocardial infarction in a parent or a long-term handicapping condition such as mental retardation or myelodysplasia in a sibling). Each parent should be asked specifically about his or her own health, the kind of pain experienced in the past or currently and whether he is seeing a physician or taking medicine. The child should also be asked about complaints and illnesses in each of his parents, grandparents and siblings.
　　b. Parents or siblings may unrealistically and secretly be regarded by the child as vulnerable to a premature death owing to an accident or a sudden illness.
　2. Psychological symptoms and disorders in the family (e.g., anxiety, depression, alcoholism or psychosis). Helpful exploratory questions include: "Who's the nervous one in your family?" or "Who does the worrying around your house?"
　3. Parental hypochondriasis or preoccupation with illness
C. Marital discord is obviously a major stressor for children.
D. Lack of mutuality in parent-child interactions (e.g., over-expectation, over-restriction, unfavorable comparison with a sibling or the child's awareness that his parents are disappointed in him)
E. The child may be hesitant to show anger in the belief that such feelings are wrong. This is especially difficult for the child whose parent is chronically or seriously ill or whose family suppresses the direct expression of anger.
F. The child's inability to make and keep friends
G. The adolescent's concerns about sexuality
H. School and learning problems
I. Economic distress in the family
J. An "overachieving" child's fear of impending failure in academic or other competitive activity

The child or adolescent and the parents will often spontaneously disclose these factors if they are consciously aware of them.

Indeed, it is best for the child or parent to suggest the possibility of a psychogenic etiology themselves: "Could it be his nerves?" If they pose such a question, it is usually best not to make an immediate affirmative response but to be somewhat tentative: "Well, that's an interesting idea. . . . You may have something there. I'd like to hear more of your ideas about that. . . " Otherwise, the parents may believe they have been entrapped.

During the interview, it is useful to learn why the parents have come now when the pain has been present for some time, what the parents and child think is wrong, how the pain has affected the child in daily life and what the parents and child expect the doctor to do. The physician will also need to surmise what the symptom brings in secondary gain and whether the complaint is masking school avoidance. ("How much school has this pain caused Susie to miss?")

The motivations for a visit in the presence of a recurrent or persistent complaint include the following:

1. There is a life crisis in the family (e.g., divorce, serious illness, death or economic calamity).

2. Feelings of anxiety or depression in a parent or child have caused amplification of the symptom and magnification of the worry.

3. School attendance authorities have demanded a medical appraisal because of the child's frequent absences from school.

4. A question of a serious biomedical illness has been recurrently raised by relatives or friends, or the parent has encountered information that causes her to seek reassurance.

5. The parent or child with a need to feel cared for comes to the physician for support and nurture.

6. The family has reached the limit of its tolerance for the child's symptom.

A meticulous physical examination is important not only for the detection of abnormal findings but also for reassurance. Since parents and adolescents may talk more freely during or after the physical examination, significant historical information may be volunteered at that time. A thorough examination conveys the physician's interest in the patient and his complaint.

Laboratory or x-ray examinations should be limited to those necessary to clarify the diagnosis and not be ordered simply because the parent "expects" such tests or to "reassure" him. Needless procedures tend to reinforce psychogenic pain. If examinations mentioned by the parents are not to be done, the doctor should explain why.

REFERENCES

Barsky, A. J., and Klerman, G. L.: Overview: Hypochondriasis, bodily complaints, and somatic styles. Am. J. Psychiatry 140:3, 1983.

Farrell, M. K.: Abdominal pain. Pediatrics 74:955, 1984.

Green, M.: Psychogenic pain disorders. In Green, M., and Haggerty, R. J. (eds.): Ambulatory Pediatrics III. Philadelphia, W. B. Saunders Co., 1984.

Green, M., Friedman, S. B., Korsch, B. M., Richmond, J. B., and Simmons, J. E.: When somatic complaints mask psychosocial disorders. Contem. Pediatr. 2:20, 1985.

Greene, J. W., Walker, L. S., Hickson, G., and Thompson, J.: Stressful life events and somatic complaints in adolescents. Pediatrics 75:19, 1985.

ETIOLOGIC CLASSIFICATION OF ABDOMINAL AND PELVIC PAIN

I. INTRA-ABDOMINAL CAUSES, 243
   A. Gastrointestinal tract and mesentery, 243
      1. Colic
      2. Peptic ulcer
      3. Zollinger-Ellison syndrome
      4. Dietary indiscretion
      5. Appendicitis; typhlitis
      6. Intussusception
      7. Intestinal malrotation
      8. Volvulus
      9. Intra-abdominal hernia
      10. Meckel's diverticulitis
      11. Mesenteric cyst
      12. Duplication of the intestinal tract
      13. Intestinal polyp
      14. Incarcerated hernia
      15. Intestinal obstruction
      16. Constipation
      17. Sigmoid volvulus
      18. Parasites
      19. Bacterial enteritis
      20. Aerophagia
      21. Ulcerative colitis
      22. Crohn's disease
      23. Allergic response to food
      24. Lactose intolerance
      25. Cystic fibrosis
      26. Hereditary angioedema
      27. Retractile mesenteritis
   B. Urinary tract, 246
      1. Obstruction
      2. Systemic hemorrhagic disease

Table continued on opposite page

ETIOLOGIC CLASSIFICATION OF ABDOMINAL AND PELVIC PAIN *Continued*

3. Renal calculus
4. Hypercalciuria
5. Acute glomerulonephritis
C. Liver and gallbladder, 246
   1. Infectious hepatitis
   2. Cholecystitis
   3. Cholelithiasis
   4. Passive congestion of the liver
   5. Sickle cell crisis
   6. Choledochal cyst or cystic dilatation of the gallbladder
   7. Hydrops of the gallbladder
   8. Hepatic tumor
   9. Chiari's syndrome
D. Spleen, 247
   1. Traumatic rupture
   2. Splenomegaly
   3. Congestive splenomegaly
E. Pancreas, 247
   1. Acute pancreatitis
   2. Congenital fibrosis
   3. Pancreatic pseudocyst
F. Ovaries, uterus, 248
   1. Torsion of ovarian pedicle, cyst or tumor
   2. Hematocolpos
   3. Dysmenorrhea
   4. Pelvic inflammatory disease
   5. Endometriosis
   6. Ectopic pregnancy
G. Lymph nodes, 248
   1. Mesenteric lymphadenitis
   2. Iliac adenitis
   3. Lymphoma
   4. Tuberculosis
H. Primary streptococcal or pneumococcal peritonitis, 249
I. Mesenteric vein thrombosis, 249
J. Pelvic osteomyelitis, 249
K. Superior mesenteric artery syndrome, 249
II. Extra-abdominal Causes, 249
   A. Right lower lobe pneumonia with diaphragmatic pleurisy, 249

B. Heart, 249
   1. Rheumatic fever
   2. Pericarditis
   3. Congenital endocardial fibroelastosis
C. Central nervous system, spinal cord and spine, 249
   1. Abdominal epilepsy
   2. Brain tumors or other intracranial lesion
   3. Herpes zoster
   4. Tuberculous spondylitis
   5. Spinal cord tumor in the dorsolumbar region
   6. Discitis; collapse of vertebra
D. Blood, 249
   1. Acute hemolytic or chronic hemolytic anemia
   2. Sickle cell crisis
   3. Leukemia
   4. Anaphylactoid or Schönlein-Henoch purpura
   5. Hemophilia
   6. Acute infectious lymphocytosis
E. Metabolic, 250
   1. Lead poisoning
   2. Hyperparathyroidism
   3. Addison's disease
   4. Diabetic ketoacidosis
   5. Hypoglycemia
   6. Hyperlipoproteinemia
   7. Acute porphyria
   8. Hereditary angioedema
   9. Familial paroxysmal polyserositis
F. Miscellaneous, 250
   1. Periarteritis nodosa
   2. Arachnidism
   3. Epidemic myalgia
   4. Rheumatoid arthritis
   5. Abdominal stitch
   6. Mesenteric arteritis
III. Psychogenic Abdominal Pain, 250

26 / ANOREXIA, POLYPHAGIA, POLYDIPSIA AND PICA

I. Anorexia

A complete list of the causes of anorexia would include most of the pediatric disorders. Food intake diminishes during almost every acute or chronic illness, in the presence of anemia, with urea cycle disorders in newborn infants, in endocrine diseases such as hypothyroidism and Addison's disease, in infectious hepatitis and appendicitis, with endocardial fibroelastosis and in vitamin D poisoning, diabetes insipidus, infantile renal acidosis, idiopathic hypercalcemia and lead poisoning. Because anorexia is a symptom of electrolyte depletion or hypochloremic alkalosis in infants with cystic fibrosis, serum electrolyte determinations are indicated. Anorexia may be a side effect of stimulant drugs. Infections ranging in severity from the common cold to sepsis in infants are commonly accompanied by a loss of appetite. Patients with Crohn's disease commonly have anorexia, perhaps associated with fear of the discomfort precipitated by eating. This failure to eat and weight loss may simulate anorexia nervosa.

Laughlin, J. J., Brady, M. S., and Eigen, H.: Changing feeding trends as a cause of electrolyte depletion in infants with cystic fibrosis. Pediatrics 68:203, 1981.
Roy, S., III: The chloride depletion syndrome. Adv. Pediatr. 31:235, 1984.

The physiologic mechanisms involved in the regulation of food intake are incompletely understood. *Appetite* refers to a desire for certain foods. Although appetite must have a physiologic basis, it is also determined by cultural patterns and modified by psychologic factors. Anxiety, worry, fear and resentment cause a diminution in appetite.

Hunger is caused primarily by vigorous gastric peristaltic contractions when the stomach is empty. The frequency and intensity of these contractions vary among different persons. Non-nutritive as well as nutritive substances placed in the mouth or entering the stomach can cause cessation of peristalsis. Psychologic factors can stop peristalsis or mask the sensation of hunger.

Satiety is reached when the hunger-appetite mechanism has caused a certain amount of food to be ingested. The hypothalamus determines, to some extent, when satiety is reached, but conditioning also plays an important role.

Normally, hunger determines when a person eats, appetite what he eats and satiety how much he eats. Fortunately, well infants and children generally take food at the right time and in the correct amounts if it is offered in nurturing environments. Babies also accept solid foods and feed themselves when their neuromuscular progress permits them to do so. The physician may need to help parents understand and accept normal feeding patterns of infants and children.

DEVELOPMENTAL GUIDES TO FEEDING

Periodicity of Hunger. Babies have hunger contractions shortly after birth. Within a few days, a rhythmical pattern develops in most babies. Parents can generally tell when hunger occurs because the infant shows his discomfort, at first by restlessness, then by crying—the physiologic indications that a baby is ready to eat. Some breast-fed infants, however, do not cry even though they are receiving insufficient calories. Weight loss, in addition to problems in breast feeding, may provide the clue.

The frequency of hunger contractions is an individual matter. The interval may be three hours for one baby, four hours for another. The same infant may have a three-hour interval at one time of day and a five-hour period at another; but a similar pattern occurs on successive days, except in those infants with an irregular, unpredictable kind of temperament.

Aldrich and Hewitt studied the individual hunger rhythms in 100 infants permitted a self-regulatory feeding pattern during the first year of life. In the first month after birth, the majority of infants wanted to be fed at a three-hour interval. Ten per cent, however, chose a two-hour schedule. Only two babies had irregular hunger rhythms. Not until the third month did a predominant number of infants want a four-hour schedule. One third of the babies still preferred to be fed every three hours at that time.

It is recognized that some mothers are not able to interpret their infants' needs accurately; consequently, their infants do not do well on a flexible schedule. Such mothers are more comfortable when they can follow a definite feeding schedule, which the physician can suggest. In the majority of instances, however, the self-regulatory program meets the infant's needs and presents no problem to the mother.

Rooting Reflex. When an infant's cheek or the corner of his mouth is stimulated by contact with the breast or nipple, the infant automatically turns toward the stimulus, prepared to suck.

Sucking Reflex. The presence of the sucking reflex in term and in most prematures is the neuromotor indication for liquid feedings. Some infants suck vigorously through an entire meal; others may stop several times during a feeding.

Protrusion Reflex. As a result of this reflex, solid food placed in the anterior third of the mouth in young infants is reflexly pushed out by the tongue. This reflex does not interfere with nursing, since the nipple empties into the back of the mouth and throat. It may, however, make early feeding of solid foods difficult. The protrusion reflex normally disappears between the third and fifth months of life, most commonly in the fourth month.

Appetite Development. *Hunger* is the factor that chiefly controls food intake during early infancy. *Appetite*, which may be evident by three months of age, usually does not become important until the latter half of the first year, when family dietary patterns, maternal dislike of foods offered, or unpleasantness associated with the introduction of certain foods act as conditioning factors that impair appetite. By 12 months of age, the baby demonstrates definite preferences and dislikes. He takes time to look over the foods offered and selects those he likes. At eight months, he may have seemed too hungry to care at mealtimes.

Self-feeding. At approximately four months of age, the baby begins to acquire some control of and skill in the use of his hands. He recognizes his bottle and may reach for it. At five to six months, he can put his hands around the bottle and guide it to his lips. By approximately nine to ten months of age, a baby has the ability of prehension; shortly after this he learns to chew. He can then be encouraged to feed himself a cracker or a cookie. At nine months, an empty cup may be placed on his tray for practice. At ten months, he can begin practicing with a spoon. Because the neuromuscular control needed is not as great, he becomes proficient in the use of a cup before he is skilled in handling a spoon. Shortly after 12 months of age, he can use a cup well. He works with the spoon in earnest between 12 and 14 months but is not really skilled at it until about 18 months. Self-feeding between twelve and eighteen months is apt to be a mixture of spoon-feeding, hand-feeding and cup-glass-feeding. By 18 to 21 months, babies who have been permitted to do so usually feed themselves well.

Chewing. Chewing motions usually appear by about the eighth or ninth month and are the neuromuscular indication that lumpy foods can be introduced whether teeth are present or not. The baby may initially resist a change in the consistency of his food. If this is the case, the mother may wait a few days before making another attempt. Some infants, especially children who have been chronically ill or are emotionally upset or retarded, continue to refuse lumpy foods for some time.

Emotional Development and Feeding. In addition to being related to an infant's physiologic needs and neuromuscular progress, feeding is also closely entwined with emotional development. Feeding is often the first arena for a struggle between parent and child; therefore, new foods or techniques should be introduced gradually and temporarily stopped if resistance develops. If the emotional environment is favorable, problems in the feeding sphere are usually transient. If not, the feeding problem may persist. Food is made a point of struggle.

When physiologic and developmental guides to infant feeding are persistently ignored, owing to a lack of satisfactory parent-child interaction, psychogenic anorexia may develop. Force has been used in almost every case of psychogenic anorexia. The infant resists force by not eating. Gagging and vomiting may also occur.

The history may indicate that the baby may be forced to restrict his self-feeding attempts because they are messy and to be neat before he is able. The baby's food preference may be ignored, and he may be forced to accept foods that are "good for him" or to take additional food even though his hunger-appetite mechanism is functioning normally. Some older infants and young children with psychologic anorexia limit their intake to a certain few foods and refuse or are wary of anything else. This may also be a manifestation of anxiety in young children.

Infants who receive poor emotional nurturing have little appetite and often feed poorly, perhaps because they are uncomfortable in the feeding situation and unsatisfied most of the time.

Infants maintained on prolonged total parenteral hyperalimentation or on gastrostomy feedings may refuse oral feedings.

Geertsma, M. A., Hyams, J. S., Pelletier, J. M., and Reiter, S.: Feeding resistance after parenteral hyperalimentation. Am. J. Dis. Child. 139:255, 1985.

Excessive milk intake in infants may be the result of psychogenic anorexia. The baby clings to his early feeding pattern and refuses solid foods. The milk intake is increased to meet caloric needs, and, eventually, two or more quarts of milk may be taken a day. Because of the lack of iron in this diet and blood loss in the stools owing to sensitivity to cow milk, iron deficiency anemia results and further accentuates the anorexia.

Temporary anorexia may occur during teething. Most infants and children also eat less during hot weather.

"Physiologic anorexia" may occur in the second year of life, owing to the deceleration of growth that occurs at that time. However, this is not a universal pattern.

Psychogenic anorexia in the preschool and school-age child usually represents a continuation of the feeding difficulties present during infancy. By this time the problem is difficult to treat. Even with guidance, it may persist for weeks or months. The child may have a history of delayed self-feeding or chewing, chewing but not swallowing solid foods, gagging and choking, coaxing and cajoling, and family scenes centering on the child's refusal to eat. Anorexia may be used as a means of gaining attention, as a manifestation of autonomy or as a symptom of disturbed parent-child relations. Anorexia may be highly selective in these children. Fussiness about foods is often prominent. Milk may be taken from a cup but not a glass. A child may insist on hamburgers, soda pop and ice cream. He eats these with relish and refuses to touch other foods. The child may drink large volumes of milk to meet his nutritional and caloric needs, but refuse most solid foods.

Children with psychogenic anorexia are often thin, and their body measurements frequently fall in the lower percentiles. At times, however, a mother may complain that her child has anorexia and is underweight when he is actually well-nourished or obese. The family dietary pattern in these instances may tend toward an excessive intake of food.

In the school-aged child and the adolescent, poor appetite may be a manifestation of depression.

Anorexia nervosa is a serious eating disorder. Loss of 25 per cent or more of body weight may occur owing to self-restriction of caloric intake. Menstruation either ceases or does not begin. Anorexia nervosa is most frequent in preadolescent and adolescent girls, usually from middle class families. Boys are rarely affected. The refusal to eat or rigorous dieting may begin after a friend or relative expresses concern about the adolescent's weight. A relentless pursuit of thinness follows. Because of her distorted body image, the adolescent does not see herself as too thin, even after a large weight loss. Characteristically, she denies she has a problem, strongly resists gaining weight and may be very manipulative. To avoid gaining weight, she may hide food. The patient may cook for the family but not eat the meal. A history of strenuous exercise, secret dieting or laxative abuse may be elicited. At other times, binge eating is followed by self-induced vomiting, or the latter may occur without the former. Many of these adolescents are almost constantly physically active, seemingly without fatigue. They are very concerned with control, including the conscious anxiety that they will not be able to control their eating in the face of their morbid fear of becoming obese.

Anorexia nervosa is not a specific clinical entity but is associated with a number of personality characteristics, environmental situations and parental attitudes. The families are often overprotective and enmeshed. Problems other than anorexia are initially denied. Some patients are severely emotionally disturbed, others are depressed, while others are reacting to a disturbing environmental situation and family strife.

A significant number of adolescents who are seen because of decreased caloric intake and resultant weight loss do not have the major emotional difficulties characteristic of those with anorexia nervosa. These adolescents begin to diet, initially intending to lose only 10 to 15 pounds, because they judge themselves, often correctly, to be a bit overweight. Instead of stopping at the projected weight, however, they continue to restrict their caloric intake. These patients do not have a distorted body image and can be persuaded, without much resistance, to eat a normal diet.

Bruch, H.: Eating Disorders: Obesity, Anorexia Nervosa and the Person Within. New York, Basic Books, 1973.

Minuchin, S., Rosman, B. L., Baker, L., and Liebman, R.: Psychosomatic Families; Anorexia Nervosa in Context. Cambridge, Harvard University Press, 1978.

II. Pica

Pica, the eating of non-nutritious substances such as dirt, sand, grass, clay, plaster, paint, salt and coal occurs in young children, usually in the toddler and preschool age groups. The child with pica is at risk for lead poisoning, other poisoning or visceral larva migrans. Although the etiology of pica is not clearly established, a nonnurturing environment with insufficient maternal supervision and availability, frequent moves, inadequate play opportunities, poor nutritional practices and major emotional problems in the family appear to be contributory etiologic factors. These children have a higher than usual prevalence of such oral behavior as use of a pacifier, thumbsucking, use of the bottle and sucking various objects. Discipline problems and tantrums are frequent. Iron deficiency and pica are often present in the child. Ice eating (pagophagia) occurs in some children and adolescents with iron-deficiency anemia.

Zinkham, W. H.: Visceral larva migrans. Am. J. Dis. Child. 132:627, 1978.

III. Increased Appetite, Special Food Craving, Hyperphagia and Binge Eating

A. Lesions in the hypothalamus that may lead to obesity by producing an intense craving for food include encephalitis; craniopharyngiomas; gliomas of the optic chiasm; histiocytosis X; pituitary tumors; congenital defects of the hypothalamus such as the Laurence-Moon-Biedl syndrome; and trauma, especially basal skull fractures. Hydrocephalus, pinealomas and porencephaly may also lead to obesity.

B. Central nervous system leukemia is associated with sudden weight gain and a voracious appetite.

C. The Prader-Willi syndrome is characterized by mental retardation, neonatal hypotonia, small hands and feet, hypogenitalism, understature, compulsive hyperphagia and obesity.

Holm, V. A., and Pipes, P. L.: Food and children with Prader-Willi syndrome. Am. J. Dis. Child. 130:1063, 1976.

D. Overeating may occur in response to anxiety, depression and frustration.

E. Bulimia, a chronic eating disorder, is characterized by an episodic compulsion to binge-eat, usually high calorie foods such as ice cream, and a continuing fear of being unable to control one's food intake. Food binges may be followed by self-induced vomiting, perhaps several times a day. Because the vomiting and the binge eating characteristically are highly secretive, with the patient appearing to eat normally in social situations, bulimia may escape recognition for a long time. While patients with anorexia nervosa may be conspicuously underweight, those with bulimia usually are not. The adolescent with bulimia, often anxious and depressed, will readily admit to the physician that she has a problem, in contrast to the patient with anorexia nervosa.

F. Psychosocial dwarfism. A history of bizarre polyphagia and polydipsia is uniformly present. Patients eat "two or three times" as much as their siblings, feed from garbage cans and drink water from toilet bowls and other unusual sources.

G. Hyperthyroidism. Most patients with this disorder have an increased appetite.

H. Pheochromocytoma may cause an increased appetite.

I. Cystic fibrosis. Parents may report a voracious appetite in some infants.

J. Glycogen storage disease may be characterized by a large appetite.

K. The Kleine-Levin syndrome is characterized by recurrent periods of excessive sleep and food gorging.

Stricker, E. M.: Hyperphagia. N. Engl. J. Med. 298:1010, 1978.

L. The premenstrual syndrome may be characterized by changes in appetite and craving for special foods.

IV. POLYDIPSIA

A. Diabetes insipidus, both central and nephrogenic

B. Diabetes mellitus

C. Psychogenic water drinking (primary polydipsia) occurs in young children as a result of a disturbed maternal-child relationship. The child asks for liquids almost constantly. Usually, the child has no history of dehydration, fever or growth failure. Laboratory examination reveals a normal serum sodium and osmolality and ability to concentrate urine. Rarely, psychogenic water drinking may accompany diabetes insipidus. Complications of severe psychogenic polydipsia include hyponatremia, convulsions, failure to thrive and hydronephrosis.

Adelman, R. D., Shapiro, S. R., and Woerner, S.: Psychogenic polydipsia with hydronephrosis in an infant. Pediatrics 65:344, 1980.
Linshaw, M. A., Hipp, T., and Gruskin, A.: Infantile psychogenic water drinking. J. Pediatr. 85:520, 1974.

D. Malformations of the urinary tract

E. Hypokalemia

F. Hypercalcemia

G. Sickle cell anemia

H. Renal tubular acidosis in older children; the de Toni-Fanconi syndrome

27 / RECTAL BLEEDING

Melena refers to the passage of black tarry stools owing to intestinal bleeding, presumably above the ileocecal valve. *Hematochezia* refers to the passage of brick red or red-brown colored blood from the distal small bowel or proximal colon. Occasionally, because of a rapid transit time, hematochezia occurs following a large hemorrhage from the upper gastrointestinal tract. Bleeding from the anorectum appears as bright red blood on the outside of the stool, on the toilet paper or in the toilet bowl water. The presence of blood may be documented by the stool guaiac test. With confirmed rectal bleeding, sigmoidoscopy, barium enema and angiography may be selectively indicated, in addition to the usual physical, rectal and laboratory examinations. The passage of a nasogastric tube to determine the presence or absence of blood in the stomach may help localize the bleeding site. Blood present in the gastric aspirate may arise from gastritis, esophageal varices, hiatus hernia or a gastric ulcer. If no blood is aspirated from the stomach, the site of hemorrhage is likely to be distal to the ligament of Treitz. Tarry stools may be simulated by bismuth subsalicylate preparations, iron medication, chocolate, grape juice and other foods. Red-colored stools may result from food-coloring or beets.

Flexible fiberoptic endoscopy is helpful in the diagnosis of esophagitis, varices, gastritis, gastric ulcers, polyps, ulcerative colitis, granulomatous colitis and other gastrointestinal lesions. Selective angiography of the mesenteric vessels may be diagnostically helpful in the following instances: with severe gastrointestinal hemorrhage; as an important first procedure in localizing the site of intestinal hemorrhage caused by a stress ulcer; in identifying a Meckel's diverticulum; in determining the cause of hemobilia. If this study is inconclusive, barium studies can then be conducted. Mesenteric angiography may also be indicated with a history of recurrent gastrointestinal bleeding or chronic blood loss unexplained by previous barium studies. An air contrast barium enema may be helpful in the diagnosis of polyps.

In some instances, the cause of rectal bleeding, even when massive, remains un-determined even after extensive investigation, especially in the newborn infant. Laparotomy is rarely of either diagnostic or therapeutic help. Although much blood may have been lost, bleeding stops spontaneously in most infants.

ETIOLOGIC CLASSIFICATION OF RECTAL BLEEDING

I. Swallowing of over 30 ml of Maternal Blood may result in grossly bloody stools during the first day of life. The Apt test may be used to ascertain whether or not the blood is of maternal or infant origin.

One part of stool is mixed with five to ten parts water. The stool must be red and grossly bloody, since in a tarry stool the oxyhemoglobin has already been changed to hematin. There must be a pink supernatant solution; otherwise, the subsequent color change will not be seen. This mixture is then centrifuged at 2000 rpm for 1 to 2 minutes, and the pink hemoglobin solution is decanted off. One part of 0.25 normal sodium hydroxide solution is then mixed with five parts of the hemoglobin solution. In the presence of adult hemoglobin, the solution will change to a yellow-brown color within 2 minutes; in the presence of fetal hemoglobin, which is alkali-resistant, the solution remains pink.

II. Volvulus in the Newborn, usually associated with malrotation of the bowel, may be characterized by vomiting, abdominal distention, an abdominal mass and bloody stools. In the newborn infant, this clinical presentation suggests a volvulus more than an intussusception.

III. Rectal Bleeding, along with loose stools and mucus, may occur in young infants allergic to cow's milk or soy protein. The blood, which is bright red, may be copious in amount or mixed in with the stool as tiny clots. Colicky abdominal pain is another prominent manifestation.

IV. Necrotizing Enterocolitis in the newborn is often characterized by the passage of gross blood, bloody mucus or He-matest-positive stools, in addition to other symptoms. Enterocolitis may complicate Hirschsprung's disease.

V. Melena is often a clinical manifestation in hemorrhagic disease of the newborn. Other congenital or acquired deficiencies of coagulation factors or platelets are less common causes of gastrointestinal hemorrhage.

VI. A "Red Diaper Syndrome," in which red pigmentation of soiled diapers occurs after storage in the diaper receptacle for 24 to 36 hours is caused by *Serratia marcescens* in the stools.

VII. Intussusception. While the passage of blood mixed with feces or a small amount of mucus (red currant jelly stool) occurs in the first 24 hours of this disease in about half of patients, rectal bleeding is not essential for early diagnosis. Chronic recurrent sigmoid intussusception, reported in children with chronic constipation, is characterized by small amounts of bright red blood in the stools.

VIII. Intestinal Gangrene, which may be secondary to volvulus or another lesion that compromises the blood supply, may cause massive gastrointestinal hemorrhage in infants. Clinical findings may include pain, abdominal distention, vomiting and shock. Barium examinations are contraindicated. Preoperative mesenteric arteriography may be helpful.

IX. Anal Fissure is the most common cause of blood on the stools in infants and young children.

X. Rectal Prolapse may cause blood on the stools.

XI. Chronic Occult Gastrointestinal Blood Loss may be caused by whole cow's milk, with resultant iron deficiency anemia in infants under 18 months of age.

XII. Meckel's Diverticulum is often characterized by the sudden, massive and painless passage of blood, either melena or hematochezia, in infants and young children. In the latter event, the blood may be brick or bright red with maroon-colored clots. A technetium scan may help localize the bleeding site.

XIII. Duplication of the Bowel

XIV. Hemolytic-uremic Syndrome

XV. Peptic Ulcer Disease. Stress ulcers in the stomach or duodenum owing to a central nervous system disorder, burn or anoxia may cause marked blood loss.

XVI. The Zollinger-Ellison Syndrome may cause gastrointestinal hemorrhage.

XVII. Esophageal Varices secondary to portal hypertension can be visualized on endoscopy or, at times, with careful x-ray examination. The cause of portal hypertension may be demonstrated by mesenteric arteriography or preoperative percutaneous splenoportography.

XVIII. Infectious Gastroenteritis. Bacillary or shigella dysentery may cause a bloody mucoid stool or hematochezia without diarrhea. Other bacterial infectious agents that cause the passage of gross blood or bloody diarrhea include *Salmonella*, *Campylobacter*, *Yersinia* and *Clostridium difficile* toxin.

XIX. Amebic Dysentery may cause a bloody, mucoid rectal discharge. Hookworm and whipworm disease (trichuriasis) and other intestinal parasites may cause blood in the stools.

Merritt, R. J., Coughlin, E., Thomas, D. W., Jariwaca, L., Swanson, V., and Sinatra, F. R.: Spectrum of amebiasis in children. Am. J. Dis. Child. 136:785, 1982.

XX. Hematochezia in Children is frequently caused by intestinal polyps in the colon or rectum. Instead of a copious passage of blood, intermittent and recurrent spotting, blood-stained mucus or streaks of bright red blood in the stool are reported. An air contrast study of the colon may be diagnostic. Sigmoidoscopy is always indicated. Most polyps are of the juvenile retention type. A few represent familial adenomatous polyposis of the colon, Gardner's syndrome, generalized juvenile gastrointestinal polyposis or Peutz-Jeghers syndrome. Lymphoid polyps or focal lymphoid hyperplasia of the colon may present with rectal bleeding or prolapse of the polyp.

Sachatello, C. R., Pickren, J. W., and Grace, J. T., Jr.: Generalized juvenile gastrointestinal polyposis. Gastroenterology 58:699, 1970.

XXI. Ulcerative Colitis and Crohn's Disease may be characterized at their onset by rectal bleeding without diarrhea, especially when the diseases are limited to the recto-sigmoid. Blood may be mixed with pus and mucus.

XXII. FOREIGN BODIES AND TRAUMA may cause rectal bleeding.

XXIII. HEMANGIOMA involving the bowel wall

XXIV. GASTROINTESTINAL NEUROFIBROMA-TOSIS may cause chronic blood loss.

XXV. MALIGNANCIES involving the bowel wall

XXVI. HENOCH-SCHÖNLEIN PURPURA

XXVII. TRAUMATIC HEMATOBILIA, in which bleeding occurs into the biliary tract after blunt or penetrating abdominal trauma, is characterized by colicky right upper quad-rant abdominal pain, at times radiating to the shoulder, followed by hematemesis with relief of pain. A right upper quadrant mass

and obstructive jaundice may occur. Gas-trointestinal hemorrhage may occur within hours or may be postponed for weeks or months. Abdominal angiography permits preoperative diagnosis by demonstration of a traumatic aneurysm of the hepatic artery.

Hawes, D. R., Franken, E. A., Jr., Fitzgerald, J. F., and Battersby, J. S.: Traumatic hematobilia. Angiographic diagnosis. Am. J. Dis. Child. 125:130, 1973.

XXVIII. MULTIPLE INTESTINAL TELANGIEC-TASIS associated with recurrent melena has been reported in a few patients with Turner's syndrome.

GENERAL REFERENCES

Collins, R. E. C.: Some problems of gastrointestinal bleeding in children. Arch. Dis. Child. 46:110, 1971.
Franken, E. A., Jr.: Gastrointestinal bleeding in infants and children. Radiologic investigation. JAMA 229:1339, 1974.
Hyams, J. S., Leichtner, A. M., and Schwartz, A. N.: Recent advances in diagnosis and treatment of gastrointestinal hemorrhage in infants and children. J. Pediatr. 106:1, 1985.

ETIOLOGIC CLASSIFICATION OF RECTAL BLEEDING

28 / JAUNDICE

CLINICAL CONSIDERATIONS

Jaundice refers to a yellowish discoloration of the sclera, mucous membranes and skin owing to an excess of bilirubin in the blood. Tears, nasal secretions, saliva and cerebrospinal fluid may also be stained. The level of serum bilirubin at which clinical jaundice appears varies in different age groups. Jaundice is evident in most newborn infants with a serum bilirubin concentration of 5 to 7 mg/dl; in older persons, jaundice appears when the serum bilirubin level reaches about 2 mg/dl.

Strong natural light is optimal for the clinical detection of jaundice; minimal jaundice may be missed in a darkened room. If artificial illumination is used, only white fluorescent light permits early detection. Jaundice usually is evident in the sclerae or in the mucous membrane of the hard palate before it is visible in the skin; indeed, these may be the only sites in which jaundice can be detected in darkly pigmented patients. Because the clinical detection of jaundice in newborn infants is unreliable, measurements of serum bilirubin levels are indicated when hyperbilirubinemia is suspected.

In jaundice of long-duration, the tissues are apt to have a greenish appearance owing to the oxidation of bilirubin to biliverdin. Pruritus rarely accompanies jaundice in children but may be a significant problem with obstructive jaundice. Carotenemia, a common cause of pigmentation in infants and the result of a large intake of carotene-containing foods, is to be differentiated from jaundice. The yellow skin discoloration with carotenemia does not involve the sclerae and is most evident in the nasolabial folds and on the palms and soles.

BILE PIGMENT METABOLISM

The initial steps in the transformation of hemoglobin to bilirubin occur in the reticuloendothelial cells of the bone marrow, spleen and liver. The first step is the formation of water-insoluble free bilirubin. Bilirubin at this stage is transported in the plasma attached to protein, chiefly albumin. Bilirubin can be displaced from this albumin binding by several drugs (sulfonamides, aspirin, salicylate, oxacillin, cephalothin), metabolic states (hypoxia, acidosis, hypoglycemia, hypothermia, hypoproteinemia) or a high concentration of free fatty acids (secondary to administration of soy bean fat emulsions such as Intralipid). The liver normally conjugates free bilirubin to form water-soluble bilirubin glucuronide, which is excreted in the bile. Unconjugated and conjugated bilirubin are roughly synonymous with indirect- and direct-reacting bilirubin, respectively. The conversion of bilirubin to water-soluble glucuronide apparently occurs in the hepatic parenchymal cells. Glucuronyl transferase, the enzyme that catalyzes this reaction, is relatively deficient in newborn infants, especially premature ones, and in patients with familial nonhemolytic jaundice (Crigler-Najjar syndrome). This deficiency leads to an elevated serum level of unconjugated bilirubin.

Bilirubin is excreted into the bile capillaries and the intestinal tract as a sodium salt. Under abnormal circumstances, sodium bilirubinate may regurgitate into the blood stream, where it probably circulates as a readily dissociable complex with albumin. This compound readily passes through the glomerulus. In the newborn infant, some of the conjugated bilirubin is converted to its unconjugated form, reabsorbed into the enterohepatic circulation and presented to the liver for reprocessing.

In older infants and children, as a result of bacterial action in the intestine, sodium bilirubinate is first reduced to two colorless substances, mesobilirubinogen and stercobilinogen, which are collectively designated as urobilinogen. Urobilinogen is then rapidly oxidized to two orange-yellow pigments designated as urobilin.

The stools of young infants are often green during episodes of diarrhea and in some normal breast-fed infants. These changes are apparently attributable to the direct oxidation of bilirubin to green biliverdin instead of the usual bacterial reduction to urobilinogen.

THE HEPATIC LOBULE

As blood traverses the sinusoids to the central vein, unconjugated or partially conjugated bilirubin and urobilinogen are removed by either the parenchymal or Kupffer cells. The ampulla and primary bile canaliculus, through which bile enters the biliary system, are particularly vulnerable structures that may become obstructed by surrounding edema, or increased connective tissue in liver disease or by inspissated bile.

Lymph vessels play an important role in regurgitation jaundice, and at least a part of the regurgitated bilirubin reaches the systemic circulation through these channels.

PHYSIOLOGIC CLASSIFICATION OF JAUNDICE

Two types of jaundice, retention and regurgitation, can be distinguished. Retention jaundice results from failure of the liver cells to convert bilirubin to bilirubin glucuronide at a rate that prevents accumulation of the unconjugated pigment in the blood. Bile is not present in the urine. Regurgitation jaundice results from the return of bilirubin to the blood stream after its conversion to bilirubin glucuronide. Bile is present in the urine.

Retention jaundice may occur in the presence of excessive hemolysis or pigment production or both, impaired liver uptake or defective conjugation. Complete or partial intrahepatic biliary obstruction may appear during the course of a severe hemolytic anemia, especially in infants. When intrahepatic obstruction occurs, the findings of regurgitation jaundice are added to those of retention jaundice.

Regurgitation jaundice may occur secondary to necrosis of liver cells or obstruction of the bile ducts.

Schmid, R.: Bilirubin metabolism in man. N. Engl. J. Med. 287:703, 1972.

ETIOLOGIC CLASSIFICATION OF JAUNDICE

I. RETENTION JAUNDICE

A. Hemolytic. Not all patients with hemolytic anemia become jaundiced; nevertheless, excessive hemolysis is a frequent cause.
   1. The appearance of jaundice in the first 24 to 48 hours of life or intense icterus at any time in the early neonatal period raises the possibility of hemolytic disease of the newborn owing to maternal-infant blood group incompatibility. The possibility of Rh sensitization is determined by examination of maternal blood for antibodies during the thirty-fourth week of gestation. Detection of antibodies at this time indicates that hemolytic disease may occur in the newborn infant. The diagnosis of ABO incompatibility cannot be made prenatally. Early diagnosis depends upon prompt detection of jaundice in the nursery. Blanching of the skin on the forehead by finger pressure helps make the icterus evident. Jaundice is noted first on the face, then on the chest and abdomen, and finally on the extremities.

Jaundice is not present at birth. Infants with ABO incompatibility usually are not clinically ill or pale. Rh-sensitized infants with active hemolysis at birth may demonstrate hepatomegaly, splenomegaly, pallor, petechiae and edema.

Laboratory examinations indicated in infants of Rh-sensitized mothers include serum bilirubin, hemoglobin and Rh type. If the infant is Rh-positive and the mother's serum has anti-Rh antibodies, the diagnosis of erythroblastosis is established. The direct Coombs' test, almost always positive in infants with Rh sensitization, is a further confirmatory finding. A negative Coombs' test does not exclude this possibility. The serum bilirubin should be followed at 6- to 12-hour intervals.

ABO incompatibility occurs in firstborn infants about as often as in those later-born. The criteria for a presumptive diagnosis of ABO hemolytic disease are jaundice in the first 24 hours of life, serum bilirubin values of 10 mg/dl or higher in the first 24 hours of life and a maternal-infant ABO blood group incompatibility in the presence of a negative Coombs' test. The hemoglobin may not be significantly reduced. Other procedures, such as examination of the infant's serum for incompatible anti-A or anti-B antibodies, may be performed, but these are not essential for the decision as to therapy. The maternal serum may be examined for blood group antibodies other than anti-A or anti-B. Spherocytosis and reticulocytosis are often severe in infants with ABO incompatibility.

Hemolytic disease of the newborn may be caused by other blood group incompatibilities (e.g., Kell, MNS, Kidd, and Duffy).

In severely affected infants, the stools may become acholic, and bile may appear in the urine between the sixth and twelfth days of life as a result of intrahepatic obstruction. In infants treated with exchange transfusions, jaundice rarely persists past the first week of life and never past the tenth day. Jaundice of longer duration with elevation of both direct and indirect bilirubin has been termed the inspissated bile syndrome. The cause is unknown. In infants treated with exchange transfusion, the peak level of serum bilirubin is usually reached on the second day of life.

Desjardins, L., Chintu, C., and Zipursky, A.: The spectrum of ABO hemolytic disease of the newborn infant. J. Pediatr 95:447, 1979.
Naiman, J. L.: Current management of hemolytic disease of the newborn infant. J. Pediatr. 80:1049, 1972.

2. Erythrocyte membrane abnormalities (see page 427).
3. Erythrocyte enzyme deficiencies (see page 429).
4. Alpha-thalassemia
5. Sickle cell anemia may cause acute hepatic sludging characterized by jaundice and mild right upper quadrant pain. The serum bilirubin may exceed 20 mg/dl with one half of this value unconjugated bilirubin. Symptomatic resolution usually occurs within one week.
6. The administration of large doses (10 mg or more) of water-soluble analogues of vitamin K to newborn infants, especially prematures, may cause a marked drop in the reduced glutathione content of red cells, hemolytic anemia, hyperbilirubinemia and kernicterus.
7. Oxytocin given to induce labor may contribute to hyperbilirubinemia through increased destruction of erythrocytes.

B. Nonhemolytic
1. Physiologic jaundice of the newborn owing to hepatic immaturity appears commonly in newborn infants between the second and fifth days of life. Jaundice in the first 24 hours of life in the term infant or the first 48 hours in the premature is not to be considered physiologic. Physiologic jaundice usually disappears by the fifth to eighth day, except in the premature, in whom it may persist into the second week of life. Jaundice may also persist in infants of diabetic mothers. Physiologic jaundice is of greater intensity and duration in premature than in full-term infants.

The peak of the bilirubin rise usually occurs on the third to fourth day in full-term infants and on the fourth to sixth days in prematures. The serum bilirubin level in full-term infants with physiologic jaundice generally is less than 7 mg/dl and rarely exceeds 10 mg/dl. Values over 12 mg/dl in term infants are to be regarded as pathologic. The level of direct-reacting bilirubin should not be more than 1.5 mg/dl. The total serum bilirubin level should not increase more than 5 mg/dl/day. Bilirubin values in premature infants may rise as high as 15 to 20 mg/dl or may exceed 20 mg/dl at the peak, even in the absence of maternal-infant blood group incompatibility. The upper limit of normal for serum bilirubin in premature infants is not known. Levels above 15 mg/dl probably represent an indication for investigation.

The rate of destruction of red blood cells in the first ten days of life is three times greater than in the adult. Jaundice would not occur, however, even with this degree of pigment production if hepatic function were mature. Physiologic jaundice is thought to be attributable, in part, to a deficiency of glucuronyl transferase. The resultant limitation of hepatic excretion of bilirubin leads to an accumulation of the indirect fraction in the blood. The premature infant can excrete bilirubin at the rate of only 1 or 2 per cent of the normal adult capacity. Maturation of the glucuronide conjugating system during the first days of life is thought to lead to disappearance of the jaundice, with the variable rate of maturation accounting for the intensity and duration of this symptom. The enterohepatic circulation of bilirubin from the newborn intestinal tract back to the liver may contribute to physiologic jaundice of the newborn. Hypoxia, hyaline membrane disease, hypoglycemia, acidosis, hypothermia and hypoproteinemia may be associated with hyperbilirubinemia and predispose to kernicterus at lower bilirubin levels.

Gollan, J. L., and Knapp, A. B.: Bilirubin metabolism and congenital jaundice. Hosp. Practice. 20:83, 1985.

Kivlahan, C., and James, E. J. P.: The natural history of neonatal jaundice. Pediatrics 74:364, 1984.

Maisels, M. J.: Jaundice in the newborn. Pediatr. Rev. 3:305, 1982.

McDonagh, A. F., and Lightner, D. A.: 'Like a shrivelled blood orange'—bilirubin, jaundice, and phototherapy. Pediatrics 75:443, 1985.

Odell, G. B.: Neonatal hyperbilirubinemia. New York, Grune and Stratton, 1980.

Poland, R. L., and Odell, G. B.: Physiologic jaundice: The enterohepatic circulation of bilirubin. N. Engl. J. Med. 284:1, 1971.

2. Unconjugated "physiologic" hyperbilirubinemia may persist for weeks in congenital hypothyroidism owing to delayed maturation of hepatic glucuronyl transferase.

3. Drugs such as novobiocin, chloramphenicol, and vitamin K analogues decrease conjugation because of competition for glucuronyl transferase.

4. Neonatal jaundice associated with breast feeding may appear between the sixth and eighth days of life. The serum unconjugated bilirubin may reach 15 to 25 mg/dl in the second and third weeks of life. Suspension of breast feeding for 24 to 48 hours results in a prompt decline of 2 to 4 mg/dl in the serum indirect bilirubin. The jaundice persists for several weeks but eventually subsides, even though breast feeding is continued.

Poland, R. L.: Breast milk jaundice. J. Pediatr. 99:86, 1981.

5. The Lucey-Driscoll syndrome (transient familial hyperbilirubinemia), owing to a potent inhibitor of bilirubin glucuronyl transferase in maternal and infant serum, is characterized by transient, severe unconjugated hyperbilirubinemia.

6. Hereditary hepatic dysfunction (congenital familial nonhemolytic jaundice; the Crigler-Najjar syndrome) is a congenital, familial, nonhemolytic type of jaundice that may be characterized, in part, by kernicterus. The infant is persistently jaundiced from a few days after birth. The patient is unable to conjugate bilirubin because of a congenital absence (type I) or partial deficiency (type II) of the glucuronyl transferase system. The indirect serum bilirubin level in type I is constantly elevated, commonly over 20 mg/dl. Rigidity, athetosis and an expressionless facies may appear between two weeks and three months of age. Some patients do not develop kernicterus, and neurologic findings may not appear for many years. The type II Crigler-Najjar syndrome is characterized by an unconjugated serum bilirubin concentration that ranges from normal to 22 mg/dl. Kernicterus is unusual in this form of the disorder.

7. Gilbert's syndrome (constitutional hepatic dysfunction) is characterized by a persistent slight elevation (under 6 mg/dl, but, at times, as high as 12 mg/dl) of the unconjugated bilirubin level in patients with otherwise normal liver function tests and absence of overt hemolysis. Jaundice is infrequently present.

Berk, P. B., Bloomer, J. R., Howe, R. B., and Berlin, N. I.: Constitutional hepatic dysfunction (Gilbert's syndrome). Am. J. Med. 49:296, 1970.

8. Hepatocellular disease (See discussion under regurgitation jaundice.)

9. Maternal-fetal or fetal-fetal transfusion

10. Hyperviscosity syndrome of the newborn

11. Massive internal hemorrhage (cephalohematoma, subdural hematoma, subcapsular liver hemorrhage) may rarely cause jaundice in the newborn.

12. Pyloric stenosis, duodenal atresia or annular pancreas may be associated with unconjugated hyperbilirubinemia, perhaps owing to increased enterohepatic circulation of bilirubin.

13. The use of excessive concentrations of a phenolic disinfectant detergent may cause neonatal hyperbilirubinemia.

Wysowski, D. K., Flynt, J. W., Jr., Goldfield, M., Altman, R., and Davis, A. T.: Epidemic neonatal hyperbilirubinemia and use of a phenolic disinfectant detergent. Pediatrics 61:165, 1978.

II. REGURGITATION JAUNDICE

A. Hepatocellular
   1. Viral
      a. Infectious hepatitis (hepatitis A) has been reported in premature infants in newborn intensive care units, probably as a result of blood transfusions. The infection in these infants is usually asympto-

matic. In older children, prodromal symptoms include anorexia, fatigue, headache, nausea, vomiting, fever, hepatomegaly and right upper quadrant pain. The range of severity includes hepatitis without jaundice, mild hepatitis with jaundice followed by recovery in six to eight weeks; fatal hepatitis simulating acute or subacute yellow atrophy; and chronic hepatitis. During the preicteric phase, urine urobilinogen, serum bilirubin and serum transaminase are the most helpful tests in establishing the presence of hepatocellular disease. During the icteric phase, severe hepatocellular damage is reflected by a decrease in the serum albumin and a rise in the serum bilirubin.

Fitzgerald, J. F., Angelides, A., and Wyllie, R.: The hepatitis spectrum. Curr. Probl. Pediatr. 11:3 1981.
Noble, R. C., Kane, M. A., Reeves, S. A., and Roeckel, I.: Posttransfusion hepatitis A in a neonatal intensive care unit. JAMA 252:2711, 1984.

b. Hepatitis B (HBV) is transmitted through the infusion of blood contaminated with the virus. Neonatal hepatitis may occur in some infants whose mothers develop hepatitis B late in pregnancy or are chronic HB$_s$Ag-positive carriers. The Gianotti-Crosti syndrome or papular acrodermatitis of childhood is associated with hepatitis B virus, and most of the patients become HB$_s$Ag carriers. Mild hepatomegaly, elevated liver enzyme levels and, occasionally, cholestatic jaundice occur.

Krugman, S., Overby, L. R., Mushahwar, I. K., Ling, C-M., Frosner, G. G., and Dienhardt, F.: Viral hepatitis, type B. Studies on natural history and prevention re-examined. N. Engl. J. Med. 300:101, 1979.
Sinatra, F. R., Shah, P., Weissman, J. Y., Thomas, D. W., Merritt, R. J., and Tong, M. J.: Perinatal transmitted acute icteric hepatitis B in infants born to hepatitis B surface antigen-positive and anti-hepatitis B positive carrier mothers. Pediatrics 70:557, 1982.

c. Non-A, non-B or type C hepatitis may cause hepatitis and cholestasis in infants one to two months of age.
d. Chronic active (aggressive) hepatitis occurs predominantly in girls above ten years of age. The onset may be abrupt, resembling acute infectious hepatitis, but it is more commonly insidious with progressive jaundice, anorexia, fatigue, abdominal pain, arthralgia, fever and epistaxis. Spider nevi may be present early. Episodes of jaundice, fatigue, pleural pain and colitis may be recurrent. Endocrine changes include acne, amenorrhea and hirsutism. Striae, giant hives, erythema multiforme, and splenomegaly are additional findings. The serum bilirubin is usually 5 to 10 mg/dl. The SGOT usually does not exceed 500 units. Hyperglobulinemia is also present.

Arasu, T. S., Wyllie, R., Hatch, T. F., and Fitzgerald, J. F.: Management of chronic aggressive hepatitis in children and adolescents. J. Pediatr. 95:514, 1979.

e. Infectious mononucleosis caused by the Epstein-Barr virus or cytomegalovirus. Hepatocellular damage indistinguishable from that of infectious hepatitis occurs in 10 to 15 per cent of patients with infectious mononucleosis. Differentiation is made on the basis of the peripheral blood smear, the heterophile agglutination test and EB and CMV titers.
f. Cytomegalovirus may cause hepatitis, pneumonitis, nephrosis, enteritis or meningoencephalitis in young infants. The clinical manifestations of jaundice in the first 24 hours of life, hepatosplenomegaly, petechiae and erythroblastemia may require differentiation from erythroblastosis fetalis, sepsis and neonatal hepatitis.
g. Congenital rubella is characterized by conjugated hyperbilirubinemia immediately after birth or during the first few days of life. Other findings may include thrombocytopenic purpura, failure to thrive, cataracts, microcephaly, deafness and congenital heart disease.
h. Herpes simplex may cause hepatitis in infants.
2. Spirochetal
a. Congenital syphilis: syphilitic hepatitis and late-developing syphilitic cirrhosis
b. Canicola fever (*Leptospira canicola*); Weil's disease (*Leptospira icterohaemorrhagiae*). Jaundice occurs in about 50 per cent of pa-

tients with Weil's disease and in 15 per cent of those with other forms of leptospirosis.

3. Bacterial. Severe or overwhelming infection with *Escherichia coli, Staphylococcus,* Group B streptococcus or *Listeria monocytogenes* is frequently accompanied by cholestatic jaundice in newborn infants. Salmonellosis may produce hepatitis in infants. Brucellosis may cause a mild hepatitis in older children. A severe urinary tract infection caused by gram-negative bacteria such as *E. coli* or *Proteus* or a severe pneumococcal infection may cause toxic cholestasis in young infants.

Navey, Y., and Friedman, A.: Urinary tract infection presenting with jaundice. Pediatrics 62:524, 1978.
Rooney, J. C., Hill, D. J., and Danks, D. M.: Jaundice associated with bacterial infection in the newborn. Am. J. Dis. Child. 122:39, 1971.

4. Protozoan
   a. Congenital toxoplasmosis may cause neonatal jaundice, hyperpyrexia, hepatosplenomegaly and purpura.
   b. Amebiasis may rarely produce jaundice as the result of a large solitary liver abscess or a diffuse amebic hepatitis.
5. Acute chemical poisoning may cause acute yellow atrophy; chronic intoxication may produce cirrhosis.
   a. Chloroform
   b. Carbon tetrachloride
   c. Arsenicals
   d. Gold
   e. Phosphorus
   f. Nitrobenzene and its derivatives
   g. Almost any drug may cause hepatocellular damage.
6. Mushroom poisoning
7. Cirrhosis
   a. Congenital syphilis
   b. Laennec's cirrhosis leads to anorexia, weight loss, nausea, vomiting, abdominal pain, enlargement of the abdomen, edema of the lower extremities, hematemesis, other hemorrhagic tendencies and jaundice. Acholic stools may appear in some patients. Symptoms are often insidious and may predate jaundice by some time.
   c. Indian childhood cirrhosis

Lefkowitch, J. H., Honig, C. L., King, M. E., and Hagstrom, J. W. C.: Hepatic copper overload of the Indian childhood cirrhosis in an American sibship. N. Engl. J. Med. 307:271, 1982.

8. Inborn errors of metabolism
   a. Wilson's disease may first present as hepatic disease without neurologic or ophthalmologic findings. Symptoms usually do not appear before six years of age, but younger children may be affected. Patients with chronic active hepatitis, fulminant hepatitis, portal hypertension or cirrhosis should have a serum ceruloplasmin determination and a slit lamp examination for Kayser-Fleischer rings. Fulminant hepatitis may suddenly occur with jaundice, ascites, hemolytic anemia and hepatic failure. Neurologic symptoms commonly appear after the age of 12.

Riely, C. A.: Wilson's disease. Pediatr. Rev. 5:217, 1983.

   b. Galactosemia is characterized by the accumulation of galactose-1-phosphate and other metabolic products that presumably have a toxic effect on the liver. If the affected baby is receiving a galactose-containing formula, direct-reacting hyperbilirubinemia usually develops during the first or second week of life, along with hepatomegaly, feeding difficulties, vomiting, diarrhea and failure to thrive. Ascites appears early. Cataracts may develop later. Both the one-minute and the total serum bilirubin values are elevated. Albuminuria, galactosuria and aminoaciduria are present. Since galactose reduces Benedict's solution, there is a positive Clinitest reaction but a negative reaction to a glucose oxidase dipstick (Clinistix) if the infant is receiving galactose in the formula. The diagnosis is established by galactose-1-phosphate uridyl transferase assay in erythrocytes. The clinical status improves and the jaundice promptly disappears on a lactose free diet. Infants with galactosemia are susceptible to gram-negative sepsis or meningitis.
   c. Hereditary fructose intolerance may rarely cause jaundice and the presence of a reducing substance in the urine if the infant is receiving fructose.

d. Hereditary tyrosinemia may cause conjugated hyperbilirubinemia. Other symptoms include vomiting, diarrhea, failure to thrive, rickets and hypoglycemia.

B. Hepatocanalicular. Damage to the ampullae and the primary bile canaliculi may occur in such widely dissimilar diseases as erythroblastosis fetalis and cirrhosis. The injured ductal epithelium allows leakage of fluid and sodium bilirubinate followed by concentration of the remaining solids within the lumen. The resulting intraluminal bile thrombi may introduce a secondary obstructive factor. Fibrosis or edema may also cause external obstruction of the ampullae or primary canaliculi.

C. Obstructive jaundice; cholestasis

Balistreri, W. F.: Neonatal cholestasis. J. Pediatr. 106:171, 1985.
Gartner, L. M.: Cholestasis of the newborn (obstructive jaundice). Pediatr. Rev. 5:163, 1983.
Sinatra, F. R.: Cholestasis in infancy and childhood. Curr. Prob. Pediatr. 12:6 (Oct.) 1982.

1. Congenital
   a. Congenital atresia of the extrahepatic bile ducts. Since the onset of icterus in this disorder often coincides with that of physiologic jaundice, biliary atresia is frequently not suspected until the infant is about three weeks of age. The stools are acholic but frequently have a pale yellow appearance caused by an outer pigmented ring of stained intestinal secretions and epithelial cells. Because cirrhosis develops rapidly in infants with atresia of the extrahepatic biliary tree, the cause of obstructive jaundice in the newborn is optimally established during the first and not later than the second month of life. Although so-called classic histologic and laboratory findings have been described in biliary atresia, many exceptions to this pattern occur (e.g., urobilinogen may be found in the stools or urine; the patient may have a history of normally pigmented stools; jaundice may have been persistent from the early days of life; the serum bilirubin, rather than continuing to rise, may actually fall; and the jaundice may appear to lessen). Biliary atresia may be accompanied in some cases by the polysplenia syndrome, with a midline liver, several right-sided spleens and cardiac malformations. Differentiation between biliary atresia, paucity of intrahepatic bile ducts and neonatal hepatitis may usually be accomplished by a scintigraph hepatobiliary imaging agent such as 99 MT$_c$PIPIDA, perhaps with the patient given phenobarbital (5 mg/kg/day) for five days prior to the scan, ultrasonography and a percutaneous biopsy.

Majd, M., Reba, R. C., and Altman, R. P.: Hepatobiliary scintigraphy with 99 MT$_c$-PIPIDA in the evaluation of neonatal jaundice. Pediatrics 67:140, 1981.

   b. Abnormalities in the development of hepatic bile ducts with or without an associated extrahepatic atresia (hypoplasia of intrahepatic bile ducts, paucity of intrahepatic bile ducts and intrahepatic biliary atresia).
      (1) This group of lesions, largely congenital or, in some cases, thought to be acquired, is not well-understood. Diagnosis is possible only by biopsy. Usually the findings are identical with those of congenital atresia of the major bile ducts. Occasionally, however, the intrahepatic ducts are not completely atretic, and some bilirubin may be excreted into the intestinal tract.
      (2) Arteriohepatic dysplasia (Alagille's syndrome) is a syndrome consisting of hypoplasia of the intrahepatic ducts; bilateral pulmonary arterial stenosis; growth retardation; butterfly vertebrae; short distal phalanges; and a characteristic facies with a prominent, overhanging forehead, deeply set eyes, mild hypertelorism, a straight nose and a small, pointed chin. These facial features may be absent in this syndrome, and they may be present in other cholestatic disorders. Xanthomas and pruritus are other findings.

Levin, S. E., Zarvos, P., Milner, S., and Schmaman, A.: Arteriohepatic dysplasia: Association of liver disease with pulmonary arterial stenosis as well as facial and skeletal abnormalities. Pediatrics 66:876, 1980.

(3) Caroli disease, characterized by saccular, segmental dilatation of the intrahepatic bile ducts, is usually accompanied by hepatic fibrosis. Patients may have mild jaundice but more commonly present with abdominal pain or fever owing to cholangitis or stone formation.

Hermansen, M. C., Starshak, R. J., and Werlin, S. L.: Caroli disease: The diagnostic approach. J. Pediatr. 94:879, 1979.

c. "Neonatal hepatitis" or neonatal jaundice with giant cell transformation of the hepatic parenchyma, are terms applied to a clinical and histologic pattern associated with cholestasis and obstructive jaundice in the newborn. Jaundice begins in the early weeks of life and, along with dark urine and acholic stools, may persist for months. Moderate hepatomegaly and splenomegaly are commonly found. The exact etiology is not known. Histologic examination demonstrates replacement of normal parenchyma by multinucleated giant liver cells, lack of intercellular bile canaliculi and absence of bile from efferent bile passages. Differentiation from congenital atresia of the extrahepatic biliary tree may not be possible on the basis of clinical history and physical examination (see page 267). Operative cholangiograms may offer the only means for definitive diagnosis. Giant cell transformation of the liver cells has also been described in infants with hemolytic disease of the newborn, congenital spherocytosis, herpes simplex hepatitis and cytomegalovirus disease. Both neonatal hepatitis and biliary atresia occur in the 13 or 18 trisomy syndromes.

d. The term "inspissated bile syndrome" has been applied to persistent jaundice over three weeks associated with erythroblastosis fetalis; a rise in both direct and indirect bilirubin; maternal-infant blood group incompatibility; and the presence of other clinical manifestations of hemolytic disease of the newborn. Rarely, an infant with maternal-infant blood group incompatibility shows elevation of the cord blood direct bilirubin level and evidence of biliary obstruction.

e. Cystic fibrosis may cause obstructive jaundice.

f. Alpha$_1$-antitrypsin deficiency may account for a highly variable clinical picture. Prolonged obstructive jaundice may begin in the first 10 weeks of life, occasionally the first day, with acholic stools, dark urine and hepatomegaly or hepatosplenomegaly. Some infants demonstrate only abnormal liver function tests, whereas others have no evidence of hepatic disease. Cirrhosis and portal hypertension may develop.

Latimer, J. S., and Sharp, H. L.: Alpha-1-antitrypsin deficiency in childhood. Curr. Probl. Pediatr. 10:5, 1980.
Sveger, T.: Alpha$_1$-antitrypsin deficiency in early childhood. Pediatrics 62:22, 1978.

g. Glycogenosis, Types III and IV, may cause jaundice in young infants.

h. Benign recurrent intrahepatic cholestasis, which begins in childhood or early adulthood, is characterized by intermittent periods of cholestasis that may last one to six months. Symptoms include jaundice, pruritus, anorexia and weight loss.

Heathcote, J., Deodhar, K. P., Scheuer, P. F., and Sherlock, S.: Intrahepatic cholestasis in childhood. N. Engl. J. Med. 295:801, 1976.
Riely, C. A.: Familial intrahepatic cholestasis: An update. Yale J. Biol. Med. 52:89, 1979.

i. Familial recurrent cholestasis may be accompanied by lymphedema appearing at birth or in adolescence secondary to lymph vessel hypoplasia.

Aagenaes, O.: Hereditary recurrent cholestasis with lymphoedema—two new families. Acta. Paediatr. Scand. 63:465, 1974.

j. Byler disease, a fatal familial intrahepatic cholestasis in an Amish kindred, is characterized by recurrent cholestatic jaundice, hepatosplenomegaly, steatorrhea, failure to thrive, pruritus and dwarfing. Gastrointestinal symptoms in the form of loose, foul-smelling stools antedate the onset of jaundice by one to eight months. Kayser-Fleischer rings may be present.

k. Zellweger cerebrohepatorenal syndrome, an autosomal recessive disorder, may be characterized by cholestasis, elevated liver enzymes, hypotonia, seizures, deformities of the hands and feet and a characteristic facies.

l. Congenital cystic dilatation of the common bile duct (choledochal cyst) in young infants may cause obstructive jaundice and acholic stools that simulate biliary atresia. In older infants and children, abdominal pain, a palpable mass in the right hypochondrium, and obstructive jaundice constitute other findings. These findings, which may occur singly or jointly, are usually intermittent, although occasionally they may persist. Fever occurs in the presence of cholangitis. Portal hypertension may ensue. An upper gastrointestinal series may show displacement of the duodenum to the left and anteriorly. Ultrasound examination of the gallbladder is diagnostically helpful.

Harris, V. J., and Kahler, J.: Choledochal cyst: Delayed diagnosis in a jaundiced infant. Pediatrics 62:235, 1978.

m. The common bile duct may be obstructed by a bile plug. Surgical exploration and transcholecystic cholangiography establish the diagnosis.

n. Congenital erythropoietic porphyria is a cause of anemia and conjugated hyperbilirubinemia in early infancy.

o. The Dubin-Johnson syndrome, characterized by chronic or intermittent jaundice that fluctuates in intensity, may be evident in the neonatal period or later in childhood. The serum bilirubin, which may range from 2 to 20 mg/dl, is composed of 25 to 75 per cent direct reacting bilirubin. Patients may be either asymptomatic or report vague abdominal pain, fatigue, anorexia, vomiting, diarrhea, dark urine and pale stools. The liver may be enlarged and tender. Bile and urobilinogen are found in the urine. Direct and total serum bilirubin concentrations are elevated. Liver biopsy demonstrates lipofuscin pigment in the liver cells.

p. Rotor's syndrome, a familial disorder, is similar to the Dubin-Johnson syndrome except for absence of the abnormal pigment.

q. Cholestasis occurs in newborn infants with severe hypoglycemia, congenital hypopituitarism and microphallus.

2. Biliary cirrhosis
   a. Obstructive biliary cirrhosis
   b. Congenital acholangic biliary cirrhosis
   c. Fibroxanthomatous biliary cirrhosis
   d. Biliary cirrhosis associated with cystic fibrosis
   e. Trihydroxycoprostanic acidemia is associated with neonatal cholestasis and cirrhosis.

3. Cholelithiasis is a rare cause of jaundice in children. The prevalence of gallstones in patients with sickle cell disease ranges from 5 to 35 per cent. Differentiation between abdominal crises, cholecystitis and cholelithiasis may be difficult. Ultrasound of the gallbladder is indicated in the older child with sickle cell anemia who is seen because of abdominal pain. Choledocholithiasis in infants with intrahepatic cholestasis may cause an abrupt, marked increase in the serum bilirubin.

Ariyan, S., Shessel, F. S., and Pickett, L. K.: Cholecystitis and cholelithiasis masking as abdominal crises in sickle cell disease. Pediatrics 58:252, 1976.

4. Neoplasms of the liver and bile ducts may cause jaundice through obstruction of the common hepatic or bile duct.
   a. Primary neoplasms
      (1) Adenomas may originate from parenchymal liver cells or bile duct epithelium. Cystic adenomas of bile duct epithelium may occur. "Hamartomas" comprise a disorganized mass of liver cells, bile ducts and blood vessels.
      (2) Multiple small cysts may arise from the bile ducts. Patients with polycystic kidneys also have hepatic cysts or fibrosis. Occasionally, large solitary cysts of unknown origin occur.
      (3) Hemangiomas, endotheliomas, hemangioendotheliomas, fibromas, teratomas, carcino-

mas and sarcomas are other primary hepatic neoplasms.

(4) Hodgkin's disease

b. Metastatic neoplasms: neuroblastoma

5. Inflammatory lesions
   a. Abscess: bacterial; amebic
   b. Tuberculoma

6. Parasites
   a. Amebiasis may cause cholecystitis, hepatitis or an obstructing liver abscess.
   b. *Ascaris* rarely obstructs the common duct.
   c. Echinococcus

7. Obstruction of extrahepatic bile ducts
   a. Peritoneal adhesions
   b. Leukemia may produce obstruction by enlargement of the lymph nodes at the porta hepatis.
   c. Hodgkin's disease
   d. Post-traumatic
   e. Spontaneous rupture of the bile duct with bile ascites in the newborn

8. Chlorpromazine, trimethoprim-sulfamethoxazole and other drugs may rarely cause cholestatic hepatitis in children.

9. Pancreas
   a. Annular pancreas
   b. Idiopathic fibrosis of the pancreas may cause obstructive jaundice, even in the absence of pain.

c. Pancreatic cyst or hemangioendothelioma.

10. Parenteral alimentation in low birth weight infants is frequently accompanied by cholestasis. Screening of serum bilirubin levels is indicated on a weekly basis.

Beale, E. F., Nelson, R. M., Bucciarelli, R. Z., Donnelly, W. H., and Eitzman, D.V.: Intrahepatic cholestasis associated with parenteral nutrition in premature infants. Pediatrics 64:342, 1979.

Black, D. D., Suttle, E. A., Whitington, P. F., Whitington, G. L., and Korones, S. D.: The effect of short-term parenteral nutrition on hepatic function in the human neonate: A prospective randomized study demonstrating alteration of hepatic canalicular function. J. Pediatr. 99:445, 1981.

GENERAL REFERENCES

Alagille, D., and Odievre, M.: Liver and Biliary Tract Disease in Children. New York, John Wiley & Sons, 1979.

Andres, J. M., Mathis, R. K., and Walker, W. A.: Liver disease in infants. Part I: Developmental hepatology and mechanisms of liver dysfunction. J. Pediatr. 90:686, 1977.

Mathis, R. K., Andres, J. M., and Walker, W. A.: Liver disease in children. Part II. Hepatic disease states. J. Pediatr. 90:864, 1977.

Mowat, A. P.: Liver Disorders in Childhood. London, Butterworths, 1979.

Thaler, M. M.: Neonatal hyperbilirubinemia. Semin. Hematol. 9:107, 1972.

ETIOLOGIC CLASSIFICATION OF JAUNDICE

Table continued on opposite page

ETIOLOGIC CLASSIFICATION OF JAUNDICE *Continued*

B. Hepatocanalicular, 267
C. Obstructive; cholestasis, 267
   1. Congenital
      a. Congenital atresia bile duct
      b. Paucity intrahepatic bile ducts; arteriohepatic dysplasia; Caroli disease
      c. Neonatal hepatitis
      d. Inspissated bile syndrome
      e. Cystic fibrosis
      f. Alpha-1-antitryspin deficiency
      g. Glycogenosis
      h. Benign recurrent intrahepatic cholestasis
      i. Familial recurrent cholestasis with lymphedema
      j. Byler disease

      k. Cerebrohepatorenal syndrome
      l. Choledochal cyst
      m. Bile plug
      n. Congenital erythropoietic porphyria
      o. Dubin-Johnson syndrome
      p. Rotor's syndrome
      q. Hypopituitarism
   2. Biliary cirrhosis
   3. Cholelithiasis
   4. Neoplasms
   5. Inflammatory lesions
   6. Parasitic infection
   7. Obstruction of extrahepatic bile ducts
   8. Drugs
   9. Pancreas
  10. Parenteral alimentation

29 / FAILURE TO GAIN; FAILURE TO THRIVE; WEIGHT LOSS

PATTERNS OF WEIGHT GAIN

The greatest gain in weight during fetal development occurs just before birth, owing to the deposition of subcutaneous fat during the last trimester. The physiologic weight loss occurring during the first three to four days after birth may amount to 5 to 8 per cent of birth weight in breast-fed infants but only 1 or 2 per cent in those who are formula fed. Usually the birth weight is regained by the seventh day in the latter and the tenth to the fourteenth day in the former. Premature infants may experience a relatively larger physiologic weight loss and may require somewhat longer to regain their birth weight.

Weight gain during early infancy is relatively rapid, amounting to 5 or 6 and sometimes up to 10 ounces a week. In the latter half of the first year the gain is slower, amounting to 3 to 5 ounces a week. During the first year of life, infants should demonstrate a steady weight gain. Failure to do so calls for prompt investigation. During infancy, regular weight gain and growth in length are sensitive indicators of nutritional and health status. *As a general rule, if an infant fails to gain on a formula that is quantitatively and qualitatively correct, something is wrong with the infant or the feeding situation and not with the formula.* Changing to other formulas will usually not correct this problem.

The infant's caloric requirement depends upon his basal metabolic rate, the rapidity of growth, the degree of physical activity, the amount of nonutilized food that is lost in the stools and the specific dynamic action of food. Since adipose tissue is not as active metabolically as other tissue, a malnourished infant with little or no subcutaneous fat has a higher level of metabolism relative to his weight than a normal infant of the same age or weight; thus, the caloric requirement of the undernourished child per unit of body weight is greater than that of the well-nourished infant. This requirement is also increased in malnourished infants because of the active anabolic processes that occur during recovery. Significant differences in activity among infants and children also account for variability in food requirements. The allowance for activity is much greater in active, kicking, tense infants than in those who are placid or somnolent. Crying may raise metabolic requirements 100 per cent or more above the basal metabolic level.

In the presence of diarrhea or impaired absorption, fecal loss of food may be as great as 30 or 40 per cent. Each Fahrenheit degree of elevation in body temperature increases caloric needs by about 7 per cent. In the first few days of life, the total caloric requirement is about 80 calories per kilogram per day. During the first year of life, a normal infant requires 100 to 120 calories per kilogram of body weight. This requirement decreases about 10 cal/kg during each succeeding three-year period.

These figures are an approximation; the exact requirement varies from one infant to another. Although these considerations are important in feeding, the best demonstration of caloric adequacy is regular weight gain.

During the second year of life, the rate of weight gain continues to diminish, the child gaining 2 1/2 ounces a week. Instead of a steady weight gain each week, the weight may remain constant for two or three weeks at a time. This pattern of periodic rather than constant weight gain becomes more pronounced in older children. From the age of two to five years, the increments in weight are less than at any other time in childhood. The average yearly weight gain is 4 to 5 pounds. After the age of five, the increments in weight begin to increase in contrast to the increments in height, which continue to decrease. An acceleration in weight increments occurs during the prepubertal years, with girls showing this weight acceleration about two years before boys. These different patterns of weight and height increments cause the prepubertal child to appear more stocky than the preschool child.

The pediatric interview, physical examination and observation of mother-infant interaction are of preeminent importance in the initial appraisal of failure to thrive. If those examinations suggest a psychosocial etiology, a period of observation in the hospital with a normal diet and developmentally appropriate nursing care will soon be confirmatory in that the baby will gain weight and develop rapidly. Although the differential list of diagnostic possibilities listed below contains predominantly biomedical disorders, failure to thrive in most babies is caused by psychosocial factors. If initial diagnosis is uncertain, selected laboratory procedures may be obtained, including CBC, urinalysis, serum electrolytes, calcium, BUN, creatinine, and T_4 and T_3. Other studies (e.g., urine for genetic screening,

bone age, skull films, sweat chloride, carotene) may be obtained as appears clinically appropriate.

ETIOLOGIC CLASSIFICATION OF FAILURE TO THRIVE OR LOSS OF WEIGHT

I. MOTHERING DISABILITY OR INADEQUATE NURTURING (see page 442).

II. QUALITATIVE OR QUANTITATIVE INADEQUACY OF FOOD INTAKE

A. Economic privation; starvation
  1. Inadequate caloric intake
  2. Chronic protein malnutrition. Kwashiorkor associated with poverty occurs in many developing countries, usually in children over one year of age. It is rare in the United States except among some Navajo children. In this country, protein malnutrition is not associated with poverty but may occur in infants under one year of age secondary to the withholding of protein from the baby's diet or the use of nondairy creamer as the sole source of nutrition. If the infant's caloric intake is nearly normal, the infant appears chubby ("sugar baby" kwashiorkor; urban kwashiorkor).

Lozoff, B., and Fararoff, A. A.: Kwashiorkor in Cleveland. Am. J. Dis. Child. 129:760, 1975.
Sinatra, F. R., and Merritt, R. J.: Iatrogenic kwashiorkor in infants. Am. J. Dis. Child. 135:21, 1981.

B. Anorexia owing to organic or psychologic factors
C. Feeding difficulties owing to organic factors
  1. Congenital anomalies such as glossoptosis or cleft palate
  2. Dyspnea causes difficulty in feeding.
  3. Infants and children who are developmentally retarded may feed poorly.
D. Inadequate formula intake
E. Breast-fed babies may fail to gain because of an inadequate intake of breast milk. Although some breast-fed infants who do not consume adequate calories cry because of hunger, others do not cry much and may, indeed, be lethargic. Since the baby appears satisfied, significant life-threatening dehydration and malnutrition may occur before the parents realize that a problem exists. Weight loss in excess of 15 to 25 per cent of body weight may occur by 10 to 14 days. Generally, the mothers in these

instances have been primaparas without prior nursing experience who were discharged prior to the time their milk came in and who have had insufficient help in establishing successful breast feeding. These infants have usually lost 5 to 10 per cent of their birth weight and have demonstrated suboptimal sucking prior to discharge.

Clark, T. A., Markarian, M., Griswold, W., and Mendoza, S.: Hypernatremic dehydration resulting from inadequate breast feeding. Pediatrics 63:931, 1979.

Lawrence, R. A.: Infant nutrition. Pediatr. Rev. 5:133, 1983.

Roddey, O. F., Jr., Martin, E.S., and Swetenburg, R.L.: Critical weight loss and malnutrition in breast-fed infants. Am. J. Dis. Child. 135:597, 1981.

F. Crohn's disease is characterized, in part, by weight loss owing to a marked diminution in appetite or fear of causing postprandial pain.
G. Prolonged or frequent use of oral fluid. Electrolyte-carbohydrate solution in an infant with recurrent loose bowel movements may provide inadequate caloric intake.
H. Child neglect with inadequate feeding is an important cause of failure to thrive.
I. Mothering disability or inadequate nurturing, both caloric and developmental, is the most frequent cause for failure to thrive. Indeed, periodic determination of an infant's weight, length, development and behavior offers a simple screening method to alert the clinician to maternal-infant transactional difficulties and lack of mutuality (see page 444). These infants may have an inadequate caloric intake either because they are not offered sufficient calories or because they do not eat or drink adequate quantities of what is offered.

Altemeier, W. A., O'Connor, S. M., Sherrod, K. B., and Vietze, P. M.: Prospective study of antecedents for nonorganic failure to thrive. J. Pediatr. 106:360, 1985.

Fischhoff, J., Whitten, C. F., and Pettit, M. G.: A psychiatric study of mothers of infants with growth failure secondary to maternal deprivation. J. Pediatr. 79:209, 1971.

Gardner, L. I.: The nosology of failure to thrive. Why is psychosocial deprivation, its major cause, underdiagnosed? Am. J. Dis. Child. 132:961, 1978.

Powell, G. F., and Low, J.: Behavior in nonorganic failure to thrive. Devel. Behav. Pediatr. 4:26, 1983.

Suskind, R. M., and Varma, R. N.: Assessment of nutritional status of children. Pediatr. Rev. 5:195, 1983.

III. DEFECTS IN FOOD ASSIMILATION

A. Inadequate digestion
   1. Failure to gain in spite of hunger and a large food intake is an early symptom of cystic fibrosis. Hypochloremic alkalosis caused by a formula low in chloride may be manifest clinically by anorexia, lethargy, and growth failure.

Chase, H. P., Long, M. A., and Lavin, M. H.: Cystic fibrosis and malnutrition. J. Pediatr. 95:337, 1979.

   2. The Schwachman-Diamond syndrome of pancreatic insufficiency, failure to thrive, neutropenia, dwarfism and metaphyseal chondrodysplasia
B. Inadequate absorption
   1. Celiac syndrome (see page 227)
      a. Failure to thrive is not an early symptom in patients with celiac disease or gluten-induced enteropathy. Vomiting and, perhaps, diarrhea may occur first, followed by irregular weight gain. Loss of weight is a prominent manifestation in children with untreated celiac disease. Some patients with celiac disease do not have diarrhea but rather present with failure to thrive and constipation.

McNicholl, B., and Egan-Mitchell, B.: Infancy celiac disease without diarrhea. Pediatrics 49:85, 1972.

      b. Giardiasis
      c. Gastrointestinal allergy
      d. Tuberculosis of mesenteric nodes
      e. Biliary atresia
C. Systemic infections may interfere with normal nutrient delivery to the tissues. Prenatal infections, (e.g., rubella) may cause failure to thrive.
D. Protein-losing gastroenteropathy
E. Aganglionic megacolon

IV. LOSS OF FOOD SUBSTANCES

A. Regurgitation and vomiting (see Chapter 21.)
B. Diarrhea (see Chapter 22.)

V. FAILURE OF UTILIZATION OR INCREASED METABOLISM

A. Excessive crying or activity; restlessness
B. Prolonged fever
C. Repeated acute or chronic infections
   1. Prenatal viral infection or neonatal bacterial sepsis

Hanshaw, J. B., and Dudgeon, J. A.: Viral Diseases of the Fetus and Newborn. Philadelphia, W. B. Saunders Co. 2nd ed., 1985.

2. Repeated respiratory infections
3. Tuberculosis
4. Intestinal parasites
5. Histoplasmosis
6. Urinary tract infections
7. Sepsis in newborn infants, especially prematures, may be primarily manifest by failure to thrive. Poor feeding, loss of vigor, regurgitation and irritability may be associated symptoms.
8. Congenital and acquired immunodeficiency diseases (see Chapter 53.)

D. The possibility of a malignancy such as Hodgkin's disease should always be kept in mind with a history of weight loss or unexplained listlessness.
E. Failure to gain may be the first indication of significant cardiac disease in infants. In infants with congenital heart disease who gain weight normally, the arterial oxygen saturation has not been reduced to a critical level. Failure to gain may be an early symptom of endocardial fibroelastosis or of impending or actual congestive heart failure, especially in infants with ventricular septal defects. Difficulty in feeding owing to dyspnea and cough with resultant poor weight gain may be the first manifestation of cardiac failure. Early symptoms in infants with coarctation of the aorta include anorexia, vomiting, tiring during feedings and failure to gain weight.
F. Chronic pulmonary disease; hypoxia. A roentgenogram of the chest is indicated in infants who fail to thrive.
G. Renal disease
1. Chronic renal insufficiency with metabolic acidosis
2. Renal tubular acidosis (idiopathic renal acidosis, hyperchloremic acidosis with nephrocalcinosis) is characterized by a hyperchloremic acidosis. The distal form of RTA (type I) is characterized by urine with a pH greater than 6 regardless of the degree of acidosis. The proximal form (type II) demonstrates normal acidification of the urine with a pH less than 5. Type I renal acidosis, with an onset between the fourth and sixth months of life, may be characterized by vomiting, anorexia, constipation, polyuria, polydipsia, dehydration, hypotonia and failure to gain weight. Infants with Type II RTA demonstrate growth failure and vomiting but are otherwise asymptomatic. In older children, renal tubu-

lar acidosis is characterized by understature, rickets, polyuria, polydipsia and nephrocalcinosis. Distal renal tubular acidosis may occur in children with hydronephrosis.

Nash, M. A., Torrado, A. D., Griefer, I., Spitzer, A., and Edelmann, C. M., Jr.: Renal tubular acidosis in infants and children. J. Pediatr. 80:738, 1972.

3. Other types of renal disease such as chronic pyelonephritis, chronic glomerulonephritis, obstructive uropathy, hydronephrosis or polycystic disease of the kidneys may lead to failure to thrive. Failure to gain and grow is probably the most common presenting complaint in infants with serious anomalies of the urinary tract.

H. Idiopathic hypercalcemia of infancy is characterized clinically by anorexia, vomiting, constipation, failure to thrive, irritability, thirst, fever, hypotonia and muscle weakness. The transient mild form begins between three and seven months of age. The severe form, which begins earlier, is associated with hypertension, mental retardation, azotemia, thirst and polyuria. A characteristic elfin face (Williams elfin facies) occurs in the severe form with full, pouting cheeks; large mouth; prominent upper lip; flat bridge; up-turned nose; hypertelorism; and epicanthal folds. The facies may not, however, be sufficiently characteristic to suggest the disorder. Idiopathic hypercalcemia with failure to thrive may be clinically indistinguishable from infantile renal acidosis. Hereditary parathyroid hyperplasia with hypercalcemia may also cause failure to thrive.

Goldbloom, R. B., Gillis, D. A., and Prasad, M.: Hereditary parathyroid hyperplasia: A surgical emergency of early infancy. Pediatrics 49:514, 1972.

I. Hepatic insufficiency
J. Bartter's syndrome causes severe failure to thrive in the early months of life. Clinical manifestations include vomiting, constipation, hypokalemia, hypochloremia and, at times, hypomagnesemia.

Simopoulos, A. P., and Bartter, F. C.: Growth characteristics and factors influencing growth in Bartter's syndrome. J. Pediatr. 81:56, 1972.

K. Chronic anemia
1. Iron deficiency anemia may cause poor weight gain because of ano-

rexia, altered cellular function or impaired absorption.

2. Sickle cell anemia is characterized, in part, by slow weight gain in infants, children and adolescents.

L. Endocrine disorders
1. Although patients with hyperthyroidism commonly eat a large amount of food, weight loss occurs if their caloric intake is inadequate for their increased metabolic needs.
2. Infants and children with hypothyroidism do not thrive well, in part owing to difficulty in sucking and swallowing and to lethargy. Failure to thrive may be the first symptom of congenital hypothyroidism.
3. Failure to gain weight or rapid loss of weight may be early manifestations of diabetes.
4. Diabetes insipidus
5. Pheochromocytoma may cause weight loss or failure to gain weight in spite of an increased food intake.

M. Storage diseases. These diseases increase children's appetite.
1. Glycogenosis
2. Infantile Gaucher's disease is characterized by physical and mental retardation, splenomegaly, hepatomegaly and neurologic symptoms. Niemann-Pick disease in infants is characterized by physical and intellectual retardation along with massive hepatosplenomegaly.
3. Wolman's disease is characterized by failure to thrive, steatorrhea, hepatosplenomegaly and calcification of the adrenals.

N. Inborn errors of metabolism may present with poor feeding, lethargy and failure to thrive.
1. Galactosemia. Infants with this disorder may be jaundiced during the neonatal period. Failure to thrive is an early symptom accompanied, at times, by vomiting, diarrhea, hypoglycemia, ascites, hepatomegaly, galactosemia and albuminuria. These infants are vulnerable to systemic gram-negative infections. Cataracts and mental retardation may develop if appropriate treatment is not instituted. Urine may be screened easily for galactose by finding a positive Clinitest reaction in the presence of a negative Testape or Clinistix test. The diagnosis is confirmed by assay of galactose-1-phosphate uridyl transferase activity in erythrocytes.

2. The de Toni-Fanconi syndrome is characterized by hypophosphatemia, renal hyperaminoaciduria, organic aciduria and renal glycosuria. Hyperchloremic acidosis, hypokalemia, polyuria and albuminuria may be associated findings. Cystinosis is the most common cause of the Fanconi syndrome. A number of other etiologies, such as heavy metal poisoning, may account for damage to the renal tubules. Failure to thrive is an early finding in these infants, along with polydipsia, lassitude and muscle weakness. Older children demonstrate understature, resistant rickets and, occasionally, photophobia. The diagnosis of cystinosis may be established by slit lamp examination of the cornea or bone marrow examination.
3. Kinky hair disease
4. Hypophosphatasia. Failure to thrive may occur in the first six months of life in these patients, along with anorexia, irritability, vomiting, fever and convulsions.
5. Hereditary fructose intolerance. With young children, clinical manifestations include failure to thrive, persistent or recurrent vomiting, hypoglycemia and hepatomegaly.
6. Homocystinuria
7. Hereditary tyrosinemia may have either an acute or a chronic course. The former occurs in the early months of life and the latter becomes clinically manifest after six months of age. Symptoms include failure to thrive, vomiting, diarrhea, and hepatosplenomegaly.
8. Urea cycle disorders; metabolic acidosis owing to branched-chain aminoacids and organic acidurias. Symptoms include feeding difficulties, anorexia, vomiting, failure to thrive, apnea, tachypnea, convulsions, lethargy, stupor and coma. Because of the possibility of protein intolerance, discontinuation of milk and other protein-containing foods is indicated, and a balanced electrolyte glucose solution is provided orally or intravenously. Urine should be examined for odor, reducing substances, specific gravity, pH and ketones, including a ferric chloride test. The odor of the urine (musty, maple syrup, etc.) should be checked. Electrophoresis for amino acids is indicated, along with gas chromatogra-

phy and mass spectrometry. Blood specimens should be analyzed for serum electrolytes, glucose, ammonia, lactate, quantitative amino acids, organic acids and short-chain fatty acids.

Aleck, K. A., and Shapiro, L. J.: Genetic-metabolic considerations in the sick neonate. Pediatr. Clin. North Am. 25:431, 1978.

Burton, B. K., and Nadler, H. L.: Clinical diagnosis of the inborn errors of metabolism in the neonatal period. Pediatrics 61:398, 1978.

Nyhan, W. L.: Approach to the diagnosis of overwhelming metabolic disease in early infancy. Curr. Probl. Pediatr. 7:3, 1977.

O'Brien, D., and Goodman, S. I.: The critically ill child: Acute metabolic disease in infancy and early childhood. Pediatrics 46:620, 1970.

Scriver, C., and Rosenberg, L. E.: Amino Acid Metabolism and its Disorders. Philadelphia, W. B. Saunders Co., 1973.

O. Miscellaneous
1. Vitamin A poisoning. Anorexia and malnutrition are part of the clinical manifestations of this disease process.
2. Progressive diaphyseal dysplasia. Children with this syndrome do not thrive and demonstrate muscle weakness, a waddling gait and diaphyseal changes on roentgenographic examination.
3. Most of the patients with chondrodysplasia punctata fail to thrive, and death frequently occurs in the first year of life. Some patients, however, develop normally.

Sheffield, L. J., Danks, D. M., Mayne, U., and Hutchinson, L. A.: Chondrodysplasia punctata— 23 cases of a mild and relatively common variety. J. Pediatr. 89:916, 1976.

4. Leprechaunism (Donohue's syndrome) is characterized by failure to thrive; an elfin facies with large, low-set ears, flat nasal bridge, thickened lips, and micrognathia; facial hirsutism; and prominence of the clitoris.

Summitt, R. L., and Favara, B. E.: Leprechaunism (Donohue's syndrome): A case report. J. Pediatr. 74:601, 1969.

5. Obstructive sleep apnea may cause failure to thrive.
6. Infants with severe combined immunodeficiency demonstrate severe failure to thrive.
7. Systemic lupus erythematosus may be accompanied by weight loss.

VI. Low Birth Weight Infants; Prenatal Events
A. Infants who are small for gestational age owing to chronic intrauterine malnutrition may remain growth-retarded.
B. Premature infants have an increased incidence of failure to thrive, usually owing to problems in maternal-infant interaction.
C. Fetal alcohol and anticonvulsant syndromes are characterized by failure to thrive with growth deficiency noted at birth. The infant continues to lag in postnatal growth rate. Symptoms include microcephaly, mental retardation; and facial anomalies including short palpebral fissures, short, upturned nose with hypoplastic philtrum, thinned upper vermilion border of the lip and retrognathia.

Smith, D. W.: Fetal drug syndromes: Effects of ethanol and hydantoins. Pediatr. Rev. 1:165, 1979.

VII. Neurologic

A. Infants with cerebral damage, mental retardation or cerebral palsy often do not thrive. Although children who demonstrate excessive muscular activity may have caloric needs considerably above the average, their caloric intake is often less owing to feeding difficulties.
B. Subdural hematoma should be considered in all infants who fail to thrive. Convulsions, vomiting and irritability are common associated symptoms.
C. Diencephalic syndrome, owing to intracranial neoplasms in the region of the hypothalamus and third ventricle in infants and children under two years of age, is characterized by a paradoxical alertness, euphoria, hyperactivity and emaciation in the face of normal or increased appetite. Vomiting may occur irregularly. The usual signs of intracranial hypertension are absent early, but optic atrophy is often present with searching or rotatory nystagmus.
D. Leigh's syndrome or subacute necrotizing encephalomyelopathy begins in infancy with failure to thrive; recurrent vomiting; dysphagia; ptosis; rolling eye movements; extraocular palsies; irregular, rapid and sighing respirations; sobbing; ataxia; hypotonia; and developmental regression.

Burr, I. M., Slonim, A. E., Danish, R. K., Godoth, N., and Butler, I. J.: Diencephalic syndrome revisited. J. Pediatr. 88:439, 1976.
Hirschman, G.H., and Chan, J. C. M.: Complex acid-base disorders in subacute necrotizing encephalomyelopathy (Leigh's syndrome). Pediatrics 61:278, 1978.

GENERAL REFERENCES

Goldbloom, R. B.: Failure to thrive. Pediatr. Clin. North Am. 29:151, 1982.
Sills, R. H.: Failure to thrive. The role of clinical and laboratory evaluation. Am. J. Dis. Child. 132:967, 1978.
Suskind, R. M., and Varma, R. N.: Assessment of nutritional status of children. Pediatr. Rev. 5:195, 1983.

ETIOLOGIC CLASSIFICATION OF FAILURE TO THRIVE OR LOSS OF WEIGHT

I. MATERNAL DISABILITY OR INADEQUATE NURTURING, 272
II. QUALITATIVE OR QUANTITATIVE INADEQUACY OF FOOD INTAKE, 272
   A. Economic privation, starvation, 272
      1. Inadequate caloric intake
      2. Chronic protein malnutrition (kwashiorkor)
   B. Anorexia, 273
   C. Feeding difficulties owing to organic factors, 273
      1. Congenital anomalies
      2. Dyspnea
      3. Developmental retardation
   D. Calorically inadequate formula, 273
   E. Inadequate breast milk feedings, 273
   F. Crohn's disease, 273
   G. Prolonged or frequent use of oral fluid, 273
   H. Child neglect, 273
   I. Mothering disability, 273
III. DEFECTS IN ASSIMILATION OF FOOD, 273
   A. Inadequate digestion, 273
      1. Cystic fibrosis
      2. The Schwachman-Diamond syndrome
   B. Inadequate absorption: celiac syndrome, 273
   C. Systemic infections, 274
   D. Protein-losing gastroenteropathy, 274
   E. Aganglionic megacolon, 274
IV. LOSS OF FOOD SUBSTANCES, 274
   A. Regurgitation and vomiting, 274
   B. Diarrhea, 274
V. FAILURE OF UTILIZATION OR INCREASED METABOLISM, 274
   A. Excessive crying or activity; restlessness, 274
   B. Prolonged fever, 274
   C. Repeated acute or chronic infections, 274
      1. Prenatal viral infection or neonatal bacterial sepsis
      2. Repeated respiratory infections
      3. Tuberculosis
      4. Intestinal parasites
      5. Histoplasmosis
      6. Urinary tract infections
      7. Sepsis
      8. Immunodeficiency diseases
   D. Malignancy, 274
   E. Cardiac disorders, 274
   F. Chronic pulmonary disease; hypoxia, 274
   G. Renal disease, 274
      1. Chronic renal insufficiency leading to metabolic acidosis
      2. Renal tubular acidosis
      3. Chronic pyelonephritis, chronic glomerulonephritis, hydronephrosis, polycystic disease of kidneys
   H. Idiopathic hypercalcemia of infancy, 274
   I. Hepatic insufficiency, 275
   J. Bartter's syndrome, 275
   K. Chronic anemia, 275
      1. Iron deficiency anemia
      2. Sickle cell anemia
   L. Endocrine disorders, 275
      1. Hyperthyroidism
      2. Hypothyroidism
      3. Diabetes mellitus
      4. Diabetes insipidus
      5. Pheochromocytoma
   M. Storage diseases, 275
      1. Glycogenosis
      2. Infantile Gaucher's disease
      3. Wolman's disease
   N. Inborn errors of metabolism, 275
      1. Galactosemia
      2. De Toni-Fanconi syndrome
      3. Kinky hair disease
      4. Hypophosphatasia
      5. Hereditary fructose intolerance
      6. Homocystinuria
      7. Hereditary tyrosinemia
      8. Urea cycle disorders; organic acidurias
   O. Miscellaneous, 276
      1. Vitamin A poisoning
      2. Progressive diaphyseal dysplasia
      3. Chrondrodysplasia punctata
      4. Leprechaunism
      5. Obstructive sleep apnea
VI. LOW BIRTH WEIGHT INFANTS; PRENATAL EVENTS, 276
   A. Intrauterine malnutrition
   B. Premature infants
   C. Fetal drug syndromes
   D. Chromosomal anomalies
   E. Prenatal infection
VII. NEUROLOGIC, 276
   A. Cerebral damage, mental retardation, cerebral palsy
   B. Subdural hematoma
   C. Diencephalic syndrome
   D. Leigh's syndrome

30 / UNDERSTATURE

The chief feature that sets infants, children and adolescents apart from the adult is the dynamic nature of their growth and development. Growth in height and weight are sensitive reflections of health. The periodic assessment of infants, children and adolescents permits the early detection of growth deficiencies and pathologic processes. A number of methods are available to assist the physician in evaluating growth adequacy. The best approach is a long-term one in which the patient is evaluated in terms of his own velocity or growth rate. Although all suggested techniques of growth assessment make some comparison of the individual to his age group, the criterion for the practical clinical importance of any method is how well it permits assessment of the individual in terms of his own potentiality.

MEASUREMENTS OF PHYSICAL GROWTH

A few selected measurements should be routinely obtained. In infants these include weight, head circumference and length. In older children and adolescents, these are height and weight. For the measurement of head circumference, a nonstretchable measuring tape is passed over the most prominent part of the occiput and above the supraorbital ridges. The total length is more readily and accurately obtained in children up to three years of age in the recumbent position. In young infants, it is, of course, difficult to obtain an entirely accurate measurement of length unless special measuring devices (neonatomer or infantomer) are used with the help of an assistant. The Harpenden stadiomer provides a method for accurate determination of height. The usual measuring rod attached to a weight scale is not precise. Balance scales of the beam type should be used for the determination of body weight.

Percentile curves for length or height, weight and head circumference have been developed by the National Center for Health Statistics and based on large and representative samples of children. They are included as an Appendix (page 453). Curves are available for two age groups—birth to 36 months and 2 to 18 years— with separate curves for boys and for girls. For the younger child, percentile curves include those for body weight for age, length for age, body weight for length and head circumference for age. In the older age group, curves are available for height for age and weight for age. In addition, weight for height curves are available for prepubescent boys and girls.

The curves represent the 5th, 10th, 25th, 50th, 75th, 90th and 95th percentiles. For the young child, weights are based on nude weights; in the older child or adolescent, they include a light examination garment. The length curves for the child from birth to 36 months are based on recumbent length without shoes. Height in older children and adolescents reflects stature obtained in stocking feet.

Body measurements should be evaluated according to their percentile ranking. These rankings should then be compared to each other to determine whether they fall more or less within the same percentile group. Current percentile rankings should be compared with those of previous examinations to detect any significant acceleration or deceleration in the growth rate.

National Center for Health Statistics: NCHS Growth Charts, 1976.

Monthly Vital Statistics Report, Vol. 25, No. 3, Supp. (HRA) 76–1120.

Health Resources Administration, Rockville, Maryland, June, 1976.

National Center for Health Statistics: NCHS Growth Charts, 1976.

Vital and Health Statistics, Series 11, Health Resources Administration, Rockville, Maryland, 1976.

Owen, G. M.: The assessment and recording of measurements of growth of children: Report of a small conference. Pediatrics 51:461, 1973.

OSSEOUS DEVELOPMENT

Investigation of osseous development may be helpful in the clinical evaluation of a child's growth progress. This assessment is based on the time when ossification centers appear and epiphyseal–diaphyseal union occurs. In newborn infants, roentgenogram of the knee or ankle and foot are informative. In later infancy, in childhood and in adolescence, a roentgenogram of the wrist and hand is usually adequate for appraisal of bone age.

Osseous development is or may be retarded in the presence of hypopituitarism, hypothyroidism, malnutrition, constitutional dwarfism, chronic disease, severe illness, male hypogonadism and delayed adolescence. Osseous development is accelerated in sexual precocity and frequently in patients with obesity. Bone age may be prognostically useful in that children and adolescents with understature and delayed osseous development have more growth potential than those with a skeletal age appropriate for their chronologic age.

GROWTH PATTERNS

A child or adolescent may be considered understatured when his length or height is three or more standard deviations below the mean for age or the velocity or rate of his growth is below that expected for his chronologic age. If the patient is being seen for the first time, his height may be compared to that of others by reference to a percentile growth chart. A long-term record of the child's growth, including birth length and weight, helps determine whether his present growth status is the result of a constant growth pattern or whether at some point in the past the child began to experience growth failure. The ninety-seventh and the third percentiles represent approximately two standard deviations above and below the mean. The height age of a child is the chronologic age at which his height would equal the fiftieth percentile. The rate of growth in length is best depicted on height velocity curves on which height increments in inches or centimeters per year are plotted against chronologic age.

Tanner, J. M., and Whitehouse, R. H.: Longitudinal standards for height, weight, height velocity and stages of puberty. Arch. Dis. Child. 51:170, 1976.

The general growth pattern is characterized in late fetal life and early infancy by phases of rapid growth. Growth then decelerates in rate until adolescence, at which time another growth spurt occurs. Growth in height is finally terminated by epiphyseal closure.

The fiftieth percentile for length at birth is 50 cm (20 inches). This increases to about 66 cm (26 inches) at 6 months for girls and 68 cm (27 inches) for boys; 74 cm (29 inches) for girls and 76 cm (30 inches) for boys at one year; 86 to 87 cm (34 inches) at two years of age. The velocity for growth in the first six months should be at least 16 cm in girls and 17 cm in boys. From 6 to 12 months, expected velocity is 8 cm for both boys and girls. Over the next 12 months, the lower limits of normal are 11 cm for girls and 10 cm for boys.

During the period from age two to five, growth in height decelerates, occurring at the rate of 6 to 8 cm (2 to 4 inches) a year. A rate of less than 6 cm per year during this time is subnormal. Growth does not occur at a constant rate throughout the year but is greater at certain times than others. The deceleration in rate of growth in height continues during the school age period with annual increments of about 5 cm (2 inches). A growth rate of less than 5 cm per year between the age of five years and the onset of the adolescent growth spurt is subnormal. Because the increments in weight are increasing during this time, the child's physique is more stocky than in the preschool period.

Although great variability exists among children in the time of onset, magnitude and duration of the adolescent growth spurt, sufficient constancy and predictability exist to permit generalization. Regardless of the chronologic age at which the acceleration in height and weight begins, all children follow the same general pattern. The adolescent growth spurt occurs about two years earlier in girls than in boys. The annual increment in stature reflects this growth acceleration between the ages of 9 and 12 years in the girl and 11 and 14 years in the boy; thus, between the ages of 11 and 13 years, girls may be taller than boys of the same chronologic age. Adolescents of either sex, however, may experience an early growth spurt and reach their maximal rate of growth in about one year. Others demonstrate a late and more moderate pattern. Because of early deceleration in their growth rate, adolescents who mature early may be smaller when growth in height has ceased than those whose maximal growth rate occurs late. Some adolescents will have completed their growth phase before others of the same chronologic age have begun. Boys who mature early may attain maximal growth before girls who mature slowly. The period of maximal growth and that of sexual maturation are closely related temporally. The peak height velocity in boys occurs, on the average, at age 14 and during Tanner genital stage 4. On the average, girls usually experience their greatest acceleration in height at age 12 and at Tanner stage 2—after breast budding and a year or so before the menarche. By menarche, growth in height is 98 per cent complete. Those who experience their maximal growth early usually have an early menarche.

Children who have a delayed adolescence as part of their constitutionally delayed growth and physical maturation constitute a significant proportion of those seen with the complaint of short stature. Usually these children have been relatively short throughout childhood and have a concomitant retardation in sexual development, skeletal maturation and muscular development. Clinical differentiation among delayed adolescence, hypopituitarism and primordial or constitutional dwarfism as causes for understature prior to sexual, somatic and skeletal growth at adolescence may not be possible.

SKELETAL PROPORTIONS

The relation of body length from the crown to the symphysis pubis (upper segment) and from the symphysis to the sole (lower segment) is of diagnostic value. The measurement is obtained by subtracting the value of the symphysis-to-sole measurement from the total height. The normal value of this ratio ranges from 1.8 at birth to about 1.0 at 9 years of age and 0.9 at age 18. Normal ratios are found in children with delayed adolescence, hypopituitarism (proportions of a child of the same size), and primordial dwarfism (proportions of an individual of the same age with normal height). Patients with sexual precocity and progeria demonstrate an advanced ratio. The ratio remains relatively high in young children with hypothyroidism, chondrodystrophy, other primary disorders of bone and cartilage and Turner's syndrome. The ratio is relatively low in patients with Hurler's syndrome and Morquio's disease and in some patients with hypogonadism.

FACTORS CONTRIBUTING TO UNDERSTATURE

Growth retardation occurs during many acute and chronic illnesses in childhood, but compensatory mechanisms permit growth to regain its intrinsic or constitutional pattern after recovery. Apart from the obvious effects of anorexia and fever, the deceleration or arrest of growth that occurs during

infections is unexplained. Inadequate nutrition leads to diminished cartilaginous growth and osteoblastic activity. Insufficient protein intake with resultant negative nitrogen balance interferes with deposition of organic matrix in bone.

Heredity is a main determinant of the pattern and rate of linear growth, probably through conditioning the intrinsic growth potential of skeletal and other tissue and their response to growth stimuli. The influence of heredity in any child is difficult to assess, and understature should not be too readily ascribed to "heredity" without due consideration of other possible causes. Evaluations to be considered in the short child whose growth velocity is subnormal include, in addition to the history and physical, a bone age determination, lateral skull x-ray, serum thyroxine, thyroid-stimulating hormone, BUN, creatinine, calcium, phosphorus, serum electrolytes, CBC, sedimentation rate, and urinalysis.

Pituitary growth hormone exerts its chief effect on linear growth through stimulation of somatomedin production. Deficiency or absence of the thyroid hormone leads to retardation of growth and maturation. Diminution in cellular metabolism, impairment of cardiovascular function, and anorexia all contribute to growth retardation. Chondrogenesis and osteogenesis are retarded. Estrogens in themselves apparently contribute little to statural growth.

Androgenic hormones facilitate protein anabolism and nitrogen retention. Testicular androgen probably accounts for the spurt of growth in boys at adolescence, appearance of secondary sexual characteristics and muscular development. The function of adrenal androgen as a complementary growth hormone during adolescence is not completely proved.

ETIOLOGIC CLASSIFICATION OF UNDERSTATURE

I. Normal Variant Growth Patterns

A. Normal variant short stature (familial or constitutional short stature) is a common cause of short stature. These children, who tend to be short at birth, follow the normal growth pattern but remain below the fifth percentile. The bone age is normal, and puberty is not delayed. The parents and other close family members are usually also short with a height of 5 feet (152 cm) or less. Growth in height is completed by age 15 in girls and 16 in boys. With a family occurrence of short stature and a normal bone age, additional studies are usually not necessary.

B. Normal variant constitutional delay. Although of normal length at birth, these children shift to a lower growth channel between 3 and 36 months of age. The rate of growth is then normal for their age and parallels the standard growth pattern. Over 90 per cent of these patients are boys. The onset of puberty and the adolescent growth spurt are delayed, but the pubertal processes are completed, although often not until the late teens. Bone age is moderately retarded. Normal adult height is eventually attained. A family history of a similar growth pattern is often obtained. If the growth rate remains at 4 cm or more a year, skeletal age is only modestly delayed and a family history of a similar growth variant is obtained, evaluation may be limited to careful longitudinal evaluation.

Horner, J. M., Thorsson, A. V., and Hintz, R. L.: Growth deceleration patterns in children with constitutional short stature: An aid to diagnosis. Pediatrics 62:529, 1978.
Smith, D. W., Truog, W., Rogers, J. E., Greitzer, L. J., Skinner, A. L., McCann, J. J., and Harvey, M. A. S.: Shifting linear growth during infancy: Illustration of genetic factors in growth from fetal life through infancy. J. Pediatr. 89:225, 1976.

II. SKELETAL

A. Constitutional diseases of bone (see page 130)
B. Osteogenesis imperfecta
C. Congenital and acquired defects of the spine
   1. Multiple hemivertebrae; Klippel-Feil syndrome
   2. Tuberculosis
   3. Cushing's syndrome
   4. Kyphosis, scoliosis
   5. Primary hyperparathyroidism with vertebral collapse
   6. Eosinophilic granuloma
   7. Chronic glucocorticoid treatment
D. Idiopathic juvenile osteoporosis is characterized by growth arrest, arthralgia and vertebral collapse.

Teotia, M., Teotia, P. S., and Singh, R. H.: Idiopathic juvenile osteoporosis. Am. J. Dis. Child. 133:884, 1979.

III. NUTRITIONAL. Chronic malnutrition causes a deficit in height for age. Growth failure secondary to undernutrition is preceded by failure to gain weight adequately. The weight deficiency is usually greater than that of the height.

IV. SYSTEMIC DISORDERS

A. Glycogen storage disease
B. Cystinosis
C. Galactosemia
D. Congenital heart disease

Suoninen, P.: Physical growth of children with congenital heart disease. Acta. Paediatr. Scand. 225(suppl):1, 1971.

E. Chronic renal disease is a diagnostic consideration in children who demonstrate understature. Poor nutrition, chronic acidosis, osteodystrophy, diminished somatomedin secretion and anemia may occur. Determinations of the serum creatinine, electrolytes and urinary pH are indicated in patients with possible renal tubular acidosis.

Lewy, J. E., and New, M. I.: Growth in children in renal failure. Am. J. Med. 58:65, 1975.
Stickler, G. B.: Growth failure in renal disease. Pediatr. Clin. North Am. 23:885, 1976.

F. Chronic pulmonary disease, including cystic fibrosis and severe asthma
G. Chronic hemolytic and other anemias, such as sickle cell anemia or beta-thalassemia

Platt, O. S., Rosenstock, W., and Espeland, M. A.: Influence of sickle hemoglobinopathies on growth and development. N. Engl. J. Med. 311:7, 1984.

H. Lipoid storage diseases: xanthomatosis, Niemann-Pick disease, Gaucher's disease
I. Bartter's syndrome
J. Mucopolysaccharidoses
K. Rickets
L. Infections, including intrauterine infections
M. Gastrointestinal disease
   1. Inflammatory bowel disease. Severe growth retardation owing to insufficient nutrient intake occurs more frequently in Crohn's disease than in ulcerative colitis with 15 to 30 per cent of patients with the former disease and 5 to 10 per cent with the latter disease ranking below the third percentile in height. In the former, growth retardation and understature may precede gastrointestinal symptoms by years.

Rosenthal, S. R., Snyder, J. D., Hendricks, K. M., and Walker, W. A.: Growth failure and inflammatory bowel disease: Approach to treatment of a complicated adolescent problem. Pediatrics 72:481, 1983.

2. Malabsorption syndromes. Asymptomatic celiac disease may cause short stature.
3. Hepatic cirrhosis; glycogen storage disease
N. Chronic metabolic acidosis
O. X-linked hypogammaglobulinemia may be accompanied by an isolated growth hormone deficiency.

V. GENETIC FACTORS

A. Normal growth variants: normal variant short stature; normal variant constitutional delay. See discussion above.
B. Chromosomal abnormalities
1. Trisomy 13
2. Trisomy 18
3. Trisomy 21
4. Gonadal dysgenesis: Turner's syndrome is characterized by moderate understature with 1.5 to 2 inches (4 to 5 cm) of growth each year and a mean ultimate height of 140 to 145 cm. Growth is relatively slow early in childhood and almost always subnormal by four or five years of age. The lower extremities are markedly shortened. The bone age is usually delayed. A karyotype should be obtained in short-statured phenotypic females even if they do not present the classic clinical findings of Turner's syndrome.

McDonough, P. G.: Gonadal dysgenesis and its variants. Pediatr. Clin. North Am. 19:631, 1972.
Newfeld, N. D., Lippe, B. M., and Kaplan, S. A.: Disproportionate growth of the lower extremities. A major determinant of short stature in Turner's syndrome. Am. J. Dis. Child. 132:296, 1978.

5. Chromosome deletion syndromes
    a. Cri du chat syndrome
    b. Wolf syndrome
    c. Deletion of long arm of chromosome 18 or 21
6. Bloom's syndrome consists of intrauterine growth retardation, photosensitivity, telangiectatic erythema, a tendency to chromosomal breakage, immunologic deficiency and hypogonadism.

VI. CENTRAL NERVOUS SYSTEM

A. Mental retardation
B. Craniopharyngioma with secondary hypopituitarism
C. Glioma of the optic chiasm
D. Pineal tumor
E. Xanthomatosis with involvement of the hypothalamic area and secondary hypopituitarism

VII. ENDOCRINE SYSTEM

The velocity of a child's or adolescent's growth is an important consideration in deciding whether to include an endocrine disorder in the differential diagnosis of short stature. In the presence of a normal growth rate, an endocrine etiology for short stature is unlikely. Since dental and osseous development are usually retarded with an endocrine disorder, normal bone age makes an endocrine cause less likely.

Raiti, S.: Endocrine causes of short stature. Postgrad. Med. 62:81, 1977.

A. Hypopituitarism may be caused by developmental, genetic or acquired defects in the production or action of growth hormone involving the hypothalamus, pituitary, somatomedin, cartilage or bone. The deficiency in human growth hormone secretion may be isolated or accompanied by deficiency of one or more of the other pituitary trophic hormones (e.g., congenital gonadotropic deficiency may be associated with micropenis). Polydactyly may have a higher than normal association with hypopituitarism. Acquired growth hormone insufficiency may occur secondarily to birth trauma, a hypothalamic glioma, an intrasellar or suprasellar tumor, septo-optic dysplasia, histiocytosis X, trauma, tuberculosis and radiation therapy. Children thought to have acquired growth hormone deficiency require a careful history for neurologic symptoms, funduscopic and visual field examinations and, possibly, computerized tomography.

Growth retardation in isolated human growth hormone deficiency (IGHD) may be noted in the first year of life or during early childhood. After this onset, the velocity of growth is slow, less than 4 to 5 cm annually. Differentiation between understature owing to hypopituitarism and that attributable to constitutional factors is difficult in childhood unless a lesion involving the pituitary area can be demonstrated. Pituitary dwarfs have normal or almost normal body proportions and immature, round, full "doll-like" or "cherubic" facial features with delayed development of the naso-orbital bridge. Their head circumference is consistent with their chronologic age. Obesity often involves the trunk and buttocks. Delay in dentition may be noted when the permanent teeth are to erupt. The bone age is retarded. The voice may be high-pitched and squeaky. In type I

IGHD, inherited on an autosomal recessive basis, the patient has a high-pitched voice and develops wrinkling of the skin in adult life. Type II IGHD, inherited as an autosomal dominant trait, is not accompanied by such voice or skin changes. Spontaneous hypoglycemia may be an accompanying problem in type I IGHD. With multitrophic pituitary hormone deficiency, evidence of thyroid or adrenal insufficiency may be present, and secondary sexual development may be delayed or absent. Hypoglycemia may occur. The diagnosis of hypopituitarism requires a minimum of two definitive stimulation tests of plasma growth hormone. Some slow-growing children thought to have delayed adolescence or constitutional short stature respond to stimulation tests in a borderline or low normal fashion. Other short children who meet the criteria of height below the first percentile, a growth velocity of 4 cm per year or less, bone age that is two or more years below chronologic age, normal growth hormone provocative tests and a low somatomedin C level, are thought to have an abnormal growth hormone secretory pattern. Radioimmunoassay of somatomedin C is a useful screening test for growth hormone deficiency. These children demonstrate an increase in growth velocity in response to growth hormone therapy.

Spiliotis, B. E., August, G. P., Hung, W., Sonis, W., Mendelson, W., and Bercu, B. B.: Growth hormone neurosecretory dysfunction. JAMA 251:2223, 1984.
Valenta, L. J., Sigel, M. B., Lesniak, M. A., Elias, A. N., Lewis, U. J., Friesen, H. G., and Kershnar, A. K.: Pituitary dwarfism in a patient with circulating abnormal growth hormone polymers. N. Engl. J. Med. 312:214, 1985.

Children who have undergone cranial irradiation because of leukemia may have an abnormality of growth hormone neurosecretory function and poor catch-up growth.

Laron's dwarfism, an autosomal recessive syndrome noted in the first year of life, is characterized by marked dwarfism, truncal obesity, partial anodontia, saddle nose, "setting sun" eye sign, high-pitched voice, frontal bossing and small genitalia. A high circulating level of immunoreactive growth hormone is present, but somatomedin levels are low. Spontaneous hypoglycemic episodes occur during infancy. Decreased somatomedin levels also occur in chronic protein calorie deficiency (kwashiorkor), chronic renal failure, and chronic liver disease and secondary to long-term administration of corticosteroids.

Elders, M. J., Garland, J. T., Daughaday, W. A., Fisher, D. A., Whitney, J. E., and Hughes, E. R.: Laron's dwarfism: Studies on the nature of the defect. J. Pediatr. 83:253, 1973.

B. Growth arrest or marked slowing may be the chief or only clinical manifestation of hypothyroidism acquired after age two. T_4 by radioassay may be determined initially. If this value is low, thyroid stimulation hormone may be determined to establish whether the hypothyroidism is primary or secondary to hypothalamic-pituitary dysfunction.
C. Some types of sexual precocity and virilism with premature epiphyseal fusion lead to understature.
D. With adequate replacement therapy, the growth of children with hypoadrenocorticism is normal.
E. Cushing's syndrome is characterized by cessation of growth.
F. Poorly controlled diabetes (Mauriac syndrome)

Mandell, F., and Berenberg, W.: The Mauriac syndrome. Am. J. Dis. Child. 127:900, 1974.

G. Pseudohypoparathyroidism
H. Hyperparathyroidism
I. Chronic glucocorticoid therapy

VIII. OTHER DISORDERS

A. Prader-Willi syndrome
B. Primordial dwarfism is characteristically but not always present at birth. Growth is normal except for its slow rate and the small stature finally attained. Most constitutionally understatured children demonstrate retarded bone age in infancy and early childhood but normal skeletal maturation by adolescence.
C. Intrauterine growth retardation; small for gestational age. These full-term infants weigh 2500 gm or less at birth. Genetic or prenatal environmental factors (e.g., placental insufficiency, chronic intrauterine malnutrition, prenatal infections, maternal toxemia, fetal drug syndrome, smoking or alcohol ingestion) may be etiologic.

Cruise, M. O.: A longitudinal study of the growth of low birth weight infants. I. Velocity and distance growth, birth to 3 years. Pediatrics 51:620, 1973.
Tanner, J. M., and Whitehouse, R. H.: Height and weight charts from birth to 5 years allowing for length of gestation: For use in infant welfare clinics. Arch. Dis. Child. 48:786, 1973.

D. Seckel's syndrome (bird-headed dwarfism) is characterized by a small head, narrow face, prominent beak-like nose and low-set ears.

E. Dwarfism in children with progeria is usually apparent by one year of age.

F. Cockayne's syndrome is characterized by dwarfism appearing in the second year, microcephaly, retinitis pigmentosa, optic atrophy, cataracts, deafness, mental retardation, kyphosis, joint contractures, photosensitivity, an aged appearance, intracranial calcification, renal disease and hypertension.

G. Pycnodysostosis, a genetic bone disorder, is associated with dwarfism; osteopetrosis; partial aplasia of the terminal phalanges with a widened, drumstick appearance of the fingers and toes; persistence of open fontanels and cranial sutures; frontal bossing; retention of deciduous teeth; and a parrot-like nose.

H. Cornelia de Lange's syndrome is characterized by severe mental retardation; microbrachycephaly; small nose with upturned nostrils; simian creases; flexion contracture of elbows; hypertrichosis; low hairline; heavy, confluent eyebrows; wide, thin upper lip; micrognathia; anomalies of the extremities; and digits with proximally placed thumbs.

I. Russel-Silver syndrome is characterized by short stature, unusually large anterior fontanel, enlargement of the head, triangular facies, underdeveloped muscle mass and hemihypertrophy.

Tanner, J. M., Lejarraga, H., and Cameron, N.: The natural history of the Silver-Russel syndrome: A longitudinal study of thirty-nine cases. Pediatr. Res. 9:611, 1975.

J. Marchesani's syndrome is characterized by small stature, myopia, spherical lens and brachydactyly.

K. Laurence-Moon-Biedl syndrome consists of retinitis pigmentosa, obesity, polydactyly and hypogonadism.

L. Leprechaunism (Donohue's syndrome) is characterized by retarded growth; peculiar facies with large ears, wide eyes, and sunken cheeks; and prominence of the nipples, areolae, clitoris and labia minora.

M. Pseudopseudohypoparathyroidism is the term applied to patients whose physical appearance suggests the diagnosis of pseudohypoparathyroidism in the absence of an aberration in calcium-phosphorus metabolism.

N. Congenital telangiectatic erythema of the face (Bloom's syndrome) is associated with dwarfism, sensitivity to sunlight and an increased incidence of leukemia.

O. The Rothmund-Thomson syndrome is characterized by short stature; telangiectasia and pigmentation involving the skin of the face, buttocks and extremities in the first three to six months of life; alopecia; cataracts; and hypogonadism.

P. The Williams syndrome is characterized by retardation in growth, elfin facies, mental retardation, congenital heart disease (e.g., supravalvular aortic stenosis) and, in some cases, hypercalcemia.

Jones, K. L., and Smith, D. W.: The Williams elfin facies syndrome: A new perspective. J. Pediatr. 86:718, 1975.

Q. The Dubowitz syndrome is characterized by mental retardation, mild microcephaly, eczema and small stature.

R. 3-M slender-boned nanism is characterized by familial, intrauterine dwarfism, large head, triangular facies, anteverted nostrils and full lips.

IX. PSYCHOSOCIAL ETIOLOGY

A. Psychosocial dwarfism is caused by emotional deprivation. A history of bizarre polyphagia and polydipsia is uniformly present. The child is said to have a voracious appetite, to eat "two or three times" as much as his siblings, to feed from garbage cans and to drink water from toilet bowls and other unusual sources. Recovery occurs in the hospital or other emotionally supportive and nurturing environments.

B. Inadequate caloric intake may occur because an infant or young child is not offered enough to eat because of either inadequate parenting or poverty. In early adolescence, growth retardation may occur because of self-imposed diet restrictions owing to fear of obesity.

GENERAL REFERENCES

Felson, B. (ed.): Dwarfs and other little people. Semin. Roentgenol. 8:133, 1973.
Frasier, S. D.: Short stature in children. Pediatr. Rev. 3:171, 1981.
Gotlin, R. W., and Mace, J. W.: Diagnosis and management of short stature in childhood and adolescence. Part I. Curr. Probl. Pediatr. 2:3, 1972.
Rimoin, D. L., and Horton, W. A.: Short stature. Parts I and II. J. Pediatr. 92:523, 697, 1978.
Root, A. W., Bongiovanni, A. M., and Eberlein, W. R.:

Diagnosis and management of growth retardation with special reference to the problem of hypopituitarism. J. Pediatr. 78:737, 1971.

Rosenfeld, R. G.: Evaluation of growth and maturation in adolescence. Pediatr. Rev. 4:175, 1982.

Schaff-Blass, E., Burstein, S., and Rosenfield, R. L.: Diagnosis and treatment of short stature. J. Pediatr. 104:801, 1984.

Smith, D. W.: Growth and Its Disorders. Philadelphia, W.B. Saunders Co., 1977

ETIOLOGIC CLASSIFICATION OF UNDERSTATURE

I. NORMAL VARIANT GROWTH PATTERNS, 280
   A. Normal variant short stature, 280
   B. Normal variant constitutional delay, 281

II. SKELETAL, 281
   A. Constitutional diseases of bone, 281
   B. Osteogenesis imperfecta, 281
   C. Congenital and acquired defects of spine, 281
      1. Multiple hemivertebrae; Klippel-Feil syndrome
      2. Tuberculosis
      3. Cushing's syndrome
      4. Kyphosis, scoliosis
      5. Vertebral collapse
   D. Idiopathic juvenile osteoporosis, 281

III. NUTRITIONAL, 281

IV. SYSTEMIC DISORDERS, 281
   A. Glycogen storage disease, 281
   B. Cystinosis, 281
   C. Galactosemia, 281
   D. Congenital heart disease, 281
   E. Chronic renal disease, 281
   F. Chronic pulmonary disease, 281
   G. Chronic hemolytic and other anemias, 281
   H. Lipoid storage diseases, 281
   I. Bartter's syndrome, 281
   J. Mucopolysaccharidoses, 281
   K. Rickets, 281
   L. Infections, 281
   M. Gastrointestinal disease, 281
      1. Inflammatory bowel disease
      2. Malabsorption syndromes
      3. Hepatitis; cirrhosis; glycogen storage disease
   N. Chronic metabolic acidosis, 282
   O. Hypogammaglobulinemia, 282

V. GENETIC FACTORS, 282
   A. Normal variant growth patterns, 282
   B. Chromosomal abnormalities, 282
      1. Trisomy 13
      2. Trisomy 18
      3. Trisomy 21
      4. Gonadal dysgenesis; Turner's syndrome
      5. Chromosome deletion syndromes
      6. Bloom's syndrome

VI. CENTRAL NERVOUS SYSTEM, 282
   A. Mental retardation, 282
   B. Craniopharyngioma, 282
   C. Glioma of optic chiasm, 282
   D. Pineal tumor, 282
   E. Xanthomatosis, 282

VII. ENDOCRINE, 282
   A. Hypopituitarism, 282
   B. Hypothyroidism, 283
   C. Sexual precocity and virilism, 283
   D. Hypoadrenocorticism, 283
   E. Cushing's syndrome, 283
   F. Poorly controlled diabetes, 283
   G. Pseudohypoparathyroidism, 283
   H. Hyperparathyroidism, 283
   I. Chronic glucocorticoid therapy, 283

VIII. OTHER DISORDERS, 283
   A. Prader-Willi syndrome, 283
   B. Primordial dwarfism, 283
   C. Intrauterine growth retardation, 283
   D. Seckel's syndrome (bird-headed dwarfism), 284
   E. Progeria, 284
   F. Cockayne's syndrome, 284
   G. Pycnodysostosis, 284
   H. Cornelia de Lange's syndrome, 284
   I. Russell-Silver syndrome, 284
   J. Marchesani's syndrome, 284
   K. Laurence-Moon-Biedl syndrome, 284
   L. Leprechaunism, 284
   M. Pseudopseudohypoparathyroidism, 284
   N. Congenital telangiectatic erythema of face, 284
   O. Rothmund-Thomson syndrome, 284
   P. Williams syndrome, 284
   Q. Dubowitz syndrome, 284
   R. 3-M slender-boned nanism, 284

IX. PSYCHOSOCIAL ETIOLOGY, 284
   A. Psychosocial dwarfism, 284
   B. Inadequate caloric intake owing to emotional factors, 284

31 / GIGANTISM, OVERSTATURE

I. CONSTITUTIONAL OR FAMILIAL TALL STATURE may be a concern to adolescent girls whose height is two standard deviations above the mean. "Excessively" tall is a term generally applied to girls over 180 cm (71 in.).

Gardner, L. I.: The child with "excessive" height predication. A clinical dilemma. Am. J. Dis. Child. 129:17, 1975.

Wettenhall, H. N. B., Cahill, C., and Roche, A. F.: Tall girls: A survey of 15 years of management and treatment. J. Pediatr. 86:602, 1975.

II. ACROMEGALIC GIGANTISM owing to excessive growth hormone secretion by a pituitary adenoma is extremely rare in adolescents.

III. SEXUAL PRECOCITY OR VIRILIZATION may cause temporary overstature.

IV. A PRIMARY DEFICIENCY OF PITUITARY GONADOTROPIC OR GONADAL HORMONE may rarely be the cause of gigantism; however, marked overstature is unusual. Delay in epiphyseal fusion results in disproportionately long extremities and span.

V. CEREBRAL GIGANTISM (Sotos' syndrome) is characterized by gigantism, prominent forehead, high-arched palate, hypertelorism, dolichocephaly, mental retardation (in about 80 per cent of patients), large hands and feet, pointed chin, accelerated bone age, poor fine motor control and premature eruption of teeth. These children are large at birth and grow most rapidly in the first four years of life.

Sotos, J. F., Cutler, E. A., and Dodge, P.: Cerebral gigantism. Am. J. Dis. Child. 131:625, 1977.

VI. PATIENTS WITH MARFAN'S syndrome are relatively tall. A marfanoid appearance occurs in patients with homocystinuria or multiple endocrine adenomatosis, a syndrome characterized by mucosal neuroma, medullary thyroid carcinoma and parathyroid adenomas.

VII. HYPERTHYROIDISM may be characterized by acceleration in growth, but the ultimate height of affected children is normal.

VIII. MACROSOMIA with a birth weight over 10 pounds may occur in babies born to diabetic or prediabetic mothers. Cardiac enlargement, hepatomegaly, normoblastemia, lethargy, a weak cry, respiratory distress and a round, plethoric, ruddy or cyanotic face ("tomato face") are characteristic findings. Brawny, generalized, nonpitting edema may be present.

Stevenson, D. K., Hopper, A. O., Cohen, R. S., Bucalo, L. R., Kerner, J. A., and Sunshine, P.: Macrosomia: Causes and consequences. J. Pediatr. 100:515, 1982.

IX. BECKWITH-WIEDEMANN SYNDROME, characterized in part by omphalocele and macroglossia, is a cause of neonatal gigantism. The bone age may be advanced.

X. CONGENITAL LIPODYSTROPHY, a disorder characterized by generalized loss of subcutaneous fat, insulin-resistant diabetes and hepatomegaly, is characterized by accelerated growth and bone age. The hands and feet are enlarged.

XI. CONGENITAL HEMIHYPERTROPHY is accompanied by an increased risk of Wilms' tumor, adrenocortical carcinoma, hepatoblastoma or focal nodular hyperplasia of the liver.

XII. WEAVER-SMITH SYNDROME is characterized by excessive intrauterine growth, gigantism, mental retardation and advanced bone age. Physical findings include megacephaly, widened bifrontal diameter, hypertelorism, large ears, elongated philtrum, micrognathia, campodactyly, broad thumbs and limited extension of the elbows and knees.

Weaver, D. W., Graham, C. B., Thomas, I. T., and Smith, D. W.: A new overgrowth syndrome with accelerated skeletal maturation, unusual facies and campodactyly. J. Pediatr. 84:547, 1974.

XIII. MARSHALL-SMITH SYNDROME is characterized by excessive intrauterine growth, increased length, retardation, blue sclerae, failure to thrive and early death.

Marshall, R. E., Graham, C. B., Scott, C. R., and Smith, D. W.: Syndrome of accelerated skeletal maturation and relative failure to thrive: A newly recognized clinical growth disorder. J. Pediatr. 78:95, 1971.

GENERAL REFERENCE

Reiter, E. O: The "too tall" child. Pediatr. Rev. 5:119, 1983.

32 / SYMPTOMS RELATED TO SEXUAL DEVELOPMENT

NORMAL DEVELOPMENT

The growth rate of the primary sex organs during most of infancy and childhood is extremely slow. Growth of the ovaries is minimal before the age of 8 years. Acceleration of growth then occurs and is especially rapid between 17 and 20 years of age. No significant increase in the size of the uterus occurs until preadolescence. In early life, the uterus is olive- or almond-sized. The cervix constitutes two thirds of the length of the uterus, and the corpus accounts for the remaining third. Because the corpus grows relatively more rapidly than the cervix after the age of 6 years, these relations become reversed. During adolescence the uterus nearly doubles in length. Little growth of the testis occurs before 11 years of age. Growth is rapid between the ages of 12 and 16 years. The sex organs undergo 90 per cent of their final growth during adolescence.

The Tanner criteria to be used in assessing sexual maturation are included on page 70 (breasts), page 101 (genitalia). The time of onset and the chronologic progress of sexual maturation differ not only between boys and girls, but also between adolescents of the same sex. In general, however, sexual growth follows a largely predictable pattern. Variations in timing and sequence are probably attributable to constitutional endocrine patterns.

In some adolescents sexual maturation occurs at an early age; in others, at an average time; and, in still others, relatively late. In adolescents who reach sexual maturity early, the period of maximal growth occurs early and over a short time. Osseous development is relatively advanced. The converse may be true in adolescents who mature late. A small number of normal adolescents may demonstrate an especially early sexual maturation— in girls from 8 to 9 years of age and in boys from 9 to 10 years. Although sexual development at these early ages may be within normal limits, the possibility of abnormal sexual precocity is to be considered and the adolescent observed over a period of time for central nervous system, gonadal or adrenal disorders. At the other extreme, the onset of adolescence may not occur until 16 or 17 years of age. In these instances the possibility of sexual infantilism is to be considered, as well as that of a normal but delayed adolescence.

At puberty, the gonadotropin releasing hormone (Gn-RH) is produced in increased amounts from the so-called hypothalamic *gonadostat*, which, at that time, becomes less sensitive to the negative feedback effects of circulating testosterone or estrogen. Before the onset of puberty, small amounts of these gonadal hormones suppress the hypothalamic-pituitary-gonadal axis. Intrinsic central nervous system inhibitory forces may also suppress Gn-RH synthesis and release. With the resetting of the gonadostat at puberty, release of follicle-stimulating hormone (FSH) and luteinizing hormone (LH) by the pituitary rapidly increases (gonadarche).

In the female, follicle-stimulating hormone supports granulosa cell function and ovum maturation as well as stimulates secretion of estradiol. The luteinizing hormone causes ovulation and the formation of a corpus luteum which elaborates progesterone. When failure of sexual maturation is attributable to hypothalamic or pituitary dysfunction, the excretion of gonadotropins is decreased. The excretion is relatively increased in girls with gonadal deficiency, as in Turner's syndrome, because the production of gonadotropins is not inhibited by the negative feedback produced by circulating estrogen, a hormone that is not secreted in these patients.

In the male, the luteinizing hormone LH (interstitial cell-stimulating hormone) promotes the development of the interstitial or Leydig cells and the production of testicular androgen. Testosterone, in turn, inhibits the production of LH and FSH in the male. The follicle-stimulating hormone leads to the development of the seminiferous tubules and spermatogenesis. In males, the Sertoli-cell protein, inhibin, inhibits FSH secretion. As in the female, the excretion of follicle-stimulating hormone is decreased in patients who have pituitary or hypothalamic disorders. Although often increased, the excretion of follicle-stimulating hormone may be normal or low in patients with testicular tubular deficiency.

The ovarian hormones consist of estrogen and progesterone. Produced by the theca cells of the graafian follicles in response to follicle-stimulating and luteinizing hormones, estrogen produces such female secondary sexual characteristics as development of the breasts, labia minora, uterus, ovaries, fallopian tubes, vaginal cornification, increased vaginal acidity, bone growth and skeletal maturation. Progesterone, produced by the corpus luteum after ovulation, is responsible for the secretory endometrial phase.

A vaginal smear may be examined for cornified epithelial cells as a readily available test for estrogen excretion. Estrogen excretion is increased in patients with granulosa cell tumor of the ovary, some adrenocortical carcinomas and hyperplasias, and chorionepithelioma and during pregnancy. The excretion is diminished in girls with sexual infantilism owing to hypopituitarism or ovarian deficiency.

In the male, androgenic hormones are produced by both the adrenal cortex (about two thirds) and the testes (about one third); in the female, by the adrenals and possibly by the ovaries. Testicular androgen, secreted by the interstitial or Leydig cells in response to the luteinizing hormone, begins to appear between the ages of 11 and 14 years.

The androgenic hormones account for adolescent physical growth and muscular development. In girls, the primary and secondary sexual characteristics that result from androgenic stimulation at puberty include growth of the labia majora and the clitoris, the appearance of axillary and pubic hair and the occurrence of seborrhea and acne. If adrenal androgen is deficient, sexual hair does not appear in the female. In the male, androgens account for the growth of the testes, scrotum, penis, prostate and seminal vesicles; the appearance of pubic, axillary and facial hair; increased sebaceous secretion; and laryngeal enlargement with voice change.

Rosenfield, R. L.: Androgen disorders in children: too much, too early, too little, too late. Pediatr. Rev. 5:147, 1983.

The excretory end-products of both testicular and adrenocortical androgens, known as the urinary 17-ketosteroids, are diminished in patients with hypopituitarism, severe nutritional deprivation, Addison's disease, and, to some extent, in Klinefelter's syndrome. Increased excretion occurs in patients with adrenocortical tumors or hyperplasia and testicular interstitial cell tumors. In patients with sexual precocity of the complete type, the values are increased to those normal for adolescents or adults. Administration of cortisone causes a diminution in the excretion of urinary 17-ketosteroids in patients with congenital adrenal hyperplasia but has no significant effect in the presence of an adrenal tumor.

Recent evidence demonstrates that in the first six months of life, especially in boys, the hypothalamic-pituitary-gonadal axis is active, as shown by increased levels of FSH, LH, testosterone and estrogen. At the age of approximately 7 years in girls and 8 years in boys, a substantial increase in adrenal androgens occurs owing to maturation of the androgenic zone of the adrenal cortex. Such adrenarche reaches the level that leads to the appearance of pubic hair at an average age of 12 ± 1.1 years in girls and 13.5 ± 1.2 years in boys.

Harlan, W. R., Harlan, E. A., and Grillo, G. P.: Secondary sex characteristics of girls 12 to 17 years of age. The U.S. Health Examination Survey. J. Pediatr. 96:1074, 1980.

Harlan, W. R., Grillo, G. P., Cornoni-Huntley, J., and Leaverton, P. E.: Secondary sex characteristics of boys 12 to 17 years of age: The U.S. Health Examination Survey. J. Pediatr. 95:293, 1979.

MENSTRUATION

The menarche occurs, on the average, during the twelfth year. The normal range for this event is between 9 and 16 years with the time of onset of menstruation strongly influenced by genetic factors. Most girls experience their maximal growth just before the menarche. Rapid deceleration in growth then occurs. In general, acceleration and deceleration in height and weight are greater in girls who menstruate early than in those who do so late.

Estrogen leads to endometrial proliferation during the first phase of the menstrual cycle. Ovulation and corpus luteum formation occur about the fourteenth day of the cycle. Progesterone, produced by the corpus luteum, acts synergistically with estrogen to initiate the secretory phase and to terminate the proliferative phase of the premenstrual endometrium. The concentration of progesterone is diminished during the latter part of the secretory phase owing to deterioration of the corpus luteum. Menstruation with loss of the epithelium then occurs about the twenty-eighth day.

Menstruation does not necessarily indicate that ovulation has taken place. Anovulatory periods may continue for a few years after the menarche. Irregularities in amount, (either scanty or excessive), duration or interval of menstruation are common in adolescents, and regularity may not be achieved for two years. Two or more years after the menarche, a positive feedback mechanism becomes established through which the rise in circulating estrogen produced in the maturing ovarian follicle stimulates the increased secretion of gonadotropins, especially luteinizing hormone.

Greydanus, D. E., and McAnarney, E. R.: Menstruation and its disorders in adolescence. Curr. Probl. Pediatr. 12:6, 1982.
Litt, I. F.: Menstrual problems during adolescence. Pediatr. Rev. 4:203, 1983.

AMENORRHEA; OLIGOMENORRHEA

Primary amenorrhea is characterized by failure of the menarche to occur: (1) by 16 years of age; (2) within one year of the menarchal age of the adolescent's mother or female siblings; or (3) within two years of the appearance of secondary sexual characteristics. The causes for primary amenorrhea include those for delayed sexual maturation or sexual infantilism listed on page 296, polycystic ovaries and, rarely, pregnancy. Female gymnasts, ballet dancers and patients with anorexia nervosa may have a delayed menarche.

Secondary amenorrhea is characterized by the absence of a menstrual period for three to six months after a regular cycle has been established. The causes for secondary amenorrhea include:

1. Acute weight loss, including anorexia nervosa
2. Psychologic stressors
3. Chronic illness
4. Pregnancy
5. Polycystic ovary syndrome in adolescents is usually manifest initially by oligomenorrhea or secondary amenorrhea. Acne, hirsutism, infertility and enlarged ovaries may be evident later. The serum FSH level is normal, but LH is elevated. Androgen excess may be evaluated by a morning plasma testosterone level.
6. Hypothalamic or pituitary tumors and disorders, including elevated prolactin levels, may cause secondary amenorrhea. Galactorrhea may occur.
7. Postpill amenorrhea may occur in adolescents who have used oral contraceptives before their normal hypothalamic rhythm has been established.
8. Drug-induced amenorrhea

Laboratory evaluation of amenorrhea may include T_4, TSH, a pregnancy test, serum LH, FSH and prolactin levels, bone age, sedimentation rate and skull roentgenogram.

Brown, D. M.: Multiple hypothalamic-pituitary abnormalities in an adolescent girl with galactorrhea. J. Pediatr. 91:901, 1977.
Emans, S. J., Grace, E., and Goldstein, D. P.: Oligomenorrhea in adolescent girls. J. Pediatr. 97:815, 1980.

DYSFUNCTIONAL BLEEDING

Dysfunctional bleeding is present in adolescent girls: (1) when the menstrual period lasts longer than seven days or is excessive (menorrhagia) but occurs at regular intervals; (2) when the menstrual bleeding occurs at irregular intervals (metrorrhagia); or (3) when menstruation occurs at frequent but irregular intervals (menometrorrhagia). In most cases, the dysfunctional bleeding is attributable to anovulatory cycles or absence of the preovulatory rise in luteinizing hormone so that the progesterone effect on the endometrium is minimal or absent. Irregular, excessive or prolonged menstrual flow results. Other causes of dysfunctional bleeding include a granulosa cell tumor, the polycystic ovary syndrome, systemic hemorrhagic states, (e.g., idiopathic thrombocytopenic purpura or von Willebrand's syndrome), adenocarcinoma of the genital tract, vaginal foreign body and hypothyroidism.

DYSMENORRHEA

Dysmenorrhea is characterized by lower abdominal cramping or severe pain during the menstrual period. Nausea, vomiting, headaches, muscle cramps and diarrhea may also occur. Menstruation may not be accompanied by pain during the first 4 to 18 months after the menarche, since cramps often are not experienced before the onset of ovulation. Painful menstruation may also be attributable to endometriosis, presence of an intrauterine device, pelvic inflammatory disease or a structural anomaly of the uterus.

PREMENSTRUAL SYNDROME

The signs and symptoms of the premenstrual syndrome include edema, bloating, headache, emotional lability, changes in appetite, constipation, breast swelling, breast tenderness and decreased concentration.

Vaitukaitis, J. L.: Premenstrual syndrome. N. Engl. J. Med. 311:1371, 1984.

SEXUAL PRECOCITY

The lower limits for the normal onset of puberty are eight years of age in girls and nine and one-half years in boys. Development of secondary sexual characteristics before these ages warrants investigation. Sexual precocity may be isosexual, the result of increased androgen production in the male or of estrogen in the female, or heterosexual, with virilization of the female or feminization of the male. In complete or true precocious puberty, sexual development simulates that which occurs normally at adolescence, with development of the gonads leading to spermatogenesis in the male and ovulation in the female. Rarely, a

patient with true sexual precocity may not demonstrate complete precocity.

In patients with incomplete precocity or pseudoprecocity, the uninvolved testis or ovary remains infantile in size and function. Although primary and secondary sexual characteristics develop, spermatogenesis and ovulation do not. Patients with heterosexual precocity and those with isosexual precocity owing to gonadal or adrenal lesions have incomplete precocity. In general, the androgen and estrogen levels in true or complete sexual precocity are normal for the patient's physiologic age. In the incomplete form, these values are usually excessive. Emotional development, intellectual progression and the dental age in sexually precocious children correspond more to chronologic than physiologic age.

ETIOLOGIC CLASSIFICATION OF SEXUAL PRECOCITY

I. Isosexual Male Precocity

A. Physiologic or constitutional idiopathic precocity is the most frequent type of isosexual precocity, accounting for 60 to 70 per cent of instances in boys. The mechanism responsible for the onset of adolescence and release of the pituitary gonadotropins becomes activated at an unusually early age, perhaps owing to constitutional or genetic factors. Early pubescence may represent a familial pattern. Normal pubertal growth of the genitalia occurs, secondary sexual characteristics appear, spermatozoa are produced, and normal adult stature is attained. The excretion of sex hormones reaches normal adolescent values. Although initial investigation may reveal no evidence of cerebral, adrenal or testicular disease, periodic reexaminations are indicated.

B. Central nervous system lesions lead to premature secretion of gonadotropin-releasing factor and pituitary gonadotropins and to true sexual precocity with a normal growth pattern of the primary sex organs, the appearance of secondary sexual characteristics and spermatogenesis. Early diagnosis may be difficult because the lesion is often very small and slow-growing.
1. Brain tumors such as hamartomas, gliomas, astrocytomas, ependymomas and cysts may lead to sexual precocity through direct or indirect involvement of the hypothalamus

and floor of the third ventricle. Pineal tumors may cause sexual precocity in boys.

2. Sequelae of encephalitis or meningitis
3. Congenital defects of the hypothalamus
4. Tuberous sclerosis
5. Tuberculoma involving the hypothalamus
6. McCune-Albright syndrome is characterized by bone lesions and café-au-lait spots.

C. Gonadal tumors cause incomplete sexual precocity. The uninvolved testis remains infantile in size, and spermatozoa are not prematurely produced. Secondary sexual characteristics may appear.

1. Interstitial or Leydig cell tumor of the testis, an extremely rare lesion, presents either as a firm, hard nodule in an enlarged testis or as a generalized enlargement of the testis. The excretion of 17-ketosteroids is increased. Adrenal "rest" cells present in the testes of patients with congenital virilizing adrenal hyperplasia may cause palpable testicular masses that can be mistaken for an interstitial cell tumor. Administration of cortisone causes regression of the masses and a fall in 17-ketosteroid output in the former but not the latter.
2. Teratoma of the testis has been reported as a cause of sexual precocity in one case.

D. Hypothyroidism may be an unusual cause of precocious puberty.

Hemady, Z. S., Siler-Khodr, T. M., and Najjar, S.: Precocious puberty in juvenile hypothyroidism. J. Pediatr. 92:55, 1978.

E. Adrenal lesions cause incomplete sexual precocity. The testes remain infantile in size, unless they contain aberrant adrenal tissue, and premature spermatogenesis does not occur. Usually the excretion of 17-ketosteroids is increased, but the absence of such elevation does not exclude a virilizing adrenal tumor.

1. Adrenocortical virilizing hyperplasia. The clinical characteristics of untreated congenital virilizing adrenal hyperplasia in the male include early enlargement of the penis and prostate, appearance of pubic and axillary hair, acne, rapid somatic growth, unusual muscular development, advanced bone age with early epiphyseal fusion and deepening of the voice. Although the genitalia may appear large at birth, they may not increase in size noticeably until two or three years of age.
2. The excretion of 17-ketosteroids in patients with an adrenocortical tumor does not decrease in response to cortisone administration as in patients with congenital adrenocortical hyperplasia. A large output of dehydroisoandrosterone or other 3-beta hydroxyketosteroids suggests the presence of an adrenal neoplasm.

F. Chorionic gonadotropin-producing tumors. True isosexual precocity has been described in boys with a sacrococcygeal teratoma, hepatoblastoma, intracranial teratoma, retroperitoneal carcinoma or thoracic polyembryoma.

Danon, M., Weintraub, B. D., Kim, S. H., Scully, R. E., and Crawford, J. D.: Sexual precocity in a male due to thoracic polyembroma. J. Pediatr. 92:51, 1978.

G. Precocious pseudopuberty or premature adrenarche is characterized by the appearance of sexual hair, usually pubic but at times axillary, in boys under 10 years of age. Endocrine studies are indicated to rule out a virilizing disorder. If the bone age is not advanced by more than one year, the pubarche is attributable to premature adrenarche.

Rosenfield, R. L., Rich, B. H., and Lucky, A. W.: Adrenarche as a cause of benign pseudopuberty in boys. J. Pediatr.101:1005, 1982.

H. Male limited familial precocious puberty may be characterized by extremely rapid virilization, especially manifested by enlarged penile size but with the testicular volume characteristic of early puberty. Increased gonadal testosterone secretion appears to be gonadotropin-independent.

Holland, F. J., Fishman, L., Bailey, J. D., and Fazekas, T. A.: Ketoconazole in the management of precocious puberty not responsive to LHRH-analogue therapy. N. Engl. J. Med. 312:1023, 1985.

Reiter, E. O., Brown, R. S., Longcope, C., and Beitins, I. Z.: Male-limited familial precocious puberty in three generations. N. Engl. J. Med. 311:515, 1984.

Rosenthal, S. M., Grumbach, M. M., and Kaplan, S. L.: Gonadotropin-independent familial sexual precocity with premature Leydig and germinal cell maturation (familial testotoxicosis): Effects of a potent luteinizing hormone–releasing factor agonist and medroxyprogesterone acetate therapy in four cases. J. Clin. Endocrinol. Metab. 57:571, 1983.

Wierman, M. E., et al.: Puberty without gonadotropins. N. Engl. J. Med. 312:1, 1985.

II. Isosexual Female Precocity

A. Physiologic, constitutional, idiopathic precocity. Eighty-five to 90 per cent of girls with sexual precocity may be placed in this category. Sexual precocity is complete, with normal maturation of the ovaries, ovulatory menstrual cycles and excretion of sex hormones at levels that are normal for the girl's physiologic rather than chronologic age.

B. Central nervous system lesions cause complete sexual precocity.
   1. With the exception of pineal tumors, intracranial lesions that cause isosexual precocity in the male may also lead to sexual precocity in the female.
   2. The McCune-Albright syndrome, or polyostotic fibrous dysplasia, is characterized by skin pigmentation and sexual precocity.
   3. Silver's syndrome consists of sexual precocity, hemihypertrophy, short stature and elevated gonadotropins.

C. Gonadal tumors. Sexual precocity owing to gonadal causes is not accompanied by ovulation. Secondary sexual characteristics influenced by estrogen secretion develop prematurely.
   1. Granulosa cell tumors lead to the development of secondary sexual characteristics. The sexual hair and advanced physical growth are probably attributable to adrenocortical activity, perhaps effected by the action of estrogen on the pituitary. The bone age also may be advanced. A whitish vaginal discharge, at times periodic, may be the first clinical symptom. Vaginal bleeding, which occurs later, may resemble irregular, scanty or profuse menstrual cycles. Vaginal bleeding may occur before, concomitantly with or after the development of other sexual characteristics. Estrogen excretion is increased. An abdominal or pelvic mass may be present.
   2. Follicle cysts
   3. Large luteinized ovarian cysts may cause incomplete sexual precocity or transient vaginal bleeding.
   4. Teratoma
   5. Chorionepithelioma

Towne, B. H., Mahour, G. H., Wooley, M. M., and Isaacs, H., Jr.: Ovarian cysts and tumors in infancy and childhood. J. Pediatr. Surg. 10:311, 1975.

D. Medicational precocity. Pseudoprecocious puberty may result from the accidental ingestion of stilbestrol. The areolae and nipples in such instances are deeply pigmented.

E. Hypothyroidism may be accompanied by a syndrome characterized by precocious menstruation, galactorrhea, absence of pubic hair, enlargement of the sella turcica and retarded skeletal age. Multicystic ovaries may be present. These findings disappear after thyroid therapy.

Lindsay, A. N., Voorhess, M. L., and MacGillivray, M. H.: Multicystic ovaries detected by sonography in children with hypothyroidism. Am. J. Dis. Child. 134:588, 1980.

F. Pseudoprecocious puberty
   1. Premature thelarche. See page 71.
   2. Premature pubarche is characterized by the appearance of pubic hair before eight and one-half years of age. See page 188.

DIAGNOSTIC APPROACH TO ISOSEXUAL PRECOCITY

I. History and Physical Examination

A. History and physical findings of precocious sexual development with secondary sexual characteristics, enlargement of primary sex organs and acceleration of physical and osseous development. In girls, the possibility of accidental ingestion of estrogen should be investigated.

B. Symptoms of intracranial lesions: headache, vomiting, visual disturbances, behavioral changes, polydipsia, polyphagia or obesity.

C. Signs of an intracranial lesion: papilledema, optic atrophy, visual field defects and head enlargement. A pineal neoplasm may cause strabismus, Argyll Robertson pupils and inability to look upward.

D. Other pertinent aspects of the physical examination include abdominal and rectal examination for the presence of an ovarian tumor; examination of the testes for physiologic or pathologic enlargement; and inspection of the skin for the pigmentation characteristic of the McCune-Albright syndrome.

II. Roentgenographic Examinations

A. Skull films
   1. Calcification of tumor masses. Calcification of the pineal gland may occur normally in a small number of children.

2. Spreading of sutures
3. Computerized tomography is indicated in children with isosexual precocity.
B. Bone age
C. Skeletal roentgenograms for polyostotic fibrous dysplasia
D. Intravenous pyelogram for evidence of renal displacement by an adrenal mass

III. HORMONE DETERMINATIONS. Adolescent hormone levels (gonadotropin, estrogen and 17-ketosteroids) are present in patients with complete precocity. Excessive values are noted in patients with incomplete precocity.

IV. SURGICAL EXPLORATION if the patient is thought to have a neoplasm of the gonads or adrenals. Testicular biopsy may be helpful in the differentiation between true sexual precocity and that owing to adrenal lesions. Development of interstitial cells occurs in the former but not the latter.

ETIOLOGIC CLASSIFICATION OF INTERSEXUAL DEVELOPMENT

I. FEMALE PSEUDOHERMAPHRODITISM

A. Female pseudohermaphroditism owing to congenital virilizing adrenal hyperplasia is transmitted as an autosomal recessive trait. In these sex chromatin–positive infants, the uterus, fallopian tubes and upper vagina develop as in other females; however, varying degrees of masculinization of the external genitalia occur. The phallus, which is enlarged at birth, often resembles a penis with hypospadias and chordee. Fusion of the labioscrotal folds ranges from none or minimal with separate urethral and vaginal orifices to the more common situation in which the fusion extends anteriorly, and the urethra and vagina open into a urogenital sinus. A penile urethra occurs in a few cases. When diagnosis and treatment have not been established in infancy, sexual and body hair, acne, and deepening of the voice may appear early. Physical, osseous and muscular growth is also accelerated. Because epiphyseal fusion occurs early, such children are ultimately relatively understatured.

Almost all instances of this syndrome are attributable to 21-hydroxylase deficiency. In about one third of these children, aldosterone deficiency occurs with a resultant salt-losing tendency. Dehy-dration, vomiting and circulatory collapse and, perhaps, diarrhea may occur. Hypertension has been reported as a result of increased production of 11-deoxycorticosteroids.

Differentiation between female pseudohermaphroditism owing to congenital virilizing adrenal hyperplasia and that of nonadrenal etiology should be established promptly on the basis of the urinary excretion of 17-ketosteroids and pregnanetriol or by the radioimmunoassay of plasma 17P (17alpha-hydroxy-progesterone). Early in life, the normal value for urinary 17-ketosteroid excretion may be as high as 2.5 mg per 24 hours; but after 2 weeks, it is under 0.5 mg per day. Usually, values of 2 to 5 mg per 24 hours are found in patients with congenital virilizing adrenal hyperplasia. When the 17-ketosteroid value is in the nondiagnostic range (less than 2 mg per 24 hours), demonstration of urinary pregnanetriol offers confirmation. Cortisone causes a diminution in the production of adrenal androgen and in the excretion of 17-ketosteroids.

B. Nonadrenal female pseudohermaphroditism. Partial embryonic masculinization of the external genitalia may occur in female infants whose mothers received synthetic progestogens during pregnancy. Enlargement of the phallus and varying degrees of fusion of the labioscrotal folds may be produced. Differentiation from congenital virilizing adrenal hyperplasia is based on the absence of increased excretion of urinary 17-ketosteroids and failure of progressive virilization. The buccal smear demonstrates a female chromatin pattern. When masculinization has been substantial, differentiation from true hermaphroditism may not be possible without an exploratory laparotomy. Such exploration is unnecessary when the mother's history indicates that she received androgens or synthetic oral progestogens during the early months of pregnancy. In other cases, no clear explanation for the occurrence of nonadrenal female pseudohermaphroditism is apparent.
C. Postnatal virilization during the first decade of life is usually attributable to an adrenal tumor. After the age of 10 or 12 years, virilization may be caused by either a tumor or adrenocortical hyperplasia.
D. Postnatal adrenal hyperplasia
E. Arrhenoblastoma is the most common androgen-producing tumor of the ovary.

II. MALE PSEUDOHERMAPHRODITISM

Much progress has been made in understanding male pseudohermaphroditism in recent years, but the subject remains complex. These individuals with a Y chromosome have testes and a portion or all of the müllerian (female) duct system. The external genitalia may resemble those of a female or male or may be ambiguous. The anatomic features vary widely. Except for the presence of testes, some of these children may resemble those with female pseudohermaphroditism owing to congenital virilizing adrenal hyperplasia. The scrotum may be cleft and resemble labia. Other physical findings include microphallus, undescended testes, hypospadias and partial vaginal orifice. Acceleration of physical development and bone age do not occur. The excretion of 17-ketosteroids is not increased. The secondary sexual characteristics may be either male or female. Gynecomastia is common.

A. Male pseudohermaphroditism may result from an autosomal recessive defect associated with decreased secretion of testosterone owing to deficiency of one of the five enzymes necessary for testosterone biosynthesis.

B. Testicular feminization syndrome, an X-linked recessive disorder attributable to abnormal androgen receptors, occurs in phenotypic females. Testes, which are present bilaterally, may appear as inguinal or labial masses. The uterus and cervix are absent. Breast development occurs at puberty, but pubic and axillary hair are absent or scant, and menstruation does not occur. These patients have a 46XY karyotype.

C. Persistent müllerian duct syndrome (hernia uteri inguinali), a recessive disorder owing to deficiency of anti-müllerian hormone, is characterized by female internal genitalia in otherwise normal appearing males.

D. Mixed gonadal dysgenesis, with a streak gonad on one side and a testis on the other, is associated with 45X/46XX mosaicism. The external genitalia appear only minimally masculinized at birth, but heterosexual virilization occurs at puberty. Some patients present with the Turner phenotype.

E. Other disorders of incomplete male pseudohermaphroditism, inherited as an X-linked recessive trait and resulting from a single mutant, are variably expressed along a spectrum extending from nearly complete failure of virilization to almost complete masculinization. Included in this group are the syndrome described by Lubs (which resembles testicular feminization in some respects) and those reported by Reifenstein (with perineoscrotal hypospadias), Gilbert-Dreyfus and Rosewater.

Wilson, J. D., Harrod, M. J., Goldstein, J. L., Hemsell, D. L., and MacDonald, P. D.: Familial incomplete pseudohermaphroditism, type 1. N. Engl. J. Med. 290:1097, 1974.

F. Pseudovaginal hypospadias, inherited as an autosomal recessive trait and associated with testicular 17-ketosteroid reductase deficiency, resembles the Reifenstein syndrome, except that gynecomastia does not develop.

G. Congenital gonadotropin deficiency may be associated with microphallus and hypospadias.

H. Males with a first- or second-degree hypospadias and radioulnar synostosis may have a sex chromosome abnormality.

I. Patients with pure Leydig cell aplasia appear as females with labial testes. The uterus and related anatomic structures are absent.

Eddy, A. A., and Mauer, S. M.: Pseudohermaphroditism glomerulopathy, and Wilms' tumor (Drash syndrome): Frequency in end-stage renal failure. J. Pediatr. 106:584, 1985.

Grumbach, M. M., and VanWyk, J. J.: Disorders of sex differentiation. In Williams, R. H. (ed.): Textbook of Endocrinology. 5th ed. Philadelphia, W. B. Saunders Co., 1974, pp. 423–501.

Imperato-McGinley, J., and Peterson, R. E.: Male pseudohermaphroditism: The complexities of male phenotypic development. Am. J. Med. 61:251, 1976.

Levy, D. J., Levine, L. S., and New, M. I.: Male pseudohermaphroditism. Pediatr. Rev. 3:273, 1982.

Opitz, J. M., Simpson, J. L., and Sarto, G. E.: Pseudovaginal perineoscrotal hypospadias. Clin. Genet. 3:1, 1972.

III. TRUE HERMAPHRODITISM

The external genitalia in these children may appear ambisexual. Both gonads are usually intra-abdominal. Hypospadias and cryptorchidism offer diagnostic clues. In adolescence, gynecomastia is common in true hermaphrodites, and the majority of these patients menstruate. Most are chromatin positive, but some are mosaics. The patient may have one ovary and one testis, one ovotestis, or an ovary and a testis on one side and either an ovary or a testis on the other.

DIAGNOSTIC APPROACH TO INTERSEXUAL DEVELOPMENT

The psychologic and psychosocial orientation of patients with hermaphroditism corresponds to the gender of their rearing rather than to anatomic or hormonal considerations. A decision must be made, therefore, as to the child's gender of rearing within a few days after birth, with the child's functional genital anatomy a major determinant. Careful diagnostic appraisal is indicated in infants with clearly ambiguous external genitalia, with either hypospadias or testes that cannot be palpated and in those with female external genitalia but with palpable masses in the labia or inguinal regions. Anatomic studies, including surgical exploration and biopsy of the gonads, may be indicated in infants shown not to have congenital virilizing adrenal hyperplasia.

I. PHYSICAL EXAMINATION directed toward the establishment of anatomic relations and structure through inspection of the external genitalia, abdominal palpation, palpation of the inguinal region, labia or scrotum, and rectal examination. The orifice at the base of the phallus should be examined to determine whether it represents urethral meatus or urogenital sinus and whether a communication is present between the urethra and the vagina. Urethroscopic examination may be necessary to demonstrate the vagina and cervix.

II. CHROMOSOMAL DETERMINATIONS. In the normal female newborn in the first two weeks of life, the percentage of chromatin-positive cells found may be low. Babies with congenital adrenal hyperplasia may also have low Barr body or sex chromatin counts. A buccal mucosal smear with Y fluorescence may be a helpful screening device in the study of abnormalities of sexual differentiation; however, in patients with abnormal sexual differentiation, a chromatin- or Barr body–positive pattern and absent Y fluorescence restricts diagnostic considerations to either female pseudohermaphroditism or true hermaphroditism. A chromatin-negative pattern with positive Y fluorescence is consistent with male pseudohermaphroditism. In the absence of both Barr bodies and Y fluorescence, a variant of mixed gonadal dysgenesis is present.

III. ROENTGENOGRAPHIC STUDIES

A. A genitogram is helpful in delineating the internal genital anatomy.

B. Calcification in an adrenal tumor or other neoplasm may be demonstrated.
C. An intravenous pyelogram may show displacement of the kidney downward and anteriorly by an adrenal tumor.

IV. HORMONAL DETERMINATIONS. The excretion of the 17-ketosteroids is abnormally increased in patients with adrenocortical hyperplasia or tumor. The excretion of large amounts (over 50 mg a day) of the 17-ketosteroids is presumptive but not absolute evidence for the presence of a tumor. An increase in the 3-beta-hydroxy 17-ketosteroids has a similar connotation. The finding of increased amounts of dehydroepiandrosterone in the urine is suggestive evidence for an adrenal tumor. Patients with congenital or postnatal adrenal hyperplasia demonstrate a significant reduction in 17-ketosteroid excretion within seven to ten days after the initiation of cortisone treatment. A similar sustained fall does not occur with an adrenal tumor. Radioimmunoassay of plasma 17P (17alpha-hydroxyprogesterone) is replacing urinary 17-ketosteroids in the diagnosis of congenital adrenal hyperplasia.

In other types of intersex, elevated levels of androgen or estrogen do not occur before puberty.

Testosterone response to human chorionic gonadotropin (hCG) may be used to determine the presence of functional testes.

V. SURGICAL EXPLORATION and possibly gonadal biopsy may be necessary for diagnosis.

Lippe, B. M.: Ambiguous genitalia and pseudohermaphroditism. Pediatr. Clin. North Am. 26:91, 1979.

Rosenfield, R. L., Lucky, A. W., and Allen, T. D.: The diagnosis and management of intersex. Curr. Probl. Pediatr. 10:4, 1980.

Saenger, P.: Abnormal sex differentiation. J. Pediatr. 104:1, 1984.

DELAYED SEXUAL MATURATION; SEXUAL INFANTILISM

In general, evidence of sexual development should appear in girls by the age of 15 or 16 years and in boys by 16 to 17 years. This permits a distinction to be made between a late onset of normal adolescence and true sexual infantilism. Constitutional delay in sexual development, more common in boys than girls, is accompanied by short stature, discussed on page 281, normal growth velocity and bone age commensurate with height age. The adolescent growth spurt is delayed.

ETIOLOGIC CLASSIFICATION OF DELAYED SEXUAL MATURATION: SEXUAL INFANTILISM

I. Central (Hypogonadotropic Hypogonadism)

A. The clinical picture in patients with sexual infantilism owing to hypopituitarism (panhypopituitarism, partial pituitary sufficiency; deficiency of pituitary gonadotropins) is determined by whether the deficiency is limited to the pituitary gonadotropins or other tropic hormones are involved; thus, sexual hair appears, though perhaps in diminished amount, in patients with normal adrenocorticotropic activity. The excretion of 17-ketosteroids is only moderately decreased or corresponds to what would be normal for the female. Abnormalities of the hypothalamic-pituitary axis are characterized by low serum levels of luteinizing hormone and follicle-stimulating hormone. Serum testosterone levels should be obtained in males and estradiol in females. A high concordance exists between bone age and sexual maturation. Delay in both sexual development and skeletal age suggests constitutionally delayed puberty.

Varying degrees of failure of sexual development may occur. In the male, the testes may show some development, but never reach normal mature size. Usually spermatogenesis does not appear in the male, and amenorrhea or irregular and scanty menstruation is noted in the female. Excretion of follicle-stimulating hormone is decreased or absent. If other tropic hormones are deficient, growth retardation, absence of sexual hair and hypoglycemia may be noted.

B. Involvement of the hypothalamus may lead to a deficiency of gonadotropin-releasing hormone.
1. Failure of sexual development may be attributable to a suprasellar cyst, glioma, craniopharyngioma or other intracranial tumor that involves the hypothalamus. Hypothalamic involvement may also occur with trauma, encephalitis or sarcoidosis.
2. The sexual infantilism in the Laurence-Moon-Biedl syndrome probably represents a genetically determined hypothalamic defect.
3. Kallmann's syndrome, owing to an isolated deficiency of gonadotropin-releasing factor, is characterized by hypogonadotropic hypogonadism, anosmia or hyposmia and color blindness. Small testes, eunuchoid body proportions, and a micropenis are present in the male; in girls, the external genitalia are normal, but breast development does not occur. The olfactory function should be evaluated in patients with hypogonadism.
4. The Prader-Willi syndrome consists of hypogonadism, which is presumably hypothalamic, obesity and mental retardation.
5. Midline central nervous system defects such as cleft palate and septo-optic dysplasia
6. Vasquez syndrome is characterized by hypogonadism, obesity, short stature and mental retardation.
7. Alstrom's syndrome is manifested by hypogonadism, mental retardation, obesity and understature.

C. Delayed puberty and sexual maturation associated with chronic disease and handicapping disorders
1. Hemoglobinopathies
    a. Puberty may be delayed until 15 to 17 years in girls and 16 to 18 years in boys with sickle cell disease.
    b. Puberty is usually delayed in girls with thalassemia major and may not occur in boys without appropriate use of blood transfusions.
2. Inflammatory bowel disease
3. Adolescents who are mentally retarded may experience delayed sexual development.
4. Anorexia nervosa
5. Chronic pulmonary disease such as cystic fibrosis
6. Chronic renal failure
7. Malignancy
8. Connective tissue disease
9. Hypothyroidism
10. Diabetes
11. Severe obesity
12. Chronic aggressive hepatitis

II. Gonadal (Hypergonadotropic Hypogonadism)

When gonadotropins are present in the urine of sexually immature patients, especially when the values are above normal, the secretion of pituitary gonadotropins may be considered to be adequate. The problem then is one of inadequate gonadal function as reflected in urinary and plasma levels of the sex steroids.

A. Testes

Biopsy and the determination of follicle-stimulating hormone excretion are usually required for a diagnosis of testicular deficiency. As a rule, the excretion of follicle-stimulating hormone is increased. Testicular function may be impaired in the following situations.

1. Congenital absence of testis; congenital anorchia; testicular hypoplasia
2. Congenital deficiency of the interstitial cells of Leydig
3. Surgical castration
4. Trauma
5. Hemorrhage
6. Infection, mumps
7. Torsion of the spermatic cord
8. Idiopathic fibrosis
9. Except for gynecomastia in some patients with Klinefelter's syndrome, the secondary sexual characteristics are normal. The testes are small (less than 1.5 cm) and firm. Spermatogenesis does not occur. The body habitus may be eunuchoid or normal male. Urinary gonadotropin excretion is increased. Plasma testosterone levels are intermediate between male and female values. Karyotyping should be obtained in prepubertal boys with abnormally small or hard testes, those with cryptorchidism and adolescents with gynecomastia. The most common karyotype in Klinefelter's syndrome is 47XXY. Other karyotypes are XXYY or XXXY and XXXYY or XXXXY. The most frequent mosaic pattern is XY/XXY. Generally, the more X chromosomes present in a male, the greater the degree of mental retardation. Klinefelter's syndrome is difficult to diagnose clinically before puberty.

Caldwell, P. D., and Smith, D. W.: The XXY (Klinefelter's) syndrome in childhood: Detection and treatment. J. Pediatr. 80:250, 1972.

10. Weinstein's syndrome is characterized by hyalinization of seminiferous tubules, obesity, blindness, nerve deafness and hyperuricemia.

B. Ovaries
1. Gonadal dysgenesis (Turner's syndrome) in phenotypic females is characterized by moderately short stature (less than 5 feet), primary amenorrhea, webbing of the neck, high arched palate, congenital lymphedema of the hands and feet, coarctation of the aorta, short fourth metacarpal, multiple nevi, horseshoe kidney, cubitus valgus, shieldlike chest and recurrent melena. Phenotypic females with stigmata of Turner's syndrome but with bilateral streak gonads and sexual infantilism have pure gonadal dysgenesis. Patients with a mosaic karyotype demonstrate fewer signs of Turner's syndrome. A few patients have some degree of masculinization. The typical chromosomal finding is 45X, but a number of other cytogenetic constitutions occur in these patients. The most frequent mosaicism is 45X/46XY. Some patients with Turner's syndrome may have a normal karyotype. A Barr body count, blood karyotype, including H-Y antigen and serum gonadotropin determination by RIA are indicated when the diagnosis is suspected.

Tho, P. T., and McDonough, P. G.: Gonadal dysgenesis and its variants. Pediatr. Clin. North Am. 28:309, 1981.

2. Ovarian degeneration following disease or radiation
3. Premature menopause is extremely rare.
4. The gonadotropin-resistant ovary syndrome, with elevated gonadotropin and low estrogen levels, is characterized by amenorrhea, infertility and normal secondary sexual characteristics.

C. Congenital absence of uterus or vagina or both

III. OTHER ENDOCRINE DISORDERS

A. Hypothyroidism may be characterized by hypogonadism.
B. Delay in sexual maturation is less common in patients with hyperthyroidism.
C. Cushing's syndrome may also be accompanied by sexual retardation.

CROSS-GENDER BEHAVIOR

Cross-gender behavior is usually not a presenting complaint in girls because the "masculine" interests demonstrated by the "tomboy girl" are more admired than scorned. "Effeminate" behavior in the school-aged or adolescent boy may be a reason for consultation. Some cross-gender behavior may be a normal developmental variation. In other cases, the boy openly admits his wish to be a girl, frequently dresses up in women's clothing, wears cosmetics, takes interest in women's fashions, chooses girls for playmates, avoids "boy's" games, plays with dolls and demonstrates exaggerated "feminine" mannerisms, gait and gestures.

GENERAL REFERENCES

Gardner, L. I. (ed.): Endocrine and Genetic Diseases of Childhood and Adolescence, 2nd ed. Philadelphia, W. B. Saunders Co., 1975.

Root, A. W.: Endocrinology of puberty. I. Normal sexual maturation. II. Aberrations of sexual maturation. J. Pediatr. 83:1, 187, 1973.

Rosenfeld, R. G.: Evaluation of growth and maturation in adolescence. Pediatr. Rev. 4:175, 1982.

Rosenfield, R. L.: Androgen disorders in children: Too much, too early, too little, or too late. Pediatr. Rev. 5:147, 1983.

Sizonenko, P. C.: Endocrinology in preadolescents and adolescents. I. Hormonal changes during normal puberty. Am. J. Dis. Child. 132:794, 1978.

Sizonenko, P. C.: Preadolescent and adolescent endocrinology: Physiology and physiopathology. II. Hormonal changes during abnormal pubertal development. Am. J. Dis. Child. 132:797, 1978.

ETIOLOGIC CLASSIFICATION OF SEXUAL PRECOCITY

ETIOLOGIC CLASSIFICATION OF INTERSEXUAL DEVELOPMENT

ETIOLOGIC CLASSIFICATION OF DELAYED SEXUAL MATURATION; SEXUAL INFANTILISM

I. CENTRAL, 296
  A. Hypopituitarism, 296
  B. Deficiency of gonadotropin-releasing hormone and of pituitary gonadotropins, 296
    1. Intracranial tumors involving the hypothalamus
    2. Laurence-Moon-Biedl syndrome
    3. Kallmann's syndrome
    4. Prader-Willi syndrome
    5. Midline central nervous system defect
    6. Vasquez syndrome
    7. Alstrom's syndrome
  C. Chronic disease, 296
II. GONADAL, 296
  A. Testes, 297
    1. Congenital absence; congenital anorchia; testicular hypoplasia
    2. Congenital deficiency of interstitial Leydig cells
    3. Surgical castration

    4. Trauma
    5. Hemorrhage
    6. Infection, mumps
    7. Torsion of spermatic cord
    8. Idiopathic fibrosis
    9. Klinefelter's syndrome
    10. Weinstein's syndrome
  B. Ovaries, 297
    1. Gonadal dysgenesis
    2. Ovarian degeneration
    3. Premature menopause
    4. Gonadotropin-resistant ovary
  C. Congenital absence of uterus or vagina or both, 297
III. OTHER ENDOCRINE DISORDERS, 297
  A. Hypothyroidism, 297
  B. Hyperthyroidism, 297
  C. Cushing's syndrome, 297

33 / OBESITY

Obesity, defined as excessive subcutaneous fat, is diagnosed on the basis of visual assessment or a skinfold thickness that exceeds two standard deviations above the mean for age as measured by calipers in the triceps and subscapular areas. Although present in infants and young children, obesity is more frequent at the end of the first decade and during adolescence. The subcutaneous tissue is normally thicker during infancy and adolescence than in the preschool or school-age periods. Weight for height above the 95th percentile is generally considered to characterize obesity in preschool children. In adolescents, weight for height is less helpful in defining obesity because of the effect of sexual maturation on body weight.

Garn, S. M., and Clark, D. C.: Trends in fatness and the origins of obesity. Pediatrics 57:443, 1976.

ETIOLOGIC CLASSIFICATION OF OBESITY

I. GENERAL CAUSES

A. Obesity in childhood is rarely an endocrine disorder. Obese children generally demonstrate normal or relatively accelerated growth and development, and they may experience an early adolescence.

B. The physical explanation for obesity is usually a direct one: the child's caloric intake exceeds his energy expenditure. In addition to an excessive food intake, obese children may have a rapid eating pattern. The child who gains weight excessively may be less active than children or expend less energy in other daily activities such as walking. The term *Pickwickian syndrome* may be applied to patients whose obesity is accompanied by alveolar hypoventilation, arterial hypoxemia, polycythemia and somnolence.

C. Both the parents and the child may disclaim excessive food intake because of a misconception of what constitutes an excessive amount of food.

D. No evidence exists that the specific dynamic action of food is less, that food is absorbed more easily or that fat is mobilized from the depots less readily in obese children than in others. Perhaps a constitutional or genetic tendency exists for some children to gain weight more rapidly than others on a similar diet.

E. The energy expenditure of children who are inactive because of illness or handicap may be decreased, especially if the metabolic rate is not elevated as a result of fever or infection. In obese children with motor handicaps, psychologic reasons for overeating are usually present in addition to their physical limitation of energy expenditure through motor activity.

II. ENDOCRINE DISORDERS

A. Thyroid deficiency does not lead to obesity except in rare instances. Although the decreased metabolism, activity and growth of children with hypothyroidism cause a diminution in energy expenditure, the accompanying anorexia may lead to a decreased food intake.

B. Insulinomas may be accompanied by obesity.

C. Mauriac syndrome, owing to poor control of diabetes, consists of obesity, short stature and hepatomegaly.

D. Cushing's syndrome may present with only obesity and premature cessation of longitudinal growth. The obesity is chiefly distributed in the face, the cervicodorsal area ("buffalo hump") and trunk. Acne and hirsutism are other common findings, and amenorrhea may be present. Violaceous striae may occur over the abdomen and thighs. Hypertension and muscle weakness may be noted.

McArthur, R. G., Cloutier, M. D., Hayles, A. B., and Sprague, R. G.: Cushing's disease in children. Mayo Clin. Proc. 47:319, 1972.
Streeten, D. H. P., Faas, F. H., Elders, M. J., Dalakos, T. G., and Voorhess, M.: Hypercortisolism in childhood: Shortcomings of conventional diagnostic criteria. Pediatrics 56:797, 1975.

E. Corticoid therapy

F. Polycystic ovary syndrome is a diagnostic consideration in adolescent girls with obesity, hirsutism, acne and menstrual irregularity. A morning plasma testosterone level should be obtained.

G. Obesity often involves the trunk and buttocks in pituitary dwarfs.

III. THE CENTRAL NERVOUS SYSTEM

A. Present evidence indicates that pituitary lesions, unaccompanied by involvement of the hypothalamus, do not produce obesity.

B. The Laurence-Moon-Biedl syndrome, which consists of mental retardation, retinitis pigmentosa, hypogonadism, polydactylism and obesity, is genetic in origin.

C. Lesions in the hypothalamus that may lead to obesity by producing an intense craving for food include encephalitis, craniopharyngioma, glioma of the optic chiasm, histiocytosis X, pituitary tumors, congenital defects of the hypothalamus such as the Laurence-Moon-Biedl syndrome and trauma, especially a basal skull fracture. Hydrocephalus, pinealomas and porencephaly may also lead to obesity. A suprapubic fat pad may make the genitalia appear smaller in obese children than they actually are; however, true hypogonadism may accompany obesity in some patients with hypothalamic lesions.

D. Central nervous system leukemia is associated with sudden weight gain and a voracious appetite.

E. The Prader-Willi syndrome is characterized by truncal obesity, mental retardation, neonatal hypotonia, small hands and feet, hypogenitalism and understature. Compulsive hyperphagia and obesity begins in late infancy or early childhood.

Cassidy, S. B.: Prader-Willi syndrome. Curr. Probl. Pediatr. 14:5, 1984.

F. Alstrom's syndrome consists of obesity, nerve deafness, diabetes, hypogonadism and blindness.

G. Vasquez syndrome is characterized by obesity, short stature and mental retardation in males.

H. Central nervous system lesions are rare causes of obesity; however, the history should include information as to vomiting, visual disturbances, headache, ataxia, head enlargement and polyuria. Careful neurologic and funduscopic examinations are indicated, as well as delineation of the visual fields. Roentgenograms of the skull and computerized tomography are indicated, in selected patients.

IV. SOCIAL AND PSYCHOLOGIC ASPECTS OF OBESITY

A. Social factors are inversely related to obesity, especially among girls.
B. Obese persons are very susceptible to environmental influences on eating. Food often has a special importance in some families.
C. Overeating may also occur in response to anxiety, depression and frustration.
D. Obesity leads to many secondary problems, especially in adolescents. In addition to being often taunted and ridiculed, the reluctance or inability of obese children or adolescents to engage in physical activities and sports may lead to poor muscular development and physical fitness. In addition, some obese children are not well-coordinated.

Heald, F. P., and Khan, M. A.: Teenage obesity. Pediatr. Clin. North Am. 20:807, 1973.

E. One or both parents of most overweight children are obese; however, not all the children in these families become obese.

GENERAL REFERENCES

Bruch, H.: Eating Disorders: Obesity, Anorexia Nervosa and the Person Within. New York, Basic Books, 1973.
Forbes, G. B.: Obesity. In Green, M., and Haggerty, R.J. (eds.): Ambulatory Pediatrics III. Philadelphia, W. B. Saunders Co., 1984, p. 405.
Merritt, R. J.: Obesity. Curr. Probl. Pediatr. 12:5, 1982.
Stricker, E. M.: Hyperphagia. N.Engl. J. Med. 298:1010, 1978.
Stunkard, A.: Satiety is a conditioned reflex. Psychosom. Med. 37:383, 1975.
Stunkard, A. J.: From explanation to action in psychosomatic medicine: The case of obesity. Psychosom. Med. 37:195, 1975.
Stunkard, A. J. (ed.): Obesity. Philadelphia, W. B. Saunders Co., 1980.
Vuille, J-C., and Mellbin, T.: Obesity in 10-year-olds: An epidemiologic study. Pediatrics 64:564, 1979.
Waxman, M., and Stunkard, A. J.: Caloric intake and expenditure of obese boys. J. Pediatr. 96:187, 1980.
Weil, W. B., Jr.: Obesity in children. Pediatr. Rev. 3:180, 1981.

ETIOLOGIC CLASSIFICATION OF OBESITY

34 / FAILURE TO DO WELL IN SCHOOL

The diagnosis and management of this complex problem that involves the child, the family and the school requires an interdisciplinary medical-educational approach.

ETIOLOGIC CLASSIFICATION OF FAILURE TO DO WELL IN SCHOOL

I. MENTAL RETARDATION

Children expected to achieve beyond their cognitive abilities are vulnerable to school failure; on the other hand, appropriate educational placement permits retarded or learning disabled children to achieve within the limits of their potential. Mental retardation is discussed more fully in Chapter 35.

II. SPECIFIC LEARNING DISABILITIES

The Special Education for All Handicapped Children Act of 1975 (Public Law 94-142) defines special learning disabilities as "a disorder in one or more of the basic psychological processes involved in understanding or in using spoken or written language. These may be manifested in disorders of listening, thinking, talking, reading, writing, spelling, or arithmetic. They include conditions which have been referred to as perceptual handicaps, brain injury, minimal brain dysfunction, dyslexia, developmental aphasia, etc. They do not include learning problems which are due primarily to visual, hearing, or motor handicaps, to mental retardation, emotional disturbance or, to environmental disadvantage."

Between 10 and 30 per cent of public school children, often with near-average to above average-intelligence, are estimated to have significant learning disabilities, more commonly in reading but also in writing, spelling and arithmetic. In some schools, as many as one half of the students have reading skills that are two or more years behind standard achievement levels. Environmental factors, including poor teaching, are the most common causes of such underachievement. When neurologic impairment is etio-

logic, neurologic signs are often subtle. The history, however, may be consistent with central nervous system damage and delayed development.

Specific or developmental dyslexia occurs in 5 to 15 per cent of children, predominantly males (4:1) with normal intelligence, and often on a familial basis. Generally, significant neurologic findings are not present. On the Wechsler Intelligence Scale for Children, patients with developmental dyslexia often have a low verbal I.Q. as well as low scores on the digit-span and coding subtests.

Kavanagh, J. F., and Yeni-Komshian, G.: Developmental dyslexia and related reading disorders. DHEW publication No. (NIH) 78-92, 1978.

Wender, E. H.: Learning disabilities in children. Pediatr. Rev. 3:91, 1981.

III. EMOTIONAL FACTORS

School underachievement may be secondary to emotional disorders characterized by depression, anxiety or intense anger that make it difficult for the child to attend to school work and impair his motivation to learn. Poor or diminished school function is an important criterion of depression. The precise etiologic factors need to be determined by interviews with the child, the mother, the father and the child's teachers. Children with specific learning disabilities, such as developmental dyslexia, often acquire secondary emotional and behavioral problems, including somatic complaints, depression, lying, stealing, delinquent behavior, feelings of frustration and low self-esteem. Resistance to attending school owing to emotional factors may interfere with educational progress.

IV. ENVIRONMENTAL FACTORS

A. Poor teaching and the inability of some schools to be responsive in their curricula and teaching methods to the individual needs of specific children is a frequent cause of school failure. Other factors that contribute to poor school performance include lack of praise and rewards, an unpleasant school environment, lack of personal interest by the teacher, absence of opportunities for self-responsibility, insufficient emphasis on academic mastery and lack of staff cohesiveness and collegiality.

Rutter, M.: School influences on children's behavior and development: The 1979 Kenneth Blackfan Lecture, Children's Hospital Medical Center, Boston. Pediatrics 65:208, 1980.

B. Frequent family moves may interfere with school achievement.
C. Frequent absences from school for social or emotional reasons, unless regularly compensated by homework, are a frequent cause for a child's inability to perform educationally. Such absence may be a clue to dysfunctional response to chronic illness, substance abuse, depression, parental illness or family disorganization.

Weitzman, M., Klerman, L. V., Lamb, G., Menary, J., and Alpert, J. J.: School absence: A problem for the pediatrician. Pediatrics 69:739, 1982.

D. Severely disturbed home environments generally disrupt school progress.
E. Failure of the family to convey to the child a sense of the importance of education may lead to multigenerational educational underachievement. The parental expectations for the child's school attendance and achievement may be minimal.
F. Hyperactivity, short attention span and distractability impede learning.

V. NEUROLOGIC FACTORS

A. Brain damage may be associated with a variety of learning disabilities.
B. Undetected petit mal seizures may impede learning.
C. Anticonvulsant drug toxicity may result in impaired school performance.
D. Inadequate function of a cerebrospinal fluid shunt may cause deterioration of school work.

VI. SENSORY FACTORS

A. Visual impairment
B. Hearing impairment. Even unilateral hearing impairment may contribute to school problems.

Bess, F. H., and Tharpe, A. M.: Unilateral hearing impairment in children. Pediatrics 74:206, 1984.

VII. SPEECH AND LANGUAGE DELAY in toddlers and preschool children may predict later reading problems.

VIII. DETERIORATION IN PREVIOUSLY ADEQUATE SCHOOL PERFORMANCE may be associated with

A. Emotional factors secondary to divorce, illness or other family crisis
B. Neurologic disorders
   1. Subacute sclerosing panencephalitis may be manifested by intellectual deterioration and subtle behavioral changes for months before other signs appear.
   2. Wilson's disease
   3. Other degenerative central nervous system disorders such as the juvenile form of metachromatic leukodystrophy or adrenoleukodystrophy
   4. Petit mal epilepsy
   5. Cerebral tumor
   6. Low grade hydrocephalus, (e.g., secondary to tumors of the third or fourth ventricles)
   7. Chronic cerebrospinal fluid shunt insufficiency may lead to deterioration in school performance, at times accompanied by ataxia or increased tone in the lower extremities.
   8. Neurotoxicity secondary to cranial irradiation or intrathecal methotrexate therapy to prevent or treat central nervous system leukemia may be characterized initially by diminished school performance, forgetfulness and confusion. Learning disabilities are especially a potential problem in young children who have experienced the "somnolence syndrome" four to five weeks after prophylactic cranial radiation.

Copeland, D. R., Fletcher, J. M., Pfefferbaum-Levine, B., Jaffe, N., Ried, H., and Maor, M.: Neuropsychological sequelae of childhood cancer in long-term survivors. Pediatrics 75:745, 1985.
Gangji, D., Reaman, G. H., Cohen, S. R., Bleyer, W. A., and Poplack, D. G.: Leukoencephalopathy and elevated levels of myelin basic protein in the cerebrospinal fluid of patients with acute lymphoblastic leukemia. N. Engl. J. Med. 303:19, 1980.

   9. Aluminum toxicity from aluminum-containing phosphate binders in patients with chronic renal disease
C. Hyperthyroidism; hypothyroidism. Poor academic performance may be an early symptom of hyperthyroidism.
D. Chorea
E. Acquired hearing loss

THE DIAGNOSTIC PROCESS

The diagnostic evaluation of a child who fails to do well in school generally involves several specialists including the physician, psychologist, audiologist, speech pathologist and educator.

I. THE PHYSICIAN'S ROLE

A. The physician reviews developmental progress, assesses the emotional status of the child and family and obtains other data that may help in understanding the causes for the school problem.
B. In addition to screening of visual acuity, hearing and speech, a careful neurologic examination is in order. Hard neurologic signs, (e.g., hemiparesis) or asymmetrical findings, such as differences in fine motor movements, rapid alternating movements of the hands and differences in the growth of the hands or thumb nails, are of special interest.

　　While "soft" neurologic signs may be statistically relevant in a population of children, they are so much a reflection of the developmental immaturity of the neurologic system as to be of little clinical significance in an individual child. Such findings include choreiform movements of the extended hand, brief attention span, synkinesis (mirroring of fine finger and hand movements from one side to the other), clumsiness, lack of appreciation of simultaneous face-hand touch, confusion in right-left discrimination, poor performance of rapid alternating movements, immature speech and language, impaired auditory discrimination, mirror writing and strephosymbolic errors.

Shaywitz, S. E., Shaywitz, B. A., McGraw, K., and Groll, S.: Current status of the neuromaturational examination as an index of learning disability. J. Pediatr. 104:819, 1984.

C. No simple screening tests are available that scientifically and reliably predict or detect learning disability. In the office, the physician may use a blackboard, crayons and paper, picture books, standardized reading or arithmetic problems and the Peabody Picture Vocabulary Test. The child may be asked to write, print, take dictation, draw a person and copy geometric figures. Children with a reading disability, for example, may be able to copy a sentence already printed but unable to print the same sentence if dictated. The child may read aloud slowly and with extreme effort, guess at words using the first letter or syllable of the word as a clue, make omissions and additions and be unable to convey the meaning of what he has just read.

Oberklaid, F., and Levine, M. D.: Precursors of school failure. Pediatr. Rev. 2:5, 1980.

II. SCHOOL REPORT

A school report that includes information about the child's school performance, test data, learning problems noted by the teachers and problems in adjustment is essential for the physician's evaluation. A variety of such report forms are available. A telephone call to the principal or teacher and, if possible, a physician-teacher personal conference is often helpful.

III. PSYCHOEDUCATIONAL EVALUATION

When intellectual retardation or a specific learning disability is a possibility, the most important diagnostic step is an adequate individual psychoeducational assessment. The Revised Wechsler Intelligence Scale for Children (WISC-R), which can be given to children at the age of five to six years or older and is particularly helpful in children with learning disabilities, shows a scatter in the sub-test verbal or performance scores and often a 10- or 20-point discrepancy between the verbal and performance quotients. Other evaluation instruments might include the *Wide Range Achievement Test* (WRAT), Raven Progressive Matrices, Peabody Picture Vocabulary Test, Bender Visual Motor Integration, Stanford-Binet achievement tests in reading and mathematics and the Illinois Test of Psycholinguistic Abilities (ITPA).

IV. SENSORY EVALUATIONS

A. Visual acuity
B. Audiological and speech evaluation is desirable if the child has delayed language development or dysphasia.

GENERAL REFERENCES

Culbertson, J. L., and Ferry, P. G.: Learning disabilities. Pediatr. Clin. North Amer. 29:121, 1982.
Grossman, H., and Shaywitz, B.(eds.): Symposium on learning disabilities. Pediatr. Clin. North. Am. 31:277, 1984.

ETIOLOGIC CLASSIFICATION OF FAILURE TO DO WELL IN SCHOOL

I. MENTAL RETARDATION, 302
II. SPECIFIC LEARNING DISABILITIES, 302
III. EMOTIONAL FACTORS, 302
IV. ENVIRONMENTAL FACTORS, 302
   A. Poor teaching, 302
   B. Frequent family moves, 303
   C. Frequent absences from school, 303
   D. Severely disturbed home environment, 303
   E. Family's failure to convey importance of education to child, 303
   F. Hyperactivity, short attention span and distractibility, 303
V. NEUROLOGIC FACTORS, 303
   A. Brain damage, 303
   B. Undetected petit mal seizures, 303
   C. Anticonvulsant drug toxicity, 303
VI. SENSORY FACTORS, 303
   A. Visual impairment, 303
   B. Hearing impairment, 303
VII. SPEECH AND LANGUAGE DELAY, 303

VIII. DETERIORATION IN PREVIOUSLY ADEQUATE SCHOOL PERFORMANCE, 303
   A. Emotional factors, 303
   B. Neurologic disorders, 303
     1. Subacute sclerosing panencephalitis
     2. Wilson's disease
     3. Other degenerative disorders of central nervous system
     4. Petit mal epilepsy
     5. Cerebral tumor
     6. Low-grade hydrocephalus
     7. Cerebrospinal fluid shunt insufficiency
     8. Neurotoxicity secondary to cranial irradiation or intrathecal methotrexate therapy
     9. Aluminum toxicity
   C. Hyperthyroidism; hypothyroidism, 303
   D. Chorea, 303
   E. Acquired hearing loss, 303

35 / MENTAL RETARDATION

DEFINITIONS

The American Association on Mental Deficiency defines mental retardation as "significantly subaverage general intellectual functioning existing concurrently with deficits in adaptive behavior, and manifested during the developmental period." Significant subaverage performance is defined as an I.Q. of 70 or below on standardized measures of intelligence. The upper limit is to serve only as a guideline and may be extended upward to an I.Q. of 75, especially in school settings, depending on clinical judgment. The Cattell scale and the Kuhlmann-Binet are commonly used tests for infants or severely retarded children. Since a diagnosis of mental retardation cannot be made on the basis of I.Q. alone, adaptive behavior, as reflected in the degree of independence and social responsibility the child has achieved, must also be significantly retarded.

Levels of mental retardation based on measured intelligence are defined as mild, moderate, severe and profound.

TABLE 35–1. LEVEL OF RETARDATION INDICATED BY I.Q. RANGE OBTAINED ON MEASURE OF GENERAL INTELLECTUAL FUNCTIONING

Term	I.Q. Range for Level
Mild mental retardation	50-55 to approx. 70
Moderate mental retardation	35-40 to 50-55
Severe mental retardation	20-25 to 35-40
Profound mental retardation	Below 20 or 25

The term "mildly retarded" is often used interchangeably with "educable retarded"; "moderate" retardation is equated with "trainable." The term "dependent" retarded is sometimes used for the severely retarded; "life support" level for the profoundly retarded. These terms convey some of the developmental characteristics, potential for training/education and social/vocational adequacy.

About 25 per cent of children with mental

retardation have a syndrome that is recognizable at birth or early in infancy or childhood. Most instances of mental retardation, however, are not identified until school entrance. Developmental appraisal as part of well-baby assessment may permit early detection of developmental retardation. When the degree of retardation is great, such determinations have prognostic significance. The long-term predictive value is limited when lesser discrepancies are found. Single infant developmental tests do not predict later intelligence or school performance.

Mental retardation is often accompanied by other handicaps. Adequate diagnosis often requires evaluation by multiple disciplines and periodic reassessment.

Chromosome studies are to be considered if a patient has multiple anomalies of idiopathic etiology, especially affecting the face, ears and distal extremities, or if the child is born small for gestational age. Other indications for karyotype studies may include a maternal history of repeated miscarriages, dermatoglyphic abnormalities, short stature, voracious appetite, single flexion crease on the fifth digit, males with mental retardation in whom no etiology is determined, families with X-linked recessive pattern of mental retardation, unusual facies, or a clinically recognizable genetic syndrome. Lysozymal storage diseases are suggested by regression or deterioration of motor and intellectual development, hepatosplenomegaly, skeletal dysostosis, cloudy cornea, cherry red macula, retinal degeneration and similarly affected siblings. An inborn error in amino acid metabolism is suggested by positive screening tests, unusual odors, metabolic acidosis, failure to thrive, seizures, lethargy, vomiting, unusual hair, ataxia and other neurologic symptoms.

ETIOLOGIC CLASSIFICATION OF MENTAL RETARDATION

I. CHROMOSOMAL ABNORMALITIES

A. Down's syndrome owing to trisomy 21, mosaicism or translocation (15/21; 21/22; 21/21). The diagnosis of Down's syndrome is usually readily made at birth or in early infancy on the basis of the following physical findings:
Developmental retardation
Brachycephaly
Flat occiput
Epicanthal folds
Slanting palpebral fissures
Flat nasal bridge
Speckled iris (Brushfield spots)
Loose skin in the posterior neck
Small, dysplastic ears
Hypotonia
Hyperextensibility of joints
Short, broad hands
Simian palmar creases
Dysplastic middle phalanx of fifth finger
Wide space between first and second toes
Congenital heart disease in some patients

B. Trisomy 13 (Patau's syndrome) is characterized by the following findings:
Severe developmental retardation
Minor seizures
Low birth weight
Failure to thrive
Microcephaly with sloping forehead
Holoprosencephaly-type central nervous system defect
Scalp defects in parietal-occipital area
Eye defects, including microphthalmia and coloboma of iris and retina
Epicanthal folds
Loose skin on posterior neck
Cleft lip and/or palate
Prominent nose
Low-set ears
Micrognathia
Overlapping fingers
Flexion deformity of fingers with or without overlapping
Retroflexible thumb
Ulnar deviation of hands
Single palmar crease; distal palmar axial triradii
Polydactyly
Hyperconvex nails
Prominent heels
Congenital heart disease: ventricular septal defect, patent ductus arteriosus, atrial septal defect
Short sternum
Hemangiomas, including capillary hemangioma on forehead
Renal anomalies

C. Trisomy 18 (Edwards' syndrome) is characterized by the following findings:
Severe developmental retardation
Low birth weight
Failure to thrive
Difficulty in feeding
High-pitched cry
Prominent occiput
Microphthalmia
Short palpebral fissures
Low-set ears
Micrognathia
Loose skin on posterior neck
Overlapping fingers

Flexion deformities of fingers with index finger overlapping the third; fifth finger overlapping the fourth
Retroflexible thumbs
Rocker bottom feet
Hammer toe
Prominent heels
Congenital heart disease, especially ventricular septal defect and patent ductus arteriosus
Hypoplastic muscles
Hypertonia
Single umbilical artery
Inguinal or umbilical hernias
Renal anomalies

D. 5p-syndrome (cri du chat syndrome) has the following characteristics:
Severe developmental retardation
Microcephaly
Hypertelorism
Oblique palpebral fissures
Epicanthal folds
Low set ears
Micrognathia
Failure to thrive
Hypotonia
Cat-like cry

E. 4p-syndrome (Wolf-Hirschhorn)
Developmental retardation
Failure to thrive
Midline scalp defect
Microcephaly
Low-set ears
Nasal deformity
Simian crease

F. 18 short arm deletion syndrome (18p-)
Developmental retardation
Cebocephaly
Microcephaly
Eye defects
Malformed ears
Micrognathia
Saddle nose
Webbed neck

G. 18 long arm deletion syndrome (18 q-)
Microcephaly
Hypotonia
Eye deformity
Ear deformity

H. Other structural abnormalities of the autosomes: trisomies, deletions, duplications (partial trisomies) and translocations.

I. X-linked mental retardation associated with a fragile site on the long arm of the X chromosome at Xq^{27} affects one in every 1000 to 2000 males and is characterized by mild to severe mental retardation. Physical examination may demonstrate large ears, prominent chin, pale blue irides, large head circumference, repetitive speech pattern and macro-orchidism.

Turner, G., Daniel, A., and Frost, M.: X-linked mental retardation, macro-orchidism, and the Xq^{27} fragile site. J. Pediatr. 96:837, 1980.

J. Klinefelter's syndrome

Lewandowski, R. C., Jr., and Yunis, J. J.: New chromosomal syndromes. Am. J. Dis. Child 129:515, 1975.
Yunis, J. J. (ed.): New Chromosomal Syndromes. New York, Academic Press, Inc. 1977.

II. LYSOSOMAL STORAGE DISEASES caused by a deficiency of one or more lysosomal enzymes

A. GM_1 gangliosidosis may appear at birth or in early infancy (infantile, type I) with a coarse facies, depressed nasal bridge, flexural contraction of fingers, kyphosis, hepatosplenomegaly and other features that suggest Hurler's syndrome. A cherry red macula and cloudy cornea are often present. Type II is characterized by normal development during the first 9 to 12 months of life followed by rapid neurologic deterioration and spastic quadriparesis.

B. GM_2 gangliosidosis I (Tay-Sachs disease). The infant develops normally for the first months of life but then begins to demonstrate hyperacusis, listlessness, irritability, hypotonia, seizures and developmental regression. A cherry red macula is present.

C. GM_2 gangliosidosis II (Sandhoff's disease) is clinically indistinguishable from Tay-Sachs disease.

D. Metachromatic leukodystrophy is characterized by normal development until the age of 12 to 14 months, followed by gait disturbance, ataxia, intellectual regression, loss of reflexes, seizures and bulbar signs. Terminally, rigidity, blindness, deafness, macular degeneration and hyperpyrexia develop. A cherry red spot may be present. The cerebrospinal fluid protein is regularly elevated. Patients with the late infantile form of metachromatic leukodystrophy experience walking impairment at about 17 months of age with progressive pyramidal and cerebellar signs and, perhaps, a pseudo-Hurler's appearance. The early juvenile form is characterized by the development of a gait disorder, tripping and falling between four and six years of age along with intellectual deterioration. Children with juvenile metachromatic leukodystrophy present between 6 and 10 years of age with school failure and behavioral and personality changes, followed in a few months or years by ataxia, gait problems and extrapyramidal signs.

MacFaul, R., Cavanagh, N., Lake, B. D., Stephens, R., and Whitfield, A. E.: Metachromatic leucodystrophy: Review of 38 cases. Arch Dis. Child. 57:168, 1982.

E. Krabbe's disease (globoid cell leukodystrophy) becomes evident before six months of age with irritability, persistent crying, recurrent unexplained fever and myoclonic responses to light and noise. Developmental arrest is followed by regression, decerebrate posture, optic atrophy and seizures. The cerebrospinal fluid protein is regularly elevated.

F. Niemann-Pick disease in its infantile form begins in early infancy with hepatosplenomegaly, cessation of development and mental retardation. A cherry red macular spot may be present.

G. Gaucher's disease in its acute, infantile form is characterized by failure to thrive, bulbar palsy, hepatosplenomegaly, developmental regression and spastic quadriparesis.

H. Wolman's syndrome is accompanied by hepatosplenomegaly and adrenal calcification.

I. Fucosidosis is characterized by normal development until one or two years of age when intellectual and physical deterioration begin. The skeletal characteristics, facial features, hepatosplenomegaly and joint contractures may suggest Hurler's syndrome. The fundi and corneae are normal.

J. Mannosidosis has many clinical features similar to Hurler's syndrome, (e.g., hepatosplenomegaly, mental retardation, kyphosis, cataracts and corneal clouding).

Booth, C. W., Chen, K. K., and Nadler, H. L.: Mannosidosis: Clinical and biochemical studies in a family of affected adolescents and adults. J. Pediatr. 88:821, 1976.

K. Aspartylglucosaminuria is a progressive disorder inherited on an autosomal recessive basis and characterized by a coarse facies with thick lips, broad nose, anteverted nostrils and hypotonia. Storage of glutamyl-ribose-5-phosphate may cause progressive neurologic deterioration.

L. Multiple sulfatase deficiency is manifested by slow development for the first one or two years of life followed by neurologic deterioration with myoclonic seizures, nystagmus, retinal degeneration, ichthyosis, hepatosplenomegaly and spasticity. The coarse facial features may simulate those of Hurler's syndrome.

M. Mucopolysaccharidoses
   1. MPS IH (Hurler's syndrome), an autosomal recessive disease, is characterized by severe mental retardation, macrocephaly, coarse facies, flat nasal bridge, flared nostrils, bushy eyebrows, full lips, large tongue, thoracolumbar gibbus, corneal clouding, skeletal deformities, stiff joints, hepatosplenomegaly, persistent rhinorrhea, umbilical and inguinal hernias and deafness.
   2. MPS I-S (Scheie's syndrome) is a milder variant of Hurler's syndrome without mental retardation but with involvement of the corneas and joints.
   3. MPS I-H/S (Hurler-Scheie's syndrome) is characterized by findings intermediate between Hurler's and Scheie's syndromes.
   4. MPS II (Hunter's syndrome), an X-linked recessive disorder occurring in both a mild and a severe form, is characterized by mental retardation, skeletal deformities, early deafness, subcutaneous nodules of MPH infiltration and retinal degeneration. Corneal clouding is absent.
   5. MPS III A and B (Sanfilippo's syndrome), an autosomal recessive disorder, is manifested by mental regression and behavior problems evident by four to five years of age and clinical features that simulate but are not as marked as those of MPS IH. Minimal hepatosplenomegaly and joint stiffness occur.
   6. MPS IV (Morquio's syndrome) is not accompanied by mental retardation. See page 131.
   7. MPS VI (Maroteaux-Lamy syndrome). Clinically, the severe form closely simulates Hurler's syndrome.
   8. MPS VII (beta-glucuronidase deficiency) is characterized by hepatosplenomegaly, corneal clouding, gibbus and developmental delay.
   9. MPS VIII. This disorder is characterized by physical findings that simulate Morquio's syndrome. Mental retardation is present.

N. Disorders of sialic acid metabolism
   1. Sialidosis 1 (cherry red spot–myoclonus syndrome), with an onset after eight years of age, is character-

ized by macular cherry red spots, punctate corneal opacities and myoclonus. The child's facies and intelligence are normal.

2. Sialidosis 2
   a. Infantile type (includes mucolipidosis I) is characterized by normal development for the first year of life followed by gradual intellectual deterioration. The facies are coarse and simulate Hurler's syndrome. Clinical features include moderate mental retardation, hepatosplenomegaly, myoclonus, ataxia, deafness, dysostosis multiplex, short stature, hernias and a cherry red macula.
   b. Juvenile type (Goldberg's syndrome, atypical mucolipidosis) with an onset after eight years of age, has the same clinical characteristics as the infantile type except for organomegaly.
3. Sialuria and sialic acid storage disease, infantile type, have their onset at one to two months of age with mental retardation, coarse facies, white hair, anemia and diarrhea. The diagnosis requires a specific assay for free sialic acid.
4. Sialuria
   a. Salla type has its clinical onset at one year of age with mental retardation, coarse facies and ataxia.
   b. French type, which becomes clinically apparent at age two, is characterized by mental retardation, hepatomegaly and seizures.
5. Mucolipidosis II (Leroy's syndrome, I-cell disease) presents early in infancy with many features that simulate Hurler's syndrome, (e.g., severe mental retardation, hepatosplenomegaly, a hoarse voice and tight skin). Corneal clouding does not occur.
6. Mucolipidosis III becomes manifest in the second year of life with dwarfing, thoracic deformity, joint contractures and hearing impairment. The clinical picture resembles that of Hurler's syndrome.

Gordon, N.: The pseudo-Hurler syndromes. Dev. Med. Child. Neurol. 20:383, 1978.

Kolodny, E. H.: Current concepts in genetics. Lysosomal storage disease. N. Engl. J. Med. 294:1217, 1976.

Stevenson, R. E., Lubinsky, M., Taylor, H. A., Wenger, D. A., Schroer, R. J., and Olmstead, P. M.: Sialic acid storage disease with sialuria: Clinical and biochemical features in the severe infantile type. Pediatrics 72:441, 1983.

III. OTHER CEREBRAL DEGENERATIVE DISORDERS

A. Ceroid lipofuscinosis (Batten's disease) has infantile, late infantile, juvenile and adult variants. The late infantile form becomes clinically manifest between two and six years of age with intellectual deterioration, myoclonic seizures, ataxia, retinal degeneration and optic atrophy. Skin biopsy or tissue culture fibroblasts can be used for diagnosis.
B. Spielmeyer-Vogt disease (juvenile amaurotic idiocy) begins in school age children with progressive loss of vision, myoclonic and grand mal seizures and intellectual deterioration.
C. Pelizaeus-Merzbacher disease becomes evident in early infancy with oscillating, wheeling nystagmus; unusual eye movements; and head tremor, followed by regression in motor and intellectual development, ataxia, intention tremor, choreoathetosis and spasticity.
D. Subacute sclerosing panencephalitis (SSPE or Dawson's inclusion body encephalitis) has four stages. Stage 1 begins insidiously with deterioration in intellectual and school performance and subtle personality changes that include temper outbursts, disobedience, forgetfulness, distractability, and hallucinations. In stage 2, myoclonic jerks occur along with incoordination, choreoathetosis and tremors. Personality and intellectual changes accompanied by myoclonic jerks suggest the diagnosis. Electroencephalographic findings, spinal fluid studies and measles antibody titers are confirmatory. Macular degeneration may be evident. Stage 3 is characterized by rigidity and unresponsiveness. Intermittent periods of laughing and crying occur in stage 4 along with hypothalamic dysfunction.
E. Huntington's chorea may have its onset in childhood with seizures, rigidity, chorea and learning problems.
F. Schilder's disease, which occurs in late childhood, is characterized by cortical blindness, spasticity, seizures and aphasia with the eventual onset of dementia and coma.

IV. ABNORMALITIES OF AMINO ACID METABOLISM

A. Hyperphenylalaninemia
   1. Phenylalanine hydroxylase deficiency (phenylketonuria). Eczema, seizures, a musty body and "mousey" urine odor may be noted in addition to retardation.

2. Hyperphenylalaninemia is caused by dihydropteridine deficiency or defects in the synthesis of dihydrobiopterin associated with "malignant" hyperphenylalaninemia. These patients demonstrate progressive neurologic deterioration despite adequate dietary treatment.

American Academy of Pediatrics, Committee on Nutrition: New developments in hyperphenylalaninemia. Pediatrics 65:844, 1980.
Scriver, C. R., and Clow, C. L.: Phenylketonuria: Epitome of human biochemical genetics. N. Engl. J. Med. 303:1336, 1394, 1980.

B. Hyperammonemia may cause episodic vomiting and lethargy.
C. Citrullinemia may produce severe disease in the newborn with episodic vomiting, seizures, coma and mental retardation.
D. Argininosuccinicaciduria becomes manifest in the first one to two years of life with growth redardation, trichorrhexis nodosa, hepatomegaly, seizures and ataxia.
E. Argininemia is characterized by mental retardation, seizures and spastic diplegia.
F. Maple syrup urine disease usually becomes symptomatic toward the end of the first week of life with difficulty in feeding, failure to thrive, absent Moro reflex, extreme flaccidity, irregular respirations, lethargy and myoclonic seizures. Opisthotonus and intermittent rigidity occur later. The urine has a maple syrup odor. Excessive amounts of valine, leucine and isoleucine and their alpha keto acids are present in urine and blood.
G. Hypervalinemia causes vomiting, lethargy and feeding difficulties in newborn infants.
H. Beta-alaninemia is characterized by lethargy and seizures in young infants.
I. Nonketotic hyperglycinemia is manifest by microcephaly, seizures and mental retardation.
J. In addition to mental retardation, patients with homocystinuria demonstrate fine, friable hair; dislocation of the lens; livedo reticularis; a malar flush; marked nervousness; and a Marfan-like habitus with genu valgum, pectus excavatum, kyphosis, scoliosis and arachnodactyly. Arterial or venous thrombotic episodes may occur. The cyanide-nitroprusside test represents a screening examination.
K. Saccharopinuria
L. Sarcosinemia causes a feeding problem and failure to thrive as well as mental retardation.
M. Hartnup disease is characterized by progressive mental retardation, reversible cerebellar ataxia and a pellagra-like rash on skin areas exposed to sunlight.
N. Isovaleric aciduria causes metabolic acidosis, urine with a sweaty feet odor and neurologic signs.
O. Propionic acidemia produces episodic vomiting, metabolic acidosis and ketonuria.
P. Methylmalonic aciduria is characterized by developmental retardation and infantile ketoacidosis.
Q. Lactic-pyruvic acidosis may cause metabolic acidosis in the newborn, ataxia and mental retardation.
R. Beta-methylcrotonyl-glycinuria produces mental retardation, urine with the odor of cat's urine and feeding problems.
S. Alpha-methyl-beta hydroxybutyric aciduria causes intermittent metabolic acidosis.
T. Carnosinemia is characterized by seizures and mental retardation.
U. Sulfite oxidase deficiency causes severe mental retardation, dislocation of the lens and blindness.

O'Brien, D., and Goodman, S. I.: The critically ill child: Acute metabolic disease in infancy and early childhood. Pediatrics 46:620, 1970
Scriver, C. R., and Rosenberg, L. E.: Amino Acid Metabolism and Its Disorders. Philadelphia, W. B. Saunders Co., 1973.

V. OTHER METABOLIC DISORDERS ASSOCIATED WITH MENTAL RETARDATION

A. Hypothyroidism may cause developmental delay during early infancy.
B. Idiopathic infantile hypercalcemia
C. Hypoglycemia may cause mental retardation.
D. Galactosemia, if not diagnosed and treated early, causes mental retardation.
E. Lesch-Nyhan syndrome is characterized by developmental regression, hypotonia that is eventually replaced by hypertonia, athetoid posturing and choreic movements.
F. Menkes' kinky hair syndrome or trichopoliodystrophy
G. Lowe's syndrome is characterized by severe mental retardation, glaucoma, hypotonia, cataracts, metabolic acidosis, rickets, organic aciduria and aminoaciduria.
H. Oasthouse urine disease (methionine malabsorption) is characterized by failure to thrive, seizures, hypotonia,

edema and an abnormal urinary odor (dried malt or hops).

I. Aspartylglucosaminuria becomes manifest during the school age years with coarse facial features, hypertelorism, broad nose, thick lips, large tongue, opacities of the lens, spasticity and dysarthria. Mental retardation is severe.

J. Methemoglobin diaphorase deficiency is characterized by methemoglobinemia and mental retardation.

K. Bartter's syndrome may be characterized by mental and physical retardation in addition to hypokalemic alkalosis.

L. Wilson's disease may begin with dementia and seizures.

M. Fanconi's syndrome

N. Adrenoleukodystrophy usually affects school-age boys, causing cortical blindness, impaired intellectual performance, dementia, ataxic or spastic gait and pigmentation of skin folds.

VI. CAUSATIVE INFECTIONS

A. Prenatal
   1. Cytomegalovirus
   2. Rubella
   3. Toxoplasmosis
   4. Syphilis
B. Postnatal
   1. Meningitis
   2. Encephalitis

VII. CAUSATIVE TOXIC AGENTS; DRUGS

A. Lead poisoning
B. Fetal alcohol syndrome
C. Fetal anticonvulsant syndrome
D. Maternal phenylketonuria
E. Neonatal hyperbilirubinemia
F. Carbon monoxide poisoning
G. Patients with aluminium toxicity and chronic renal failure who are receiving aluminum-containing phosphate binders may develop dementia.

Andreoli, S. P., Bergstein, J. M., and Sherrard, D. J.: Aluminum intoxication from aluminum-containing phosphate binders in children with azotemia not undergoing dialysis. N. Engl. J. Med. 310:1079, 1984.

VIII. CAUSATIVE TRAUMA; HYPOXIA

A. Perinatal hypoxia
B. Birth trauma
C. Intracranial hemorrhage
D. Head injury

IX. OTHER SYNDROMES AND DISORDERS THAT MAY BE ASSOCIATED WITH MENTAL RETARDATION

A. Cerebral malformations
   1. Hydranencephaly; porencephaly. Transillumination of the head is indicated in infants seen because of mental retardation.
   2. Primary microcephaly may be inherited on either an autosomal dominant or an autosomal recessive basis. Children with autosomal recessive microcephaly have an acutely inclining forehead, a wrinkled or furrowed scalp and severe mental retardation. Those with the autosomal dominant form are more likely to have mild or borderline mental retardation.

Haslam, R. H. A., and Smith, D. W.: Autosomal dominant microcephaly. J. Pediatr. 95:701, 1979.

   3. Holoprosencephaly
B. Aicardi syndrome, which occurs in females, consists of mental retardation, agenesis of the corpus collosum, infantile spasms and chorioretinopathy.
C. Cerebral palsy may be accompanied by mental retardation. Accurate appraisal of the child's intellectual ability is often difficult in the presence of severe motor and, at times, sensory handicaps.
D. Tuberous sclerosis may be accompanied by mental retardation.
E. Sturge-Weber-Dimitri syndrome
F. Neurofibromatosis may be accompanied by mild to moderate mental retardation.
G. Laurence-Moon-Biedl syndrome consists of mental retardation, obesity, hypogenitalism, retinitis pigmentosa and polydactylism.
H. Cornelia de Lange's syndrome is characterized by bradycephaly; a pathognomonic facies with hyperconvex forehead, hypoplasia of the supraorbital ridges and zygomatic arches; small nose; depressed nasal root; flaring nostrils; micrognathia and low-set ears. The eyebrows are bushy and confluent in the midline and the eyelashes long and delicate. Scalp hair extends low on the forehead, which is covered by fine, lanugo hair. There is general hypertrichosis. The fingers are short and tapering, and a simian palmar crease is often present along with proximal insertion of the thumb, clinodactyly of the little finger and poor development of the thenar muscles. Extension of the elbows is limited. Retardation is moderate to severe.
I. The Rubinstein-Taybi syndrome is characterized by mental retardation and short, broad terminal phalanges of the thumbs and great toes. Other features

include high arched palate, slight anti-mongoloid palpebral fissures and a prominent nose.

J. Prader-Willi syndrome
K. Incontinentia pigmenti
L. Smith-Lemli-Opitz syndrome
M. Cerebral gigantism
N. Cerebrohepatorenal syndrome of Zellweger is a genetic disorder associated with the absence of peroxisomes and characterized by mental retardation, severe hypotonia, hepatomegaly, jaundice, failure to thrive and facies characterized by a high forehead, brachycephaly, persistent metopic suture, hypertelorism, hypoplastic supraorbital ridges, micrognathia and low set ears. Eye findings may include glaucoma, corneal clouding, epicanthal folds, Brushfield spots and nystagmus. Epiphyseal stippling and elevated liver enzymes may be present.

Danks, D. M., Tippett, P., Adams, C., and Campbell, P.: Cerebro-hepato-renal syndrome of Zellweger. J. Pediatr. 86:382, 1975.

O. Canavan's disease is characterized by marked head enlargement in early infancy, sutures splitting, spasticity, progressive intellectual deterioration and blindness.
P. Alexander's disease is characterized by macrocephaly, muscle weakness, contractures and mental retardation.

X. INFANTILE AUTISM has an insidious onset before 30 months of age. In some, abnormal behavior is noted in the first year of life; in others, between 2 and 2 1/2 years of age. Autistic children may be retarded or borderline in their general intelligence or social functioning. The disorder is characterized by a marked and continuing social distance and lack of appropriate social responsiveness with, in some cases, reluctance to be held or cuddled. Some autistic children may cling to their mother but without emotional warmth. Little or brief eye contact may occur, and the child seems to look through, rather than at, other persons. Splinter skills, such as rote memory or puzzle solving may be present at a level much above the general mental age of the child's other achievements. Activity often consists of stereotyped, compulsive and repetitive move-ments such as rocking, bouncing, tapping, swinging, whirling, spinning objects or staring at his own hands. The patient may become furious if his activities are interrupted. A severe sleep problem may be present. Toe-walking is another common clinical characteristic. Either speech is absent or the child demonstrates a secret language, gibberish, echolalia or a limited vocabulary. Pronouns may be misused. The clinical manifestations of phenylketonuria may simulate those of childhood autism.

Aug, R. G., and Ables, B. S.: A clinician's guide to childhood psychosis. Pediatrics 47:327, 1971.
DeMyer, M. K.: Infantile autism: patients and their families. Curr. Probl. Pediatr. 12:6, 1982.
Rutter, M., and Schopler, E. (eds.): Autism—A Reappraisal of Concepts and Treatments. New York, Plenum Press, 1978.

XI. CULTURAL-FAMILIAL FACTORS are the most common cause for retardation and for a disparity between a child's actual performance and his innate abilities. Insufficient physical, social and emotional stimulation from a mother or mother-substitute may lead to retarded behavior in infants and young children. Children who are economically or socially disadvantaged are over-represented in this group.

Haywood, H. C. (ed.): Social-Retardation. New York, Appleton-Century-Crofts, 1970.

XII. SENSORY DEFICITS such as hearing and visual impairment if undetected or treated

GENERAL REFERENCES

Beaudet, A. L.: Genetic diagnostic studies for mental retardation. Curr. Probl. Pediatr. 7:3, 1978.
Grossman, H. J., (ed.): Manual on Terminology and Classification in Mental Retardation. Washington, D.C., American Association on Mental Deficiency, Special Publication Series No. 2., Revised, 1973.
Grossman, H. S.: Mental retardation. In Green, M., and Haggerty, R.J. (eds.): Ambulatory Pediatrics III. Philadelphia, W. B. Saunders Co., 1984, p. 492.
Holmes, L. B., Moser, H. W., Halldorsson, S., Mack, C., Pant, S. S., and Hatzilevich, B.: Mental Retardation: An Atlas of Diseases with Associated Physical Abnormalities. New York, The Macmillan Co., 1972.
Smith, D. W., and Simons, F. E. R.: Rational diagnostic evaluation of the child with mental deficiency. Am. J. Dis. Child. 129:1285, 1975.

ETIOLOGIC CLASSIFICATION OF MENTAL RETARDATION

I. CHROMOSOMAL ABNORMALITIES, 306
   A. Down's syndrome, 306
   B. Trisomy 13 (Patau's syndrome), 306
   C. Trisomy 18 (Edwards' syndrome), 306
   D. 5p-syndrome (cri du chat syndrome), 307
   E. 4p-syndrome (Wolf-Hirschhorn syndrome), 307
   F. 18 short arm deletion syndrome (18p-), 307
   G. 18 long arm deletion syndrome (18q-), 307
   H. Other autosomal abnormalities, 307
   I. X-linked mental retardation and Xq fragile chromosome, 307
   J. Klinefelter's syndrome, 307
II. LYSOSOMAL STORAGE DISEASE, 307
   A. GM_1 gangliosidosis, 307
   B. GM_2 gangliosidosis I (Tay-Sachs disease), 307
   C. GM_2 gangliosidosis II (Sandhoff's disease), 307
   D. Metachromatic leukodystrophy, 307
   E. Krabbe's disease (globoid cell leukodystrophy), 308
   F. Neimann-Pick disease, 308
   G. Gaucher's disease, 308
   H. Wolman's disease, 308
   I. Fucosidosis, 308
   J. Mannosidosis, 308
   K. Aspartylglucosaminuria, 308
   L. Multiple sulfatase deficiency, 308
   M. Mucopolysaccharidoses, 308
     1. MPS IH (Hurler's syndrome)
     2. MPS I-S (Scheie's syndrome)
     3. MPS I-H/S (Hurler-Scheie syndrome)
     4. MPS II (Hunter's syndrome)
     5. MPS III A and B (Sanfilippo's syndrome)
     6. MPS IV (Morquio's syndrome)
     7. MPS VI (Maroteaux-Lamy syndrome)
     8. MPS VII
     9. MPS VIII
   N. Disorders of sialic acid metabolism, 308
     1. Sialidosis 1
     2. Sialidosis 2
       a. Infantile type
       b. Juvenile type
     3. Sialuria and sialic acid storage disease, infantile type
     4. Sialuria
       a. Salla type
       b. French type
     5. Mucolipidosis II
     6. Mucolipidosis III
III. OTHER CEREBRAL DEGENERATIVE DISORDERS, 309
   A. Ceroid lipofuscinosis (Batten's disease), 309
   B. Spielmeyer-Vogt disease (juvenile amaurotic idiocy), 309
   C. Pelizaeus-Merzbacher disease, 309
   D. Subacute sclerosing panencephalitis, 309
   E. Huntington's chorea, 309

   F. Schilder's disease, 309
IV. ABNORMALITIES OF AMINO ACID METABOLISM, 309
   A. Hyperphenylalaninemia, 309
     1. Phenylketonuria
     2. Malignant hyperphenylalaninemia
   B. Hyperammonemia, 310
   C. Citrullinemia, 310
   D. Argininosuccinicaciduria, 310
   E. Argininemia, 310
   F. Maple syrup urine disease, 310
   G. Hypervalinemia, 310
   H. Beta-alaninemia, 310
   I. Nonketotic hyperglycinemia, 310
   J. Homocystinuria, 310
   K. Saccharopinuria, 310
   L. Sarcosinemia, 310
   M. Hartnup disease, 310
   N. Isovaleric aciduria, 310
   O. Propionic acidemia, 310
   P. Methylmalonic aciduria, 310
   Q. Lactic-pyruvic acidosis, 310
   R. Beta-methylcrotonyl-glycinuria, 310
   S. Alpha-methyl-betahydroxybutyric aciduria, 310
   T. Carnosinemia, 310
   U. Sulfite oxidase deficiency, 310
V. OTHER METABOLIC DISORDERS ASSOCIATED WITH MENTAL RETARDATION, 310
   A. Hypothyroidism, 310
   B. Idiopathic infantile hypercalcemia, 310
   C. Hypoglycemia, 310
   D. Galactosemia, 310
   E. Lesch-Nyhan syndrome, 310
   F. Menkes' kinky hair syndrome, 310
   G. Lowe's syndrome, 310
   H. Oasthouse urine disease, 310
   I. Aspartylglycosaminuria, 311
   J. Methemoglobin diaphorase deficiency, 311
   K. Bartter's syndrome, 311
   L. Wilson's disease, 311
   M. Fanconi's syndrome, 311
   N. Adrenoleukodystrophy, 311
VI. CAUSATIVE INFECTIONS, 311
   A. Prenatal, 311
     1. Cytomegalovirus
     2. Rubella
     3. Toxoplasmosis
     4. Syphilis
   B. Postnatal, 311
     1. Meningitis
     2. Encephalitis
VII. CAUSATIVE TOXIC AGENTS; DRUGS, 311
   A. Lead poisoning, 311
   B. Fetal alcohol syndrome, 311
   C. Fetal anticonvulsant syndrome, 311
   D. Maternal phenylketonuria, 311
   E. Neonatal hyperbilirubinemia, 311
   F. Carbon monoxide poisoning, 311

Table continued on following page

36 / GIFTEDNESS

The Marland report entitled *Education of the Gifted and Talented* classified gifted and talented children as those with demonstrated achievements or potential in one or more of the following areas: general intellectual ability, specific academic aptitude, creative and productive thinking, leadership ability and the visual or performing arts. Most programs for gifted children are concerned with those whose mental abilities are within the upper 2.5 to 3 per cent of the population and whose I.Q. score is 130 or above.

Although intelligence tests offer a convenient method for categorization, they do not necessarily identify the potential for creativity or outstanding achievement.

Children of high intelligence often begin to read before the age of five, frequently without instruction. They characteristically have unusually large vocabularies, a facility of expression, a strikingly retentive memory, an early interest in games, a limitless supply of questions, a wide range of interests, an insatiable curiosity, an interest in experimenting, a sense of humor and a great interest in time relations, e.g., calendars and clocks. They generally have persistent, goal-directed behavior, a large amount of general and advanced knowledge, a high level of abstract thinking and the ability to apply knowledge to new situations.

Paradoxically, gifted children may be seen by the physician because they may appear hyperactive, have a poor or failing school performance or are reported to have behavior problems at school. The differential diagnosis of school underachievement and behavioral difficulties includes the possibility that the patient has high intellectual ability but is bored and has lost motivation.

GENERAL REFERENCES

Gallagher, J.: Teaching the Gifted Child. Boston, Allyn and Bacon, 1975.
Marland, S.: Education of the Gifted and Talented. Participants in the National Student Symposium on the Education of the Gifted and Talented: On Being Gifted. Sponsored by The American Association for Gifted Children, 1978.
Miller, B. S., and Prile, M. (eds.): The Gifted Child, The Family and The Community. New York, Walker and Co., 1981.
Webb, J. T., Meckstroth, E. A., and Tolan, S. S.: Guiding the Gifted Child. A Practical Source for Parents and Teachers. Columbus, Ohio, Psychology Publishing Co., 1982.

37 / HYPERACTIVITY; ATTENTIONAL DEFICIT

Hyperactivity is a common, nonspecific symptom of many etiologies. "Hyper" or "hyperactive" has come to be an adjective used by parents to describe almost any behavioral symptom in a child, including oppositional behavior or the symptoms characteristic of a conduct disorder. The child seen because of "hyperactivity" may, in fact, have normal behavior that has been misinterpreted as abnormal by an inexperienced parent. Occasionally, the complaint may be made by an unseasoned teacher who cannot maintain discipline, especially in an open classroom. Other children reported to be hyperactive have a constitutionally high level of motor activity. Most commonly, however, hyperactive or overactive behavior is a manifestation of anxiety or depression secondary to environmental and situational stresses such as not doing well in school; having a sibling who is handicapped or ill with a serious disorder such as leukemia; family financial problems; marital discord; divorce; parental illness, including alcoholism; maternal depression; death of a relative; crowding; a chaotic living situation; or developmentally inappropriate care with too little or too much stimulation. The boundless curiosity of some gifted young child may cause them to be regarded as hyperactive.

Possible etiologies for hyperactivity and attention deficit include brain damage secondary to central nervous system infections such as encephalitis or meningitis, head injury, cerebral hypoxia or lead intoxication. Hyperactivity, distractibility, headache, vertigo, difficulty in controlling anger and sleep problems may be part of a post-traumatic syndrome following head injury. Some neurologically impaired children demonstrate a mixed clinical picture that consists of hyperactivity, developmental retardation, brain damage and autistic behavior. Children receiving phenobarbital for prophylaxis against febrile seizures may be hyperactive and irritable. Hyperactivity may occur in children with neurofibromatosis, hyperthyroidism, urea cycle disorders and the fetal alcohol syndrome. Infants small for gestational age may be hyperactive. Increased motor activity may be seen in gifted children who are bored in school or in children with learning disabilities. Patients with anorexia nervosa may demonstrate periods of overactivity. The narcotic withdrawal syndrome is characterized by hyperactivity with the infant kicking, squirming and moving about. When maternal depression is a problem, the child's hyperactivity is often worse on those days when the mother is most depressed.

Fergusson, D. M., Horwood, L. J., and Shannon, F. T.: Relationship of family life events, maternal depression, and child-rearing problems. Pediatrics 73:773, 1984.

Attentional deficit disorder with hyperactivity (ADDH) is the most recent name applied to a group of behavioral symptoms that occur before seven years of age, persist for at least six months and include developmentally inappropriate inattention, impulsiveness, and motor hyperactivity.

I. THE CHILD WITH ADDH IS UNABLE TO SIT STILL AND IS ALWAYS ON THE GO. He may constantly move about, fidget, squirm, aimlessly pick up objects, open drawers, climb on chairs, touch everything in sight, bother others, and be unable to sit through a television program or a story. Disorders of sleep and eating may have been present since infancy.

II. THE SHORT ATTENTION SPAN AND EASY DISTRACTIBILITY cause failure to complete tasks, sloppy school work, disorganization and inability to remember instructions and assignments. The child does not seem to listen. These behaviors are usually less marked in one-on-one or structured situations in relatively stimulus-free environments.

III. THE CHILD SHOWS IMPULSIVE MOTOR AND VERBAL BEHAVIOR, commonly interrupting others, blurting out in school and having trouble waiting his turn.

IV. THE CHILD EXHIBITS OVEREXCITABILITY. Stimulating or exciting situations such as parties, guests, shopping centers, amusement parks and crowds tend to make the behavior worse. Temper tantrums or crying are precipitated by trivial affronts.

V. SOCIALIZATION PROBLEMS EXIST. The child often bothers or comes crashing in on other children as well as adults. He has poor peer relations, fights frequently and is overly aggressive and demanding. Older children with ADDH may suffer from low self-esteem.

VI. OTHER EMOTIONAL AND BEHAVIORAL SYMPTOMS may include fire-setting, disobedience, defiance, destructiveness and mood swings.

VII. SCHOOL PROBLEMS may be secondary to the child's short attention span and distractibility or to concomitant learning disorders.

THE PHYSICAL EXAMINATION

Many children seen because of hyperactivity or the attention deficit syndrome do not display abnormal behavior in the one-on-one office setting. The neurologic examination may disclose a number of nondiagnostic "soft" signs that usually represent a maturational lag in motor development. Occasionally, hyperreflexia or asymmetry of the deep tendon reflexes and extensor plantar reflexes occurs.

APPROACH TO DIAGNOSIS

The diagnosis of hyperactivity is based on clinical judgment since no specific test or array of diagnostic studies is available. Observation of the child in the office on one visit may be misleading. Reports from the parents and teachers regarding the child's behavior in a variety of settings, perhaps using standardized questionnaires such as those developed by Connors, and a review of possible contributing environmental factors are diagnostically helpful. Genetic factors may play an etiologic role. The family assessment should include recent stressors such as the death of a person close to the child; marital discord; divorce; and long-term family vicissitudes, such as alcoholism, mental illness and chaotic, crowded living arrangements. An electroencephalogram is indicated only if the history or physical examination suggests a convulsive disorder. Psychoeducational and language evaluation is appropriate in children thought to have a learning disorder. A variety of parent and teacher rating scales are available for evaluating the child's attention span and social adjustment. Electronic devices that are worn on a belt are now being investigated and may be helpful in quantifying motor activity.

GENERAL REFERENCES

Eisenberg, L.: Hyperkinesis revisited. Pediatrics 61:319, 1978.

Miller, J. S.: Hyperactive children: A ten-year study. Pediatrics 61:217, 1978.

Sandberg, S. T., Rutter, M., and Taylor, E.: Hyperkinetic disorder in psychiatric clinic attenders. Dev. Med. Child. Neurol. 20:279, 1978.

Schmitt, B. D.: The minimal brain dysfunction myth. Am. J. Dis. Child. 129:1313, 1975.

Schmitt, B. D.: Guidelines for living with a hyperactive child. Pediatrics 60:387, 1977.

Shaywitz, S. E., and Shaywitz, B. A.: Diagnosis and management of attention deficit disorder: A pediatric perspective. Pediatr. Clin. North Am. 31:429, 1984.

Weiss, G., and Hechtman, L.: The hyperactive child syndrome. Science 205:1348, 1979.

PHYSIOLOGY OF SLEEP

Except in the newborn period and early infancy, when the cycles are less defined, normal sleep consists of regular cycles of rapid eye movement (REM) and non-rapid eye movement (NREM) sleep. After the age of two years, the sleep pattern is similar to that in the adult, with approximately five sleep cycles occurring each night and about three fourths of the night occupied in NREM sleep. The ratio of REM to NREM sleep in infants is 1:1, whereas in adults it is 1:4. The REM-NREM sleep cycle in infants is 50 to 60 minutes; in adults it is 90 to 100 minutes. REM sleep is characterized by rapid, synchronous eye movement and marked brain activity. Most dreaming occurs during REM sleep. NREM sleep during which rapid eye movements are absent and the brain assumes a resting phase, is composed of four stages: stage 1 or transitional; stage 2, during which sleep spindles are noted; and stages 3 and 4, which are characterized by high-amplitude slow waves.

ETIOLOGIC CLASSIFICATION OF SLEEP PROBLEMS

I. HYPERSOMNIAS

A. Narcolepsy, a disorder of REM sleep, most frequently has its onset between 15 and 25 years of age. A history of excessive sleepiness during the daytime in childhood and early adolescence is frequently reported. Excessive daytime sleepiness begins three or four hours after awakening and is manifest in micro-sleep episodes, some 5 to 15 seconds in duration, during which the adolescent has a glassy look. The overpowering sleepiness causes the patient to fall asleep. Because of the numerous brief sleep episodes, the adolescent may experience considerable difficulty in learning.

Associated symptoms may also appear. Cataplexy, characterized by sudden weakness or loss in muscle tone that lasts from seconds to minutes, may be precipitated by laughter, anger or surprise. During these episodes, the patient may experience a jaw drop, feel weak in the knees, fall and be unable to move. Consciousness is maintained. Cataplexy may precede the sleep attacks. Sleep paralysis, which occurs either while the patient is falling asleep or awakening, is a brief attack of flaccid paralysis, perhaps accompanied by intense fear or by visual and auditory hypnagogic hallucinations.

Zarcone, V.: Narcolepsy. N. Engl. J. Med. 288:1156, 1973.

B. The Kleine-Levin syndrome, or periodic hypersomnia and bulimia, a disorder limited to males, is characterized by episodes of excessive sleep and overeating. The episodes occur from two to four times a year and last several days to weeks. During an episode, the child usually sleeps continuously, awakening only to go to the bathroom or to gorge himself with food. The cause is unknown. Spontaneous remission usually occurs after two or three years.

Frank, Y., Braham, J., and Cohen, B. E.: The Kleine-Levin syndrome. Am. J. Dis. Child. 127:412, 1974.

C. Depression is the most common cause of hypersomnia in adolescents, and excessive sleepiness owing to diminished duration of stages 3 to 4 NREM sleep and early awakening. The depressed adolescent may also have trouble falling asleep. This pattern is to be differentiated from the normal practice of many adolescents to sleep late on week-ends, perhaps owing, in part, to a chronic sleep deficit that had begun in the preadolescent years.

D. Sleep apnea-hypersomnia syndrome is an important cause of daytime hypersomnolence, with the child falling asleep frequently during the day and complaining of headache on arising, fatigue and poor school performance. The child's sleep, characterized by periods of loud snoring, retractions and use of the accessory muscles of respiration, is repeatedly interrupted by apnea and partial awakening, at times with an abrupt jump. The apnea spells, which appear chiefly during NREM sleep and may interrupt over half the sleep period, cause hypoxemia, hypercapnia and mild acidosis. These episodes may be precipitated by a sleep-induced intermittent hypotonia of the tongue muscles that causes partial or complete upper airway obstruction, marked enlargement of the tonsils and adenoids, glossoptosis in the Pierre-Robin syndrome, and extreme obesity (the obesity-hypoventilation or pickwickian syndrome). Obstructive sleep apnea also occurs in achondroplasia, arthrogryposis multiplex congenita and in the following syndromes: Prader Willi, Scheie's, Down's, Morquio's, Larsen's, Arnold-Chiari and Crouzon. Sleep apnea may also follow surgical correction of velopharyngeal incompetence. Patients with a history suggestive of sleep apnea should be examined while asleep.

Brouillette, R. T., Fernbach, S. K., and Hunt, C. E.: Obstructive sleep apnea in infants and children. J. Pediatr. 100:31, 1982.
Frank, Y., Kravath, R. E., Pollack, C. P., and Weitzman, E. D.: Obstructive sleep apnea and its therapy: Clinical and polysomnographic manifestations. Pediatrics 71:737, 1983.
Gilleminault, C., Eldridge, F. L., Simmons, F. B., and Dement, W. C.: Sleep apnea in eight children. Pediatrics 58:23, 1976.
Kravath, R. E., Pollak, C. P., and Borowiecki, B.: Hypoventilation during sleep in children who have lymphoid airway obstruction treated by nasopharyngeal tube and T and A. Pediatrics 59:865, 1977.
Simpser, M. D., Streider, D. J., Wohl, M. E., Rosenthal, A., and Rockenmacher, S.: Sleep apnea in a child with the Pickwickian syndrome. Pediatrics 60:290, 1977.

E. Children who stay up late at night to watch television may be sleepy during the daytime.

F. Postencephalitic sleep disorder may be characterized by sleep reversal or hypersomnia.

G. Sleep disorders may be part of the posttraumatic syndrome after a head injury.

H. Prescribed or street drugs are an important, and often overlooked, etiology of excessive sleepiness in the classroom. Children who receive phenobarbital prophylaxis for febrile seizures may experience somnolence or frequent awakening at night.

I. Child abuse. Prolonged sleeping episodes may be caused by intentional poisoning of a child. Unless suspected and identified, such poisoning may continue in the hospital during parental visits.

Shnaps, Y., Frand, M., Rotem, Y., and Tirosh, M.: The chemically abused child. Pediatrics 68:119, 1981.

J. A *somnolence syndrome* may occur four to eight weeks after prophylactic cranial irradiation in patients, especially young children. Symptoms may persist for up to two weeks and be followed, in some cases, by a learning disability.

II. DISORDERS OF AROUSAL related to emergence from stage 3 or 4 NREM sleep (parasomnias)

A. Somnambulism, or sleep walking, is estimated to occur at least once in 15 per cent of school age children and to be persistent or recurrent in 1 to 6 per cent of the population. It occurs most frequently in boys within the first three hours of sleep during the transition from stage 3 or 4 NREM sleep to more superficial levels preceding the first REM sleep cycle period. The child suddenly awakens, sits up, climbs out of bed and walks about, poorly coordinated, with his eyes open but uncomprehending. He may give mumbled and monosyllabic responses to questions. Unless protected, the sleep walker may injure himself. The child does not remember the episodes, which last from seconds to 30 minutes. One to four episodes may occur per week. The cause of somnambulism is not clear, but the most likely etiology is a developmental one, as sleep walking tends to be outgrown within a few years. Complex partial (psychomotor) seizures are another diagnostic consideration.

B. Night terrors (pavor nocturnus) occur during arousal from stage 3 to 4 NREM sleep early in the night, usually 90 to 100 minutes after going to sleep. Most frequent in the 3 to 8 year age group, night terrors also occur in older infants and adolescents. The child suddenly sits up, screams in terror, appears intensely anxious with tachycardia, sweating and agitation and cannot be consoled. Episodes last from a few seconds to 10 to 30 minutes and are not remembered by the child. Night terrors probably are a developmental phenomenon, as they disappear with further maturation of the central nervous system. Occasionally, a stressful environmental event is a precipitating cause.

C. Nightmares are frightening dreams that occur during REM sleep. The child is more easily aroused from a nightmare than from a night terror. He usually awakens fully and vividly recalls the dream. An occasional nightmare is within normal limits, but persistent or frequent episodes suggest a developmental disturbance.

D. Enuresis, discussed more fully in Chapter 39, occasionally occurs as the child arouses from stage 3 or 4 NREM sleep prior to entering the first REM sleep period one to three hours after going to sleep.

E. Somniloquy or talking while asleep occurs during periods of arousal from REM sleep.

III. DEVELOPMENTAL/PSYCHOLOGICAL. The prevalence of these problems is high.

A. Colic may interfere with an infant's sleep pattern, usually with going to sleep.

B. Infants between the ages of six and nine months may resist going to sleep. Since sleep is a separation experience, it is understandable that infants of this age may be uncomfortable or anxious about going to sleep. If the parent is unable to set limits or fears that the baby's crying will disturb the neighbors, the problem may persist and develop into a chronic disorder. Sleep resistance is frequent in infants of depressed mothers.

C. Beginning at about nine months, infants awaken in the middle of the night and then refuse to go back to sleep (sleep or night awakening). The problem is compounded when the child is able to crawl out of his crib. The frequency of night waking in infants between 6 and 12 months of age ranges from 25 to 50 per cent. These episodes often begin during an illness. If the parent is firm about the expectation that the baby go to sleep, the problem will be a transient one; however, if the parent is not firm or attempts to remedy the problem by taking the baby into the parent's bed, sleep awakening may persist. Since one of the parents often also has a sleep problem, an appropriate question is, "Who else in your family has trouble sleeping?" Awakening during the night is a frequent manifestation in infants of depressed mothers.

Lozoff, B., Wolf., A. W., and Davis, N. S.: Co-sleeping in urban families with young children in the United States. Pediatrics 74:171, 1984.
Schmitt, B. D.: Infants who do not sleep through the night. Dev. Behavor. Pediatr. 2:20, 1981.

D. Sleep problems are common in the vulnerable child syndrome. The child often sleeps in the parents' bedroom, either with the mother, with both parents, or in his own crib or bed that is kept next to the mother and in her direct line of vision. The parents may report that the baby does not sleep well, but a closer inquiry often reveals that it is the parent who awakens several times a night to check on the child, often managing to arouse him to be sure that he is alive. The interview may reveal that the mother is unable to sleep at night unless she feels the baby is safe and sound. It becomes apparent that many such mothers unwittingly keep the baby awake through a series of visual, auditory and tactile stimuli that convey her insistence that the baby not fall asleep, probably because of her fear that she would again feel the baby was dead.

E. Night-time rocking and head banging. Some babies may normally rock themselves to sleep. If this habit is exaggerated, possible environmental factors should be reviewed.

Sallustro, F., and Atwell, C. W.: Body rocking, head banging, and head rolling in normal children. J. Pediatr. 93:704, 1978.

F. Night-time wandering. Some preschool-age children seen because of hyperactivity, destructiveness or autism are reported to climb out of bed during the night, wander around the house, turn on the electric or gas range and start fires. Since these children usually have major emotional disturbances, psychiatric help is generally required.

G. Children with the attention deficit syndrome may sleep poorly.

IV. INSOMNIA OR DISORDERS OF INITIATING AND MAINTAINING SLEEP. Adolescents with persistent insomnia may be tense, worried, moody or depressed. As many as 5 to 12 per cent of adolescents report trouble sleeping. Those who are depressed may find it difficult to fall asleep or they may awaken during the night or early morning. Stimulant drugs may cause insomnia.

Price, V. A., Coates, T. J., Thoresen, C. E., and Grinstead, O. A.: Prevalence and correlates of poor sleep among adolescents. Am. J. Dis. Child. 132:583, 1978.
Young people who sleep badly. Editorial. Brit. Med. J. 2:1450, 1978.

V. SLEEP REVERSALS occur in some children with hepatic failure or as a postencephalitic sequela. Delirious children may be drowsy during the daytime and unable to sleep at night.

VI. COMPLEX PARTIAL (PSYCHOMOTOR) SEIZURES are a rare diagnostic possibility in children with night terrors or somnambulism.

VII. GRAVES' DISEASE may be characterized by restless sleep and insomnia.

VIII. NARCOTIC WITHDRAWAL in a newborn infant may cause him to sleep very little.

IX. JUVENILE PRIMARY FIBROMYALGIA is often accompanied by restless sleep with frequent awakening.

GENERAL REFERENCES

Anders, T. F.: Night-waking in infants during the first year of life. Pediatrics 63:860, 1979.
Kales, A., and Kales, J. D.: Sleep disorders. N. Engl. J. Med. 290:487, 1974.
Lozoff, B., Wolf, A. W., and Davis, N. S.: Sleep problems seen in pediatric practice. Pediatrics 75:477, 1985.
Mark, J. D., and Brooks, J. G.: Sleep-associated airway problems in children. Pediatr. Clin. North Am. 31:907, 1984.
Rabe, E. F.: Recurrent paroxysmal nonepileptic disorders. Curr. Probl. Pediatr. 4:3, 1974.

ETIOLOGIC CLASSIFICATION OF SLEEP PROBLEMS

39 / ENURESIS

Several studies have demonstrated that 10 per cent or more of children have nocturnal enuresis at age five, but that by the end of adolescence, the incidence is less than 1 per cent. The delay in achieving nighttime bladder control often has a familial background. While relapse or secondary enuresis often occurs after psychologically upsetting events and stressors such as separation, divorce, a move or a family death, there is little evidence that psychological factors are of major importance in primary enuresis.

Organic disorders that may cause involuntary urination include obstructive uropathy, a pelvic mass, diabetes mellitus, diabetes insipidus, and psychogenic water drinking. Children with myelomeningocele and a neurogenic bladder frequently have urinary incontinence, as may those who are mentally retarded.

Urinary incontinence is discussed on page 414.

DIAGNOSIS

As with other developmental symptoms, diagnosis and treatment should proceed simultaneously, with the interview serving as the principal tool to collect data and to establish a constructive relationship among the doctor, the child and the family. Through the interview, the physician clarifies for himself and for the patient the multiple etiologic possibilities and determines the familial incidence of enuresis, the family and the child's understanding of the problem, their interest in overcoming the symptom, the methods that have already been tried, and their notions about what might work. The frequency of dry nights or periods of several nights during which enuresis has not occurred has some predictive value as to the spontaneous cessation of the symptom. Observation of the boy's urinary stream by the physician may be indicated to determine whether he has difficulty in initiating urination or an interrupted urinary stream.

Diurnal or daytime enuresis presents a different problem than nocturnal enuresis, although they may coexist. Most children are dry during the day by the age of two and one-half years except for the occasional time when they do not want to interrupt their play to void. In addition to the causes listed above for nocturnal wetting, organic etiologies for diurnal enuresis include an ectopic ureter, urinary tract infection, urethritis in girls owing to bubble bath products, and fecal impaction. Giggle incontinence may rarely occur in girls when they laugh vigorously. Daytime wetting may occasionally be caused by bouts of bladder spasm in adolescent girls. Diurnal enuresis is usually secondary to anxiety associated with such environmental stressors as marital discord, separation, divorce, parental illness, death of a relative, maternal depression, or inappropriate parenting (e.g., harsh punishment or abuse).

LABORATORY EVALUATION

The laboratory investigation of children with enuresis should include a urinalysis for specific gravity, glycosuria, proteinuria, pyuria and, in girls, a urine culture, although this examination is rarely positive. In the presence of a normal urinalysis and urine culture, normal physical examination (including the external genitalia) and absence of a neurological abnormality, routine radiologic studies need not be obtained. Symptoms such as frequency, urgency, dribbling, dysuria, hesitancy in beginning or straining on urination, a poor urinary stream, a history of previous urinary tract infections and a preponderance of daytime wetting suggest true urinary incontinence or obstructive urologic disease and indicate the need for dynamic urinary tract studies, excretory urography and voiding cystourethrography.

GENERAL REFERENCES

Committee on Radiology, American Academy of Pediatrics: Excretory urography for evaluation of enuresis. Pediatrics 65:644, 1980.

McLain, L. G.: Childhood enuresis. Curr. Probl. Pediatr., 9:4, 1979.

Schmitt, B. D.: Daytime wetting (diurnal enuresis). Pediatr. Clin. North Am., 29:9, 1982.

Schmitt, B. D.: Nocturnal enuresis: An update on treatment. Pediatr. Clin. North Am. 29:21, 1982.

Shelov, S. P., et al.: Enuresis: A contrast of attitudes of parents and physicians. Pediatrics 67:707, 1981.

Smith, L. R.: Nocturnal enuresis. Pediatr. Rev. 2:183, 1980.

40 / CONVULSIONS

Convulsive seizures affect an estimated 7 per cent of children under age five. The underlying pathophysiologic cause of convulsive seizures is not known. Classification of convulsive seizures cannot, therefore, be based on fundamental considerations. Instead, it must be based on factors such as the patient's age, the clinical pattern of the seizure, electroencephalographic (EEG) findings, anatomic localization and the clinical disorders that may be accompanied by this symptom. The classification given here, intended as a guide to diagnostic considerations in children with convulsive seizures, relates to a number of these etiologic factors. Some of these processes may account either for isolated seizures or for recurrent episodes. A patient may demonstrate more than one type of seizure. A detailed description of the seizure and possible precipitating events may be helpful diagnostically.

ETIOLOGIC CLASSIFICATION OF CONVULSIONS

I. FEBRILE CONVULSIONS. Not infrequently, convulsive seizures accompany acute febrile illnesses in children under the age of three years, especially in the first two years, and more commonly in boys. In children under the age of five years, these episodes have been estimated to occur with an incidence of between 3.5 and 4 per cent. Febrile seizure is not to be considered as an initial diagnostic possibility to explain convulsions in infants who are less than three months of age.

The febrile seizure, either generalized with tonic and clonic components or focal, usually follows a rapid rise in temperature to 39.4° C (103° F) or above. The seizure may be brief (one to ten minutes) and mild, or long (over one half hour) and severe.

A number of relationships exist between fever and convulsive seizures. Fever, in itself, may be the direct cause of a convulsion; on the other hand, severe convulsive seizures may cause some elevation of body temperature as a result of vigorous muscular activity. The seizure may be caused primarily by an infectious or other disease and

not by the fever itself; therefore, a careful effort should be made to determine the primary cause of the fever and the seizure in each child with a "febrile" convulsion. Elevation of body temperature may act as a precipitating event in a child destined to have idiopathic epilepsy. Rarely, fever may, in itself, be an epileptic manifestation.

Most children who have one or two febrile convulsions never experience another; however, about one third have a subsequent febrile seizure, and 2 to 3 per cent have recurrent nonfebrile seizures. Although it is impossible to prognosticate, children with seizures that are focal, persist over 30 minutes or are followed by neurologic findings such as hemiparesis are more likely to have later convulsions. Children who have a history of repeated seizures with only slight temperature elevation are also likely to have future difficulty. Other high-risk factors include a family history of seizures without fever and pre-existing neurologic impairment in the child. The usefulness of the EEG in the diagnostic study of febrile seizures remains controversial.

Fishman, M. A.: Febrile seizures: The treatment controversy. J. Pediatr. 94:177, 1979.

Freeman, J. M.: Febrile seizures: An end to confusion. Pediatrics 61:806, 1978.

Nelson, K. B., and Ellenberg, J. H.: Prognosis in children with febrile seizures. Pediatrics 61:720, 1978.

Verity, C. M., Butler, N. R., and Golding, J.: Febrile convulsions in a national cohort followed up from birth. Br. Med. J. 290:1307, 1311, 1985.

II. GENERALIZED SEIZURES

A. Absence seizures (petit mal). Absence episodes, which are most common between four and eight years of age, are characterized by transient (5 to 30 seconds) lapses of consciousness. The patient has a blank, staring expression, or his eyes may roll up. He either becomes immobile or demonstrates rhythmic movements or stereotyped automatisms, such as blinking; lip smacking; chewing movements; nodding or jerking of the head, extremities or trunk; truncal swaying; twitching about the eyes or mouth; and finger snapping. The child may walk in circles. The patient does not fall, but he may drop whatever he is holding. The seizure begins and ends abruptly with no aura or postictal symptoms. Only a few seizures, or as many as a hundred, may occur per day. Petit mal episodes can often be precipitated by hyperventilation for three minutes. Differentiation from brief complex partial seizures may be difficult. Absence status may cause the child to remain in a confused, groggy, daydream-like state for hours. In addition to lethargy, the child with absence status may have facial twitches and muscle jerks or may stagger about.

Moe, P. G.: Spike-wave stupor. Petit mal status. Am. J. Dis. Child. 121:307, 1971.

Atypical absence (petit mal variants, Lennox-Gestault) seizures begin in the second or third year and are associated with a poor outcome. The patients are usually mentally retarded. Clinical manifestations include tonic seizures, atypical absences and myoclonic or atonic seizures.

B. Tonic-clonic seizures (grand mal). About half the children who have grand mal epilepsy experience a motor, sensory or visceral aura before the convulsion. Abdominal pain is a common aura. Other presentations include a peculiar sensation in the throat, an unusual taste or smell, chewing motions or turning of the head.

The actual seizure begins suddenly with loss of consciousness. The child may cry out. If standing, he falls. The first or tonic phase, which lasts about one-half to one minute, is characterized by stiffening of the body owing to tonic muscle contraction, rolling of the eyes, tongue biting, cyanosis and drooling. Involuntary urination and defecation may occur. This period is followed by the clonic phase, which is characterized by violent jerking movements of the trunk and extremities that may last a few seconds or several minutes before they become accentuated but less frequent and then gradually cease. The seizure is followed by sleep from which the child is not easily aroused. On awakening, he may appear confused and complain of a severe headache. Occasionally, transient paresis of an extremity or hemiparesis may develop (Todd's paralysis).

C. Myoclonic seizures
1. Massive myoclonic seizures of infancy (lightning seizures, infantile spasms, West syndrome) are brief convulsive episodes in infants (sa-laam convulsion, head dropping or jackknifing) characterized by flexion and adduction or upward and outward movement of the upper extremities, flexion of the head on the chest, jackknife flexion of the thighs on the abdomen, generalized quivering and rolling of the eyes. Occasionally, extension of the head and lower extremities occurs. The baby may also cry out. The seizures, which may number a hundred or so in one day, often follow in close succession. Infants with this seizure pattern usually have extensive brain damage and are both microcephalic and retarded. The term "hypsarrhythmia" refers to the characteristic electroencephalographic pattern.

2. Myoclonic seizures in older children are characterized by sudden, spasmodic contractions of the muscles of the trunk or extremities, most commonly the flexors of the arms. The contractions last only a few seconds. Extensor spasms may also occur. When marked, the flexor spasms may cause the child to pitch forward so violently as to injure his face and head. Disorders associated with myoclonic seizures in infants and children include tuberous sclerosis, Menkes' kinky hair disease, pyridoxine dependency or deficiency, phenylketonuria, maple syrup urine disease, cytomegalic inclusion disease, toxoplasmosis, congenital malformations of the brain, subacute sclerosing panencephalitis, gangliosidosis, other degenerative central nervous system disorders and Unverrichtlundborg progressive familial myoclonic epilepsy.

3. Benign myoclonus of early infancy is the term applied to a small group of infants in whom myoclonic seizures, especially involving the extensors and flexors of the neck or adversive jerking or turning of the head (cephalic myoclonus), stop spontaneously a few weeks or months after their onset.

Livingston, S.: Diagnosis and treatment of childhood myoclonic seizures. Pediatrics 53:542, 1974.
Lombroso, C. T., and Fejerman, N.: Benign myoclonus of early infancy. Ann. Neurol. 1:138, 1977.

4. In myoclonic encephalopathy of infants (Kinsbourne dancing eye syndrome), the affected infant demonstrates jerking movements of the

head, trunk and extremities; ataxia; and dancing movements (opso-clonus) of the eyes.

5. In sensory precipitation epilepsy, myoclonic seizures may be precipitated by tapping or touching.

6. Sleep myoclonus refers to the sudden jerk, either generalized or localized to the extremities that may normally occur when a child is falling asleep.

D. Akinetic epilepsy (drop fits) are characterized by a sudden loss of muscle tone, with the child nodding or slumping to the floor. Generalized seizures and staring spells may also occur. Many of these children are retarded.

E. Tonic seizures are characterized primarily by tonic contractions of major muscle groups of the trunk and extremities with a clonic component absent or minimal. Extensor posturing in infants with gastroesophageal reflux may simulate a tonic seizure.

F. Clonic seizures are without a tonic phase.

G. Atonic seizures are characterized by a sudden loss of muscle tone.

H. Status epilepticus is characterized by repeated or unrelenting convulsive seizures that persist for at least 30 minutes. Such seizures are usually tonic-clonic in character, but absence or complex partial status may also occur.

I. Sensory-precipitated seizures may be caused by a variety of sensory stimuli. Photoconvulsions, the most common sensory-precipitated type of seizure, are usually precipitated by watching television. They may also be self-induced by waving fingers before the eyes or blinking while looking at a bright light. Other precipitating stimuli are music (musicogenic epilepsy), brushing the teeth, touching, tapping and reading.

J. Apneic episodes, occurring either during sleep or while awake, may represent a convulsion in infants.

III. PARTIAL SEIZURES (FOCAL, LOCAL)

A. Simple partial seizures, which do not alter consciousness, may be either motor or sensory or a mixture of both. Jacksonian seizures begin with unilateral twitching around the eye or mouth and spread over the face, or they may begin in the thumb and "march" up the arm. They may involve only one side of the body or progress to a generalized seizure. Partial motor or adversive seizures may be characterized by contraversive movement of the head and eyes and lifting of the contralateral upper extremity. Focal motor seizures, which may occur during or on awakening from sleep, may be accompanied by rolandic or midtemporal spikes (benign epilepsy of childhood with rolandic or centrotemporal spikes). Attacks of paroxysmal choreoathetosis with their sensory and motor components may simulate a simple partial seizure (see page 121). Occipital seizures may cause transient blindness. Focal seizures may occur secondary to a brain tumor, cerebral abscess, hemorrhage, trauma, vaso-occlusive crisis or encephalitis. These disorders may also cause generalized rather than focal seizures; on the other hand, systemic disorders such as hypoglycemia may cause focal or partial seizures.

Focal sensory seizures may cause paresthesias, tingling, numbness, burning, or a variety of visual, auditory or olfactory sensations. Seizures with autonomic manifestations may be characterized by episodes of flushing, pallor, dizziness, hypertension, dilatation of one or both pupils, lacrimation, perspiration, tachycardia, salivation, vomiting, masticatory movements, paroxysmal abdominal pain, fever or headache.

B. Complex partial seizures (psychomotor, temporal lobe), which are associated with alteration of consciousness, have highly varied symptoms. The manifestations may be chiefly automatisms, such as rubbing, chewing, lip smacking, drooling, spitting, hissing, muttering, swallowing, sucking, staring, grimacing, blinking, muscle jerks, laughing (gelastic epilepsy), shouting, pulling at clothes or body parts, searching through desk drawers, purposeless wandering and running (cursive epilepsy). Others may be *autonomic* with salivation, vomiting, pallor or flushing or *psychic* in the form of confused, dream-like states; fugues; hallucinations; fearfulness; manic, aggressive or psychotic behavior; and temper outbursts. Still other manifestations may be *sensory* with numbness, tingling, impaired vision, blindness, hearing loss and dizziness. Visual illusions in which objects appear small and far away or unusually large or distorted may be reported. Episodes usually last a few seconds or minutes, although rarely they may continue for hours or progress to a generalized tonic-clonic convulsion.

Irritability, hyperactivity, headache and altered appetite may be noted hours or days before episodes. Auras include epigastric discomfort or heaviness that moves up to the throat, fear, buzzing sensations, dizziness, visual or auditory illusions, repetitious sounds and peculiar smells.

Complex partial seizures may begin with a simple partial seizure followed by an alteration in consciousness. The patient may or may not have amnesia for the seizure. The electroencephalogram may be normal or demonstrate a focal seizure pattern. Differentiation between a severe behavior disorder, schizophrenia and complex partial seizures may be difficult, and they may coexist. They may also simulate absence seizures. The Alice in Wonderland syndrome in juvenile migraine may simulate a partial seizure.

Geschwind, N.: Behavioral change in temporal lobe epilepsy. Arch. Neurol. 34:453, 1977.
Gold, A. P.: Psychomotor epilepsy in childhood. Pediatrics 53:540, 1974.

IV. METABOLIC FACTORS

A. Hypocalcemia
1. Newborn. Symptoms associated with hypocalcemia (serum calcium less than 7 mg/dl) in the newborn include jitteriness, tremor, irritability, laryngospasm and seizures. The infant may also appear lethargic or may vomit or fail to feed.
    a. Birth to 72 hours
        1. Maternal factors
            a. Hyperparathyroidism. The maternal serum calcium and phosphorus should be determined.
            b. Toxemia of pregnancy
            c. Diabetes mellitus
        2. Perinatal factors
            a. Placenta previa, abruptio placentae
            b. Low birth weight; prematurity or small for gestational age
            c. Cesarean section
            d. Birth trauma with cerebral injury
            e. Asphyxia
            f. Respiratory distress syndrome
            g. Sepsis
            h. Hyperbilirubinemia
    b. After 72 hours
        1. High phosphate intake in infants given cow's or soybean milk or other formula that has a high phosphate:calcium ratio

2. Hypomagnesemia
3. Hypoparathyroidism
2. Hypoparathyroidism
    a. Transient idiopathic
    b. Familial
    c. DiGeorge's syndrome may be associated with seizures owing to hypocalcemia in the first months of life. Other findings include congenital heart disease, especially interrupted aortic arch or truncus arteriosus and dysmorphic facies with hypertelorism, anteverted nostrils, micrognathia and low-set, pointed ears.

Conley, M. E., Beckwith, J. B., Mancer, J. K. K., and Teckhoff, L.: The spectrum of DiGeorge's syndrome. J. Pediatr. 94:883, 1979.

    d. Acquired
    e. Pseudohypoparathyroidism
3. Rickets owing to vitamin D deficiency or metabolic defect

Root, A. W., and Harrison, H. E.: Recent advances in calcium metabolism II. Disorders of calcium homeostasis. J. Pediatr. 88:177, 1976.

4. Pediatric sodium dihydrogen phosphate enemas may cause hypocalcemia secondary to hyperphosphatemia. Tetany, coma and dehydration may result.

Sotos, J. F., Cutler, E. A., Finkel, M. A., and Doody, D.: Hypocalcemic coma following two pediatric phosphate enemas. Pediatrics 60:305, 1977.

B. Hypomagnesemia. Serum magnesium concentrations should be obtained in infants with tetany.
C. Hypoglycemia
1. Symptomatic neonatal hypoglycemia occurs with a frequency of 2 to 3 per 1000 live births. Many other infants have subclinical hypoglycemia. Blood glucose determinations (Dextrostix or blood sugar) need to be repeated frequently in infants at risk, as well as in those with signs and symptoms such as irritability, tremors, convulsions, apnea, cyanosis, listlessness, poor feeding, rolling eye movements, high-pitched cry, unstable body temperature, pallor, absent Moro reflex or limpness. A blood sugar determination is indicated whenever a newborn infant seems ill. The diagnostic criteria for hypoglycemia are two or more determinations under 20 mg/dl in infants under 2500 grams; under 30 mg in term newborn infants; and under 40 mg in older infants and children.

Hypoglycemia may occur early and subclinically in infants of diabetic mothers and in those with hemolytic disease of the newborn before and after exchange transfusion. Secondary hypoglycemia may follow such perinatal stressors as hypoxia, sepsis, respiratory distress, hypothermia, central nervous system impairment, hyperviscosity and multiple congenital anomalies. Transient neonatal hypoglycemia tends to be severe and to recur in infants, especially males, who are small for gestational age; with toxemia of pregnancy; and in the smaller of twins. The metabolic, endocrine and enzymatic disorders listed below may also cause neonatal hypoglycemia. In the older infant and child, the manifestations of hypoglycemia include "wilting" spells, blank stares, rolling of the eyes, episodes of pallor, periods of unexplained irritability and crying, stiffening, limpness, twitching and generalized convulsions.

Cowett, R. M.: Pathophysiology, diagnosis, and management of glucose homeostasis in the neonate. Curr. Probl. Pediatr. 15(3): March, 1985.

2. Hyperinsulinemia
    a. Beta-cell hyperplasia; Beckwith-Wiedemann syndrome
    b. Beta-cell tumors
    c. Nesidioblastosis
    d. Functional beta-cell defects
3. Ketotic hypoglycemia, which usually becomes apparent between the ages of 18 months and 5 years and undergoes spontaneous cessation by 10 years of age, is probably the most common cause of hypoglycemia beyond the newborn period. In addition to hypoglycemia, the patient demonstrates ketonuria and ketonemia.
4. Endocrine disorders
    a. Hypopituitarism
    b. Isolated ACTH deficiency
    c. Addison's disease
    d. Hypothyroidism
5. Hepatic enzyme deficiencies
    a. Glycogenosis
        1. Glucose-6-phosphatase (glycogenosis Type I) causes marked ketosis, hypoglycemia, lactic acidosis, hepatomegaly and failure to thrive in young infants.
        2. Amylo-1,6-glucosidase
        3. Defects of the phosphorylase enzyme system

    b. Disorders of gluconeogenesis
        1. Fructose-1,6-diphosphatase. The presenting signs and symptoms are indistinguishable from those owing to deficiency of glucose-6-phosphatase.
        2. Pyruvate carboxylase
    c. Other enzymatic defects
        1. Glycogen synthetase
        2. Galactose-1-phosphate uridyl transferase (galactosemia)
        3. Fructose-1-phosphate aldolase (hereditary fructose intolerance) is characterized by hypoglycemia and vomiting after fructose ingestion.
6. Other inborn errors of metabolism
    a. Maple syrup urine disease
    b. Congenital lactic acidosis
    c. Lysosomal acid phosphatase deficiency

Cornblath, M., and Schwartz, R.: Disorders of Carbohydrate Metabolism in Infancy. 2nd ed. Philadelphia, W. B. Saunders Co., 1976.

Guterlet, R. L., and Cornblath, M.: Neonatal hypoglycemia revisited, 1975. Pediatrics 58:10, 1976.

Lubchenco, L. O., and Bard, H.: Incidence of hypoglycemia in newborn infants classified by birth weight and gestational age. Pediatrics 47:831, 1971.

Pagliara, A. S., Karl, I. E., Haymond, M., and Kipnis, D. M.: Hypoglycemia in infancy and childhood. Parts I and II. J. Pediatr. 82:365, 558, 1973.

Schwartz, J. F., and Zwiren, G. T.: Islet cell adenomatosis and adenoma in an infant. J. Pediatr. 79:232, 1971.

Stanley, C. A., and Baker, L.: Hyperinsulinism in infants and children: Diagnosis and therapy. Adv. Pediatr. 23:315, 1976.

D. Since hyponatremia and hypo-osmolarity may occur in children with acute infections of the central nervous system, determination of the serum electrolytes is indicated in such patients who have an otherwise unexplained seizure. Water intoxication may occur in normal infants less than 6 months of age who are offered dilute formula or water alone.

David, R., Ellis, D., and Gartner, J. C.: Water intoxication in normal infants: Role of antidiuretic hormone in pathogenesis. Pediatrics 68:349, 1981.

E. Uremia
F. Poisoning is an etiologic possibility in children with an unexplained convulsive seizure. Seizures owing to lead encephalopathy, more common in the summer, may first occur during an

acute infection and be mistakenly ascribed to the illness, to fever or to idiopathic epilepsy. Early symptoms of lead poisoning include vomiting, constipation, irritability and lethargy. Although parents should be specifically asked about pica, especially chewing of paint-covered surfaces, denial of such exposure does not eliminate the possibility. Qualitative determination of urine coproporphyrins is a preliminary screening test. A more significant finding is increased free erythrocyte protoporphyrin. The peripheral blood may demonstrate hypochromic microcytic stippled erythrocytes. Radiopaque material may be seen in the gastrointestinal tract on a plain film of the abdomen. Glycosuria and aminoaciduria may be noted. Examination of the cerebrospinal fluid may demonstrate increased pressure and protein concentration. Early, the latter may be present without the former.

Piomelli, S., Rosen, J. F., Chisolm, J. J., Jr., and Graef, J. W.: Management of childhood lead poisoning. J. Pediatr. 105:523, 1984.

Other poisons that cause convulsive seizures include:
    Strychnine
    Arsenic
    Sodium fluoride
    Camphor
    Pyrethrum
    Kerosene
    Gasoline sniffing
    Volatile oils
    Poisonous plants
    Salicylate poisoning

G. Pyridoxine (vitamin B_6) deficiency or dependency in young infants may cause irritability, hyperacusia, colic, regurgitation and convulsive seizures.
H. Hypoxemia
    1. Asphyxia
    2. Carbon monoxide poisoning. Convulsions may occur when the level of carboxyhemoglobin reaches 40 to 60 per cent.
    3. Near-drowning
    4. Breath-holding spells are common in infants, especially during the latter part of the first year and the early months of the second year, and may persist in unusual situations until the age of four years. Episodes may be triggered by some injury, often trivial; a reprimand; sudden fright; anger; or frustration. Vigorous crying is the first manifestation. After a variable period, the child gasps suddenly or holds his breath until he becomes blue or pale, unconscious and limp. Rigidity, convulsive movements, or opisthotonus may rarely follow if unconsciousness is prolonged. Some children, especially those who experience large numbers of these episodes, may only gasp or cry briefly before holding their breath.

The presenting complaint is usually convulsions or blacking out rather than breath-holding or syncope. The history and sequence of events are so characteristic that the differential diagnosis generally presents no problem; however, when the precipitating event seems extremely trivial, when no triggering circumstance is apparent, when the child is said to cry or hold his breath for only a short time, or when the convulsive movements are a prominent clinical feature, differentiation from epilepsy may require an electroencephalogram and further observation.

Some babies seem especially prone to have these spells, and a familial incidence may be noted. Although in some cases no contributory disturbance in the home or in the mother-infant relationship is apparent, these possibilities need to be explored. Immature parents, maternal depression, parental inability to set limits, the child's manipulativeness and other difficulties in maternal-infant interaction need to be dealt with if the spells are to be prevented. Many of these children have an iron deficiency anemia that appears to be an associated rather than a causative disorder.

Livingston, S.: Breathholding spells in children. A differentiation from epileptic attacks. JAMA 212:2231, 1970.

    5. Respiratory failure
    6. Seizure-like states, hot flashes and episodes of weakness may be presenting complaints in children with primary pulmonary hypertension.
I. Phenothiazine tranquilizers may precipitate or increase seizures in patients with epilepsy.
J. Newborn infants may demonstrate narcotic withdrawal symptoms such as respiratory distress, restlessness, trembling, irritability, convulsions and a shrill, high-pitched cry.
K. Phenylketonuria may be characterized by seizures.

L. Other inborn errors of metabolism that cause metabolic acidosis or hyperammonemia

M. Elevated theophylline levels may cause seizures in infants.

V. CEREBRAL FACTORS

A. Trauma
   1. Cerebral concussion; contusion; laceration; focal or generalized edema of the brain. During the week following hospitalization for head trauma, a few children have a seizure. Approximately 25 per cent of those who experience this complication develop post-traumatic epilepsy.
   2. Extradural hematoma; subdural hematoma
   3. Whiplash injury in an infant, caused by abusive shaking, may be characterized by convulsions, retinal hemorrhage, bulging fontanel and vomiting.

B. Infections of the central nervous system
   1. Toxoplasmosis is an important diagnostic consideration with convulsive seizures in newborn and young infants. Congenital toxoplasmosis must be differentiated from the Aicardi syndrome. The latter occurs in females and is characterized by infantile spasms, mental retardation, agenesis of the corpus callosum and a pathognomonic chorioretinopathy with discrete yellow-white holes representing atrophy of the pigment epithelium.

Willis, S., and Rosman, N. P.: The Aicardi syndrome versus congenital infections: Diagnostic considerations. J. Pediatr. 96:235, 1980.

   2. Encephalitis. Herpes simplex encephalitis may cause seizures with temporal lobe localization.
   3. Convulsions may be an important clinical manifestation of meningitis.
   4. Subdural effusion complicating bacterial meningitis is to be considered in the presence of persistent fever after 72 hours, a positive cerebrospinal fluid culture after 48 hours, general or focal convulsions, vomiting during the convalescent period, neurologic abnormalities, hemiparesis, opisthotonus, bulging fontanel, head enlargement, impaired consciousness, persistent irritability or an otherwise unsatisfactory clinical course.
   5. Intracranial abscess may initially present with a seizure.
   6. Rabies
   7. Cerebral cysticercosis, owing to eating the ova of the pork tapeworm and endemic in Central and South America and in parts of Asia and Africa, may present with a generalized convulsive seizure. Computerized tomography may be diagnostically helpful.

Percy, A. K., Byrd, S. E., and Locke, G. E.: Cerebral cysticercosis. Pediatrics 66:967, 1980.

C. Intracranial hemorrhage
   1. Generalized, unilateral or focal convulsions are a common manifestation of a subdural hematoma.
   2. Extradural hematoma
   3. Subarachnoid hemorrhage owing to rupture of a congenital aneurysm of the circle of Willis is a rare cause of seizures in older children.
   4. Hemorrhagic diseases such as hemophilia or thrombocytopenic purpura may be complicated by an intracranial hemorrhage.

D. Thrombosis of cerebral vessels
   1. Children with cyanotic heart disease and polycythemia may develop cerebral thrombosis, especially when they are dehydrated. Syncope, coma and severe, persistent convulsions may result.

Phornphutkul, C., Rosenthal, A., Nadas, A. S., and Berenberg, W.: Cerebrovascular accidents in infants and children with cyanotic congenital heart disease. Am. J. Cardiol. 32:329, 1973.

   2. Sickle cell anemia may produce seizures, strokes and altered states of consciousness owing to a vaso-occlusive crisis. The seizures are usually generalized, but they may be focal.

Portnoy, B. A., and Herion, J. C.: Neurological manifestations in sickle cell disease with a review of the literature and emphasis on the prevalence of hemiplegia. Ann. Intern. Med. 76:643, 1972.

   3. Occlusion of the venous sinuses and the cerebral veins may be caused by severe dehydration in infants and young children, trauma, infection and acute lymphoblastic leukemia. Clinical manifestations include impaired consciousness and convulsive seizures.
   4. Acute infantile hemiplegia in infants and young children is caused by a sudden vascular accident, such as embolism or thrombosis of the middle cerebral artery. It almost always has a sudden onset with a severe convulsion, usually unilateral but oc-

casionally generalized, followed by fever, coma and hemiparesis. Convulsions continue for one to five days, and coma may persist for seven to ten days.

Solomon, G. E., Hilal, S. K., Gold, A. P., and Carter, S.: Natural history of acute hemiplegia of childhood. Brain 93:107, 1970.

E. Neurocutaneous syndromes
   1. Seizures in the Sturge-Weber syndrome may be generalized or limited to the contralateral side.
   2. Tuberous sclerosis may present with seizures as the initial complaint. Infants may experience infantile spasms or myoclonic seizures.
F. Psychologic factors
   1. Breath-holding spells
   2. Self-induced seizures may be precipitated by children who have a low threshold to photic stimulation by blinking or waving their fingers in front of their eyes. Other children may produce seizures by hyperventilation. Patients with self-induced seizures are usually mentally retarded or emotionally disturbed.
   3. Emotional factors may increase the frequency of seizures.
   4. Pseudoseizures have a superficial resemblance to true seizures, especially to tonic-clonic or partial epileptic convulsions with complex symptomatology. Opisthotonic posturing, tremulousness, thrashing about, rhythmic and coordinated movements, yelling, cursing, crying, combativeness and absence of postictal symptoms or urinary incontinence suggest a pseudoseizure. Both true and pseudoseizures may occur in the same child. EEG telemetry and videotaping may be diagnostically helpful.

Holmes, G. L., Sackellares, J. C., McKiernan, J., Ragland, M., and Dreifuss, F. E.: Evaluation of childhood pseudoseizures using EEG telemetry and video tape monitoring. J. Pediatr. 97:554, 1980.

   5. Dissociative reactions in psychotic children may simulate a seizure disorder.
G. Encephalopathy
   1. Postpertussis vaccine encephalopathy may be characterized by a high-pitched cry, convulsions and a shock-like state.
   2. Pertussis may cause convulsions owing to cerebral hemorrhage, encephalitis or anoxia.

   3. Hypertensive encephalopathy may cause convulsive seizures.
   4. Toxic encephalopathy with seizures and impairment of consciousness may occur during severe systemic diseases such as bacillary dysentery.
   5. Seizures may occur with lupus erythematosus.
   6. Infectious mononucleosis may rarely cause seizures.
   7. Convulsions may be a complication of corticosteroid treatment, especially in lupus erythematosus.
   8. The hemolytic-uremic syndrome may be characterized by seizures, alterations of consciousness and transient hemiparesis.

Bale, J. F., Jr., Brasher, C., and Siegler, R. L.: CNS manifestations of the hemolytic-uremic syndrome. Am. J. Dis. Child. 134:869, 1980.

   9. Reye's syndrome in infants may be accompanied by seizures. A convulsion may be the presenting complaint.
   10. Gasoline or other solvent sniffing
H. Degenerative diseases
   1. Demyelinating encephalopathies may first become manifest with a convulsion; however, seizures are not a regular occurrence.
   2. GM_1 gangliosidosis (type II or late infantile) becomes manifest in the second or third year with retardation and seizures. Juvenile GM_1 gangliosidosis is characterized by ataxia, seizures and intellectual deterioration.
   3. Metachromatic leukodystrophy becomes symptomatic at about the end of the first year of life with ataxia followed later by intellectual deterioration and seizures.
   4. Infantile sialidosis or the cherry red spot–myoclonus syndrome
   5. Convulsive seizures are a late manifestation in Tay-Sachs disease.
   6. Other cerebromacular degenerative diseases
   7. Niemann-Pick disease
   8. Infantile Gaucher's disease
   9. Subacute sclerosing panencephalitis (SSPE) is initially manifested by subtle personality changes and deterioration in school performance. Behavioral changes include forgetfulness, temper outbursts, distractability, hallucinations and insomnia. Myoclonic seizures involving the head, trunk and extremities, which appear late, may initially simulate ataxia. Eventually, the episodes occur every

5 to 15 seconds without loss of consciousness. The diagnosis may be made at this stage by characteristic electroencephalographic, spinal fluid and measles antibody findings. With progression of the disorder, the myoclonic jerks become exaggerated and intellectual deterioration occurs.

Noronha, M. J.: Cerebral degenerative disorders of infancy and childhood. Dev. Med. Child. Neurol. 16:228, 1974.

I. Brain tumors. Generalized convulsive seizures may occur with supratentorial tumors as the initial symptom unaccompanied by signs of increased intracranial pressure. Convulsions are less commonly the initial symptom in patients with infratentorial tumors. Increased pressure in the posterior fossa may produce "cerebellar fits" characterized by decerebrate rigidity, opisthotonus, respiratory difficulty and cyanosis. Patients with unexplained, especially focal, seizures should be followed carefully with repeated neurologic examinations. In addition, changes in behavior, school performance, response to medication or type and frequency of seizures warrant diagnostic consideration of a brain tumor.

J. Tetanus
K. Hyperexplexia is a hereditary disorder characterized by an excessive startle response, generalized muscle stiffness and sudden falling.

CONVULSIONS IN NEWBORN INFANTS

Seizures in the newborn and young infant may be subtle and require special diagnostic alertness. Focal clonic convulsions, which may either move rapidly from one part of the body to another or remain localized, are the most frequent. Multifocal clonic (moving from one part of the body to another), tonic and myoclonic seizures may also occur. Other manifestations of neonatal seizures include pallor, cyanosis, apnea, repetitive sucking, abrupt posturing of an arm or leg, eyelid fluttering, drooling, ocular deviation, extensor or decerebrate posturing, episodes of limpness, laughter and stereotyped repetitive movement of an extremity. The seizure may or may not be accompanied by unconsciousness. Tonic spasms are rarely seen. Even in metabolic disorders, the seizures are focal or localized to one-half of the body. In the newborn, true seizures require differentiation from the normal jitteriness precipitated by handling or startling. Such normal tremors, unaccompanied by abnormal eye movements and stimulus-sensitive, are characterized by an equal rate and amplitude and cease when the extremity is held. Benign myoclonic jerks, present chiefly during sleep, may involve the face or parts of an extremity. Neonatal seizures, on the other hand, are usually clonic with both slow and fast components, may be accompanied by eye rolling, and are not stimulus-responsive.

ETIOLOGIC CLASSIFICATION OF CONVULSIONS IN NEWBORN INFANTS

I. CENTRAL NERVOUS SYSTEM DISORDERS

A. Infants subjected to hypoxia are often apathetic, floppy and jittery. Seizures owing to hypoxia usually begin 6 to 24 hours after birth.
B. Intracranial hemorrhage
   1. Periventricular or intraventricular hemorrhage is a common complication of prematurity. However, it may occur in some term newborns as well. The hemorrhage may be suddenly manifest immediately after birth or in the first 24 to 72 hours with a bulging fontanel, seizures, stupor, coma, apnea, opisthotonus and other signs of a catastrophic event. In other infants, symptoms or signs of an intracranial hemorrhage may not occur until days or weeks later, and some infants remain asymptomatic.
   2. Subarachnoid hemorrhage may produce focal seizures in a previously well infant. Examination of the spinal fluid demonstrates increased protein and xanthochromic supernatant fluid.
   3. Subdural hematoma
C. Cerebral contusion owing to birth trauma may cause seizures on the first day of life.
D. Developmental cerebral malformations
E. Infections
   1. Prenatal
     a. Toxoplasmosis
     b. Cytomegalovirus

c. Rubella
d. Herpes simplex encephalitis may occur in the newborn in the absence of mucocutaneous lesions.
2. Meningitis
3. Tetanus neonatorum

II. METABOLIC DISORDERS

A. Hypoglycemia or hyperglycemia may cause seizures on the first day of life.
B. Hypocalcemia (see page 325)
C. Hypomagnesemia
D. Hyponatremia
E. Hypernatremia
F. Narcotic withdrawal in newborns is an uncommon cause of neonatal seizures. Tremors occur in nearly all affected infants.

Fricker, H. S., and Segal, S.: Narcotic addiction, pregnancy, and the newborn. Am. J. Dis. Child. 132:360, 1978.

G. Fetal alcohol syndrome may be characterized by seizures.
H. Inborn errors of metabolism (e.g., urea cycle disorders, maple syrup urine disease, nonketotic hyperglycinemia)
I. Pyridoxine deficiency or dependency may account for seizures in the first 24 hours of life.
J. Neonatal drug intoxication owing to administration of a local anesthetic agent (mepivacaine) in maternal paracervical, pudendal, epidural or local episiotomy anesthesia may cause seizures in the first six hours of life. Accompanying symptoms include bradycardia, apnea, hypotonia, mydriasis, absent doll's eyes maneuver and loss of the pupillary light reflex. Puncture marks or linear scratches may be present on the infant's scalp.
K. Neonatal polycythemia and hyperviscosity
L. Hyperbilirubinemia
M. Hyperthermia

III. SEPSIS

Brown, J. K.: Convulsions in the newborn period. Dev. Med. Child. Neurol. 15:823, 1973.
Brown, J. K., Cockburn, F., and Forfar, J. O.: Clinical and chemical correlates in convulsions of the newborn. Lancet 1:135, 1972.
Freeman, J. M.: Neonatal seizures—diagnosis and management. J. Pediatr. 77:701, 1970.
Myers, G. J., and Cassady, G.: Neonatal seizures. Pediatr. Rev. 5:67, 1983.
Rose, A. L., and Lombroso, C. T.: Neonatal seizure states. Pediatrics 45:404, 1970.

Volpe, J.: Neonatal seizures. N. Engl. J. Med. 289:413, 1973.

DIAGNOSTIC APPROACH TO CONVULSIVE SEIZURES

The history, including a detailed description of the seizure, is of great diagnostic help. Special attention should be given to the perinatal period and developmental progress. Information should also be obtained about the possibility of head trauma, pica, accidental ingestion of drugs or poisons, previous seizures and concurrent symptoms such as fever.

The physical examination should include a careful developmental and neurologic evaluation. The funduscopic examination and determination of the blood pressure should be performed in every child with convulsive seizures. Transillumination of the skull is indicated in infants with seizures. The following diagnostic procedures include those that may be indicated in patients with convulsive seizures, depending on the clinician's diagnostic impressions.

I. BLOOD

A. Serum calcium, phosphorus
B. Blood urea nitrogen, serum creatinine
C. Blood sugar
D. Serum electrolytes
E. Free erythrocyte protoporphyrin. Examination of erythrocytes for basophilic stippling
F. Blood and other cultures if infection is suspected
G. Complete blood count
H. Complement fixation and neutralization tests if encephalitis is thought to be present
I. "TORCH" screen if prenatal viral infection is suspected
J. Toxic screen

II. LUMBAR PUNCTURE is not routinely indicated but is reserved for those instances when meningitis or other intracranial lesion is suspected. Spinal taps are indicated in newborn and young infants with seizures.

III. A SUBDURAL TAP may be indicated in infants with otherwise unexplained convulsive seizures.

IV. THE ELECTROENCEPHALOGRAM is of great value in diagnosing the type and location of the seizure and as a guide to therapy and prognosis.

V. SKULL ROENTGENOGRAMS AND CT SCANS

in patients thought to have a focal lesion, increased intracranial pressure, head trauma or prenatal infection. Skull roentgenograms are not routinely indicated in patients with an uncomplicated initial seizure.

VI. URINALYSIS

VII. CRANIAL ULTRASOUND in the newborn

VIII. BLOOD AND URINE STUDIES for inborn errors of metabolism

GENERAL REFERENCES

Dodson, W. E., Prensky, A. L., DeVivo, D. C., Goldring, S., and Dodge, P. R.: Management of seizure disorders. Selected aspects. Parts I and II. J. Pediatr. 89:527, 695, 1976.

Golden, G. S.: Vascular diseases of the brain and tics, twitches and habit spasms. Curr. Probl. Pediatr. 8:3, 1978.

ETIOLOGIC CLASSIFICATION OF CONVULSIONS IN OLDER INFANTS AND CHILDREN

I. FEBRILE CONVULSIONS, 322
II. GENERALIZED SEIZURES, 322
  A. Absence seizures, 322
  B. Tonic-clonic seizures, 323
  C. Myoclonic seizures, 323
    1. Massive myoclonic seizures of infancy
    2. Myoclonic epilepsy of older children
    3. Benign myoclonus of early infancy
    4. Myoclonic encephalopathy
    5. Sensory precipitation epilepsy
  D. Akinetic epilepsy, 324
  E. Tonic seizures, 324
  F. Clonic seizures, 324
  G. Atonic seizures, 324
  H. Status epilepticus, 324
  I. Sensory-precipitated seizures, 324
  J. Infantile apnea, 324
III. PARTIAL SEIZURES (FOCAL, LOCAL), 324
  A. Simple partial seizures, 324
  B. Complex partial seizures (psychomotor; temporal lobe), 324
IV. METABOLIC FACTORS, 325
  A. Hypocalcemia, 325
    1. Newborn
    2. Hypoparathyroidism
    3. Rickets
    4. Sodium dihydrogen phosphate enemas
  B. Hypomagnesemia, 325
  C. Hypoglycemia, 325
    1. Infants of diabetic mothers; hemolytic disease before and after exchange transfusion; perinatal stressors
    2. Hyperinsulinemia
    3. Ketotic hypoglycemia
    4. Endocrine disorders
    5. Hepatic enzyme deficiencies
    6. Other inborn errors of metabolism
  D. Hyponatremia, 326
  E. Uremia, 326
  F. Poisoning, 326
  G. Pyridoxine deficiency or dependency, 327
  H. Hypoxemia, 327
    1. Asphyxia
    2. Carbon monoxide poisoning
    3. Near-drowning
    4. Breath-holding spells

    5. Respiratory failure
    6. Primary pulmonary hypertension
  I. Phenothiazine tranquilizers, 327
  J. Infants of narcotic-addicted mothers, 327
  K. Phenylketonuria, 327
  L. Other inborn metabolic errors, 328
  M. Elevated theophylline levels, 328
V. CEREBRAL FACTORS, 328
  A. Trauma, 328
    1. Cerebral concussion; contusion; laceration; focal or generalized edema of the brain
    2. Extradural hematoma; subdural hematoma
    3. Child abuse. Whiplash injury
  B. Infections of the central nervous system, 328
    1. Toxoplasmosis
    2. Encephalitis
    3. Meningitis
    4. Subdural effusion
    5. Intracranial abscess
    6. Rabies
    7. Cerebral cysticercosis
  C. Intracranial hemorrhage, 328
    1. Subdural hemorrhage
    2. Extradural hematoma
    3. Subarachnoid hemorrhage
    4. Systemic hemorrhagic diseases
  D. Thrombosis of cerebral vessels, 328
    1. Congenital heart disease
    2. Sickle cell anemia
    3. Severe dehydration
    4. Sudden vascular accident (acute infantile hemiplegia)
  E. Neurocutaneous syndromes, 329
    1. Sturge-Weber syndrome
    2. Tuberous sclerosis
  F. Psychologic factors, 329
    1. Breath-holding spells
    2. Self-induced seizures
    3. Emotional factors
    4. Pseudoseizures
    5. Dissociative psychotic episodes
  G. Encephalopathy, 329
    1. Postpertussis vaccine encephalopathy
    2. Pertussis encephalopathy

Table continued on opposite page

ETIOLOGIC CLASSIFICATION OF CONVULSIONS IN OLDER INFANTS AND CHILDREN *Continued*

3. Hypertensive encephalopathy
4. Bacillary dysentery
5. Lupus erythematosus
6. Infectious mononucleosis
7. Corticosteroid treatment
8. Hemolytic-uremic syndrome
9. Reye's syndrome
10. Gasoline or other solvent sniffing
H. Degenerative diseases, 329
1. Demyelinating encephalopathies
2. GM_1 gangliosidosis, type II

3. Metachromatic leukodystrophy
4. Infantile sialidosis
5. Tay-Sachs disease
6. Other cerebromacular degenerative diseases
7. Neimann-Pick disease
8. Infantile Gaucher's disease
9. Subacute sclerosing panencephalitis
I. Brain tumors, 330
J. Tetanus, 330
K. Hyperexplexia, 330

ETIOLOGIC CLASSIFICATION OF CONVULSIONS IN NEWBORN INFANTS

I. CENTRAL NERVOUS SYSTEM DISORDERS, 330
A. Hypoxia, 330
B. Intracranial hemorrhage, 330
1. Periventricular or intraventricular
2. Subarachnoid
3. Subdural hematoma
C. Cerebral contusion owing to birth trauma, 330
D. Cerebral malformations, 330
E. Infection, 330
1. Prenatal
2. Meningitis
3. Tetanus neonatorum
II. METABOLIC DISORDERS, 331

A. Hypoglycemia; hyperglycemia, 331
B. Hypocalcemia, 331
C. Hypomagnesemia, 331
D. Hyponatremia, 331
E. Hypernatremia, 331
F. Narcotic withdrawal, 331
G. Fetal alcohol syndrome, 331
H. Inborn errors of metabolism, 331
I. Pyridoxine deficiency or dependency, 331
J. Maternal local anesthesia, 331
K. Polycythemia and hyperviscosity, 331
L. Hyperbilirubinemia, 331
M. Hyperthermia, 331
III. SEPSIS, 331

41 / DELIRIUM

Delirium represents a reversible toxic or metabolic encephalopathy characterized by a disturbance in consciousness that ranges from extreme hyperactivity to coma. Symptoms of delirium characteristically fluctuate widely but are generally worse at night. Since the sleep-wakefulness cycle is commonly disturbed, the child may be excessively alert and unable to fall asleep at night or unusually drowsy during the day. The delirious patient's ability to sustain his attention is limited, and his conversation may skip abruptly from one topic to another. At one moment the child may seem to be in complete contact with his environment, while a few seconds later he obviously does not clearly perceive or understand what is going on. At times, the impairment in consciousness is persistent and does not fluctuate.

The delirious child may demonstrate great excitement and hyperactivity—running about the examining room, trying to open the door, struggling and thrashing around the examining table or bed. Anxiety, fear, anger, depression, euphoria and apathy may be displayed. The child may pull at his fingertips, reach for imaginary objects or pick at his clothes. Motor incoordination, incoherent speech, inability to write, tremulousness and ataxia may be noted. Auditory and visual hallucinations and illusions lead the child to misinterpret shadows (e.g., he may see large bugs on his bed or on the walls). Cognitive function, short-term memory and comprehension are impaired. The confused older child may be unable to answer orientation questions, attend to a task such as sequentially subtracting 7 or 3 from 100, repeat backwards a series of digits or respond correctly to other components of a mental status examination (e.g., date, time and place).

ETIOLOGIC CLASSIFICATION OF DELIRIUM

I. INFECTIOUS DISORDERS

A. Any acute, febrile disease, especially the exanthemas, may cause delirium.
B. Pneumococcal or other bacterial pneumonia. In some instances, delirium and fever may be the only presenting symptoms.
C. Inflammatory diseases of the central nervous system such as meningitis or encephalitis.
D. Reye's syndrome is characterized by a prodromal illness. Protracted vomiting, lethargy, disorientation, irrational behavior, hallucinations, combativeness, stupor and coma may follow. Elevated levels of SGOT, SGPT and blood ammonia are found.
E. Typhoid fever
F. Rabies may be characterized by periods of hyperactivity, combativeness and disorientation alternating with intervals of normal mental status.
G. Toxic shock syndrome may be accompanied by confusion, disorientation, agitation and somnolence.
H. Infectious hepatitis may produce signs of delirium owing to impending hepatic failure.

II. DRUGS AND POISONING

A careful search for possible poisoning is indicated in all children with acute delirium, including a review of the contents of medicine cabinets, night tables and all medications taken currently or in the past by the parents or other adults in the household. In the absence of a history of drug ingestion, a blood and urine screen for toxic substances should be pursued. The possibility of intentional poisoning of children should be kept in mind.

A. Barbiturates
B. Antihistamines taken orally or contained in preparations for cutaneous application
C. Theophylline poisoning may lead to extreme restlessness.
D. Corticosteroids
E. Isoniazid
F. Jimson weed poisoning. The seeds or leaves of the Jimson weed contain hyoscyamine and other belladonna alkaloids, and their ingestion may produce delirium. Convulsions are also a common complication. Symptoms, which may begin in minutes or a few hours, initially include visual illusions, dryness of the mouth, extreme thirst, incoherent speech, confusion, disorientation, combative behavior, stupor, coma, incoordination and hyperactivity. The pupils are dilated and fixed, and the skin is flushed and dry. Opisthotonus may develop. A diffuse erythematous rash may be present. The temperature may be as high as 40.6° C (105° F). Recovery usually occurs in 24 to 48 hours. Imipramine poisoning may cause similar symptoms.

Nghiem, Q. X., Randel, R. C., and Leach, T. L.: Imipramine poisoning. Pediatr. Rev. 1:317, 1980.
Rumach, B. H.: Jimsonweed abuse. Pediatr. Rev. 5:141, 1983.

G. Atropine poisoning may occur after conjunctival instillation.
H. Amphetamine intoxication
I. LSD, psilocybin, mescaline, or other psychedelic agents. Delirium that persists for several days may be caused by phencyclidine ("angel dust") intoxication. Hypertension and urinary retention may also be present.

Cohen, S.: The "angel dust" states: phencyclidine toxicity. Pediatr. Rev. 1:17, 1979.

J. Gasoline sniffing
K. Alcohol may produce delirium and other manifestations of delirium.

Drugs that cause psychiatric symptoms. Med. Lett. 26:75, 1984.
Silber, T. J., and D'Angelo, L.: Psychosis and seizures following the injection of penicillin G procaine. Am. J. Dis. Child. 139:335, 1985.

III. HYPOXEMIA (e.g., carbon monoxide poisoning or respiratory failure) may cause confusion.

IV. METABOLIC (e.g., uremia, hypoglycemia, hepatic failure).

V. Burn Encephalopathy, characterized by delirium, personality changes, seizures or coma, may occur with acute burns owing to hypovolemia, sepsis or hyponatremia.

Antoon, A. Y., Volpe, J. J., and Crawford, J. D.: Burn encephalopathy in children. Pediatrics 50:609, 1972.

VI. Head Trauma

VII. Complicated Migraine

A. Acute confusional state is characterized by restlessness, hyperactivity, confusion, combativeness, agitation, or stupor. Episodes may persist for hours.

B. Alice in Wonderland syndrome, occurring immediately or several days before a headache, could simulate delirium, with aberration of time perception, distortions in body image, visual illusions and trancelike states.

VIII. Heat Stroke may produce incoherent speech and disorientation before progressing to stupor and unconsciousness.

ETIOLOGIC CLASSIFICATION OF DELIRIUM

---

42 / LETHARGY AND COMA

Alterations in the state of consciousness in infants and children include delirium, stupor and coma. *Delirium* is marked by confusion, disorientation, irrationality and, perhaps, excitability. *Lethargy* is characterized by drowsiness and disinterest in the environment. *Obtundation* refers to an increase in the depth of the lethargy. *Stupor*, a state of unconsciousness from which the child may be momentarily aroused, often precedes coma. *Coma* represents prolonged and profound unconsciousness.

ETIOLOGIC CLASSIFICATION OF COMA

I. Central Nervous System Disturbances

A. Trauma. Since the following traumatic lesions have similar neurologic findings, their clinical differentiation may not be possible. The most important finding to be carefully followed is the patient's state of consciousness in terms of his responsiveness to questions and to visual, auditory or sensory stimuli.

1. Cerebral concussion, contusion or laceration may be followed immediately by unconsciousness that persists for minutes or hours. Post-traumatic amnesia may be accompanied by retrograde amnesia. With slight head trauma, the symptoms may be limited to mild lethargy, perhaps one or more episodes of vomiting, and, occasionally, transient blindness. Post-traumatic headaches may occur after a mild concussion.

2. Subdural hematoma is a prominent diagnostic possibility in patients who continue to do poorly after a head injury. Headache, unilateral pupillary dilatation and localizing neurologic signs may be present. While symptoms may appear in a few hours, coma may not ensue until days or weeks later. Chronic subdural hematoma, which may cause head enlargement, vomiting, failure to thrive, convulsions and other neurologic signs, is not regularly characterized by coma, except terminally.

3. In infants and children with an extradural hematoma, the following physical findings occur, usually within several minutes to a few hours after injury: scalp swelling, hemiparesis, drowsiness progressing to stupor, positive Babinski's sign, unequal pupils with dilatation of the pupil on the involved side, coma, decerebrate posture, convulsions, strabismus and papilledema. Occasionally, these symptoms may be delayed in their onset for a few days. Less commonly, a period of unconsciousness immediately after the injury is followed first by a lucid interval and then by a gradual reappearance of coma. Similar physical findings may be noted in patients with cerebral contusion, laceration or hemorrhage and with an acute subdural hematoma. A skull fracture may be present. A definitive diagnosis may not be possible until surgical exploration. Blood loss of as much as 100 to 150 ml into the extradural space accounts for the acute anemia and shock that may appear in some of these infants, even in the absence of neurologic findings.

4. Localizing neurologic signs, convulsions and hemiparesis may occur within minutes to a few hours after head injuries in children owing to focal and generalized edema of the brain. Spontaneous recovery occurs within a few hours.

DeVivo, D. C., and Dodge, P. R.: The critically ill child: Diagnosis and management of head injury. Pediatrics 48:129, 1971.
Singer, H. S., and Freeman, J. M.: Head trauma for the pediatrician. Pediatrics 62:819, 1978.

B. Disturbances in circulation
1. Hemorrhage
    a. Subdural hematoma. The symptoms of posterior fossa subdural hemorrhage in the newborn may resemble those of an intracerebellar hemorrhage.

Serfontein, G. L., Rom, S., and Stein, S.: Posterior fossa subdural hemorrhage in the newborn. Pediatrics 65:40, 1980.

    b. Intraventricular and periventricular hemorrhages occur commonly in premature infants and infrequently in full-term and somewhat older infants. Factors that appear to predispose to this complication include hypoxemia, acidosis and hypernatremia. While some affected infants are asymptomatic, others follow a catastrophic course over minutes to hours with nonreactive pupils, seizures, bulging fontanel, decerebrate posturing, respiratory deterioration, deep stupor or coma. On the other hand, the course may be a gradual and intermittent one over hours or days with alteration in level of consciousness, hypotonia and abnormal eye movements. Diagnostic procedures include ultrasonography and computed tomography.

Bejar, R., Curbelo, V., Coen, R. W., Leopold, G., James, H., and Gluck, L.: Diagnosis and follow-up of intraventricular and intracerebral hemorrhages by ultrasound studies of infant's brain through the fontanelle and sutures. Pediatrics 66:661, 1980.
Mitchell, W., and O'Tuama, L. O.: Cerebral intraventricular hemorrhages in infants: A widening age spectrum. Pediatrics 65:35, 1980.
Volpe, J. J.: Intraventricular hemorrhage in premature infants. Pediatr. Rev. 2:145, 1980.

    c. Subarachnoid hemorrhage due to rupture of an intracranial arterial aneurysm has a sudden onset with severe suboccipital or frontal headache, perhaps pain in the neck or back, screaming, vomiting, the rapid appearance of coma and, perhaps, convulsions. The child may suddenly become unconscious and fall. Signs of meningeal irritation occur with nuchal rigidity and a positive Kernig's sign. The deep tendon reflexes are increased, and the cerebrospinal fluid is bloody. Localizing neurologic signs are not present if the hemorrhage is entirely subarachnoid. Often, however, intracortical hemorrhage also occurs, and the patient may have focal findings.

Shucart, W. A., and Wolpert, S. M.: Intracranial arterial aneurysms in childhood. Am. J. Dis. Child. 127:288, 1974.

d. Acute infantile hemiplegia is discussed on page 125 and below.
e. Hemorrhagic diseases such as thrombocytopenic purpura or hemophilia may be complicated by an intracranial hemorrhage.
f. Intracranial hemorrhage is an infrequent complication of pertussis.
g. Coma may be produced by a sudden hemorrhage into an intracranial tumor, such as a malignant cerebral glioma. If the symptoms follow head trauma, the possibility of an intracranial neoplasm may be overlooked because the trauma is a distractor.
h. Intraparenchymal cerebral hemorrhage may be produced by vigorous abusive shaking of an infant. Retinal hemorrhages may be noted.
2. Cerebral vascular occlusions
a. Thrombosis
1. Cerebral thrombosis occurs not uncommonly in children who have polycythemia secondary to cyanotic congenital heart disease. Clinical manifestations include convulsive seizures, impaired consciousness and monoplegia or hemiplegia.
2. Occlusion of the venous dural sinuses and the cerebral veins occurs in severely dehydrated infants and young children. Numerous small cerebral thrombi may also form during the course of acute infectious diseases. Thrombosis of the sagittal sinus is manifested by coma, convulsions, para-

plegia, and distention of the scalp veins. Cavernous sinus thrombosis produces proptosis, papilledema, conjunctival and retinal hemorrhages and ophthalmoplegia owing to paresis of the third, fourth and sixth cranial nerves.
3. Coma may occur in children with sickle cell anemia, presumably owing to cerebral thrombosis.
4. Thrombotic thrombocytopenic purpura
b. Embolism
1. Bacterial endocarditis
2. Congenital heart disease with right-to-left shunt
3. Pulmonary or other abscess
4. Fat embolism following fractures
C. Acute infantile hemiplegia, a disorder of unknown etiology, begins suddenly with a severe convulsive seizure, usually unilateral but occasionally generalized, followed by coma and hemiparesis. Fever may also occur. Convulsions recur for one or two days, and coma may persist for a week or ten days. The cerebrospinal fluid is normal. Gradual improvement in the hemiparesis may ensue with flaccidity replaced by spasticity. Cerebral arteriography may demonstrate occlusion of the middle cerebral artery.
D. Central nervous system infections
1. An intracranial abscess may develop secondary to otitis media, mastoiditis or purulent lesions elsewhere. Children with cyanotic heart disease and polycythemia are especially vulnerable to this complication. Although not a common symptom, coma occasionally occurs in patients with an intracranial abscess.
2. The classic signs of purulent meningitis may not be present in young infants, so the diagnosis must be suspected on the basis of such vague symptoms as failure to feed or vomiting. A history of unusual irritability or drowsiness may be an indication for cerebrospinal fluid examination. Alterations in the state of consciousness in patients with bacterial meningitis range from hyperexcitability and delirium to stupor and coma. Patients with aseptic meningitis have no disturbance of consciousness.
3. Symptoms attributable to encephalitis include drowsiness, disorienta-

tion, stupor, coma, irritability, convulsions, headache, nuchal rigidity, hemiparesis, paralysis of cranial nerves, tremor, choreiform or athetoid movements, rigidity, aphasia and ataxia. These findings may also be caused by an intracranial neoplasm or abscess. Clinical diagnosis is difficult unless the symptoms accompany a recognized infectious disease. Examination of the cerebrospinal fluid may show an increase in the number of cells, mostly lymphocytes, and an elevation in protein. Complement fixation and neutralization tests may be diagnostically helpful. Encephalitis may precede, accompany or follow the acute exanthematous diseases of childhood. Encephalopathy may follow pertussis vaccination. Coma due to encephalitis may occasionally occur in children with mumps or pertussis. Encephalitis accompanied by unexplained lymphadenopathy may be caused by cat-scratch disease. Herpes encephalitis tends to demonstrate localization in the temporoparietal area with focal electroencephalographic findings. Brain biopsy is required for definitive diagnosis.

4. Infectious mononucleosis may be characterized by disorientation, drowsiness, stupor, coma, headache, nuchal rigidity, diplopia and an increased number of cells in the cerebrospinal fluid.

5. Toxic encephalopathy may occur during severe systemic diseases, especially those characterized by high fever and general toxicity. In the absence of diarrhea, the meningismus, disorientation, coma and convulsions in patients with *Shigella* dysentery may initially suggest encephalitis.

6. Burn encephalopathy may be characterized by delirium, seizures and coma.

7. Reye's syndrome should be considered in a child who during recovery from chickenpox, influenza or other viral illness develops repeated or persistent vomiting, irritability, confusion, delirium, combative behavior, lethargy, stupor and coma. Hyperventilation, apnea, seizures and diarrhea may occur in infants. Reye's syndrome may be classified in five stages: Stage I is characterized by vomiting, lethargy, sleepiness, hepatic dysfunction (SGOT, glucose, blood ammonia) and a type 1 EEG;

stage II is manifested by delirium, combativeness, hyperventilation, hyperactive reflexes, responsiveness to painful stimuli, liver dysfunction and type 2 EEG; stage 3 is characterized by stupor or coma, hyperventilation, decerebrate rigidity, positive pupillary light reaction, liver dysfunction and a type 2 EEG; stage IV is accompanied by deepening coma, decerebrate rigidity, loss of the doll's eye reflex, large and fixed pupils, minimal hepatic dysfunction and type 3 or 4 EEG; and stage V is characterized by seizures, loss of deep tendon reflexes, type 4 EEG and respiratory arrest.

Lovejoy, F.H., et al.: Clinical staging in Reye's syndrome. Am. J. Dis. Child. 128:36, 1974.

E. Brain tumors. Hemorrhage into an intracranial neoplasm may cause the sudden onset of coma. Blockage of the ventricular circulation with increase in the intracranial pressure may also result in unconsciousness. Tumors of the brain stem may be accompanied by coma, even without increased intracranial pressure. Coma occasionally occurs in children with leukemia owing to involvement of the central nervous system. The Dandy-Walker syndrome may be associated with recurrent episodes of lethargy, irritability and sudden coma.

F. Hypertensive encephalopathy may result in impaired consciousness as well as convulsive seizures.

G. Postconvulsion coma. A period of unconsciousness, usually not prolonged, may follow convulsive seizures in children. Coma is more persistent in patients in status epilepticus.

H. Obstruction of a cerebrospinal fluid shunt may cause acute lethargy and vomiting.

II. METABOLIC DISORDERS

A. Metabolic acidosis may lead to lethargy, stupor and coma.
    1. Diabetic ketoacidosis
    2. Branched-chain amino acids or organic acidemias

B. Ammonia encephalopathy
    1. Disorders of the urea cycle. Lethargy, stupor, apnea, tachypnea, seizures, vomiting and coma occur in newborn infants with hyperammonemia. In older children, these symptoms may be preceded by irritability and hyperactivity. Urea cycle disorders include

carbamyl phosphate synthetase deficiency, ornithine transcarbamoylase deficiency, citrullinemia, argininosuccinic aciduria, argininemia and ornithinemia.

Batshaw, M. L.: Hyperammonemia. Curr. Probl. Pediatr. 14:6, 1984.
Campbell, A. G. M., Rosenberg, L. E., ᵗ ;rass, P. J., and Nuzum, C. T.: Ornithine ti arbamoylase deficiency. N. Engl. J. Me(288:1, 1973.
Snyderman, S. E.: Clinical aspects of disorders of the urea cycle. Pediatrics 68:284, 1981.

2. **Other disorders in the neonatal period.** Hyperammonemia in newborn infants may be caused by severe perinatal asphyxia or hepatic failure associated with sepsis. Transient hyperammonemia of prematurity, which occurs in the first 48 hours of life, is characterized by respiratory distress, convulsions and lethargy progressing to coma.

Ballard, R. A., Vinocur, B., Reynolds, J. W., Wennberg, R. P., Merritt, A., Sweetman, L., and Nyhan, W. L.: Transient hyperammonemia of the preterm infant. N. Engl. J. Med. 299:920, 1978.

3. **Hepatic coma** may occur as a complication of Reye's syndrome, fulminant viral hepatitis, cirrhosis or other cause of hepatic failure. Initial symptoms include clouding of the sensorium, apathy, confusion, emotional lability and slurred speech. Coma may occur abruptly, but more commonly it evolves gradually. Asterixis, a flapping tremor, may be present.
4. **Valproic acid therapy** has been associated with stupor and coma.

Coulter, D. L., and Allen, R. J.: Hyperammonemia with valproic acid therapy. J. Pediatr. 99:317, 1981.

5. **Increased production of ammonia** may occur in patients with marked dilation of the urinary tract who acquire an infection with urease-producing organisms.

Samtoy, B., and DeBeukelaer, M. M.: Ammonia encephalopathy secondary to urinary tract infection with *Proteus mirabilis*. Pediatrics 65:294, 1980.

C. **Leigh's syndrome,** or subacute necrotizing encephalomyelopathy, may be characterized by lethargy and coma.

Grover, W. D., Auerbach, V. H., and Patel, M. S.: Biochemical studies and therapy in subacute necrotizing encephalomyelopathy (Leigh's syndrome). J. Pediatr. 81:39, 1972.

D. **Hypoglycemia.** Coma caused by insulin overdosage may persist for days, even though the blood sugar level has been restored to normal.
E. **Renal insufficiency**
F. **Hypoxemia**
   1. Near-drowning
   2. **Carbon monoxide poisoning.** Coma develops when the level of carboxyhemoglobin is 60 to 70 per cent.

Zimmerman, S. S., and Truxal, B.: Carbon monoxide poisoning. Pediatrics 68:215, 1981.

   3. Congestive cardiac failure
   4. Loss of consciousness lasting from a few minutes to two or three hours may occur during episodes of paroxysmal dyspnea in infants with cyanotic congenital heart disease. Although coma may be preceded by cyanosis and dyspnea, this is not always the case.
   5. **Adams-Stokes attacks** may be associated with atrioventricular heart block in children. Symptoms may include vertigo, syncope, coma or convulsions.
   6. Acute respiratory failure may cause stupor or coma.
   7. High altitude pulmonary edema without dyspnea or cough may present with somnolence or coma in children.
G. **Tetany** may lead to unconsciousness. Coma may also be attributable to hypercalcemia in patients with hyperparathyroidism. Tetany and coma may be complications of pediatric sodium dihydrogen phosphate enemas.

Sotos, J. F., Cutler, D. A., Finkel, M. A., and Doody, D.: Hypocalcemic coma following two pediatric phosphate enemas. Pediatrics 60:305, 1977.

H. **Addison's disease** during a crisis
I. **Systemic carnitine deficiency** may cause a recurrent Reye's syndrome–like disorder following an upper respiratory tract infection. Hyperammonemia, elevated serum transaminases, hepatomegaly, hypoglycemia and coma may occur.

Chapoy, P. R., Angelina, C., Brown, W. J., Stiff, J. E., Shug, A. L., and Cederbaum, S. D.: Systemic carnitine deficiency—a treatable inherited lipid-storage disease presenting as Reye's syndrome. N. Engl. J. Med. 303:1389, 1980.

J. Acute hyponatremia; water intoxication. Hypernatremia; hyperosmolarity
K. Hyperviscosity syndrome in the newborn is characterized by lethargy.
L. Heat stroke, heat exhaustion
M. Kawasaki disease may be characterized, in some patients, by lethargy or coma during the febrile period.
N. Septic shock may cause stupor or coma owing to a compromise of the cerebral blood flow.
O. Hemolytic-uremic syndrome may be accompanied by lethargy, coma and seizures.

Bale, J. F., Brasher, C., and Siegler, R. L.: CNS manifestations of the hemolytic-uremic syndrome. Am. J. Dis. Child. 134:869, 1980.

III. DRUGS, POISONS. Stage 1 coma following drug ingestion is manifest by drowsiness, with the patient responsive to verbal command; stage 2 is characterized by coma with response to mildly painful stimuli; stage 3 denotes coma responsive only to deeply painful stimuli; and stage 4 is present when the patient is unresponsive and areflexic. *Poisoning is a possibility in every patient with unexplained coma.*

A. Barbiturates, phenothiazines, benzodiazepines, propoxyphene, pentazocine, tricyclic antidepressants.
B. Surreptitious drug administration to children with resultant severe lethargy or coma may represent child abuse or Munchausen's syndrome by proxy. Symptoms may include prolonged sleep, confusion, ataxia, seizures and coma.

Dine, M. S., and McGovern, M. E.: Intentional poisoning of children—an overlooked category of child abuse: Report of seven cases and review of the literature. Pediatrics 70:32, 1982.

C. Narcotics. Miosis is classically present in noncomatose patients who have taken narcotics. Patients who have ingested barbiturates, phenothiazines or ethanol also demonstrate increased miosis as their coma deepens. Other drug ingestion should be suspected if pupillary dilatation does not follow administration of the narcotic antagonist naloxone in a comatose patient suspected of narcotic ingestion.

Mitchell, A. A., Lovejoy, F. H., Jr., and Goldman, P.: Drug ingestions associated with miosis in comatose children. J. Pediatr. 89:303, 1976.

D. Lead poisoning. Alteration of lethargy or stupor with lucid periods is suggestive of impending lead encephalopathy, especially in a vomiting child in the summertime.
E. Ethanol ingestion may be accompanied by an overdose of other sedatives.

Moss, M. H.: Alcohol-induced hypoglycemia and coma caused by alcohol sponging. Pediatrics 46:445, 1970.

F. Salicylate poisoning, especially oil of wintergreen
G. Inhalation of carbon tetrachloride, gasoline or other fluids used in cleaning
H. Mushroom poisoning
I. Kerosene poisoning
J. Organic phosphate (parathion) poisoning
K. Lomotil may cause respiratory depression, lethargy and coma in young children.

Rumack, B. H., and Temple, A. R.: Lomotil poisoning. Pediatrics 53:495, 1974.

L. Hexachlorophene toxicity

IV. INTUSSUSCEPTION. Altered consciousness manifest by acute drowsiness, lethargy, apathy or stupor may be an early sign in intussusception.

Margolis, B.: Apathy as an early manifestation of intussusception. Am. J. Dis. Child. 137:701, 1983.

V. NARCOLEPSY is characterized by excessive and abnormal sleepiness. Cataplexy, which may be an associated symptom, refers to muscular weakness or paralysis precipitated by emotions such as laughter or anger. Excessive sleepiness may be caused by lesions in the pituitary and hypothalamic regions.

VI. A CONVERSION REACTION may account for the patient who is seemingly unresponsive.

PHYSICAL EXAMINATION OF COMATOSE PATIENTS

The depth of the coma and the status of the tendon, corneal and pupillary reflexes are usually of little diagnostic value. Those reflexes, along with swallowing and cough, are progressively depressed as the coma deepens. Because of the absence of voluntary motor activity in comatose patients, paralysis may not be readily evident. Comatose patients should be examined for signs of meningitis and cranial trauma and for leakage of blood or cerebrospinal fluid from cranial orifices. Funduscopic examination for papilledema or retinal hemorrhage should be performed and the blood pressure determined.

DIAGNOSTIC PROCEDURES

A. In newborn and older infants suspected of having a urea cycle disorder or a metabolic acidosis owing to branched-chain amino acids or organic acidemias, milk and other protein-containing foods should be discontinued, and a balanced electrolyte-glucose solution started orally or intravenously. The urine should be examined for odor, reducing substances, specific gravity, pH and ketones. A ferric chloride test should also be obtained. The odor of the urine (musty, maple syrup, etc.) should be checked. Electrophoresis for amino acids should be performed, along with gas chromatography and mass spectrometry. Blood specimens should be analyzed for serum electrolytes, glucose, ammonia, lactate, quantitative amino acids, organic acids and short-chain fatty acids.

B. In other patients with coma:
1. Urinalysis: Microscopic. Chemical for albumin, acetone, glycosuria, salicylates. Glycosuria may be present in patients who have meningitis or other central nervous system disease.
2. Blood examinations:
   Complete blood cell count
   Evaluation of clotting mechanism
   Examination of blood smear for sickling or stippling
   Blood glucose
   Blood ammonia
   Hepatic enzymes
   Blood nonprotein nitrogen; serum creatinine
   Serum bicarbonate, chloride, sodium
   Serum calcium
   Salicylate level
   Spectrophotometry for carbon monoxide and methemoglobin
   Heterophile antibodies
   Blood cultures
3. Examination of the cerebrospinal fluid is an important diagnostic procedure in patients with coma of unknown etiology. Possible contraindications to lumbar puncture include increased intracranial pressure and shock.
4. Unless the patient is in shock, roentgen examination or computed tomography of the head should be obtained if a head injury is suspected or confirmed. Changes in the sella turcica, intracranial calcification or separation of the suture lines may be evident.
5. If the possibility of poisoning exists, gastric lavage may be indicated for diagnostic as well as therapeutic reasons.
6. In patients thought to have encephalitis, neutralization and complement fixation studies are obtained.
7. An electroencephalogram may be indicated in patients with unexplained stupor or coma.

ETIOLOGIC CLASSIFICATION OF COMA

Table continued on following page

43 / FAINTING

Fainting or syncope refers to brief, usually sudden, periods of unconsciousness, loss of postural tone, and falling due to cerebral ischemia. Generally, the history is the most helpful diagnostic tool. Special attention must be given to the circumstances in which the syncope occurred; possible precipitating factors; prodromal symptoms and signs; the suddenness of onset; the duration of the episode; and the occurrence of convulsive movements.

Friedberg, C. K.: Syncope: Pathological physiology: Differential diagnosis and treatment. Mod. Concepts Cardiovasc. Dis. 40:55, 61, 1971.

ETIOLOGIC CLASSIFICATION OF FAINTING

I. VASODEPRESSOR SYNCOPE (SIMPLE FAINT). Vasodepressor syncope due to a sudden and marked fall in blood pressure is the most common cause of fainting in adolescents. Fainting may occur when the patient becomes suddenly frightened or threatened by some real or imagined danger. It may also represent a reaction to severe pain or other unpleasant stimulus such as the sight of blood or a needle puncture. Syncope is especially likely to occur in hot, humid, close quarters; after prolonged motionless standing; when the patient is fatigued; and after fasting. In patients with emotionally induced syncopal attacks, anxiety may be overt or reported in frightening dreams. Psychologic factors may cause recurrent fainting spells, especially those not precipitated by apparent cause.

Simple faints almost always begin with the patient standing. Prodromal symptoms include a feeling of great weakness, generalized numbness, pallor, nausea, excessive salivation, warmth, sweating, lightheadedness, yawning, sighing, blurring of vision and epigastric discomfort. The antecedent complaints may either suddenly terminate in the faint or be aborted spontaneously or by assumption of the head-low position. The interruption of consciousness in a syncopal episode usually lasts only a few seconds, but it may persist for several minutes. Clonic movements may ensue if the patient remains unconscious longer than 15 to 20 seconds. Symptoms may recur if the patient sits or stands up too quickly.

II. CONVERSION REACTION. Syncope may also be a symbolic expression of unconscious, repressed instinctual impulses, usually of a sexual or hostile nature and often directed toward a member of the family. Such episodes, most common in adolescent girls, may also be precipitated by a real or fantasied sexual experience. The patient may have a history of repeated episodes of syncope as well as other manifestations of a conversion disorder. It is postulated that conversion of the consciously unacceptable impulse to physical expression in the form of syncope permits a partial discharge of these feelings and helps avoid the anxiety that would be engendered by the conscious expression or direct gratification of the impulse.

Whereas overt anxiety is frequently noted with vasodepressor syncope, the patient with hysterical syncope shows little concern. These episodes characteristically occur in the presence of others and are not preceded or accompanied by prodromal symptoms such as nausea, weakness, pallor and sweating. Patients with conversion syncope may slump or fall in a dramatic fashion, but they avoid injury. They may faint while sitting or recumbent, an unusual sequence in vasodepressor syncope. During the episode, the patient's eyes may flutter or remain open or tightly closed. Moaning, groaning or other sounds may be noted. Unusual positions and movements may be assumed. The patient may slip in and out of unconsciousness or have less impairment of consciousness. Interruption of consciousness may persist for seconds or hours.

III. EPILEPSY. Differentiating by history between vasodepressor syncope, breath-holding spells and epilepsy is occasionally difficult, since the first two disorders may be accompanied by clonic movements. Syncope due to epilepsy usually lasts longer (generally over 30 seconds) and is more likely to occur with the patient recumbent than is characteristic of simple syncope. An electroencephalogram and other studies may be necessary for differentiation.

IV. CARDIAC CAUSES. A history of fainting during, rather than after, exercise may be associated with an aberrant left coronary artery. Occasionally, syncope occurs with exertion in patients with a marked isolated pulmonic stenosis. Primary pulmonary hypertension may be characterized by episodes of syncope, especially on effort, and syncope may be the presenting complaint. Mitral valve prolapse may be characterized by precordial pain, arrhythmias or syncopal episodes. Congenital or acquired heart block or cardiac arrhythmias may decrease cardiac output sufficiently to produce unconsciousness. Severe aortic stenosis may cause syncope, especially after physical exertion. Idiopathic hypertrophic subaortic stenosis or hypertrophic obstructive cardiomyopathy in adolescents may produce slight dyspnea and angina on exertion and syncope. A systolic ejection murmur is heard along the upper right sternal border. Attacks of paroxysmal dyspnea in infants with congenital heart disease, (e.g., tetralogy of Fallot) may terminate in syncope. Episodes of palpitation, weakness, faintness and syncope may occur with paroxysmal supraventricular tachycardia and with sudden obstruction of the mitral orifice by a left atrial myxoma.

V. TUSSIVE (COUGH) SYNCOPE. Loss of consciousness, usually of short duration and owing to cerebral hypoxia, may occur after severe paroxysms of coughing.

Katz, R. M.: Cough syncope in children with asthma. J. Pediatr. 77:48, 1970.

VI. ANEMIA. Severe anemia may be accompanied by lightheadedness, giddiness and, occasionally, syncope.

VII. HYPOGLYCEMIA. Although hypoglycemia does not lead to true syncope, the patient may complain of faintness and exhibit pallor and sweating. A meticulous history (e.g., relation of the syncope to meals and careful description of other symptoms) is of diagnostic help.

VIII. HYPERVENTILATION SYNDROME. Hyperventilation may cause lightheadedness ("dizziness"), generalized weakness, chest pain, palpitations, tingling and numbness of the hands, tetany or syncope. Adolescent patients are more likely to report "blacking-out" spells, seizures, sensations of smothering, choking or shortness of breath; overbreathing; or tingling and numbness of the hands. A panic attack may be characterized by hyperventilation along with other symptoms. Direct questioning or an attempt to replicate the symptoms by having the patient hyperventilate for a couple of minutes may be necessary.

IX. BREATH-HOLDING. Breath-holding spells are common in infants, especially during the latter part of the first year and the early months of the second year. Less frequent in younger or older children, breath-holding may persist until the age of four years. The episodes are triggered by some injury, often trivial, or by the child's suddenly becoming angry or frustrated. Vigorous crying is the first manifestation. After a variable period, the child suddenly gasps or holds his breath until he becomes blue or pale, unconscious and limp. Convulsive movements or opisthotonus may ensue if the period of unconsciousness is prolonged.

The presenting complaint is usually convulsions or blacking-out rather than breath-holding or syncope. The history and sequence of events are so characteristic that the differential diagnosis generally presents no problem; however, when the precipitating event seems extremely trivial, when no triggering circumstance can be identified, when the child is said to cry or hold his breath for only a short time, or when the convulsive movements are a prominent clinical feature, differentiation from epilepsy may require an electroencephalogram and further observation.

Some babies seem especially prone to have breath-holding spells, and a familial incidence may exist. Although in some cases no contributory disturbance in the home or in the mother-infant relation is apparent, these areas should be explored carefully. Immature parents, maternal depression, inability to set limits, and similar difficulties in the maternal-infant interaction also should be explored if the spells are to be prevented. Many of these children have an iron deficiency anemia as an associated, rather than causative, disorder.

X. OTHER DISORDERS ASSOCIATED WITH FAINTING

A. Attacks of syncope lasting from a brief faint to unconsciousness for 5 to 10 minutes are rarely associated with congenital deafness, prolonged Q-T interval and large T waves on the electrocardiogram. Sudden death has been described in the full surdocardiac syndrome or in the partial syndrome without deafness. Episodes may be precipitated by emotional stress or physical exertion.

Frank, J. P., and Friedberg, D. A.: Syncope with prolonged QT interval. Am. J. Dis. Child. 130:320, 1976.

B. Attacks of unconsciousness may occur in patients with fused cervical vertebrae.
C. Sudden unconsciousness may be precipitated by needle puncture of the pleural space and by drainage of fluid from the pleural or peritoneal cavities. The mechanism is probably similar to that underlying vasodepressor syncope.
D. Postural or orthostatic hypotension, an unusual cause of syncope in pediatrics, may occur when a child or adolescent has stood motionless for a long time in a military or parade formation. Orthostatic hypotension causing syncope may occur in the toxic shock syndrome.
E. Takayasu's disease (primary aortitis) may cause syncope.
F. Carbon monoxide poisoning causes syncope at a carboxyhemoglobin level of 40 to 60 per cent.
G. Hyperventilation and syncope may occur after an intense physical effort in an athletic contest.

Smith, N. J.: Medical issues in sports medicine. Pediatr. Rev. 2:229, 1981.

ETIOLOGIC CLASSIFICATION OF FAINTING

44 / VERTIGO; DIZZINESS

Vertigo, or dizziness, implies a sense of rotation or motion of the patient or his environment. Since vertigo is a subjective symptom, the clinician has to decide whether the complaint accurately describes the child's symptoms. Often the patient will inaccurately use the term "dizziness" to describe the lightheadedness or faintness that characterizes such disorders as the hyperventilation syndrome or primary pulmonary hypertension. The specific cause for vertigo is often difficult to establish. Investigation should include a neurologic appraisal, particularly of the cranial nerves, audiometric evaluation and examination of vestibular functioning. Vertigo in infants and young children may be expressed as irritability.

ETIOLOGIC CLASSIFICATION OF VERTIGO

I. LABYRINTHINE DISORDERS may give rise to paroxysmal, brief episodes of vertigo. The onset may be explosive, accompanied by tinnitus, decreased auditory acuity, nystagmus, nausea and vomiting. Nystagmus that persists for several days is usually central rather than labyrinthine in origin. Toxic labyrinthitis may be caused by mumps or encephalitis. Vestibular neuronitis and vertigo may occur secondary to upper respiratory and middle ear infections.

Meniere's disease (hydrops of the labyrinth) may occur rarely in children as attacks of severe vertigo, nystagmus and a sensorineural hearing loss. Complete recovery tends to occur between episodes.

II. CENTRAL DISORDERS such as brain tumors may be accompanied by gradually increasing dizziness that is usually less severe and more continuous than that due to labyrinthine disease. Cerebellopontine angle, supratentorial, temporal lobe and midbrain tumors may be accompanied by vertigo. Benign positional vertigo may occur a few days or weeks after cerebral concussion as part of the post-traumatic headache syndrome.

Episodes of vertigo may be a sequela of meningitis. Transient dizziness may also represent a prodromal symptom of epilepsy or migraine headaches. Vertigo is a frequent symptom in basilar artery migraine. Vertiginous seizures arising from the temporal lobe cortex may cause paroxysmal episodes of vertigo, headache, nausea, vomiting and unconsciousness. Vertigo may also be a symptom of more widespread seizure activity accompanied by to-and-fro or lateral swaying of the body, falling, unconsciousness and seizures.

III. MOTION SICKNESS may represent hyperreactivity to labyrinthine stimuli.

IV. PSYCHOGENIC FACTORS may give rise to the complaint of dizziness. Hyperventilation syndrome is characterized by complaints of dizziness, headaches, chest pain, lightheadedness and "smothering" spells.

V. POSTURAL VERTIGO, IMBALANCE AND HEADACHE may be initiated by trigger areas in the sternocleidomastoid muscle.

VI. BENIGN PAROXYSMAL VERTIGO is characterized by recurrent episodes, sudden in onset and a few seconds to minutes in duration, in which the child, usually between the ages of one to five years, appears frightened, cries out, clings for support, staggers or falls. Accompanying findings include torticollis, pallor, sweating and nystagmus. Torticollis may persist for hours or days. The electroencephalogram is normal, but the caloric stimulation test is often abnormal. The child may later develop classic migraine.

Dunn, D. W., and Snyder, C. H.: Benign paroxysmal vertigo of childhood. Am. J. Dis. Child. 130:1099, 1976.

VII. DRUGS, including kanamycin and aminoglycosides such as gentamicin, may cause vertigo.

VIII. CARBON MONOXIDE POISONING may cause dizziness, nausea and headaches.

IX. HYPERTROPHIC OBSTRUCTIVE CARDIOMY-
OPATHY may cause dizziness, easy fatigability and syncope.

X. DIZZINESS is a prodromal symptom of
heat stroke.

XI. DIZZINESS is a symptom of solvent or
gasoline sniffing.

GENERAL REFERENCE

Eviatar, L., and Eviatar, A.: Vertigo in children: Differential
diagnosis and treatment. Pediatrics 59:833, 1977.

ETIOLOGIC CLASSIFICATION OF VERTIGO

---

45 / HEADACHES

Chronic, recurrent headaches, like abdominal pain, represent a pediatric problem
that may have both organic and psychologic
etiologic possibilities.

ETIOLOGIC CLASSIFICATION OF HEADACHES

I. MUSCLE CONTRACTION HEADACHES (TEN-
SION HEADACHES)

A. Muscle contraction, presumably secondary to tension, is the most common
cause of chronic, recurrent or persistent
headache in childhood. In some instances the discomfort begins in the
muscles of the neck, shoulders or occiput
and migrates anteriorly to the frontal
region, but the headache is usually generalized. At times described as a "tight
band around the head," "a heavy weight
on the head," "a pressure from the outside" or persistent aching, the headache
may continue for days or weeks. In fact,
a persistent headache is almost always
psychogenic owing to anxiety or depression. Nausea, vomiting, dizziness or nervousness may occur concurrently in
some cases. Severe headaches of any
cause are frequently accompanied by
spasm of the neck and shoulder muscles.
Both migraine and muscle contraction
headaches may be precipitated by stressors (e.g., arguments between the child
and someone close to him). They may
also be associated with disappointment,
rejection, intense excitement, anxiety,
and fear of failure in school examinations, auditions, recitals or contests.
Children and adolescents and, at times,
their families who experience either
muscle contraction or migraine headaches may have difficulty with the acceptance or expression of assertiveness,
anger, or resentment, especially toward
significant persons. Unaware of a relationship between headaches and feelings, they are unlikely to spontaneously
volunteer such an association. Because
they are often unconscious, these feelings may be denied. Although muscle
contraction or migraine headaches may
be precipitated by events that immediately evoke anger, the patient who is
chronically inhibited from its direct
expression by strong parental disap-

proval, personal discomfort, or guilt may carry a burden of intense resentment. It is appropriate to ask the child or adolescent what kinds of things make him angry, how he deals with anger, and how he would like to manage his anger. Similar information should be obtained from the parents. The presence of anxiety and depression in the child should also be explored.

B. Occipital neuralgia due to instability of the first and second cervical segments is characterized by headaches in the occipital or suboccipital area secondary to muscle spasm, scalp pain, tenderness and paresthesia involving the second cervical dermatome.

II. VASCULAR HEADACHES

A. Common or classic migraine headaches, not uncommon in the pediatric age group, have an incidence of 2 to 4.5 per cent. Although children above the age of seven may experience migraine headaches similar to those in adults, in very young children the headaches may be generalized rather than unilateral, and cyclic vomiting may be the preeminent symptom. Prodromal or accompanying symptoms may include photophobia, nausea, vomiting, abdominal pain, pallor, sweating, facial flushing, transient blindness, eyelid edema and mood changes. Scintillating scotomata, hemianopsia, zigzag lines, random blind spots, blurred vision or paresthesias are less frequent in children than in adults.

Classically, the migraine headache is periodic, unilateral and present in the retro-orbital, frontal or temporal region. Initially throbbing, pounding or pulsating and unilateral, the headache usually becomes constant and generalized. The duration of the episode is generally two to three hours, but some attacks persist as long as 48 hours or more. A migraine headache may be followed by a period of sleep, or it may awaken a child from sleep. Most children have only infrequent migraine headaches, but a few have several a week. A family history of migraine is present in about 70 per cent of cases. Patients with migraine headaches report numerous precipitating factors, including excessive noise, confusion, illness, foods (cheese, chocolate, citrus fruits, hot dogs, salami or bacon), alcohol, menstruation, oral contraceptives, extreme exertion, stress, fasting, loss of sleep, prolonged sleep, bright and flashing lights, and lengthy viewing of television or movies. Migraine-like headaches may occur in patients with lupus erythematosus.

Brown, J. K.: Migraine and migraine equivalents in children. Devel. Med. Child Neurol. 19:683, 1977.
Prensky, A. L., and Sommer, D.: Diagnosis and treatment of migraine in children. Neurology 29:500, 1979.
Shinnar, S., and D'Souza, B.: Migraine in children and adolescents. Pediatr. Rev. 3:257, 1982.

B. Complicated migraine
1. Ophthalmoplegic migraine, usually involving the oculomotor and less frequently the abducens nerve, is a rare form of the migraine syndrome in early childhood. Twelve to 24 hours after the onset of the headache, the following signs develop: eye pain; nausea; vomiting; sudden, usually unilateral ptosis; pupillary dilatation; and reduced eye mobility. These findings may last for days or weeks.
2. Hemiplegic migraine, at times familial, is characterized by neurologic deficits such as aphasia, paresthesias, hemiparesis or hemisensory loss that may last for hours to days. Headache usually follows on the contralateral side.

Verret, S., and Steele, J. C.: Alternating hemiplegia in childhood: A report of eight patients with complicated migraine beginning in infancy. Pediatrics 47:675, 1971.

3. Acute confusional states lasting 10 minutes to 24 hours may be the initial or later manifestation of a migraine episode in later childhood and adolescence. Since the accompanying symptoms may include agitation, apprehension and combativeness, this form of complicated migraine is to be differentiated from other causes of delirium. See page 334.

Ehyai, A., and Fenichel, G. M.: The natural history of acute confusional migraine. Arch. Neurol. 35:368, 1978.
Emery, E. S.: Acute confusional state in children with migraine. Pediatrics 60:110, 1977.

4. Basilar artery migraine begins suddenly with vertigo, ataxia, dysarthria, tinnitus, transient blindness, blurred vision, drop attacks, oculomotor abnormalities, other cranial nerve deficits and paresthesias around the mouth and the distal extremities. Severe bifrontal, temporal or occipital headache and vomiting follow. Although most episodes last less than

three to four hours, others last longer. The headache may be bifrontal, bitemporal or occipital.

Lapkin, M. L., and Golden, G. S.: Basilar artery migraine. Am. J. Dis. Child. 132:278, 1978.

5. The Alice in Wonderland syndrome is characterized by olfactory, gustatory and auditory hallucinations, micropsia, metamorphopsia; distortions of time, space, and body image; lethargy; or hyperactivity. Confusion, disorientation, apraxia, agnosia, speech and language disorders, feelings of déjà vu and trance or dreamlike states may also occur. These episodes may be an immediate prodrome or may occur several days before the migraine headache.

Golden, G. S.: The Alice in Wonderland syndrome in juvenile migraine. Pediatrics 63:517, 1979.

C. Cluster headaches, characterized by bursts of one to three headaches a day over a period of weeks, are uncommon in children. In addition to severe headaches, the patient may develop unilateral conjunctival injection, rhinorrhea, lacrimation, flushing and sweating.

III. COMBINED MIGRAINE AND MUSCLE CONTRACTION HEADACHES may occur simultaneously.

IV. TRACTION HEADACHES result from traction on intracranial contents, especially vascular structures.

A. Headache is less commonly a presenting symptom of intracranial tumors in children than in adults, in part because of the early separation of sutures and spontaneous decompression that occur in the young patient. Headache, an uncommon manifestation of supratentorial neoplasms, is more frequent with cerebellar tumors. Although the headache associated with a brain tumor usually occurs in the morning shortly after arising and disappears after a brief time, it may be reported at other times of the day and may awaken the child from sleep. Headaches may be precipitated by sudden exacerbations of intracranial pressure caused by coughing, sneezing, straining with a bowel movement or position change. Traction headaches are usually described as dull, deep and intermittent, although occasionally steady. They may also be intense and incapacitating. That the headache may be temporarily relieved by aspirin or other mild analgesic does not rule out a brain tumor. Temporary lessening of the headache may be attributable to separation of the sutures. Diplopia may occur. Headaches with the following characteristics suggest the possibility of a brain tumor or other cause of increased intracranial pressure: always occur in the same area; are sudden in onset, severe, incapacitating and unresponsive to medication; undergo a change in quality, frequency or pattern; and are accompanied by changes in personality or vomiting.

Honig, P. S., and Charney, E. B.: Children with brain tumor headaches. Am. J. Dis. Child. 136:121, 1982.

B. Brain abscess may be accompanied by headache, fever, nausea, vomiting and leukocytosis.

Fischer, E. G., McLennan, J. E., and Suzuki, Y.: Cerebral abscess in children. Am. J. Dis. Child. 135:746, 1981.

C. Rupture of an intracranial aneurysm may be accompanied by excruciating headache, photophobia, meningeal signs and impaired consciousness.
D. Arteriovenous malformations may produce a sudden headache, obtundation, focal neurologic defect, signs of meningeal irritation and increased intracranial pressure.
E. Pseudotumor cerebri is characterized by intermittent, severe, usually generalized headaches that are worse in the morning. In addition to severe headache, patients may have blurring of vision, diplopia, nausea, vomiting and papilledema. The neurologic examination and CT scan are normal. Symptoms may persist for weeks. Conditions associated with pseudotumor cerebri include hypoparathyroidism, adrenal insufficiency, corticosteroid administration or withdrawal, hypervitaminosis A, tetracycline administration, oral contraceptives, initiation of thyroid replacement therapy and iron deficiency anemia.

Weisberg, L. A., and Chutorian, A. M.: Pseudotumor cerebri of childhood. Am. J. Dis. Child. 131:1243, 1977.

F. Neurofibromatosis may cause headaches.
G. Central nervous system leukemia causes headaches, vomiting, irritability, diplopia, polyphagia and rapid weight gain.
H. Obstruction of a cerebrospinal fluid

shunt may produce headache, irritability, lethargy and vomiting.

I. Subdural hematoma is a diagnostic consideration in children with headaches of recent origin.

V. MENINGITIS OR ENCEPHALITIS may cause severe headache.

VI. POST-TRAUMATIC HEADACHE. Headaches that occur in children after a severe head injury, especially an injury accompanied by unconsciousness, may persist for months or years. The patient with a post-traumatic syndrome may also complain of dizziness, nervousness, heightened sensitivity to noise, withdrawal, inability to concentrate, hyperactivity, sleep disturbances and difficulty controlling anger. Whereas the child may have experienced an unusually severe emotional reaction to the injury, his emotional adjustment prior to the trauma and current environmental stresses should be explored. Pending litigation following the child's involvement in an accident seems to contribute to the symptoms' persistence in some cases. A chronic subdural hematoma needs to be included in the differential diagnosis.

Rune, V.: Acute head injuries in children. Acta Paediatr. Scand. (Suppl.)209:122, 1970.

VII. OCULAR DISORDERS. Headache may be caused by eyestrain due to uncorrected refractive errors, astigmatism, muscle imbalance or impaired convergence. Other ocular symptoms may include burning, tearing, conjunctival hyperemia, blurring and dizziness. Because photophobia and conjunctival injection may accompany severe headache of any cause, these signs do not necessarily imply eye disease.

VIII. SINUSITIS or inflammation and engorgement of the nasal turbinates are infrequent causes of severe headache in children.

IX. HYPERTENSION. Although it is an unusual cause of chronic headache in children, hypertension should be included in the differential diagnosis. Hypertensive encephalopathy is manifested by severe headache, retinal findings, nausea, vomiting, confusion, seizures and transient, focal neurologic findings. Headache, characteristically pounding in character, commonly occurs in patients with pheochromocytoma.

X. "GOGGLE" HEADACHE is caused by compression of the supraorbital nerve within the supraorbital notch by tight-fitting swimming goggles.

XI. ACUTE MOUNTAIN SICKNESS may cause an intense headache accompanied by nausea and vomiting.

XII. Since CARBON MONOXIDE POISONING may cause a headache, the possibility of a gas leak, faulty flue or other environmental exposure should be explored to account for a persistent headache accompanied by anorexia and dizziness.

XIII. PSYCHOGENIC HEADACHES

A. Psychogenic headaches may have the same etiologic factors as recurrent abdominal pain. See page 251.

B. Conversion reaction

C. Depression in children may present as a severe headache that persists for days or weeks.

Ling, W., Oftedal, G., and Weinberg, W.: Depressive illness in childhood presenting as severe headache. Am. J. Dis. Child. 120:122, 1970.

D. Hypochondriasis is characterized by headache and multiple other somatic complaints.

XIV. The PREMENSTRUAL SYNDROME may be accompanied by headaches.

XV. HEADACHES OF UNKNOWN ORIGIN. In some cases it may be impossible to determine the exact cause of a headache, even after thorough study.

DIAGNOSIS

The pediatric interview is the most helpful diagnostic tool in understanding the cause of headaches. Organic disease and emotional problems may coexist. Children with either migraine or tension headaches commonly have relatives, especially parents, with similar symptoms. Headaches of psychogenic origin are especially likely to represent identification with a relative or other significant person.

The physical examination should include careful funduscopy, testing of visual fields, screening of visual acuity, ability to converge and phorias. Reevaluation is indicated periodically, especially in the first four to six months after onset of the headaches.

A headache is not usually the only manifestation of a seizure disorder, so an electroencephalogram is rarely helpful. Since most headaches in children are muscle contrac- tion or migraine in etiology, laboratory procedures such as computed tomography, electroencephalogram or skull roentgenograms are rarely necessary. A thoughtful history, negative physical examination, and a therapeutic trial, if indicated, reliably make the diagnosis most of the time.

ETIOLOGIC CLASSIFICATION OF HEADACHES

---

46 / IRRITABILITY

Irritability may accompany almost any pediatric illness. Unusual irritability occurs in the following disorders with or without other symptoms.

ETIOLOGIC CLASSIFICATION OF IRRITABILITY

I. METABOLIC DISORDERS

A. Disturbances in water and electrolyte metabolism
  1. Changes in serum sodium concentration
    a. Irritability may be heightened in patients with hypernatremia so that the child demonstrates a marked reaction to touch, sound and light stimuli.
    b. Restlessness, irritability and convulsions may occur with hyponatremia.

Schueman, J.: Infantile water intoxication at home. Pediatrics 66:119, 1980.

  2. Changes in serum calcium concentration
    a. Hypercalcemia
    b. Hypocalcemia

3. Hypokalemia
4. Diabetes insipidus in infancy
B. Hypoglycemia produces irritability in the newborn. Older infants may develop episodes of limpness, pallor, flushing, twitching or tremors.
C. Urea cycle disorders with hyperammonemia may initially cause irritability, hyperactivity and poor feeding. Vomiting, seizures, lethargy and coma may follow.
D. Reye's syndrome is characterized early by irritability, lethargy and confusion.
E. Nutritional disturbances
1. Underfeeding. Protein malnutrition (Kwashiorkor)
2. Scurvy
3. Celiac disease
4. Iron deficiency is an important cause of irritability. A diminution of such irritability may be the first sign of response to iron therapy.
5. Zinc deficiency secondary to prolonged parenteral alimentation may cause irritability with unconsolable crying.

Sivasubramanian, K. N., and Henkin, R. I.: Behavioral and dermatologic changes and low serum zinc and copper concentrations in two premature infants after parenteral alimentation. J. Pediatr. 93:847, 1978.

F. Endocrine disorders
1. Hyperthyroidism may cause irritability and nervousness.
2. Premenstrual syndrome may be characterized by irritability or emotional lability.

II. NEUROLOGIC DISORDERS

A. Subdural hematoma
B. Subdural effusion may account for persistent irritability during treatment of bacterial meningitis.
C. Unusual irritability in a young infant, especially if associated with other changes in sensorium, suggests the possibility of meningitis.
D. Encephalitis
E. Brain tumor
F. Neurologically impaired infants may demonstrate excessive irritability and "colic." Hydrencephaly may be characterized by rage reactions.
G. Central nervous system degenerative disorders such as Krabbe's and Batten's disease may be characterized early by unusual irritability and persistent crying.
H. Whiplash-shaken, abused infants, may demonstrate hyperirritability, a bulging fontanelle, forceful vomiting, retinal hemorrhages and convulsions.

Caffey, J.: The whiplash shaken syndrome: Manual shaking by the extremities with whiplash-induced intracranial and intra-ocular bleedings, linked with permanent brain damage and mental retardation. Pediatrics 54:396, 1974.

I. Increased intracranial pressure owing to head trauma, subdural hematoma, brain tumor or obstruction of cerebrospinal fluid shunts leads to irritability, lethargy, headache and vomiting.
J. Migraine headaches are often accompanied by irritability. In rare instances, irritability in a toddler may represent a migraine headache.

III. CARDIAC DISORDERS

A. Paroxysmal atrial tachycardia
B. Irritability may be an early symptom of cardiac failure in infants, along with anorexia and easy tiring on feeding.
C. Although the onset of endocardial fibroelastosis may be acute and fulminant, irritability, anorexia and failure to thrive may be present for some time before dyspnea and cyanosis appear.
D. In tetralogy of Fallot, episodes of irritability or crying may be associated with periods of hypoxemia.

IV. RESPIRATORY FAILURE characterized by hypoxemia and hypercapnia

V. HEMATOLOGIC DISORDERS

A. Anemia
B. Leukemia
C. Infectious mononucleosis may cause irritability, anxiety and depression.

VI. DRUGS, POISONS, TOXINS

A. Lead poisoning may be characterized early by extreme irritability, lethargy, drowsiness, fearfulness and unexplained crying.
B. Gasoline sniffing may produce irritability, anorexia, tremor, vomiting and delirium.

Boeckx, R. L., Postl, B., and Coodin, F. J.: Gasoline sniffing and tetraethyl lead poisoning in children. Pediatrics 60:140, 1977.

C. Vitamin A poisoning may occur in infants and young children. In addition to irritability, findings include pruritus, hepatomegaly, alopecia and painful swelling of the extremities.
D. The fetal alcohol and hydantoin syn-

dromes may be characterized by withdrawal symptoms such as irritability, tremors and seizures.

Iosub, S., Fuchs, M., Bingolin, N., and Gromisch, D. S.: Fetal alcohol syndrome revisited. Pediatrics 68:475, 1981.

E. Irritability is the most common manifestation of neonatal narcotic withdrawal. Other signs include a high-pitched, screeching and raucous cry, restlessness, tremors, purposeless movements, jitteriness, convulsions, vomiting, drowsiness, poor feeding, muscular hypertonicity, hyperactivity, nasal congestion, sneezing, dyspnea, yawning, frantic sucking, sweating, tachypnea, fever and convulsions. Symptoms may begin within the first 12 hours or be delayed until three to four days of age. Withdrawal symptoms from methadone may be delayed until two weeks of age in some infants.

Sweet, A.Y.: Narcotic withdrawal syndrome in the newborn. Pediatr. Rev. 3:285, 1982.

F. Theophylline overdose in an infant may cause extreme irritability.
G. Phenobarbital may cause irritability and hyperactivity in some children. Infants born to mothers who have taken barbiturates throughout pregnancy may manifest withdrawal symptoms.

Desmond, M. M., Schwanecke, R. P., Wilson, G. S., Vasunaga, S., and Burgdorff, I.: Maternal barbiturate utilization and neonatal withdrawal symptomatology. J. Pediatr. 80:190, 1972.

VII. PSYCHOSOCIAL FACTORS

A. Mothering disabilities. Excessive irritability in an infant may be attributable to psychologic factors, (e.g., situations in which the baby's nurturing needs are inadequately met, underfeeding, overfeeding and restriction of movement). Maternal depression or excessive tension in the home may cause irritability in an infant.
B. Childhood depression with dysphoric mood may be characterized by irritability, whininess, truculence or temper outbursts.

VIII. OTHER DISORDERS ACCOMPANIED BY IRRITABILITY

A. Atopic eczema
B. Cow's milk allergy
C. Unrecognized skeletal trauma
D. Inguinal hernia
E. Unrecognized ingestion of a foreign body such as an open safety pin
F. Gastroesophageal reflux may be accompanied by extreme irritability owing to esophagitis.
G. Unrecognized deafness
H. Otitis media with effusion
I. Infantile cortical hyperostosis
J. Discitis in young children is manifested by irritability, low-grade fever, vague extremity pains, and, perhaps, refusal to walk or sit up. Symptoms improve when the child lies flat.

Fisher, G. W., Popich, G. A., Sullivan, D. E., Mayfield, G., Mazat, B. A., and Patterson, P. H.: Discitis: A prospective diagnostic analysis. Pediatrics 62:543, 1978.

K. Pheochromocytoma may cause marked irritability.
L. Persistent irritability occurs with the Smith-Lemli-Opitz syndrome.
M. Anal fissures are an important cause of crying and irritability in young infants.
N. Teething
O. Colic, a syndrome of many etiologies, is characterized by the episodic occurrence of vigorous and persistent crying. The infant appears to be in pain with his hands clenched, arms and thighs flexed, face beet red, and abdomen distended. Some infants have colic almost every evening or night for two to three months. Usually no specific cause can be established. Poor feeding technique may be etiologic in some instances. Emotional tension in the home may be related in a few cases. Cow's milk allergy may be a factor in a few other babies. In general, however, the cause is obscure.

Carey, W. B.: "Colic"—primary excessive crying as an infant-environment interaction. Pediatr. Clin. North Am. 31:993, 1984.

P. Irritability in the newborn may be a symptom of bacterial or viral infections. Marked irritability occurs during the acute phase of Kawasaki disease and may persist for one to two weeks after resolution of the fever.
Q. Motion sickness in toddlers may be manifest as irritability rather than vomiting.
R. A child who has difficulty having his needs understood because of highly unintelligible speech or other communication problem may become highly frustrated and irritable.

ETIOLOGIC CLASSIFICATION OF IRRITABILITY

47 / RESPIRATORY DISTRESS; DYSPNEA; APNEA

CLINICAL CONSIDERATIONS

Dyspnea is a subjective feeling of respiratory discomfort. In the infant and young child, the term *dyspnea* is probably not semantically correct and *respiratory distress* may be preferable. Orthopnea is a form of dyspnea that is present in the recumbent position but absent when the patient sits up. In infants, respiratory distress is usually accompanied by tachypnea with a respiratory rate greater than 60 per minute. Normally, the newborn infant has an average respiratory rate of 40, with a range of 35 to 50. A fall in the respiratory rate implies that the tachypnea is improving or that the in-

TABLE 47–1. APGAR SCORE

Sign	0	1	2
Heart rate	Absent	Slow (below 100)	Over 100
Respiratory effort	Absent	Slow, irregular	Good, crying
Muscle tone	Flaccid	Some flexion of extremities	Active motion
Reflex irritability	No response	Grimace	Vigorous cry
Color	Blue, pale	Body pink, extremities blue	Completely Pink

fant is beginning to experience respiratory failure.

Downes, J. J., Fulgencio, T., and Raphaely, R. C.: Acute respiratory failure in infants and children. Pediatr. Clin. North Am. 19:423, 1972.
Haddad, G. G., and Mellins, R. B.: The role of airway receptors in the control of respiration in infants. A review. J. Pediatr. 91:281, 1977.
Polgar, G.: Practical pulmonary physiology. Pediatr. Clin. North Am. 20:303, 1973.

Asphyxiation of the newborn should be evaluated immediately at birth by the Apgar score (Table 47–1). A score of 0 to 3 implies severe distress and is an indication for immediate resuscitation. Apgar scores of 4 to 7 indicate moderate respiratory distress. With a score of 7 to 10, continued observation is all that is required. When the respiratory problem is urgent and intervention cannot wait until one and five minute Apgar scores have been obtained, only the respiratory effort and heart rate may be evaluated. If respiratory effort is good and heart rate is above 100, continued observation is appropriate. If respiration is inadequate or labored and the heart rate is over 100 per minute, oxygen by mask or positive pressure by Ambu bag may be used. If the heart rate is under 100, intubation and positive pressure ventilation is indicated. Respiratory failure in children may be characterized by hypoxemia with normal P_{CO_2} or hypocapnia (Type I), caused usually by an imbalance of ventilation and perfusion; hypercapnia with hypoxemia (Type II) owing largely to alveolar hypoventilation; or a mixture of both types.

Pagtakhan, R. D., and Chernick, V.: Respiratory failure in the pediatric patient. Pediatr. Rev. 3:247, 1981.

ETIOLOGIC CLASSIFICATION OF RESPIRATORY DISTRESS

I. NEONATAL RESPIRATORY DISORDERS associated with respiratory distress

A. Atelectasis, either asymptomatic or extensive enough to cause retractions and intermittent cyanosis, exists normally at birth and may persist for days. Atelectasis or pneumonitis of the right upper lobe may occur with esophageal atresia. Factors that limit pulmonary expansion in newborn infants include a poorly developed, weak and yielding thoracic skeleton and musculature and incoordination of the respiratory movements secondary to damage or immaturity of the respiratory centers.

Purves, M. J.: Onset of respiration at birth. Arch. Dis. Child. 49:333, 1974.

B. Respiratory distress syndrome (hyaline membrane disease) is caused by surfactant deficiency associated either with (1) immaturity and an inadequate number of type II pneumocytes or surfactant-producing cells or (2) stress, e.g., asphyxia, hypovolemia, acidosis, hypothermia, hypoglycemia, sedation and maternal hemorrhage that impairs the surfactant-producing pneumocytes. A history of fetal distress is common. The respiratory distress syndrome is more common in premature than in full-term infants, with the greatest incidence in infants who weigh between 1000 and 2000 gm. The second of a set of twins is more likely than the first to have hyaline membrane disease.

Clinical features are suggestive but not diagnostic. Expiratory grunting, rapid respiratory rate, flaring of the alae nasi, inspiratory retractions and cyanosis may be noted in the delivery room or shortly thereafter. The full syndrome is apparent within 6 to 12 hours after birth. The respiratory rate may be greater than 100 per minute. Edema, especially of the hands and feet, may develop.

Respiratory failure in an infant with respiratory distress syndrome is present when greater than a 50 to 60 per cent inspired oxygen concentration is required to maintain arterial oxygen tension at 50 mm Hg. Respiratory acidosis, reflected by an increasing Pa_{CO_2} or apnea, are other indications for mechanical ventilation. If supplemental oxygen is not required for a period exceeding 24 hours, hyaline membrane disease is not present.

A characteristic diffuse reticulogranular appearance with air bronchograms and hypoaeration is noted on the chest roentgenogram. A patent ductus arteriosus may complicate the course of respiratory distress syndrome, producing a need for augmented oxygen therapy and ventilation. Group B beta-hemolytic streptococcus or other bacterial pneumonia may simulate or complicate the respiratory distress syndrome. Differences frequently noted between the two include (1) the diminished lung volume in hyaline membrane disease in contrast to the normal volume with pneumonia and (2) the patchy infiltrates, pleural effusion and fluid in the fissure in pneumonia. Respiratory distress syndrome may be complicated by a patent ductus arteriosus.

Ablow, R. C., Driscoll, S. G., Effmann, E. L., Gross, I., Jolles, C. J., Kauy, R., and Warshaw, J. B.: A comparison of early onset group B streptococcal neonatal infection and the respiratory distress syndrome of the newborn. N. Engl. J. Med. 294:65, 1976.

C. Transient tachypnea of the newborn occurs in both premature and full-term infants. Symptoms begin shortly after birth with respiratory distress manifested chiefly by tachypnea but, at times, also by grunting, flaring of the alae nasi, retractions and mild cyanosis. The respiratory rate, often 80 to 140 per minute, may remain elevated for two to five days. Recovery usually occurs within 48 hours. The chest film shows slight cardiomegaly, an increased lung volume, hyperinflated peripheral lung fields with accentuated central vascular markings or patchy infiltrates, edematous interlobar septa, an increased anteroposterior chest diameter and, possibly, a pleural effusion. PCO_2 and blood pH are compatible with normal alveolar ventilation. The mother's history may indicate heavy maternal medication, anesthesia, caesarean section or maternal diabetes.

D. Meconium aspiration syndrome, a largely preventable complication, occurs in term or post-term infants who have experienced hypoxia owing to intrauterine distress or placental insufficiency. The amniotic fluid is meconium-stained. The clinical findings are caused by plugging of the distal airways by meconium-containing amniotic fluid. Roentgenographic chest examination demonstrates an uneven pattern of atelectasis, consolidation and emphysema. The lung fields may appear hyperinflated and the anteroposterior diameter increased. Interstitial emphysema or pneumomediastinum may also be noted. Right-to-left shunting occurs, and ventilation-perfusion is abnormal. The infant has a high risk of pneumonia.

Bacsik, R. D.: Meconium aspiration syndrome. Pediatr. Clin. North Am. 24:463, 1977.

E. Pulmonary hemorrhage, manifested by respiratory distress and hemoptysis, may be associated with hemolytic disease of the newborn, central nervous system trauma, pneumonia, sepsis, hemorrhagic disease of the newborn and other neonatal disorders.

F. Bronchopulmonary dysplasia, the most common chronic respiratory disease of infants who have been treated with mechanical ventilation and supplemental oxygen, is characterized by cyanosis when the infant cries in the absence of supplemental oxygen and by fine, diffuse rales.

Edwards, D. K., Dyer, W. M., and Northway, W. H., Jr.: Twelve years experience with bronchopulmonary dysplasia. Pediatrics 59:839, 1977.

G. Pulmonary interstitial emphysema may be a complication of mechanical ventilation in infants with respiratory distress syndrome.

Levine, D. H., Trump, D. S., and Waterkotte, G.: Unilateral pulmonary interstitial emphysema: A surgical approach to treatment. Pediatrics 68:510, 1981.

H. Mikity-Wilson syndrome may develop insidiously in premature infants after the first week of life. Symptoms, which include recurrent episodes of respiratory distress and cyanosis, reach their maximal severity in four to eight weeks, then clear slowly over a period of months. Apnea occurs frequently late in the course of the disease. The chest x-ray is distinctive, with diffuse, streaky infiltrates and small cystic areas present initially, followed by basilar hyperaeration with residual upper lobe stranding.

Mikity, V. G., and Taber, P.: Complications in treatment of respiratory distress syndrome: Bronchopulmonary dysplasia, oxygen toxicity, and the Wilson-Mikity syndrome. Pediatr. Clin. North Am. 20:419, 1973.

I. Pneumonia

1. Group B streptococcus pneumonia may be confused with hyaline membrane disease. The presence of pleural effusion in the former and its absence in the latter may be diagnostically helpful. Premature rupture of the membranes or maternal fever may be noted in the history. Symptoms usually begin suddenly a few hours after birth with apnea, grunting respiration, retraction, cyanosis and shock. The white blood count is often less than 5000 per mm. *Haemophilus influenza* type B may cause a similar clinical picture.

Baker, C. J.: Group B streptococcal infections in neonates. Pediatr. Rev. 1:5, 1979.

Lilien, L. D., Yeh, T. F., Novak, G. M., and Jacobs, N. M.: Early-onset *Hemophilus* sepsis in newborn infants: Clinical roentgenographic and pathologic features. Pediatrics 62:299, 1978.

2. Acquired cytomegalovirus infection in premature infants who have received blood transfusions may become clinically manifest at four to six weeks of age with an abrupt respiratory failure, gray pallor and signs of sepsis.

Ballard, R. A., Drew, L., Hufnagle, K. G., and Riedel, P. A.: Acquired cytomegalovirus infection in preterm infants. Am. J. Dis. Child. 133:482, 1979.

3. Pneumonia owing to *Chlamydia trachomatis* may begin in the second and third weeks of life with a distinctive pertussis-like cough and respiratory rates above 50 to 60.

4. Pulmonary fungal infections in very low birth weight infants present with respiratory deterioration, abdominal distention and guaiac-positive stools.

Baley, J. E., Kliegman, R. M., and Fanaroff, A. A.: Disseminated fungal infections in very low-birth-weight infants: Clinical manifestations and epidemiology. Pediatrics 73:144, 1984.

J. Hyperviscosity syndrome

K. Congenital anomalies

1. Micrognathia with glossoptosis, and a high arched and cleft palate are present in the Pierre Robin syndrome. The cerebrocostomandibular syndrome is characterized by cerebral maldevelopment, gaps in the dorsal segments of the ribs and cleft palate, as well as micrognathia and glossoptosis. Respiratory distress dates from birth with stridor, cyanosis, retractions and, at times, opisthotonus. Feeding is difficult, and the infant fails to thrive. Complications may include cardiomegaly, cor pulmonale and pulmonary edema. The Pierre Robin syndrome is present in some patients with the Stickler syndrome consisting of myopia, cleft palate and spondyloepiphyseal dysplasia. Characteristic x-ray changes may be present in the distal tibial epiphyses.

Schreiner, R. L., McAlister, W. H., Marshall, R. E., and Shearer, W. T.: Stickler syndrome in a pedigree of Pierre Robin syndrome. Am. J. Dis. Child. 126:86, 1973.

2. Macroglossia

3. Atresia of the posterior nasal choanae. Since infants usually sleep with their mouths closed and are obligate nose breathers during the first four months of life, patent airways are important for normal respiration. Obstruction owing to congenital occlusion of the posterior nares may lead to irritability, intermittent cyanosis, and dyspnea, especially during feedings.

4. Tracheoesophageal fistula with esophageal atresia is characterized by excessive mucus, choking and intermittent cyanosis. Similar symptoms may be produced by a pseudodiverticulum of the esophagus.

5. Pulmonary hypoplasia may occur unilaterally or bilaterally along with other findings such as diaphragmatic hernia, fetal hydrochylothorax, renal disease, thoracic dystrophy and persistent fetal circulation.

Swischuk, L. E., Richardson, C. J., Nichols, M. M., and Ingman, M. J.: Primary pulmonary hypoplasia in the neonate. J. Pediatr. 95:573, 1979.

6. Primary mediastinal cyst

7. Congenital pulmonary cyst; cystic adenomatoid hyperplasia

8. Asphyxiating thoracic dystrophy

9. Lobar emphysema owing to massive overinflation of a single pulmonary lobe is a diagnostic consideration in newborn and young infants who present with tachypnea and dyspnea, often intermittent, in the absence of a preceding respiratory infection or disease. Involvement is limited to the upper or middle lobes. About half of the patients

have symptoms on the first day or two of life. Respiratory distress, which often worsens rapidly, may be accompanied by wheezing, coughing and cyanosis. Physical examination may demonstrate hyperresonance and decreased breath sounds over the affected side. Lobar emphysema is confirmed on roentgenographic examination.

Eigen H., Lemen, R. J., and Waring, W. W.: Congenital lobar emphysema: Long-term evaluation of surgery and conservatively treated children. Am. Rev. Respir. Dis. 113:823, 1976.

10. Congenital vascular ring may cause episodes of dyspnea and cyanosis. Respiratory symptoms may also be produced by compression of bronchi by pulmonary arteries or the left atrium.
11. Pulmonary sequestration may cause respiratory distress in the newborn or older infant. The extralobar form of sequestration usually occurs on the left side in association with a diaphragmatic hernia. The intralobar sequestration is present in the posterior basal segment of a lower lobe, usually the left.

deParedes, C. G., Pierce, W. S., Johnson, D. G., and Waldhausen, J. A.: Pulmonary sequestration in infants and children: A 20-year experience and review of the literature. J. Pediatr. Surg. 5:136, 1970.
Pearl, M.: Sequestration of the lung. Am. J. Dis. Child. 124:706, 1972.

12. Diaphragmatic hernia or diaphragmatic eventration owing to hypoplasia, atrophy or paralysis secondary to unilateral phrenic nerve injury is a diagnostic consideration in newborn and young infants with respiratory distress. Most instances of phrenic nerve paralysis are associated with Erb's palsy. A scaphoid abdomen in an infant with respiratory distress suggests a diaphragmatic hernia. In infants with a hernia on the right, the ipsilateral lung may be hypoplastic. In the presence of a defect in the cervicodorsal spine, a jejunal enteric canal extending into the chest, a neuroenteric cyst or a thoracic kidney are to be considered. Fluoroscopy with barium swallow and an intravenous pyelogram are indicated.

Neuhauser, E. B. D.: Right diaphragmatic hernia with thoracic kidney. Postgrad. Med. 48:57, 1970.

13. Congenital bronchobiliary fistula causes recurrent aspiration pneumonia, atelectasis and bile-stained sputum.
L. A small pneumothorax in the newborn may be asymptomatic or cause only mild apnea, irritability or restlessness. With larger amounts of pleural air, distress may be extreme, with marked tachypnea, cyanosis, grunting, restlessness and collapse. Pneumothorax is a diagnostic consideration whenever respiratory distress suddenly occurs in a newborn infant with the respiratory distress syndrome, especially on a ventilator; severe renal malformation (including total renal agenesis); and the meconium aspiration syndrome. Frequent determination of the vital signs and blood gases help identify the onset of a pneumothorax. The blood pressure, heart rate, respiratory rate and Po_2 are usually decreased. An association exists between intraventricular hemorrhage and pneumothorax in the premature infant.

Chernick, V., and Reed, M. H.: Pneumothorax and chylothorax in the neonatal period. J. Pediatr. 76:624, 1970.
Hill, A., Perlman, J. M., and Volpe, J. J.: Relationship of pneumothorax to occurrence of intraventricular hemorrhage in the premature newborn. Pediatrics 69:144, 1982.
Ogata, E. S., Gregory, G. A., Kitterman, J. A., Phibbs, R. H., and Tooley, W. H.: Pneumothorax in the respiratory distress syndrome: Incidence and effect on vital signs, blood gases, and pH. Pediatrics 58:177, 1976.
Stern, L., Fletcher, B. D., and Dunbar, J. S.: Pneumothorax and pneumomediastinum associated with renal malformations in newborn infants. Am. J. Roentgenol. 66:785, 1972.

M. Pneumomediastinum. Spontaneous pneumomediastinum may be a complication of the respiratory distress syndrome, especially in infants on ventilators. Symptoms include dyspnea and, perhaps, cyanosis. Pneumomediastinum is a diagnostic consideration in every newborn infant with otherwise unexplained respiratory distress.
N. Spontaneous chylothorax.

Van Aerde, J., Campbell, A. N., Smyth, J. A., Lloyd, D., and Bryan, M. H.: Spontaneous chylothorax in newborns. Am. J. Dis. Child. 138:961, 1984.

II. PULMONARY FACTORS

A. Pneumonia (see Chapter 49)
1. Viral
2. Bacterial

3. Protozoan. *Pneumocystis carinii* pneumonia most commonly presents with respiratory distress followed by fever and nonproductive cough.
4. Mycobacterial
5. Fungal

Imbeau, S. A., Cohen, M., and Reed, C. E.: Allergic bronchopulmonary aspergillosis in infants. Am. J. Dis. Child. 131:1127, 1977.

B. Interstitial pneumonitis may present with symptoms of dyspnea, tachypnea and cough either with exercise or at rest. Lung biopsy may be necessary for diagnosis. The cause of the various histological variants of interstitial pneumonitis is unknown. A considerable overlap exists between interstitial pneumonitis and other pulmonary disorders listed below in other categories, e.g., respiratory tract infections, hypersensitivity pneumonitis, pulmonary vasculitis and others.

Hilman, B. C.: Interstitial and hypersensitivity pneumonitis and their variants. Pediatr. Rev. 1:229, 1980.

1. Unusual interstitial pneumonitis (UIP) is a progressive disorder accompanied by fibrosis. Symptoms include cough, chest pain, cyanosis and clubbing of the fingers.
2. Desquamative interstitial pneumonia (DIP) with a proliferation and desquamation of alveolar pneumocytes is manifested by gradually progressive dyspnea, nonproductive cough, anorexia, weight loss and easy fatigability. The respiratory rate is increased. Chest roentgenographic changes are not specific. Lung biopsy may be necessary.

Howatt, W. F., Heidelberger, K. P., LeGoven, D. P., and Schnitzer, B.: Desquamative interstitial pneumonia. Am. J. Dis. Child. 126:346, 1973.

3. Giant cell interstitial pneumonitis (GIP)
4. Lymphoid interstitial pneumonitis (LIP)

O'Brodovich, H. M., Moser, M. M., and Lu, L.: Familial lymphoid interstitial pneumonia: A long-term follow-up. Pediatrics 65:523, 1980.

5. Bronchiolitis obliterans with interstitial pneumonia and possible sequela of unilateral hyperlucent lung
6. Plasma cell interstitial pneumonitis (PIP)

C. Drug-related pulmonary disease
1. Nitrofurantoin
2. Methotrexate; cyclophosphamide. Chemotherapeutic agents may cause an interstitial pneumopathy and pulmonary fibrosis.
D. Pulmonary infiltrates with eosinophilia (PIE) syndrome
1. Simple pulmonary eosinophilia (Löeffler's syndrome) is characterized by recurrent respiratory illness with wheezing, pulmonary infiltrates and marked eosinophilia.
2. Cryptogenic pulmonary eosinophilia
3. Pulmonary vasculitis may occur with periarteritis nodosa, lupus erythematosus and Goodpasture's syndrome.
4. Pulmonary eosinophilia with asthma
E. Pulmonary alveolar proteinosis generally occurs in infants under one year of age. Initially, the symptoms may be gastrointestinal in character with diarrhea and vomiting. Dyspnea, cyanosis, cough and clubbing soon ensue.

Colon, A. R., Lawrence, R. D., Milis, S. D., and O'Connell, E. J.: Childhood pulmonary alveolar proteinosis (PAP). Am. J. Dis. Child. 121:481, 1971.

F. Hypersensitivity pneumonitis
1. Lycoperdonosis owing to inhalation of large quantities of spores from the puffball mushroom

Strand, R. D., Neuhauser, E. B. D., and Sornberger, C. F.: Lycoperdonosis. N. Engl. J. Med. 277:88, 1976.

2. Pigeon-breeder's lung caused by hypersensitivity to pigeon dust, is characterized by severe interstitial pneumonia with progressive dyspnea, fever, chest pain, chronic cough, cyanosis and weight loss.

Chandra, S., and Jones, H. E.: Pigeon fancier's lung in children. Arch. Dis. Child. 47:716, 1972.

3. Hypersensitivity to cow's milk (Heiner's syndrome) may cause recurrent pulmonary infiltrates, chronic cough, wheezing, pulmonary hemosiderosis, eosinophilia and iron-deficiency anemia.

Boat, T. F.: Hyperreactivity to cow milk in young children with pulmonary hemosiderosis and cor pulmonale secondary to nasopharyngeal obstruction. J. Pediatr. 87:23, 1975.
Lee, S. K., Kniker, W. T., Cook, C. D., and Heiner, D.C.: Cow's milk–induced pulmonary disease in children. Adv. Pediatr. 25:39, 1976.

G. Pulmonary edema associated with left ventricular failure or an obstruction to pulmonary venous flow is characterized by tachypnea with respiratory rates over 60. Rales may not be evident until considerable fluid is present in the alveoli. In infants, head retraction and grunting respirations occur when the edema is marked. Differentiation from dyspnea owing to primary pulmonary disease may be difficult. Rales and rhonchi may be heard in both situations, and the chest film may not be differentially helpful. Pulmonary edema may also occur as a complication of croup and epiglottitis, heroin overdose, head trauma and other disorders characterized by an acute increase in intracranial pressure, as well as in susceptible children a day or two after rapid ascent to a high altitude. Symptoms include pallor, fatigue, cyanosis, dyspnea, cough, hemoptysis, wheezing and chest pain. Physical and roentgenographic findings are characteristic of pulmonary edema. Acute mountain sickness is characterized by headache, anorexia, dyspnea and flu-like symptoms.

Frates, R. C., Jr., Harrison, G. M., and Edwards, G. A.: High-altitude pulmonary edema in children. Am. J. Dis. Child. 131:687, 1977.

Milley, J. R., Nugent, S. K., and Roger, M. C.: Neurogenic pulmonary edema in childhood. J. Pediatr. 94:706, 1979.

Rios, B., Driscoll, D. J., and McNamara, D. G.: High-altitude pulmonary edema with absent right pulmonary artery. Pediatrics 75:314, 1985.

Travis, K. W., Todres, I. D., and Shannon, D. C.: Pulmonary edema associated with croup and epiglottitis. Pediatrics 59:695, 1977.

H. Chronic obstructive pulmonary disease owing to alpha-1-antitrypsin deficiency. Emphysema, lethal in infancy, occurs in the syndrome of cutis laxa, ligamentous laxity and delayed development.

Taiamo, R. C., Levison, H., Lynch, M. J., Hercz, A., Hyslop, N. E., Jr., and Bain, H. W.: Symptomatic pulmonary emphysema in childhood associated with hereditary alpha-l-antitrypsin and elastase inhibitor deficiency. J. Pediatr. 79:20, 1971.

I. Pulmonary sarcoidosis may be manifested by dyspnea, cough, pleuritic pain, wheezing, fever and malaise. Pulmonary function tests reveal restrictive lung disease and decrease in pulmonary function.

Merten, D. F., Kirks, D. R., and Grossman, H.: Pulmonary sarcoidosis in childhood. Am. J. Roentgenol. 135:673, 1980.

J. Pleural effusion, empyema, hemothorax, chylothorax

K. Pneumomediastinum may complicate the respiratory distress syndrome, pneumonia, measles, pertussis, asthma, acute laryngotracheobronchitis or foreign body aspiration.

L. Pneumothorax may occur in the newborn, in infants with staphylococcal pneumonia, in an adolescent with cystic fibrosis or spontaneously for an unknown reason.

M. Acquired pneumatoceles, usually asymptomatic, may occur during the course of pneumonia, especially when the *Staphylococcus, Streptococcus* or *Klebsiella* organisms are the etiologic agents. Sudden enlargement of a pneumatocele may cause acute respiratory distress. Most lesions regress spontaneously over a period of weeks. Interstitial pulmonary emphysema occurs in some infants with respiratory distress syndrome, especially those on ventilatory support. Chest roentgenograms demonstrate either large cysts surrounded by normal pulmonary parenchyma or diffuse multicystic involvement of all lobes.

Stocker, J. T, and Madewell, J. E.: Persistent interstitial pulmonary emphysema: Another complication of the respiratory distress syndrome. Pediatrics 59:847, 1977.

N. Pulmonary lymphangiectasia is a congenital abnormality that is often symptomatic at birth with respiratory distress and cyanosis. In one form, complex cardiac disease and obstructed pulmonary venous return are associated anomalies. Some children with non–cardiac-associated pulmonary lymphangiectasia may appear normal and have an unremarkable chest roentgenogram before the delayed onset of the disorder. The x-ray findings may resemble those of stage III bronchopulmonary dysplasia.

Felman, A. H., Rhatigan, R. M., and Pierson, K. K.: Pulmonary lymphangiectasia. Am. J. Roentgenol. 66:548, 1972.

O. Asthma and reactive airway disease

P. Obstruction to airways (see Chapter 48 on Stridor and Wheezing.)

Q. Smoke inhalation. Respiratory complications may be delayed up to 24 hours in patients subjected to smoke inhalation. Serious respiratory damage may occur in the absence of facial burns. Symptoms include tachypnea, stridor, hoarseness, retractions and cough. Auscultation reveals decreased breath sounds, wheezes and rales.

Mellins, R. B., and Park, S.: Respiratory complications of smoke inhalation in victims of fires. J. Pediatr. 87:1, 1975.

R. Baby powder aspiration
S. In carbon monoxide poisoning, exertional dyspnea is present at a 10 to 20 per cent level of carboxyhemoglobin.
T. Idiopathic pulmonary hemosiderosis is characterized by episodes of coughing, occasionally with blood-tinged sputum; slight exertional dyspnea; pallor; failure to gain weight; and easy fatigability. Acute episodes are manifested by dyspnea, tachycardia, cough, hemoptysis, hematemesis, pallor and fever. Bilateral perihilar, patchy infiltration is noted on the chest roentgenogram. Sputum or gastric washings may contain hemosiderin-laden macrophages, a diagnostic finding in the absence of other causes of pulmonary passive congestion.
U. The acute chest syndrome, a common complication of sickle cell anemia, may be caused by pulmonary infarction, embolization or infection owing to *Diplococcus pneumoniae*. Symptoms include acute fever, pain on respiration and dyspnea.

Barrett-Connor, E.: Pneumonia and pulmonary infarction in sickle cell anemia. JAMA 224:997, 1973.
Powars, D. R.: Natural history of sickle cell disease—the first ten years. Semin. in Hematol. 12:267, 1975.

V. Rheumatic pneumonia is characterized by extreme tachypnea and marked pulmonary consolidation.

Serlin, S. P., Rimsza, M. E., and Gay, J. H.: Rheumatic pneumonia: The need for a new approach. Pediatrics 56:1075, 1975.

W. Cystic fibrosis

MacLusky, I., McLaughlin, F. J., and Levison, H.: Cystic fibrosis: Parts I and II. Curr. Probl. Pediatr. 15(6-7):3, 1985.
Wang, E. E. L., Prober, C. G., Manson, B., Corey, M., and Levison, H.: Association of respiratory viral infections with pulmonary deterioration in patients with cystic fibrosis. N. Engl. J. Med. 311:1653, 1984.

X. Pulmonary leukemia may simulate diffuse interstitial pneumonia in the absence of other evidence of relapse. Open lung biopsy is required for diagnosis.

Wells, R. J., Weetman, R. M., Ballantine, T. V. N., Grosfeld, J. L., and Baehner, R. L.: Pulmonary leukemia in children presenting as diffuse interstitial pneumonia. J. Pediatr. 96:262, 1980.

Y. The adult respiratory distress syndrome (ARDS, "shock lung") may be caused by severe hypoxia, near-drowning, near-strangulation, sepsis, trauma, head injury, shock and burns. It is characterized by pulmonary edema, ventilation-perfusion abnormalities, shunting and hypoxemia.

Pfenninger, J., Gerber, A., Tschappeler, H., and Zimmerman, A.: Adult respiratory distress syndrome in children. J. Pediatr. 101:352, 1982.

Z. Chemical pneumonitis

III. CARDIOVASCULAR FACTORS

A. Congenital heart disease. Depending upon the degree of hypoxemia associated with the cardiac lesion, dyspnea on exertion may range from mild to severe. Infants with congenital heart disease of the cyanotic type, especially those with extreme pulmonary stenosis, may experience attacks of paroxysmal dyspnea owing to an increase in right-to-left shunting or an increased peripheral demand for oxygen. During these episodes, the cyanosis becomes much more intense, the infant gasps for breath, and unconsciousness may ensue. Although the attacks may be spontaneous, they are often precipitated by feeding, bathing, crying or defecation. When dyspnea occurs with the minimal exertion of nursing, adequate nutrition may be difficult to maintain. Anomalous origin of the left coronary artery, among other cardiac lesions of the noncyanotic type in infants, may be characterized by dyspnea, at times paroxysmal in character. Children who have an isolated pulmonary stenosis with an intact interventricular septum may have dyspnea on exertion. Respiratory distress syndrome is frequently complicated by a patent ductus arteriosus, and congestive heart failure may augment the respiratory problem.
B. Congestive cardiac failure in infants may be initially manifested by dyspnea, especially during nursing, and tachypnea, with respiratory rates of 50 to 100 during sleep. These episodes of respiratory distress may last several hours, often occur with only mild cyanosis, and may be misdiagnosed as pneumonia, asthma or bronchiolitis.

Goldring, D., Hernandez, A., and Hartmann, A. F., Jr.: The critically ill child: Care of the infant in cardiac failure. Pediatrics 47:1056, 1971.
Tripp, M. E.: Congestive cardiomyopathy of childhood. Adv. Pediatr. 31:179, 1984.

C. Persistence of the fetal circulation may present with mild to severe pulmonary distress and central cyanosis.

D. Chronic constrictive pericarditis

E. Paroxysmal tachycardia

F. Myocarditis in infants and children may have dyspnea as a prominent manifestation. Tachycardia, a change in the quality of heart sounds and enlargement of the liver may be noted. Because of the severity of the respiratory distress, the diagnosis of myocarditis is sometimes overlooked because the child is thought to have pneumonia.

G. Endocardial fibroelastosis may become symptomatic in the first six months of life with dyspnea, irritability, cough, anorexia and failure to thrive. Respiratory distress, cyanosis, tachycardia and vomiting may appear abruptly, followed by a fulminant downhill course; on the other hand, the symptoms may occur intermittently. Abdominal pain may appear to be present during these episodes.

H. Moderate to severe anemia may cause dyspnea on exertion. Shortness of breath may appear during a hemolytic crisis.

I. Pulmonary embolism may follow an elective abortion.

J. Fat embolism may cause acute dyspnea, tachypnea and cyanosis.

Shulman, S. T., and Grossman, B. J.: Fat embolism in childhood. Am. J. Dis. Child. 120:480, 1970.

K. Dyspnea may also occur in patients in shock and in those with acute adrenal insufficiency.

L. Primary pulmonary hypertension may be characterized by dyspnea, especially on exertion, easy fatigability and, at times, cyanosis and episodes of syncope. Primary pulmonary hypertension may occur in children who live at high altitudes.

M. Congenital pulmonary arteriovenous aneurysm may be characterized by dyspnea, usually on exertion, as well as by cyanosis, polycythemia and clubbing of the fingers. Symptoms may begin in childhood.

IV. MECHANICAL FACTORS

A. Because of the poorly developed and yielding thoracic skeleton and musculature in premature and some term infants, contraction of the diaphragm may be accompanied by retraction of the thoracic wall instead of a simultaneous elevation of the ribs and expansion of the chest.

B. In patients with chronic obstructive lung disease and in certain other dyspneic states, expiration is an active, rather than largely a passive, process.

C. Ascites

D. Abdominal distention in infants may cause dyspnea, tachypnea and cyanosis. The respiratory distress becomes especially noticeable in the presence of pneumonitis or patchy atelectasis.

E. Large abdominal tumor

F. Peritonitis. Respiratory movements in these patients are chiefly thoracic. Grunting may occur because of the pain associated with abdominal respiration.

G. Rhabdomyolysis with respiratory involvement may cause dyspnea and respiratory failure.

H. Marked kyphoscoliosis

I. Thickened secretions after anesthesia and surgery

J. Mediastinal tumor

K. Osteogenesis imperfecta

V. ACIDOSIS AND OTHER METABOLIC FACTORS. Chemoreceptors in the medullary respiratory center respond to acidosis or lowering of the blood pH with an increase in the depth and, to a lesser extent, in the rate of respiration. Severe acidosis has a depressing, rather than an excitory, effect on respiration and may cause respiratory failure.

A. Diabetic ketoacidosis

B. Salicylate poisoning should be suspected in a child who presents with hyperventilation, even in the absence of a history of salicylate ingestion. Hyperpnea occurs three to eight hours after ingestion of salicylates in toxic amounts. The ferric chloride urine test may be useful. A burgundy-red color persists after boiling in the presence of salicylate, but not in the case of acetoacetic acid.

C. Acidosis or hyperammonemia associated with inborn errors of metabolism, (e.g., glycogenosis, congenital lactic acidosis, fructose-1,6 diphosphatase deficiency, organic acidemias and disorders in the urea cycle).

D. Silo filler's disease owing to inhalation of nitrogen dioxide in fumes from freshly filled silos may cause an episode of bronchitis or moderately severe dyspnea, cough and chest pain. A relapse may occur in about ten days and lead to death from pulmonary edema and bronchiolitis obliterans.

E. Unremitting gasping respirations have been described with benzyl alcohol poisoning in premature infants.

F. The narcotic withdrawal syndrome in newborns is accompanied by tachypnea.

VI. NEUROLOGIC FACTORS

A. Immaturity of the respiratory center
B. Depression of respiratory centers owing to intrauterine hypoxemia, anesthesia, barbiturates, morphine, carbon dioxide intoxication and anoxia
C. Brain tumors and other causes of increased intracranial pressure may cause neurogenic hyperventilation secondary to midbrain-pontine herniation.
D. Cerebral hemorrhage
E. Cerebral edema
F. Encephalitis, meningitis
G. Reye's syndrome, especially in infants under one year of age, may be accompanied by hyperventilation owing to stimulation of the medullary respiratory centers.
H. Unilateral congenital diaphragmatic paralysis following injury to the phrenic nerve
I. Poliomyelitis or the Guillain-Barré syndrome. Early diagnosis of intercostal or diaphragmatic paralysis or both is important if mechanical ventilation is to be used promptly to prevent fatigue and hypoxemia. Early findings in patients with respiratory paralysis include irregular, shallow respiration; perhaps an increase in the respiratory rate; use of the accessory muscles of respiration; dilatation of the alae nasi; slight grunting; unwillingness to talk; interrupted or monosyllabic speech; restlessness; anxiety; fear of falling asleep; mental confusion and disorientation. Decreased vital capacity may be demonstrated by asking the patient to count rapidly to ten. Patients with respiratory difficulty cannot do this. A vital capacity of less than 12 ml/kg and a Pao_2 of less than 70 mm Hg in air are physiologic criteria for respiratory failure. Cyanosis is a late symptom, as is the forced use of the accessory muscles of respiration with gasping for each breath. With involvement of the deltoid muscles, the diaphragm may also be paralyzed, either unilaterally or bilaterally. Fluoroscopy may be helpful in determining the extent of this paralysis. The diaphragm on the involved side is elevated and demonstrates paradoxical movement, moving upward during inspiration. A shift of the mediastinum may occur toward the contralateral side. In patients with intercostal muscle weakness, splinting of the abdomen by the examiner accentuates the use of accessory respiratory musculature; conversely, splinting of the chest wall in patients with diaphragmatic involvement leads to overt dyspnea.
J. Myasthenia gravis
K. Diphtheritic neuritis
L. Werdnig-Hoffmann's disease
M. Acute parathion poisoning is manifested by the rapid onset of respiratory distress owing to muscle paralysis or impairment of the central respiratory center. Clinical features include excessive salivation, constricted pupils, muscle tremors and weakness, cough, wheezing, dyspnea and pulmonary edema.
N. Bulbar paralysis. The pooling of saliva in the pharynx leads to respiratory difficulty.
O. Botulism

VII. PSYCHOLOGIC FACTORS

A. Hyperventilation syndrome is to be considered in adolescents, especially girls, who complain of shortness of breath, "smothering" spells, inability to breathe, dizziness, light-headedness, generalized weakness, tingling and numbness of the hands, headache, chest pain, palpitations, blackout episodes or fainting. Tetany or syncope may ensue. The complaint of rapid breathing is virtually never volunteered. Some children experience numerous episodes of hyperventilation syndrome owing to anxiety. Direct questioning or an attempt to have the patient reproduce the symptoms by hyperventilating for a minute or two may be diagnostically helpful.

Magarian, G. J.: Hyperventilation syndromes: Infrequently recognized common expressions of anxiety and stress. Medicine 61:219, 1982.
Missri, J. C., and Alexander, S.: Hyperventilation syndrome. JAMA 240:2093, 1978.

B. Hyperventilation may be a manifestation of a suicidal drug overdose with ingestion of aspirin or sympathomimetics such as amphetamines.

GENERAL REFERENCES

Avery, M. E., and Fletcher, B. D.: The Lung and Its Disorders in the Newborn Infant. 3rd ed. Philadelphia, W. B. Saunders Co., 1974.
Kendig, E. L., Jr., and Chernick, V. (eds.): Disorders of the Respiratory Tract in Children. 3rd ed. Philadelphia, W. B. Saunders Co., 1977.
McBridge, J. T., and Wohl, M. E. B.: Pulmonary function tests. Pediatr. Clin. North Am. 26:537, 1979.
Taussig, L. M., and Lemen, R. J.: Chronic obstructive lung disease. Adv. Pediatr. 26:343, 1979.

ETIOLOGIC CLASSIFICATION OF RESPIRATORY DISTRESS

APNEA

I. APNEIC EPISODES in the newborn

A. Significant apnea is defined as cessation of respiration for 20 or more seconds or for briefer time periods if accompanied by bradycardia, cyanosis or pallor. The differential diagnosis includes immaturity, maternal oversedation, seizure disorder, hypothermia, intraventricular hemorrhage and hypoxic brain damage. Severe infections, including pneumonia, meningitis and sepsis, are important considerations when apnea occurs in the first 24 hours of life. Group B streptococcus sepsis, for example, frequently causes severe apnea on the first day of life.

Apnea is also associated with severe respiratory distress syndrome and with pulmonary hemorrhage, anemia, patent ductus arteriosus, hypotension, gastroesophageal reflux, acidosis, hypoglycemia, hypocalcemia, hypomagnesemia, hyper- and hyponatremia, upper airway obstruction, hyperviscosity, neonatal drug intoxication owing to local anesthesia administered to the mother, hyperammonemia, pneumothorax, necrotizing enterocolitis, anticonvulsant overdosage, impaired regulation of breathing and activation of posterior pharyngeal reflexes by suction catheters or nipple. Recurrent, abrupt apnea of prematurity occurs in most infants who weigh less than 1000 gm at birth and in up to 25 per cent of those who weigh less than 2500 gm at birth. Cyanosis and bradycardia may accompany the apnea.

Kattwinkel, J.: Neonatal apnea: Pathogenesis and therapy. J. Pediatr. 90:342, 1977.

B. Periodic breathing, characterized by respiratory pauses of 5 to 10 seconds, occurs frequently in premature and some term infants during sleep in the first weeks of life. The cause is unknown.

Rigatto, H., and Brady, J. P.: Periodic breathing and apnea in preterm infants I and II. Pediatrics 50:202, 219, 1972.

C. Congenital central alveolar hypoventilation syndrome (Ondine's curse) is characterized by failure of automatic control of ventilation during sleep, perhaps owing to defective central chemoreceptors. Assisted ventilation is required.

Guilleminault, C., McQuitty, J., Ariagno, R. L., Challamel, M. J., Korobkin, R., and McClead, R. E., Jr.: Congenital central alveolar hypoventilation syndrome in six infants. Pediatrics 70:684, 1982.

II. SUDDEN INFANT DEATH SYNDROME, the leading cause of death in infants after the first week of life, occurs most frequently between the second and fourth months of life, usually during sleep, with 90 per cent of instances occurring by six months of age. The incidence is increased in males, low birth weight infants and lower socioeconomic groups.

III. INFANTILE APNEA EPISODES, which may occur while an infant is asleep or awake, are accompanied by limpness, stiffness, cyanosis or pallor. The apneic episodes may be accompanied by an absence of respiratory effort and air movement or by apparent respiratory efforts without air movement or sound. Patients with infantile apnea require appropriate cardiorespiratory and neurophysiologic studies and home-monitor observation. The frequency of such apneic spells is greatest during episodes of nasopharyngitis.

Ariagno, R. L., Guilleminault, C., Korobkin, R., Owen-Boeodiker, M., and Baldwin, R.: "Near-miss" for sudden infant death syndrome infants: A clinical problem. Pediatrics 71:726, 1983.
Kelly, D. H., and Shannon, D. C.: Episodic complete airway obstruction in infants. Pediatrics 67:823, 1981.
Rosen, C. L., Frost, J. D., Jr., and Harrison, G. M.: Infant apnea: polygraphic studies and follow-up monitoring. Pediatrics 71:731, 1983.
Steinschneider, A.: Nasopharyngitis and prolonged sleep apnea. Pediatrics 56:967, 1975.

IV. BRIEF PAUSES IN BREATHING lasting from 5 to 15 seconds occur in many normal infants, often preceded by a sigh.

V. APNEA, CHOKING, WHEEZING AND LARYNGOSPASM may occur in infants with gastroesophageal reflux.

VI. CHOKING may cause a brief episode of apnea, stridor and a transient skin color change.

VII. APNEIC EPISODES AND HYPERVENTILATION may occur in Reye's syndrome, especially in infants under one year of age.

VIII. ARNOLD-CHIARI MALFORMATION

IX. APNEA AND SUDDEN UNEXPECTED DEATH may occur in infants with achondroplasia.

X. The DANDY-WALKER SYNDROME may result in apneustic type of breathing and respiratory failure.

Tal, Y., Freigang, B., Dunn, H. G.., Durity, F. A., and Moyes, P. D.: Dandy-Walker syndrome: Analysis of 21 cases. Dev. Med. Child. Neurol. 22:189, 1980.

XI. RESPIRATORY SYNCYTIAL VIRUS INFECTION may cause apnea, especially in premature infants.

XII. APNEA may represent a seizure disorder with or without staring, eye movement or change in tone. The electroencephalogram may be normal except during apneic spells.

Watanabe, K., Hara, K., Hakamada, S., Negoro, T., Suigiura, M., Matsumoto, A., and Maehara, M.: Seizures with apnea in children. Pediatrics 79:87, 1982.

XIII. CARDIAC DYSRHYTHMIAS

XIV. LEIGH'S SYNDROME

XV. OBSTRUCTIVE SLEEP APNEA

A. Extreme obesity may be associated with alveolar hypoventilation and airway obstruction during sleep. The sleep deprivation caused by repeated apnea and recurrent awakening leads to excessive somnolence. Periodic breathing, cyanosis and secondary polycythemia may also occur.

Simpser, M. D., Strieder, D. J., Wohl, M. E., Rosenthal, A., and Rockenmacher, S.: Sleep apnea in a child with the pickwickian syndrome. Pediatrics 60:290, 1977.

B. Apnea may result from sleep-induced functional upper airway obstruction. Cinefluoroscopic examination may demonstrate intermittent functional airway obstruction during sleep. Symptoms include loud nocturnal snoring, retractions, labored breathing, and periodic apnea with cessation of snoring, although respiratory effort continues. The apneic episodes, which may be numerous, are followed by resumption of snoring and arousal of the patient. Because of the frequent interruptions of sleep, the child is excessively sleepy during the day. Etiologic factors include chronic upper airway obstruction owing to enlarged tonsils and adenoids, micrognathia, glossoptosis, facial maldevelopment or surgical correction of velopharyngeal incompetence.

Brouillette, R. T., Fernbach, and Hunt, C. E.: Obstructive sleep apnea in infants and children. J. Pediatr. 100:31, 1982.
Guilleminault, C., Eldridge, F. L., Simmons, F. B., and Dement, W. C.: Sleep apnea in eight children. Pediatrics 58:23, 1976.
Kravath, R. E., Pollak, C. P., Borowiecki, B., and Weitzman, E. D.: Obstructive sleep apnea and death associated with surgical correction of velopharyngeal incompetence. J. Pediatr. 96:645, 1980.
Mathew, O. P.: Maintenance of upper airway patency. J. Pediatr. 106:863, 1985.

ETIOLOGIC CLASSIFICATION OF APNEA

48 / STRIDOR, NOISY BREATHING, SNORING, WHEEZING

CLINICAL CONSIDERATIONS

Stridor is a harsh, vibratory, high-pitched, sometimes shrill, crowing noise, usually most distinct during inspiration. Clinical manifestations of respiratory obstruction include hoarseness, dyspnea, inspiratory retractions, brassy cough, tachycardia, apprehensiveness, increased respiratory rate and use of the accessory muscles of respiration. Restlessness, an early indication of hypoxia, occurs before overt cyanosis. Increasing restlessness in an infant or child with respiratory obstruction may indicate the need for a tracheostomy or ventilatory support. Sedative medication is contraindicated in children in respiratory distress, as it may mask the manifestations of hypoxemia and inhibit needed accessory respiratory efforts. Once an adequate airway has been established, restlessness is followed almost dramatically by sleep.

That the incidence of respiratory obstruction is relatively greater in infants than in older children may, in part, be ascribed to three anatomic features: the small size of the infant larynx, the presence of loose submucous connective tissue in the supraglottic and subglottic regions, and the rigid encirclement of the subglottic area by the cricoid cartilage. The triangular glottic opening of the infant larynx is approximately 7 mm in length and 4 mm in width at the base. The degree of inflammatory edema that produces signs of respiratory obstruction in infants would, in the adult, result only in hoarseness. The laryngeal mucosa is loosely fixed to the epiglottis anteriorly and along the aryepiglottic folds laterally. Edema in the supraglottic spaces secondary to inflammation causes downward pressure on the epiglottis and laryngeal obstruction. A similar process may occur in the narrow subglottic area with swelling of the submucosal tissue and acute respiratory obstruction. Since this space is completely encircled by the cricoid cartilage, swelling owing to edema impinges upon the airway.

ETIOLOGIC CLASSIFICATION OF STRIDOR

I. INTRINSIC OBSTRUCTION OF AIRWAYS

A. Congenital anomalies
   1. Inspiratory laryngeal collapse (congenital laryngeal stridor, laryngomalacia) generally becomes symptomatic at birth or in the first weeks of life and continues to be symptomatic until the end of the first year. This disorder, caused by flaccidity of the epiglottis, aryepiglottic folds and arytenoids, is characterized by retractions and stridor that is usually inspiratory but, occasionally, also expiratory. The stridor, which may appear only with excitement or crying, often diminishes or disappears when the infant lies in the prone position.
   2. A congenital laryngeal mucous membrane web across the anterior half to two thirds of the vocal cords or around the glottis may produce signs of respiratory obstruction and absence of a cry. The stridor may be biphasic.
   3. Enlargement of a laryngeal cyst may produce progressive respiratory obstruction.
      a. Cyst of laryngeal ventricle
      b. Cyst of aryepiglottic fold
   4. Congenital subglottic stenosis, a relatively common laryngeal abnormality, is characterized by inspiratory and expiratory stridor, a barking cough and, perhaps, cyanosis.
   5. Tracheal stenosis
   6. Absence of or defect in tracheal cartilaginous rings
   7. Calcification of laryngeal and tracheal cartilage may cause congenital stridor.

Smith, R. J. H., and Catlin, F. E.: Congenital anomalies of the larynx. Am. J. Dis. Child. 138:35, 1984.

B. Laryngeal paralysis
1. Bilateral laryngeal paralysis in the newborn may be unsuspected in the presence of a normal though weak cry, but severe inspiratory and expiratory stridor are generally present. With unilateral paralysis, the cry is usually weak or absent. Inspiratory stridor, dyspnea and intercostal retractions are present; on the other hand, the symptoms may be minimal. Left-sided unilateral paralysis may be associated with a cardiovascular or pulmonary disorder, whereas right vocal cord paralysis is usually an isolated finding.
2. Congenital cardiovascular anomalies may produce unilateral recurrent nerve paralysis, usually on the left, with minimal laryngeal obstruction. Hoarseness and slight stridor may occur.
3. Birth trauma
4. Bilateral abductor vocal cord paralysis causing severe stridor may occur suddenly in infants with increased intracranial pressure associated with Arnold-Chiari malformation and hydrocephalus. Since the paralyzed cords are flaccid, the cry is normal.

Holinger, P. C., Holinger, L. D., Reichert, T. J., and Holinger, P. H.: Respiratory obstruction and apnea in infants with bilateral abductor vocal cord paralysis, meningomyelocele, hydrocephalus, and Arnold-Chiari malformation. J. Pediatr. 92:368, 1978.

C. Tumors
1. Laryngeal papilloma may cause croupy cough, hoarseness or aphonia. The occurrence of stridor and retractions depends upon the degree of laryngeal obstruction. Although symptoms may appear in young infants, they are most common between the ages of two and four years.
2. Fibrolipoma
3. Hemangioma of the trachea is a common cause of subglottic obstruction in the first six months of life. The lesion may be covered by mucosa and difficult to visualize.
D. Trauma
1. Repeated or inexpert tracheal aspiration may cause laryngeal edema.
2. Dislocation of the cricothyroid or cricoarytenoid articulations during birth may cause partial inspiratory obstruction.
3. Subglottic stenosis may be a complication of neonatal intubation. Stridor may appear from six weeks to a few months of age.

E. Croup syndrome
1. Acute viral laryngitis, laryngotracheitis or infectious croup usually occurs between 6 months and 3 years of age. Most episodes of laryngotracheitis are of viral etiology, with parainfluenza virus type 1 the most common cause. Other viral etiologic agents include parainfluenza 2 and 3, influenza A and B, respiratory syncytial virus and adenoviruses. *Mycoplasma pneumoniae* along with the influenza virus may cause croup in children above the age of five to six years. Occurring usually during an acute viral upper respiratory tract infection, symptoms begin gradually with increasing stridor that is usually inspiratory but, at times, expiratory, a barking or brassy cough, and, perhaps, a low-grade fever.

Denny, F. W., Murphy, T. F., Clyde, W. A., Jr., Collier, A.M., and Henderson, F. W.: Croup: An 11-year study in a pediatric practice. Pediatrics 71:871, 1983.

2. Acute bacterial croup (membranous croup; acute bacterial tracheitis) is characterized initially by a course similar to that of viral croup, but then the patient becomes more seriously ill with fever, toxicity and progressive respiratory failure. Copious mucopus or adherent thick, inspissated mucus and inflammatory debris are present below the subglottic swelling. Etiologic agents include *Haemophilus influenzae* type B, *Staphylococcus aureus* and group A *Streptococcus*.

Denneny, J. C., and Handler, S. D.: Membranous laryngotracheobronchitis. Pediatrics 70:705, 1982.
Jones, R., Santos, J. L., and Oveall, J. C., Jr.: Bacterial tracheitis: A new syndrome. JAMA 242:721, 1979.
Nelson, W. E.: Bacterial croup: A historical perspective. J. Pediatr. 105:52, 1984.

3. Epiglottitis, a medical emergency, occurs usually in children between the ages of two and eight years. The etiologic agent is almost always *Haemophilus influenzae* type B. The onset of epiglottitis is abrupt with severe sore throat, high fever, toxicity, dysphagia, drooling, stridor, dyspnea and a muffled voice. Very ill, anxious, and complaining of pain on swallowing, the child sits with his

mouth open, tongue protruded, head forward and neck slightly flexed. The inflamed and edematous epiglottis may look like a bright red cherry or raspberry sitting at the base of the tongue; however, the use of a tongue depressor to see the epiglottis is contraindicated, since forceful depression of the tongue may cause respiratory arrest. A portable lateral roentgenogram of the neck is diagnostic, but the child's posture of comfort should not be compromised by having him lie down or undergo other manipulations during this examination.

    4. Acute spasmodic laryngitis usually begins suddenly during the night with acute and often alarming symptoms that include hoarseness; a tight, barking, brassy, sepulchral cough; stridor; and suprasternal and infrasternal retractions. Acute spasmodic laryngitis occurs almost exclusively during the preschool age period. Some children experience many episodes.

F. Laryngeal edema
    1. Angioedema
    2. Trauma owing to foreign body or laryngeal intubation
    3. Corrosives, such as lye
    4. Nephrosis
    5. Infectious mononucleosis

G. Laryngospasm
    1. Tetany
    2. Acute infantile Gaucher's disease

H. A foreign body in the respiratory tract must be considered in the differential diagnosis of respiratory obstruction and unexplained pulmonary lesions. A laryngeal foreign body may simulate laryngitis. Symptoms include hoarseness or aphonia; persistent, perhaps barking cough; wheezing; dyspnea; hemoptysis; and, at times, cyanosis. The parent may find the infant placing safety pins in his mouth or suddenly miss a small object; however, a history of choking or gagging at the time of aspiration is often not obtained. In some cases the child may have a history of recurrent pneumonia. Usually a foreign body does not remain lodged in the larynx, but progresses to the trachea or is coughed back into the pharynx. Egg shell is the most common laryngeal foreign body. Signs of a tracheal foreign body include stridor, wheezing and retractions.

Cotton, E., and Yasuda, K.: Foreign body aspiration. Pediatr. Clin. North Am. 31:937, 1984.

I. Rarely, an esophageal foreign body may cause only stridor. A foreign body in the hypopharyngeal region may occlude the glottal opening.

Tauscher, J. W.: Esophageal foreign body: An uncommon cause of stridor. Pediatrics 61:657, 1978.

J. Cri du chat syndrome is characterized by an inspiratory stridor and a characteristic cry. Other symptoms and signs include microcephaly, hypertelorism, hypotonia, epicanthal folds and severe mental retardation.

K. Cricoarytenoid arthritis associated with juvenile rheumatoid arthritis may cause stridor.

Jacobs, J. C., and Hui, R. M.: Cricoarytenoid arthritis and airway obstruction in juvenile rheumatoid arthritis. Pediatrics 59:292, 1977.

L. Laryngeal candidiasis may cause inspiratory stridor.

II. EXTRINSIC OBSTRUCTION OF AIRWAY

A. Congenital anomalies
    1. In infants with stridor, the base of the tongue should be palpated for a thyroglossal duct cyst that may produce respiratory obstruction by forcing the epiglottis into the laryngeal aperture.
    2. Micrognathia with glossoptosis
    3. Macroglossia
    4. Diaphragmatic hernia
    5. Compression of the trachea by a vascular anomaly is a diagnostic consideration in infants who present with wheezing, stridor, apnea, rattling and gurgling respiratory noises, hyperextension of the head, inspiratory retractions, a history of recurrent pneumonia, and hesitancy in swallowing, especially solid foods. Feedings may cause an exaggeration of respiratory symptoms and cyanosis.
       a. Double aortic arch usually produces symptoms in the first six months of life.
       b. Right aortic arch with left ligamentum arteriosum may not cause symptoms until the end of the first year or later.
       c. Anomalous innominate artery
       d. Anomalous left common carotid artery
       e. Aberrant subclavian artery
       f. The pulmonary artery "sling" or aberrant left pulmonary artery

Rheuban, K. S., Ayres, N., Still, J. G., and Alford, B.: Pulmonary artery sling: A new diagnostic tool and clinical review. Pediatrics 69:472, 1982.

B. Infections
   1. Retropharyngeal abscess
   2. Infections of the closed spaces of the neck
C. Tumors
   1. Thyroid tumor
   2. Cystic hygroma
   3. Mediastinal mass or lymphadenopathy
   4. Lymphomas: lymphosarcoma, leukemia, Hodgkin's disease
D. Organ enlargement
   1. Mediastinal lymphadenopathy—tuberculosis, sarcoidosis or chronic inflammatory disease
   2. Congenital goiter

III. SLIGHT STRIDOR is not uncommon during periods of vigorous crying in many normal babies.

IV. STRIDOR may occur on a conversion basis.

Smith, M. S.: Acute psychogenic stridor in an adolescent athlete treated with hypnosis. Pediatrics 72:247, 1983.

DIAGNOSTIC STUDIES

Roentgenographic Studies. Anteroposterior and lateral soft tissue roentgenograms or fluoroscopy of the neck and chest may be helpful in patients with respiratory obstruction.

Foreign Bodies. Opaque foreign bodies may easily be visualized. Nonopaque objects may also be detected in left anterior oblique chest films if they create a defect in the column of radiolucent air or if obstructive atelectasis or emphysema is evident. Anteroposterior and lateral films in both full inspiration and expiration may be helpful. Fluoroscopy, lung scan, computed tomography and bronchoscopy may also be indicated if foreign body aspiration is possible or in the presence of persistent wheezing, stridor or cough.

Vascular Anomalies. Plain lateral films of the chest may demonstrate narrowing and forward displacement of the trachea. Fluoroscopy with barium swallow reveals posterior esophageal compression at the level of the third or fourth thoracic vertebra. Arteriography may be diagnostically helpful.

Laryngoscopy. Direct visualization of the larynx is indicated if respiratory obstruction cannot otherwise be explained.

NOISY BREATHING AND SNORING

Snoring or snorting noises occasionally arise from the nasopharynx in young infants, perhaps owing to imperfect functioning of the soft palate. Noisy breathing may also occur in infants with stenosis of the posterior choanae. Children with sleep apnea also snore loudly at night.

Guilleminault, C., Eldridge, F. L., Simmons, F. B., and Dement, W. C.: Sleep apnea in eight children. Pediatrics 58:23, 1976.

The stertorous breathing that occurs in some children with cerebral palsy is caused by narrowing of the airway secondary to tonic contractions of the muscles at the base of the tongue and in the posterior pharynx. Stertorous breathing while asleep may be associated with upper airway obstruction owing to enlarged tonsils and adenoids. In time, alveolar hypoventilation, pulmonary hypertension and congestive heart failure may develop secondary to the obstruction.

WHEEZING

Wheezing may occur in the following disease states:
1. Asthma; reactive airway disease. Wheezing and cough may be induced by exercise.

Bierman, C. W., Kawabori, I., and Pierson, W. E.: Incidence of exercise-induced asthma in children. Pediatrics 56:847, 1975.

2. Infants with viral pneumonia or acute bronchiolitis may demonstrate expiratory wheezing, respiratory distress and, perhaps, cyanosis. Infants who have recurrent episodes of wheezing usually have asthma.
3. Aspiration pneumonitis
4. Cystic fibrosis may present with a history of recurrent wheezing.
5. Lobar emphysema
6. Extrabronchial pressure owing to enlarged hilar and mediastinal nodes or tumor. Endobronchial tuberculosis or nontuberculous mycobacterial endobronchitis may be manifested clinically by persistent coughing or wheezing.

Powell, D. A., and Walker, D. H.: Nontuberculous mycobacterial endobronchitis in children. J. Pediatr. 96:268, 1980.

7. Aspiration of a foreign body, especially vegetal foreign bodies. An asymptomatic latent period may occur after aspiration of a foreign body.

8. Compression of the trachea by vascular anomalies. An anomalous course of the left pulmonary artery (pulmonary artery "sling") may cause compression of the right main stem bronchus, resulting in respiratory distress in newborn infants. Tracheomalacia may also be present. Symptoms include prolongation of expiration, wheezing and suprasternal and subcostal retractions. The right lung is emphysematous. Barium swallow reveals indentation or constriction of the anterior esophagus and right main stem bronchus.

9. An isolated tracheoesophageal fistula may cause wheezing.

10. Wheezing may occur secondary to pulmonary congestion in patients with large left-to-right shunts.

11. Audible wheezing may occur in patients with left heart failure owing to transudate in the bronchioles. The symptoms may simulate bronchiolitis with obstructive airway disease.

12. Visceral larva migrans may be characterized by recurrent wheezing, dyspnea, pulmonary infiltration, eosinophilia and hepatomegaly.

13. The middle lobe syndrome, characterized by wheezing, cough, and atelectasis of the right middle lobe, occurs most commonly in children with reactive airway disease. Atelectasis of the right middle lobe may also be associated with recurrent food aspiration, cystic fibrosis or IgA deficiency.

14. Conversion reaction

Christopher, K. L., Wood, R. P., II, Eckert, R. C., Blager, F. B., Raney, R. A., and Souhrada, J. F.: Vocal-cord dysfunction presenting as asthma. N. Engl. J. Med. 308:1566, 1983.

15. Wheezing, dyspnea on exertion, lower respiratory tract infections and chronic cough may occur in infants who have had bronchopulmonary dysplasia.

Smyth, J. A., Tabachnik, E., Duncan, W. J., Reilly, B. J., and Levison, H.: Pulmonary function and bronchial hyperreactivity in long-term survivors of bronchopulmonary dysplasia. Pediatrics 68:336, 1981.

16. Interstitial and hypersensitivity pneumonitis

17. Bronchial hyperreactivity may occur in infants after surgical correction of a tracheoesophageal fistula, bronchiolitis or hydrocarbon pneumonitis.

Kattan, M.: Long-term sequelae of respiratory illness in infancy and childhood. Pediatr. Clin. North Am. 26:525, 1979.

18. Wheezing may be associated with recurrent aspiration secondary to gastroesophageal reflux.

19. Esophageal achalasia may present with wheezing after exercise along with cough and sputum production owing to compression of the trachea and aspiration.

20. Pulmonary sarcoidosis

21. Wheezing may occur in children with chronic myelogenous leukemia owing to peribronchial cuffing with immature granulocytes.

GENERAL REFERENCES

Howard, W. A.: Differential diagnosis of wheezing in children. Pediatr. Rev. 1:239, 1980.

Levinson, H., Tabachnik, E., and Newth, C. J. L.: Wheezing in infancy, croup, and epiglottitis. Curr. Probl. Pediatr. 12:7, 1982.

ETIOLOGIC CLASSIFICATION OF STRIDOR

I. INTRINSIC OBSTRUCTION OF AIRWAYS, 366
  A. Congenital anomalies, 366
    1. Inspiratory laryngeal collapse
    2. Congenital laryngeal web
    3. Laryngeal cyst
    4. Subglottic stenosis
    5. Tracheal stenosis
    6. Absence of or defect in tracheal cartilaginous rings
    7. Calcification of laryngeal and tracheal cartilage
  B. Laryngeal paralysis, 367
    1. Bilateral laryngeal paralysis
    2. Cardiovascular anomalies
    3. Birth trauma
    4. Bilateral abductor vocal cord paralysis

  C. Tumors, 367
    1. Laryngeal papilloma
    2. Fibrolipoma
    3. Hemangioma
  D. Trauma, 367
    1. Repeated and inexpert tracheal aspiration
    2. Dislocation of the cricothyroid or cricoarytenoid articulations
    3. Subglottic stenosis secondary to intubation
  E. Croup syndrome, 367
    1. Acute viral laryngitis, laryngotracheobronchitis
    2. Acute bacterial croup
    3. Epiglottitis
    4. Acute spasmodic laryngitis
  F. Laryngeal edema, 368

Table continued on opposite page

ETIOLOGIC CLASSIFICATION OF STRIDOR *Continued*

1. Angioedema
2. Foreign body or laryngeal intubation
3. Corrosives
4. Nephrosis
5. Infectious mononucleosis
G. Laryngospasm, 368
   1. Tetany
   2. Acute infantile Gaucher's disease
H. Foreign bodies in the respiratory tract, 368
I. Esophageal foreign body, 368
J. Cri du chat syndrome, 368
K. Cricoarytenoid arthritis, 368
L. Laryngeal candidiasis, 368
II. EXTRINSIC AIRWAY OBSTRUCTION, 368
A. Congenital anomalies, 368
   1. Thyroglossal duct cyst
   2. Micrognathia with glossoptosis
   3. Macroglossia

4. Diaphragmatic hernia
5. Compression of trachea by vascular anomalies
B. Infections, 369
   1. Retropharyngeal abscess
   2. Infections of closed spaces of neck
C. Tumors, 369
   1. Thyroid tumor
   2. Cystic hygroma
   3. Mediastinal mass
   4. Lymphomas: lymphosarcoma, leukemia, Hodgkin's disease
D. Organ enlargement, 369
   1. Mediastinal lymphadenopathy
   2. Congenital goiter
III. PERIODS OF CRYING IN NORMAL BABIES, 369
IV. CONVERSION REACTION, 369

49 / RESPIRATORY INFECTIONS

CLINICAL CONSIDERATIONS

Respiratory infections are the most frequent childhood illnesses for which physicians are consulted, accounting for 50 per cent of sick child visits. Diseases of the respiratory tract produce a number of signs and symptoms, including fever, stridor, tachypnea, dyspnea, cough, failure to thrive and cyanosis.

ETIOLOGIC CLASSIFICATION OF UPPER RESPIRATORY TRACT INFECTIONS

I. ACUTE NASOPHARYNGITIS (THE COMMON COLD) causes well-known symptoms. In infants, the first evidence of a cold may be sudden anorexia; otherwise, clinical manifestations are usually mild but may persist somewhat longer than in older children and adults. Nasal obstruction owing to rhinitis may make it difficult for the infant to nurse.

Children experience, on the average, eight colds during the second year of life with the frequency decreasing to three or four a year by adolescence. Some children, however, appear to have a cold almost constantly during the winter. Children under two years of age who attend a day care center have more days with respiratory symptoms and more febrile illnesses than those who remain at home. Complications of the common cold, especially during infancy and early childhood, include otitis media, cervical adenitis, sinusitis, laryngitis, acute spasmodic laryngitis and pneumonia. Viral etiologic agents include rhinoviruses, respiratory syncytial virus, coronaviruses, influenza, parainfluenza and some adenoviruses and enteroviruses.

Carson, J. L., Collier, A. M., and Shih-Chin, S. H.: Acquired ciliary defects in nasal epithelium of children with acute viral upper respiratory infections. N. Engl. J. Med. 312:463, 1985.

Strangert, K.: Respiratory illness in preschool children with different forms of day care. Pediatrics 57:191, 1976.

Symptoms simulating those of the common cold may occur in the prodromal phases of measles and pertussis. Frequent or chronic colds may occur with seasonal or perennial allergic rhinitis, repeated exposure to infectious contacts, sinusitis and cystic fibrosis.

II. ACUTE SINUSITIS may be accompanied by high or spiking fever, periorbital edema, cellulitis, nasal discharge, obstruction, localized pain and tenderness, cough and headache. Chronic sinusitis may be characterized by "frequent colds," cough, nasal obstruction, fatigue and anorexia. In addition to bacterial pathogens (e.g., Group A beta-hemolytic *Streptococcus, Haemophilus influenzae, Staphylococcus* and pneumococcus), respiratory viral agents may be etiologic. Ethmoid sinusitis may occur during the newborn period or later. Maxillary sinusitis usually does not occur before 18 to 24 months of age. Sinusitis may occur in patients with Kartagener's syndrome, the immotile cilia syndrome (primary ciliary dyskinesia) and cystic fibrosis. In children with primary or acquired immunodeficiency disorders, sinusitis may be caused by mucormycosis, aspergillosis or candidiasis. See also the discussion of sinusitis on page 46.

Greenstone, M., and Cole, P. J.: Primary ciliary dyskinesia. Arch. Dis. Child. 59:704, 1984.
Rachelefsky, G. S., Katz, R. M., and Siegel, S. C.: Diseases of paranasal sinuses in children. Curr. Probl. Pediatr. 12:6, 1982.

III. ACUTE PHARYNGITIS AND TONSILLITIS are probably the most common causes of fever in children. Clinical differentiation between bacterial, mycoplasmal and viral pharyngitis cannot be made on physical examination alone. Tonsillar exudates, which occur in viral, bacterial and mycoplasmal pharyngitis, range from pinpoint to pinhead in size and from a thin, translucent membrane, easily missed on superficial examination, to thick, crumpled, opaque patches. The presence of a scarlatiniform rash or palatine petechiae are suggestive of Group A beta-hemolytic streptococcal infection. A specific diagnosis can be made only by throat culture. Only 5 to 15 per cent of instances of pharyngitis with fever are caused by the Group A beta-hemolytic *Streptococcus.* Streptococcal antibodies may not develop for 7 to 10 days. A streptococcal etiology can be proven by culture within 24 hours. About 50 per cent of patients with pharyngitis and a positive streptococcus culture without an antibody response are likely to be chronic carriers with the symptoms caused by a different etiologic agent. With streptococcal carriers, fewer streptococcal colonies grow out.

Kaplan, E. L.: The group A streptococcal upper respiratory tract carrier state: An enigma. J. Pediatr. 97:337, 1980.
Rapid office diagnostic tests for streptococcal pharyngitis. Med. Letter 27:49, 1985.

Pharyngitis is not always accompanied by the complaint of a sore throat, especially in preschool children. Instead, the child may simply refuse to eat. Complications of pharyngitis include otitis media, cervical adenitis, retropharyngeal abscess, peritonsillar abscess, acute glomerulonephritis and rheumatic fever. Accepted indications for tonsillectomy or adenoidectomy or both include cor pulmonale secondary to chronic, severe upper airway obstruction (tonsillectomy or adenoidectomy); enlargement of the tonsils sufficient to cause difficulty (tonsillectomy); nasal obstruction causing speech distortion and difficulty breathing (adenoidectomy); and chronic or recurrent otitis media. Nasopharyngeal obstruction and hypertrophy of adenoid tissue cause mouth breathing and may, over a period of time, produce bony distortion of the face, maxilla, palate and chest. The child often has a poor appetite and some feeding difficulty, sleeps poorly, and becomes easily fatigued and irritable.

Paradise, J. L., et al.: History of recurrent sore throat as an indication for tonsillectomy. N. Engl. J. Med. 298:409, 1978.
Paradise, J. L., and Bluestone, C. D.: Toward rational indications for tonsil and adenoid surgery. Hosp. Pract. 11:79, 1976.

A. Viral
1. Pharyngitis may be caused by the adenovirus, parainfluenza, influenza, coxsackieviruses A and B, ECHO, respiratory syncytial and Epstein-Barr viruses. The tonsillitis may be characterized, perhaps not until several hours after the onset of fever, by grayish or yellow-white, pinhead-sized or larger, discrete areas of exudate on the tonsils. Enlargement of the cervical lymph nodes may occur in some cases. Viral pharyngitis usually lasts three or four days.
2. Herpangina owing to Coxsackie and ECHO viruses is a disorder that occurs in the summertime and is characterized by papulovesicular pharyngeal lesions, dysphagia and a mildly sore throat. The lesions, few in number, appear chiefly on the anterior tonsillar pillars, occasionally on the

tonsils and the soft palate and more unusually on the tongue. They range in size from 1 to 4 mm, are surrounded by a zone of intense erythema and leave grayish-yellow ulcers on rupture. The pharynx may be diffusely injected, but the buccal mucosa and gingivae are not involved.

3. Infectious mononucleosis may be characterized by a diffusely red pharynx, follicular tonsillitis, a pharyngeal membrane or ulcerative pharyngitis. Streptococcal pharyngitis not uncommonly accompanies infectious mononucleosis.

Andiman, W. A.: The Epstein-Barr virus and EB virus infections in childhood. J. Pediatr. 95:171, 1979.

4. Pharyngoconjunctival fever, an epidemic disease caused by type 3 adenovirus, is characterized by low-grade fever, follicular conjunctivitis, sore throat and cervical lymphadenopathy.

B. Bacterial pharyngitis
1. Group A beta-hemolytic *Streptococcus* pharyngitis may be characterized by exudate on the tonsils and enlarged, tender cervical nodes.

Peter, G., and Smith, A. L.: Group A streptococcal infections of the skin and pharynx. N. Engl. J. Med. 297:311, 365, 1977.

2. Pneumococcus
3. *Staphylococcus* is not a primary etiologic agent in acute pharyngitis except in immunocompromised children.
4. *Haemophilus influenzae*
5. Pharyngeal diphtheria is characterized by one or more dirty gray or yellowish-white, moderately thick, adherent, membranous, tonsillar patches that may become confluent and spread to the contiguous soft palate and pharynx. Removal of the membrane causes oozing from the underlying mucous membrane.
6. Gonococci may cause acute pharyngitis.

C. *Mycoplasma pneumoniae* is an infrequent cause of pharyngitis in early adolescence.

IV. OTITIS MEDIA in infants and young children occurs frequently as a complication of the common cold. Bacterial otitis media is also a frequent finding in the newborn intensive care unit. Etiologic agents in the premature and term newborn infant include *Staphylococcus aureus, Escherichia coli,* group B *Streptococcus* and *Klebsiella pneumoniae.* In infants and young children, bacterial etiologic organisms include the Group A beta-hemolytic *Streptococcus*, pneumococcus, *Staphylococcus* and *Haemophilus influenzae.* Other etiologic agents include *Mycoplasma pneumoniae,* coxsackievirus B, and respiratory syncytial viruses, influenza, parainfluenza, enterovirus, adenovirus and rhinoviruses. The relatively high incidence of otitis media in infants may be explained, in part, by their short, almost horizontal, relatively wide eustachian tubes. This anatomic feature may facilitate progression of infection from the nasopharynx to the middle ear, a process augmented by the proximity of abundant lymphoid tissue to the eustachian orifices in the nasopharynx. Complications of otitis media may include mastoiditis, petrositis, meningitis, arachnoiditis, lateral sinus thrombosis, brain abscess, facial nerve paralysis and hearing impairment. See also page 42.

Berman, S. A., Balkany, T. J., and Simmons, M. A.: Otitis media in the neonatal intensive care unit. Pediatrics 62:198, 1978.

ETIOLOGIC CLASSIFICATION OF UPPER RESPIRATORY DISEASE

ETIOLOGIC CLASSIFICATION OF LOWER RESPIRATORY DISEASE

I. Croup Syndromes (see page 367)

A. Acute laryngotracheitis (infectious croup), which occurs chiefly in infants and young children, usually has a viral etiology, especially parainfluenza type 1. Other viral agents include parainfluenza types 2 and 3, influenza A and B, respiratory syncytial virus, adenovirus and the same agents that cause nasopharyngitis.
B. Acute bacterial croup
C. Acute epiglottitis
D. Acute spasmodic croup

II. Acute Tracheobronchitis may occur in patients with measles or pertussis and as an extension of upper respiratory tract infections, especially during the first years of life. Rhinoviruses, influenza, parainfluenza virus type 3, coxsackieviruses, respiratory syncytial virus and adenovirus may be etiologic agents. Persistent bronchitis may be present with chronic sinusitis, respiratory allergy, bronchiectasis, cystic fibrosis and typhoid fever. The incidence of pneumonia and bronchitis in the first year of life is increased by passive exposure to parental smoking.

Colley, J. R. T., Holland, W. W., and Corkhill, R. T.: Influence of passive smoking and parental phlegm on pneumonia and bronchitis in early childhood. Lancet 2:1031, 1974.

III. Acute Bronchiolitis, Wheezing-Associated Respiratory Infections (WARI) and Asthmatoid Bronchitis, disorders that occur most frequently in the first two years of life, are characterized by cough, wheezing and severe expiratory dyspnea owing to the bronchiolar obstruction caused by mucosal edema and mucus. The respiratory syncytial virus is the most common cause. Other agents include parainfluenza virus types 1 and 3, influenza A, adenovirus, rhinoviruses and, in school age children, *Mycoplasma pneumoniae*.

Henderson, F. W., Clyde, W. A., Jr., Collier, A. M., Denny, F. W., Senior, R. J., Sheaffer, C. I., Conley, W. G., III, and Christian, R. M.: The etiologic and epidemiologic spectrum of bronchiolitis in pediatric practice. J. Pediatr. 95:183, 1979.
Wohl, M. E. B., and Chernick, V.: Bronchiolitis. Am. Rev. Respir. Dis. 118:759, 1978.

IV. Pneumonia. Clinical differentiation between viral and bacterial pneumonia is difficult or impossible. In the newborn infant, pneumonia may be part of a transplacental infection caused by rubella, cytomegalovirus, type II *Herpesvirus, Treponema pallidum*, toxoplasmosis, influenza virus or listerosis. Group B beta-hemolytic *Streptococcus* is a major cause of pneumonia in newborn infants. A little later, *Staphylococcus aureus, Chlamydia trachomatis* and *Klebsiella pneumoniae* are etiologic agents. In older children, about 95 per cent of pneumonias have a viral etiology.

The alveolar spaces may be principally involved, as in bacterial or viral pneumonia, or the interstitial tissues, as in pneumonia caused by viral agents, *Mycoplasma, Chlamydia,* pneumocystis, Q fever and legionellosis. Pneumonia occurs frequently in the course of treatment of acute lymphoblastic leukemia, especially during the initial four months. Opportunistic pulmonary infections may be associated with the acquired immune deficiency syndrome.

Siegel, S. E., Nesbit, M. E., Baehner, R., Sather, H., and Hammond, G. D.: Pneumonia during therapy for childhood acute lymphoblastic leukemia. Am. J. Dis. Child. 134:28, 1980.

The onset is usually more sudden and the child likely to be more toxic and in greater respiratory distress with bacterial than with viral infections. Bacterial pneumonia may also be accompanied by pleural effusion or empyema. Slight pleural effusion may occur with mycoplasma pneumonia but not with viral pneumonia. Lobar or segmental consolidations are predominantly caused by the pneumococcus and less likely by *Klebsiella* or group A streptococci. Blood cultures may permit identification of the etiologic bacterial agent. Bone marrow cultures may be useful in patients thought to have histoplasmosis.

Bronchoscopy and culture of aspirated secretions for bacteria and fungi are usually reserved for patients who have chronic pneumonitis or who are not responding to therapy. Bronchial secretions may also be inoculated into guinea pigs if tuberculosis is suspected. Tuberculin, blastomycin or coccidioidin skin tests may be indicated.

The physical findings on percussion and auscultation may be normal in some infants with pneumonia. Pneumonia is a likely diagnosis in the presence of rapid, shallow breathing, flaring of the alae nasi, decreased pulmonary excursions, a short inspiratory phase and expiratory grunting. The child may attempt to splint his chest, perhaps by lying on the involved side, is disinclined to talk and may use monosyllabic speech.

Eichenwald, H. F.: Pneumonia syndromes in children. Hosp. Pract. 11:89, April 1976.

A. Bacterial pneumonia
1. Pneumococcal is the most frequent type of bacterial pneumonia in infants and children. Children with sickle cell anemia have an increased risk of pneumococcal pneumonia.
2. Staphylococcal pneumonia, which has its greatest incidence in early infancy, may be characterized by a paroxysmal, pertussiform cough and severe dyspnea. Pyopneumothorax may develop suddenly. Multiple pulmonary abscesses and bacteremia may also occur.
3. Tuberculosis is always a diagnostic consideration in infants and children with pulmonary disease.
4. Group A beta-hemolytic streptococcal pneumonia occurs in children above the age of five or six. The onset is abrupt and the symptoms severe. In addition to fever, chills, lethargy, myalgia, dyspnea, cough, chest pain and hemoptysis, cyanosis occurs in more than 50 per cent and empyema in 100 per cent of patients. Streptococcal pharyngitis may occur concomitantly. Fever and chest pain persist for 8 to 10 days.

Molten, R. A.: Group A beta-hemolytic streptococcal pneumonia. Am. J. Dis. Child. 131:1366, 1977.

5. *Haemophilus influenzae* type B pneumonia in infants may be complicated by pleural effusion and meningitis. A lumbar puncture may be indicated in infants when a diagnosis of *Haemophilus influenzae* type B pneumonia is established.

Ginsburg, C. M., Howard, J. B., and Nelson, J. D.: Report of 65 cases of *Haemophilus influenzae* b pneumonia. Pediatrics 64:283, 1979.

6. Pseudomonas
7. Friedlander's bacillus
8. *Klebsiella* pneumonia usually occurs in infants, but it may also develop in an older immunodeficient child. Characteristic radiologic findings include bulging of the lung fissures, absence of pleural effusion and presence of lung abscesses or pneumatoceles.
9. Children with cystic fibrosis have frequent episodes of pneumonia. In the early episodes, the hemolytic *Staphylococcus aureus* is usually the etiologic agent.
10. Tularemia
11. Pneumonia caused by nocardiosis may occur in immunocompromised children.
12. Legionnaires' disease may cause pneumonia, especially in immunocompromised children.
13. *Proteus*
14. *Escherichia coli*
B. Viral pneumonia has a varied symptomatology. Cough may be a prominent feature. Dyspnea, cyanosis, inspiratory retractions and expiratory wheezing may be present in infants. The chest x-ray often demonstrates more extensive involvement than that suspected on physical examination, and the involvement tends to be more interstitial than alveolar. Hyperinflation, not seen with bacterial pneumonias, may be present. Clinical differentiation of viral and mycoplasmal pneumonia may not be possible.
1. Adenovirus, especially types 3, 7 and 21, may cause a severe necrotizing bronchopneumonia with chronic sequelae such as bronchiectasis, bronchiolitis obliterans and lobar emphysema.

James, A. G., Lang, W. R., Liang, A. Y., Mackay, R. J., Morris, M. C., Newman, J. N., Osborne, D. R., and White, P. R.: Adenovirus type 21 bronchopneumonia in infants and young children. J. Pediatr. 95:530, 1979.

2. Parainfluenza virus, types 1, 2 and 3. Type 3 causes viral pneumonia in infants.
3. Respiratory syncytial virus is an etiologic agent in infants under one year of age.
4. Rhinoviruses
5. Influenza A and B usually occurs with epidemic incidence.
6. Infectious mononucleosis
7. Measles, chickenpox

Siegel, M. M., Walter, T. K., and Ablin, A. R.: Measles pneumonia in childhood leukemia. Pediatrics 60:38, 1977.

8. Psittacosis, ornithosis
9. Lymphocytic choriomeningitis
10. Giant cell pneumonia (Hecht's disease), a chronic, interstitial pneumonia, may develop in patients with measles or as an isolated disease.
11. Cytomegalovirus infection may be characterized by a chronic interstitial pneumonia. Gastrointestinal symptoms or hepatosplenomegaly may also be present. In infants, the clinical, radiologic and laboratory findings may be indistinguishable

from a *Chlamydia* or *Pneumocystis* infection.

Stagno, S., Brasfield, D. M., Brown, M. B., Cassell, G. H., Pifer, L. L., Whitley, R. J., and Tiller, R. E.: Infant pneumonitis associated with cytomegalovirus, *Chlamydia, Pneumocystis, and Ureaplasma:* A prospective study. Pediatrics 68:322, 1981.

12. *Ureaplasma urealyticum*

C. *Mycoplasma pneumoniae* is the chief cause of pneumonia in school age children. Headache is usually severe. Other symptoms include sore throat, anorexia, malaise, fever, chills and a paroxysmal, dry cough. Physical findings are generally minimal. The chest roentgenogram reveals interstitial pneumonitis.

Denny, F. W., Clyde, W. A., Jr., and Glezen, W. P.: *Mycoplasma pneumoniae* disease: Clinical spectrum, pathophysiology, epidemiology and control. J. Infect. Dis. 123:74, 1971.

D. *Chlamydia trachomatis* is a frequent etiologic agent in young infants with pneumonia. Symptoms generally begin in the fourth to twelfth week with tachypnea and a pertussis-like staccato cough as the principal manifestations. Nasal congestion and discharge may also be present. Coughing paroxysms may be followed by cyanosis and vomiting. Inspiratory crepitant rales are usually present. The patient is afebrile. Hyperexpansion with diffuse interstitial and patchy alveolar infiltrates is noted on the chest x-ray. Serum immunoglobulins G and M are elevated, and peripheral eosinophilia may be present.

Tipple, M. A., Beem, M. O., and Saxon, E. M.: Clinical characteristics of the afebrile pneumonia associated with *Chlamydia trachomatis* infection in infants less than 6 months of age. Pediatrics 63:192, 1979.

E. Congenital syphilis may be accompanied by pneumonitis.
F. Rickettsial
   1. Q fever
   2. Rocky Mountain spotted fever
   3. Typhus
G. Fungal infections are a diagnostic consideration with persistent pneumonia.
   1. Histoplasmosis
   2. Moniliasis
   ·3. Blastomycosis

Laskey, W. K., and Sarosi, G. A.: Blastomycosis in children. Pediatrics 65:111, 1980.

   4. Coccidioidomycosis
   5. Aspergillosis
   6. Sporotrichosis
   7. Actinomycosis
H. Protozoan
   1. Toxoplasmosis
   2. *Pneumocystis carinii* pneumonia occurs in immunosuppressed or immunodeficient patients. Dyspnea is the most common presenting symptom, followed by fever, cough, tachycardia, cyanosis and chest pain. Except, perhaps, for intercostal retractions, physical findings are minimal or absent. Rales are absent. The chest x-ray shows bilateral, diffuse haziness or patchy interstitial infiltrates. The disease may be fulminant. Diagnosis is best made by open-lung biopsy.

Hughes, W. T.: *Pneumocystis carinii* pneumonia. N. Engl. J. Med. 297:1381, 1977.
Walzer, P. D., et al.: *Pneumocystis carinii* pneumonia in the United States. Epidemiologic, diagnostic, and clinical features. Ann. Intern. Med. 80:83, 1974.

I. Aspiration
   1. Lipoid
   2. Kerosene or hydrocarbon poisoning. Respiratory distress following the ingestion of furniture polish containing mineral seal oil is usually more severe than that caused by other hydrocarbon products.
   3. Recurrent pneumonia may be caused by a foreign body.
   4. Aspiration pneumonia may occur after repair of an esophageal atresia or be a complication of gastroesophageal reflux.

Berquist, W. L.: Gastroesophageal reflux—associated recurrent pneumonia and chronic asthma in children. Pediatrics 68:29, 1981.
Whitington, P. F., Shermeta, D. W., Seto, D. S. Y., Jones, L., and Hendrix, T. R.: Role of lower esophageal sphincter incompetence in recurrent pneumonia after repair of esophageal atresia. J. Pediatr. 91:550, 1977.

   5. Milk and other food substances. Persistent pneumonia may occur in infants with a tracheoesophageal fistula, in infants who are severely retarded and in children with cerebral palsy who aspirate because of their inability to swallow normally.
J. Eosinophilic infiltration
   1. Löffler's syndrome or eosinophilic pneumonia may be asymptomatic or cause severe cough and respiratory distress.

2. Visceral larva migrans in infants and young children is characterized by eosinophilia, leukocytosis, elevation of serum globulins, pulmonary infiltration and hepatomegaly.
K. Familial dysautonomia is characterized by frequent episodes of pulmonary disease. Chest roentgenograms show widespread changes that simulate those of cystic fibrosis.
L. Lupus erythematosus may cause an interstitial pneumonitis.
M. Asthma is a frequent cause of persistent or recurrent pneumonia.

Eigen, H., Laughlin, J. J., and Homrighausen, J.: Recurrent pneumonia in children and its relationship to bronchial hyperreactivity. Pediatrics 70:698, 1982.

V. PLEURISY

A. Acute or fibrinous pleurisy
1. Pleurisy may accompany upper respiratory tract infections.
2. The pneumococcus may cause fibrinous pleurisy.
3. Rheumatic fever
4. Rheumatoid arthritis
5. Tuberculosis
B. Pleurisy with effusion
1. Serofibrinous
a. Tuberculosis is the most common cause of serofibrinous pleurisy.

b. Rheumatic fever
c. Lupus erythematosus also may be accompanied by a dry pleurisy.
2. Purulent empyema
a. Pneumococcus
b. *Staphylococcus*
c. Group A beta-hemolytic *Streptococcus.* The effusion is initially serous, then serosanguineous and finally fibrinopurulent.
d. *Haemophilus influenzae* type B
e. *Escherichia coli*
3. *Mycoplasma pneumoniae*
4. Adenovirus

Freis, B. J., Kusmiesz, H., Nelson, J. D., and McCracken, G. H., Jr.: Parapneumonic effusions and empyema in hospitalized children: A retrospective review of 227 cases. Pediatr. Infect. Dis. 3:578, 1984.

C. Pleural effusions caused by malignancies
   Diagnostic measures include a pleural tap with culture, smear (gram and methylene blue), cell count, protein determinations and cell block.

GENERAL REFERENCES

Lipow, H. W.: Respiratory tract infections. In Green, M., and Haggerty, R. J. (eds.): Ambulatory Pediatrics III. Philadelphia, W. B. Saunders Co., 1984, p. 111.
Rubin, B. K.: The evaluation of the child with recurrent chest infections. Pediatr. Infect. Dis. 4:88, 1985.

ETIOLOGIC CLASSIFICATION OF LOWER RESPIRATORY DISEASE

I. CROUP SYNDROME, 374
   A. Acute viral laryngitis, laryngotracheobronchitis, 374
   B. Acute bacterial croup, 374
   C. Acute epiglottitis, 374
   D. Acute spasmodic croup, 374
II. TRACHEOBRONCHITIS, 374
III. BRONCHIOLITIS OR WHEEZING-ASSOCIATED RESPIRATORY INFECTIONS, 374
IV. PNEUMONIA, 374
   A. Bacterial pneumonia, 375
      1. Pneumococcal
      2. Staphylococcal
      3. Tuberculosis
      4. Group A beta-hemolytic *Streptococcus;* group B beta-hemolytic *Streptococcus*
      5. *Haemophilus influenzae*
      6. *Pseudomonas*
      7. Friedlander's bacillus
      8. *Klebsiella*
      9. Cystic fibrosis
      10. Tularemia
      11. Nocardiosis
      12. Legionnaires' disease

      13. *Proteus*
      14. *Escherichia coli*
   B. Viral pneumonia, 375
   C. *Mycoplasma pneumoniae*, 376
   D. *Chlamydia trachomatis*, 376
   E. Spirochetal, 376
   F. Rickettsial, 376
      1. Q fever
      2. Rocky Mountain spotted fever
      3. Typhus
   G. Fungal infection, 376
      1. Histoplasmosis
      2. Moniliasis
      3. Blastomycosis
      4. Coccidioidomycosis
      5. Aspergillosis
      6. Sporotrichosis
      7. Actinomycosis
   H. Protozoan, 376
      1. Toxoplasmosis
      2. *Pneumocystis carinii*
   I. Aspiration, 376
      1. Lipoid
      2. Kerosene or hydrocarbon poisoning

Table continued on following page

ETIOLOGIC CLASSIFICATION OF LOWER RESPIRATORY DISEASE *Continued*

3. Foreign bodies
4. Recurrent aspiration pneumonia
5. Milk and other foods
J. Eosinophilic infiltration, 376
   1. Löffler's syndrome
   2. Visceral larva migrans
K. Familial dysautonomia, 377
L. Lupus erythematosus, 377
M. Asthma, 377
V. PLEURISY, 377
A. Acute or fibrinous, 377

1. Upper respiratory tract infections
2. Pneumococcus
3. Rheumatic fever
4. Rheumatoid arthritis
5. Tuberculosis
B. Pleurisy with effusion, 377
   1. Serofibrinous
   2. Purulent empyema
   3. *Mycoplasma pneumoniae*
   4. Adenovirus
C. Pleural effusions caused by malignancies, 377

50 / COUGH AND HEMOPTYSIS

CLINICAL CONSIDERATIONS

Coughing begins with a short inspiratory phase followed by closure of the glottis and a forceful expiration. With opening of the glottis, air is suddenly released under pressure, and the child coughs. This process is controlled by a medullary cough center. Excitatory stimuli arise from respiratory, central or other extrapulmonary sources. Afferent impulses from the pharynx, larynx, trachea (especially at the bifurcation), bronchi of the first and second order, and from the pleura are transmitted through the vagi. Stimuli from the ear traverse the same pathway (auricular branch of the vagus, Arnold's nerve). The glossopharyngeal nerve may transmit some of the impulses that arise in the pharynx. The efferent arc of the cough reflex is through the motor innervation of the respiratory and laryngeal musculature.

Afferent stimuli occur secondary to an alteration in the respiratory secretions or mucosal changes. Not all portions of the respiratory tree have a uniform stimulus threshold. Cough may be absent, at times, even with a foreign body in the tracheobronchial tree. Tolerance or decreased reflex excitability may also develop.

In general, cough is an important defense mechanism that excludes infected secretions from the tracheobronchial tree and dislodges and removes secretions, exudates and foreign bodies. The elongation and widening of the tracheobronchial tree during inspiration alternates with shortening and narrowing during expiration to propel secretions from the periphery to the larger bronchi. This expiratory compression is even more forceful during cough.

Although cough is usually an important physiologic mechanism, and therapy is best designed to enhance its effectiveness, persistent coughing causes fatigue, interrupts sleep, interferes with feeding and may precipitate vomiting.

The cough reflex is absent in very young infants. Effective coughing may also be impossible in emaciated children, in those whose respiratory musculature is weak or paralyzed and in those with massive ascites.

ETIOLOGIC CLASSIFICATION OF COUGH

I. RESPIRATORY

A. Infections
   1. The profuse nasal discharge of the common cold may cause pharyngeal irritation and a cough that is worse at night.

2. Chronic sinusitis with a postnasal mucous drip is a common cause for nasal discharge and a persistent cough, especially on arising and after going to bed. The cough may be caused more by the drying and inflammation of the pharynx and larynx associated with mouth breathing than by the postnasal drip.

Rachelefsky, G. S., Katz, R. M., and Siegel, S. C.: Diseases of paranasal sinuses in children. Curr. Probl. Pediatr. 12:5, 1982.

3. Hypertrophy of adenoid tissue and nasopharyngeal obstruction may prevent normal warming and moistening of inspired air so that laryngeal irritation and cough may occur.
4. Pharyngitis may cause an irritative cough.
5. Croup is characterized by a tight, hoarse, barking and brassy cough.
6. Tracheobronchitis, bronchitis. The cough in these patients is deep and often paroxysmal.
   a. Bronchitis may accompany upper respiratory tract infections, especially sinusitis.
   b. Measles. A hoarse, barking or hacking, non-productive cough may be present in patients with measles.
   c. Pertussis is classically characterized by paroxysms of hacking, expiratory cough followed by a sudden, deep, tight, crowing inspiration or whoop. The child's face may become suffused or cyanotic during these episodes, especially in young infants. Vomiting of stringy mucoid material may occur after the paroxysms of coughing. In young infants the episodes may consist more in choking than in coughing. The severity and frequency of cough vary widely in individual patients. Some older infants and children do not vomit or whoop, and the atypical symptomatology may be misdiagnosed as persistent bronchitis. Since atypical forms of the disease are difficult to diagnose clinically, the physician has to rely on a history of exposure, the white blood cell count (lymphocytosis) and fluorescent antibody staining of nasopharyngeal smears. False-positive smears may occur if the technician is not experienced.

The cough usually begins to diminish after three or four weeks, but paroxysmal episodes may continue for weeks or months.
   d. Parapertussis
   e. Adenoviruses may be associated with a pertussis-like syndrome, perhaps reflecting concurrent infections or reactivation of a latent adenoviral infection by *Bordetella pertussis.*

Keller, M.A., Aftandelians, R., and Connor, J.D.: Etiology of pertussis syndrome. Pediatrics 66:50, 1980.

   f. Typhoid fever
   g. Scarlet fever
   h. Reactive airway disease accompanying respiratory infections
7. Cystic fibrosis is a diagnostic consideration in infants with a persistent cough or frequent respiratory infections. The cough may be paroxysmal and resemble that of pertussis.

Shwachman, H.: Cystic fibrosis. Curr. Probl. Pediatr. 8:5, 1978.
Waring, W.W.: Current management of cystic fibrosis. Adv. Pediatr. 23:401, 1976.

8. Pneumonia. Because of the accompanying chest pain, cough may be a distressing symptom in older children with pneumonia. Cough may be absent, especially in young infants; however, with staphylococcal, *Ureaplasma urealyticum,* cytomegalovirus and *Pneumocystis carinii* pneumonia, coughing may be paroxysmal and resemble that of pertussis. Chlamydia pneumonia in young infants is characterized by tachypnea and a pertussis-like staccato cough. In the school and adolescent age group, *Mycoplasma pneumoniae* may be the most common infectious cause of cough with paroxysms occurring over a period of weeks or months. Interstitial pneumonitis is another important cause of a persistent cough.
9. Tuberculosis
10. Fungus infections
    a. Histoplasmosis
    b. Candidiasis
    c. Coccidioidomycosis
11. Lung abscess
12. Because of pain, the child with pleurisy may attempt to suppress coughing.
13. The hyperimmunoglobulin E recurrent infection (Job's) syndrome

causes recurrent bronchitis with productive cough.

B. Parasitic infections
1. Ascariasis
2. Strongyloidiasis
3. Hookworm infection
4. In young children with a history of pica, visceral larva migrans may present with a chronic cough, often paroxysmal and worse at night; wheezing; and irritability. Fever, leukocytosis, eosinophilia and hepatomegaly may also occur.

Schantz, P. M., and Glickman, L. T.: Toxocaral visceral larva migrans. N. Engl. J. Med. 298:436, 1978.

C. Congenital or acquired disorders
1. Bronchiectasis secondary to cystic fibrosis, agammaglobulinemia or endobronchial tuberculosis may cause a paroxysmal cough that may be initiated or accentuated by postural changes.

Davis, P. B., Hubbard, V. S., McCoy, K., and Taussig, L. M.: Familial bronchiectasis. J. Pediatr. 102:177, 1983.
Lewiston, N. J.: Bronchiectasis in childhood. Pediatr. Clin. North Am. 31:865, 1984.

2. Immotile cilia syndrome (ciliary dyskinesia; Kartagener's syndrome), which consists of bronchiectasis, otitis media, chronic sinusitis, situs inversus and sperm immotility, is frequently accompanied by productive cough.

Turner, J. A. P., Corkey, C. W. B., Lee, J. Y. C., Levison, H., and Sturgess, J.: Clinical expressions of immotile cilia syndrome. Pediatrics 67:805, 1981.

3. Middle lobe syndrome
4. Intralobar bronchopulmonary sequestration is associated with chronic cough, recurrent pneumonia, hemoptysis and roentgenographic evidence of a mass in the basilar segments of the lower lobe.

Durnin, R. E., Lababidi, Z., Butler, C., Selke, A., and Flege, J. B.: Bronchopulmonary sequestration. Chest 57:454, 1970.

5. Diaphragmatic hernia
6. A brassy cough may be present for several months after surgical correction of esophageal atresia with tracheoesophageal fistula.

D. Allergy; bronchial hyperreactivity
1. Allergic rhinitis with a postnasal drip
2. A deep, annoying cough may occur during asthmatic episodes. When a chronic nonproductive cough is nocturnal, exercise-induced or precipitated by exposure to cold, a metacholine or treadmill running challenge test for bronchial hyperreactivity may be indicated. Wheezing may not have been reported or noted on auscultation in these instances.
3. Bronchial hyperreactivity, manifest in infants by cough or wheezing, may persist after bronchial mucosal injury caused by croup, viral respiratory infections or bronchopulmonary dysplasia. Later, viral infections may cause wheezing and cough owing to an acquired airway hyperreactivity. In the school age child and adolescent, cough may persist for weeks after a viral upper respiratory tract infection because of increased bronchial reactivity.

Cloutier, M. M., and Loughlin, G. M.: Chronic cough in children: A manifestation of airway hyperreactivity. Pediatrics 67:6, 1981.
Morgan, W. J., and Taussig, L. M.: The chronic bronchitis syndrome in children. Pediatr. Clin. North Am. 31:851, 1984.
Taussig, L. M., Smith, S. M., and Blumenfeld, R.: Chronic bronchitis in childhood: What is it? Pediatrics 67:1, 1981.

4. Persistent coughing during the winter months may be caused by irritation from dry heated air.

E. Pulmonary edema; congestive cardiac failure
F. Idiopathic pulmonary hemosiderosis is characterized by iron deficiency anemia and recurrent mild hemoptysis. A chest film may suggest the diagnosis.
G. Pulmonary alveolar proteinosis may be suspected in infants with failure to thrive, cough and increasing dyspnea. A fine perihilar increase in pulmonary density is noted on the chest roentgenogram. The diagnosis is established by cytologic examination of the sputum.
H. Interstitial and hypersensitivity pneumonitis. See page 358.
I. Pulmonary sarcoidosis
J. Mechanical obstruction
1. Intrinsic
a. Foreign body. The initial symptoms produced by foreign bodies in the air and food passages, which include paroxysms of coughing, choking and gagging, may be followed by a symptomfree period lasting from hours to years. A laryngeal foreign body may cause cough and wheezing with aphonia. Anteroposterior and lateral chest roentgenograms in

both phases of respiration are indicated if a foreign body is suspected. Fluoroscopy represents another helpful diagnostic procedure.

Blazer, S., Navey, Y., and Friedman, A.: Foreign body in the airway. Am. J. Dis. Child. 134:68, 1980.

  b. Copious secretions associated with bronchiectasis and cystic fibrosis
  c. Atelectasis
  d. Children with an isolated tracheo-esophageal fistula may cough, choke and, perhaps, become cyanotic during feedings, especially liquid feedings.
  e. Middle lobe syndrome, which occurs most commonly in young children with allergic airway disease, is characterized by recurrent or persistent coughing and wheezing.
  f. Congenital bronchopulmonary-foregut malformation, in which accessory lung tissue communicates with the gastrointestinal tract, can cause cough during feedings.
  g. Recurrent bronchitis with cough, especially on lying down at night or after eating, wheezing, choking, apnea and laryngospasm, may be caused by recurrent bronchitis and aspiration pneumonitis secondary to gastroesophageal reflux.

Danus, O., Casar, C., Larrain, A., and Pope, C. E., II: Esophageal reflux—an unrecognized cause of recurrent obstructive bronchitis in children. J. Pediatr. 89:220, 1976.

  h. Tuberculous or nontuberculous mycobacterial endobronchitis

Powell, D. A., and Walker, D. H.: Nontuberculous mycobacterial endobronchitis in children. J. Pediatr. 96:268, 1980.

  i. Cigarette smoking
    1. Smoking is an important cause of chronic, productive cough in adolescents.
    2. Increased bronchial reactivity occurs in infants subjected to passive cigarette smoke inhalation.
  2. Extrinsic
  a. Retropharyngeal abscess
  b. Mediastinal tumor
  c. Enlargement of mediastinal lymph nodes owing to infection

or lymphoma may cause a persistent, nonproductive, brassy cough.
  d. Pleurisy with effusion; empyema
  e. A vascular ring may cause a brassy cough.

II. EXTRARESPIRATORY

A. Ear. The auricular branch of the vagus nerve (Arnold's nerve) may be stimulated by impacted cerumen, foreign body or external otitis.
B. Esophageal duplication
C. Esophageal achalasia owing to compression of the trachea and aspiration of secretions
D. Psychogenic
  1. Psychogenic cough tic accounts for recurrent, severe paroxysms of coughing occurring every few seconds or minutes in older children and adolescents. Paroxysms do not occur during sleep. The nonproductive cough is explosive, loud, deep, barking, brassy, honking or seal-like.

Cohlan, S. Q., and Stone, S. M.: The cough and the bedsheet. Pediatrics 74:11, 1984.

  2. Cough tics also occur in the Gilles de la Tourette's syndrome.

GENERAL REFERENCES

Eigen, H.: The clinical evaluation of chronic cough. Pediatr. Clin. North Am. 29:67, 1982.
Irwin, R. S., Rosen, M. J., and Braman, S. S.: Cough. A comprehensive review. Arch. Intern. Med. 137:1186, 1977.

HEMOPTYSIS

Massive pulmonary hemorrhage may occur in hypoxemic low birth weight infants and in infants with neonatal hyperammonemia.

Sheffield, L. J., Danks, D. M., Hammond, J. W., and Hoogenraad, N. J.: Massive pulmonary hemorrhage as a presenting feature in congenital hyperammonemia. J. Pediatr. 88:450, 1976.

Bloody sputum or hemoptysis always raises the possiblity of a foreign body in the airway (e.g., Timothy grass or pine needles).
Group A beta-hemolytic Streptococcus pneumonia
Pertussis, after severe paroxysms of coughing
Bronchiectasis
Cystic fibrosis in adolescents and young

adults may be a cause of massive hemoptysis. Bronchial arteriography may be helpful in localizing the bleeding site.

Stern, R. C.: Treatment and prognosis of massive hemoptysis in cystic fibrosis. Am. Rev. Respir. Dis. 117:825, 1978.

Although rare in children, the possibility of a bronchogenic tumor such as bronchial adenoma, papilloma or hemangioma enters the differential diagnosis of cough and hemoptysis. Chest x-rays and bronchoscopy are diagnostically helpful.

De Paredes, C. G., Pierce, W. S., Gruff, D. B., and Waldhausen, J. A.: Bronchogenic tumors in children. Arch. Surg. 10:574, 1970.

Plasma cell granuloma, a postinflammatory pseudotumor, may cause cough or hemoptysis in infants and children.

Pearl, M., and Wooley, M. M.: Pulmonary xanthomatous post inflammatory pseudotumors in children. J. Pediatr. Surg. 8:255, 1973.

Lung abscess
Tuberculosis
Foreign body in the laryngotracheobronchial tree
Esophageal duplication
Idiopathic pulmonary hemosiderosis is characterized by the production of blood-stained sputum.

Hemorrhagic disorders
Extreme pulmonic stenosis (chiefly tetralogy with outflow atresia); enlarged bronchial arteries
Pulmonary vascular obstructive disease: primary pulmonary hypertension; Eisenmenger reaction in right-to-left shunt or single ventricle; following systemic-pulmonary anastomosis.

Haroutunian, L. M., and Neill, C. A.: Pulmonary complications of congenital heart disease: Hemoptysis. Am. Heart J. 84:540, 1972.

Mitral stenosis
Fungus infection involving bronchus
Wegener's granulomatosis
Goodpasture's syndrome, rare in children, is characterized by hemoptysis, pulmonary infiltration, anemia and renal failure.
Lupus erythematosus may be characterized, in part, by pulmonary hemorrhage.
Pulmonary artery hypoplasia, a cause of the hyperlucent lung syndrome, may be accompanied by cough, hemoptysis and wheezing.
Hemoptysis is a common complaint in the Munchausen's syndrome.

PERSISTENT HICCOUGHS

Acute renal failure

ETIOLOGIC CLASSIFICATION OF COUGH

I. Respiratory, 378
  A. Infections, 378
    1. Common cold
    2. Chronic sinusitis
    3. Hypertrophy of adenoid tissue and nasopharyngeal obstruction
    4. Pharyngitis
    5. Croup
    6. Tracheobronchitis, bronchitis
    7. Cystic fibrosis
    8. Pneumonia
    9. Tuberculosis
    10. Fungal infections
    11. Lung abscess
    12. Pleurisy
    13. Hyperimmunoglobulin E recurrent infection (Job's) syndrome
  B. Parasitic infections, 380
    1. Ascariasis
    2. Strongyloidiasis
    3. Hookworm infection
    4. Visceral larva migrans
  C. Congenital or acquired disorders, 380
    1. Bronchiectasis
    2. Immotile cilia syndrome
    3. Middle lobe syndrome
    4. Intralobar bronchopulmonary sequestration

    5. Diaphragmatic hernia
    6. Esophageal atresia with tracheoesophageal fistula
  D. Allergy; bronchial hyperreactivity, 380
    1. Allergic rhinitis with postnasal drip
    2. Asthma
    3. Airway reactivity
    4. Drying effects of hot air
  E. Pulmonary edema; congestive heart failure, 380
  F. Idiopathic pulmonary hemosiderosis, 380
  G. Pulmonary alveolar proteinosis, 380
  H. Interstitial and hypersensitivity pneumonitis, 380
  I. Pulmonary sarcoidosis, 380
  J. Mechanical obstruction, 380
    1. Intrinsic
    2. Extrinsic
II. Extrarespiratory, 381
  A. Ear, 381
  B. Esophageal duplication, 381
  C. Esophageal achalasia, 381
  D. Psychogenic, 381
    1. Psychogenic cough tic
    2. Gilles de la Tourette's syndrome

51 / CYANOSIS

CLINICAL CONSIDERATIONS

Cyanosis refers to a bluish skin color, attributable, in most cases, to an abnormally large amount of reduced hemoglobin (5 gm/dl) in the capillaries. Methemoglobin acts similarly when its concentration exceeds 15 per cent of the total hemoglobin. Carboxyhemoglobin, formed as a result of carbon monoxide intoxication, produces a reddish, rather than a bluish, skin discoloration.

The presence of cyanosis may, at times, be difficult to ascertain clinically. Because cyanosis is more easily seen in bright light, newborn infants should be placed in a well-lighted room during the initial observation period. Most newborn infants are cyanotic during the first few minutes of life, and cyanosis may persist for more than 10 minutes in a few of them.

Cyanosis may be *central* (tongue, mucous membranes and peripheral skin) owing to arterial desaturation or an abnormal hemoglobin. *Peripheral* cyanosis, confined to the extremities, is caused by an increased arteriovenous oxygen difference in the presence of normal arterial saturation. Precise differentiation between central and peripheral cyanosis may depend upon the determination of arterial oxygen saturation or Pao_2. The cyanosis may be considered central if the Pao_2 is under 75 mm Hg at one day of age or if the oxygen saturation is under 94 per cent.

Cyanosis is first apparent and most evident where the epidermis is thin, pigmentation minimal and capillaries numerous (e.g., the tips of the fingers and toes [nail beds], ear lobes, tip of the nose, lips, tongue and buccal mucous membrane). In deeply pigmented persons, cyanosis may be apparent only in the tongue and mucous membranes. In patients in whom arterial unsaturation is not severe, redness, rather than blueness, may be noted in the lips, cheeks, nose and fingers. In polycythemia or hyperviscosity syndrome of the newborn, the cyanosis may appear bluish-red and have a blotchy, rather than uniform, distribution. The color of true cyanosis disappears if blood is expressed from the capillaries by diascopic pressure.

PHYSIOLOGY OF CYANOSIS

In the newborn infant, central cyanosis may be noted in the tongue and mucous membranes with only 3 grams of reduced hemoglobin and an arterial saturation of 75 to 88 per cent. An anemic patient with less than 5 gm/dl of hemoglobin cannot become cyanotic since 5 gm. of reduced hemoglobin per deciliter of capillary blood is necessary. Owing to the high affinity of fetal hemoglobin for oxygen and the large amount of such hemoglobin in the newborn, serious degrees of anoxia may be present in the absence of cyanosis.

Duc, G.: Assessment of hypoxia in the newborn. Suggestions for a practical approach. Pediatrics 48:469, 1971.

ETIOLOGIC CLASSIFICATION OF CYANOSIS

Please also see chapters on respiratory distress and respiratory disease. Some of the disorders discussed there also produce cyanosis.

I. CYANOSIS OWING TO ABNORMAL FORMS OF HEMOGLOBIN. The diagnosis in these cases depends upon a careful history and spectrophotometry.

A. Familial methemoglobinemia may be due to either an abnormality of erythrocyte energy-dependent mechanisms for reducing methemoglobin or inherited defects in hemoglobin structure, as in the hemoglobin M group. Methemoglobin diaphorase deficiency and deficiency of cytochrome b_5 reductase is characterized by both methemoglobinemia and mental retardation. With methemoglobinemia, the blood is chocolate brown when drawn and does not become red when mixed.

Vichinsky, E. P., and Lubin, B. H.: Unstable hemoglobins, hemoglobins with altered oxygen affinity, and M-hemoglobins. Pediatr. Clin. North Am. 27:421, 1980.

B. Methemoglobinemia may be caused by well-water (nitrate) ingestion in young infants, especially those with diarrhea and with coliform organisms in the upper intestine. Vegetables with a known high nitrate content (beets, cabbage and spinach) may lead to methemoglobinemia under special circumstances. The nitrates are converted to nitrites by bacteria. With absorption of nitrite, methemoglobin is produced.

Keating, J. P., Lell, M. E., Strauss, A. W., Zarkowsky, H., and Smith, G. E.: Infantile methemoglobinemia caused by carrot juice. N. Engl. J. Med. 288:824, 1973.
Report of the Committee on Nutrition of the American Academy of Pediatrics: Infant methemoglobinemia: The role of dietary nitrate. Pediatrics 46:475, 1970.

C. Methemoglobinemia in young infants has been caused by aniline dyes used in marking shirts and diapers. Ingestion of wax crayons has caused methemoglobinemia in older children. Methemoglobinemia has also been attributed to benzocaine ointment or rectal suppositories.
D. Low oxygen affinity hemoglobin variants, (e.g., hemoglobin Kansas) are associated with cyanosis.
E. Cyanosis owing to carbon monoxide poisoning.

II. CYANOSIS OWING TO ABNORMAL AMOUNTS OF REDUCED HEMOGLOBIN

A. Cyanosis in which the primary factor is an increased amount of hemoglobin passing in reduced form through aerated portions of the lung. The essential change is an increase in the value for arterial oxygen unsaturation in the blood returning from the lungs. If inhalation of 100 per cent oxygen increases the partial pressure of oxygen in the alveoli and aids diffusion, arterial oxygen unsaturation is diminished and cyanosis improved. Cyanosis does not appear until alveolar ventilation has been reduced.
 1. Decreased alveolar ventilation owing to failure of the respiratory center secondary to prematurity, intrauterine hypoxia, intracranial hemorrhage, drug administration or Ondine's curse.
 2. Decreased alveolar ventilation owing to obstruction of the respiratory tract
   a. Congenital obstructive lesions
     1. Atresia of the posterior nasal choanae
     2. Macroglossia
     3. Hypoplasia of the mandible

with glossoptosis (Pierre Robin syndrome). Posterior displacement of the tongue in these babies causes airway obstruction and may precipitate episodes of cyanosis.
     4. Thyroglossal duct cyst
     5. Laryngeal web or cyst
     6. Congenital absence of the cartilaginous rings of the trachea; tracheal stenosis
     7. Congenital vascular ring
   b. Acquired intrinsic obstruction
     1. Nasal mucus in the newborn. The young infant may lack the ability to open his mouth reflexly during sleep.
     2. Meconium aspiration
     3. Bilateral paresis of the vocal cords owing to intracranial hemorrhage at birth
     4. Damage to the cricothyroid or cricoarytenoid cartilages during birth
     5. Retropharyngeal abscess; infections of the deep spaces of the neck
     6. Acute laryngotracheobronchitis; acute epiglottitis; spasmodic croup
     7. Laryngeal edema; angioedema; serum sickness; nephrotic syndrome
     8. Laryngospasm
     9. Foreign body in the larynx or trachea
     10. Laryngeal neoplasm: papilloma, hemangioma, fibrolipoma
     11. Cystic fibrosis
     12. Acute bronchiolitis
   c. Acquired extrinsic obstruction
     1. Pneumomediastinum
     2. Congenital goiter
     3. Cystic hygroma
     4. Enterogenous cyst in the chest
     5. Lymphadenopathy: lymphoma, tuberculosis, sarcoidosis
 3. Decreased alveolar ventilation owing to structural changes in the lungs, diffusion impairment, ventilation/perfusion unevenness and shunting
   a. Cystic fibrosis
   b. Asthma
   c. Interstitial pneumonitis. See page 358.
   d. Congenital pulmonary cysts
   e. Pulmonary interstitial emphysema
   f. Diaphragmatic hernia

g. Respiratory distress syndrome
h. Transient tachypnea of the newborn
i. Bronchopulmonary dysplasia
j. Atelectasis in the newborn
k. Aspiration pneumonitis. An isolated tracheoesophageal fistula is a diagnostic consideration when cyanotic episodes accompany feedings in infancy. A history of choking and repeated episodes of aspiration pneumonia may be obtained. Meconium aspiration.
l. Pneumonia. Since the blood is shunted to aerated portions of the lung in patients with pneumonia, only a small portion of the total hemoglobin is exposed to unaerated, consolidated lung. Group B beta-hemolytic streptococcal pneumonia is a special consideration in the newborn.
m. Pulmonary edema. In cardiac failure, pulmonary edema may interfere with the diffusion of gases.
n. Idiopathic pulmonary hemosiderosis may be characterized by repeated attacks of cyanosis, pallor, dyspnea, cough and fatigue, along with iron-deficiency anemia.
o. Congestive heart failure
p. Pneumothorax. Since blood is shunted to the remaining aerated lung, cyanosis may not appear if the lung collapse is unilateral.
q. Empyema; pyopneumothorax; hemothorax; chylothorax; pleural effusion
r. Pulmonary hypoplasia, perhaps in association with renal agenesis or diaphragmatic hernia
s. Abdominal distention with pressure on the diaphragm may cause cyanosis.
t. Pulmonary hemorrhage
u. Congenital cystic adenomatoid malformation of the lung may cause cyanosis and tachypnea in infants. The mediastinum is displaced to the opposite side. Roentgenographic examination demonstrates a mass of soft-tissue density and scattered radiolucent areas.
v. Congenital lobar emphysema
w. Pulmonary lymphangiomatosis
x. Wilson-Mikity syndrome
y. *Pneumocystis carinii* pneumonia
4. Decreased alveolar ventilation owing to neuromuscular dysfunction
5. Breath-holding spells
6. Decreased alveolar exchange owing to lowered barometric pressure. Rapid ascent to high altitudes may cause pulmonary edema in susceptible children.
7. The pickwickian or cardiopulmonary syndrome associated with obesity may cause cyanosis owing to alveolar hypoventilation. Secondary polycythemia, periodic breathing, right ventricular hypertrophy and somnolence.

B. Cyanosis in which the primary factor is the amount of hemoglobin passing in reduced form through unaerated, venoarterial shunts from the right side of the heart to the arterial blood in the lungs or through the foramen ovale or the ductus arteriosus. The essential change is an increased arterial oxygen unsaturation in the systemic arteries. The value for arterial oxygen unsaturation in blood returning from the lungs is normal.

The inhalation of 100 per cent oxygen will cause only a slight diminution in the cyanosis in these patients because the hemoglobin passing through the lungs is normally oxygenated. Inhalation of 100 per cent oxygen increases the oxygenation of pulmonary blood only 1/2 to 1 volume per 100 ml in normal persons. An additional 2 volumes per 100 ml may be dissolved in the plasma, but this oxygen is slowly released and has little effect on the amount of reduced hemoglobin. The minimal decrease in arterial oxygen unsaturation gained by oxygen therapy is usually not sufficient to counteract the effect of a large amount of venous blood shunted into the arterial circulation. In most of these patients, the extent of oxygen unsaturation is further increased with exercise. In infants with increased pulmonary vascular resistance, however, there may be a direct effect of oxygen to dilate the pulmonary vessels and reduce venoarterial shunting.

1. Cyanotic congenital heart disease
   a. Transposition of the great vessels is the most frequent cause of cyanotic congenital heart disease in infants. Severe cyanosis is usually present within two to three days after birth. Pulmonary vascular markings are increased. If oxygenated blood is shunted to the systemic circulation through a persistent ductus, the hands are more cyanotic than the feet, since the ductus arteriosus enters the aorta distal to the origin of the arteries to the arms.

b. Tricuspid atresia with a nonfunctioning, rudimentary right ventricle is associated with severe cyanosis from birth and decreased pulmonary vascular markings.

c. Pseudotruncus arteriosus, a severe form of tetralogy with pulmonary atresia, is a cause of neonatal cyanosis. Pulmonary vascular markings are decreased.

d. Pulmonary atresia causes severe cyanosis during the first week of life. Pulmonary vascular markings are decreased.

e. Hypoplastic left heart syndrome causes cyanosis and congestive failure in the first 24 to 48 hours of life. Pulmonary vascular markings are increased.

f. Persistent pulmonary hypertension of the newborn infant (persistent fetal circulation syndrome) owing to continuing postnatal pulmonary hypertension is characterized by abnormal right-to-left shunting through a patent foramen ovale or patent ductus arteriosus. This hemodynamic pattern may occur in full term infants with pulmonary disease, hypoglycemia, polycythemia, or asphyxia or for unknown reasons. The infant, usually term or near term, may appear normal at birth but then develops cyanosis accompanied by tachypnea and acidemia in the first 24 hours of life. The second pulmonic sound is often loud. The chest x-ray shows normal pulmonary parenchymal markings. Simultaneously obtained blood samples from the right radial or temporal artery and the umbilical artery catheter may demonstrate a Pao_2 difference greater than 10 torr. Transcutaneous double site monitoring may also be utilized.

Drummond, W. H.: Persistent pulmonary hypertension of the neonate (persistent fetal circulation syndrome). Adv. Pediatr. 30:61, 1983.

Fox, W. W., and Duara, S.: Persistent pulmonary hypertension in the neonate: Diagnosis and management. J. Pediatr. 103:505, 1983.

g. The cardiac anomaly of a single ventricle may not be accompanied by early cyanosis. Pulmonary vascular markings are increased.

h. Truncus arteriosus is characterized by a delayed appearance of cyanosis. Pulmonary vascular markings are increased.

i. Tetralogy of Fallot consists of pulmonary stenosis or atresia, a ventricular septal defect, a dextroposed aorta that overrides the septal defect and right ventricular hypertrophy. Pulmonary vascular markings are decreased. Although cyanosis is present at birth in about one third of these patients, in most instances it does not appear or become persistent until the child begins to walk or run. Cyanosis is accentuated by exercise or exertion.

j. Pulmonary stenosis, if sufficiently severe, may be accompanied by cyanosis. Pulmonary vascular markings are decreased.

k. Ebstein's malformation of the tricuspid valve is accompanied by decreased pulmonary vascular markings.

l. Total anomalous pulmonary venous return is characterized by an increase in pulmonary vascular markings. The infant frequently is asymptomatic during the first month of life.

m. Pulmonary hypertension and patent ductus arteriosus. When the pressure in the pulmonary circulation exceeds that in the systemic circulation, the descending aorta receives blood from the pulmonary artery. As a result, cyanosis is greater in the feet than in the hands. Because of its proximity to the ductus arteriosus, the subclavian artery may also receive venous blood from the pulmonary artery. As a result, cyanosis may be greater in the left than in the right hand.

n. Primary pulmonary hypertension owing to an abnormality in the pulmonary vascular bed may be characterized by cyanosis, dyspnea and fatigue. Cyanosis may result from a right-to-left shunt through a patent foramen ovale secondary to elevation of the pressure in the right ventricle and atrium. In other children, cyanosis has occurred in the absence of a septal defect. Some of these instances may be attributable to an arteriovenous aneurysm or pulmonary shunt. Primary pulmonary hypertension may occur in children who live at high altitudes.

o. Eisenmenger complex. Cyanosis frequently does not appear until adolescence.

p. A preductile coarctation of the aorta with a patent ductus arteriosus may be associated with differential cyanosis between the upper and lower extremities, blood from the right ventricle being shunted through the ductus.

Nadas, A. S., and Fyler, D. C.: Pediatric Cardiology. 3rd ed. Philadelphia, W. B. Saunders Co., 1972.
Rudolph, A.: Congenital Diseases of the Heart. Chicago, Year Book Medical Publishers, 1974.

2. Cyanosis owing to a pulmonary arteriovenous fistula. With this lesion, unoxygenated blood is shunted from the pulmonary arteries to the pulmonary veins. The degree of cyanosis and dyspnea depends upon the extent of the shunt. Symptoms usually begin in childhood. A murmur may be audible over the shunt. Polycythemia and clubbing of the fingers gradually develop.
3. Respiratory disease syndrome produces hypoxia because of alveolar hypoventilation and right-to-left shunts.
4. Cyanosis owing possibly to portopulmonary anastomoses or pulmonary arteriovenous fistulas in patients with chronic hepatic disease and portal hypertension.
5. Intermittent cyanosis may occur in the cardiorespiratory syndrome of obesity. In addition to extreme obesity, symptoms and findings include dyspnea, polycythemia, somnolence, right ventricular hypertrophy and right-sided heart failure. The exact cause of the cyanosis is unknown.

C. Cyanosis in which the primary factor is the amount of hemoglobin converted to the reduced form while passing from the arteries to veins, (e.g., the extent of deoxygenation in the capillaries). This is usually attributable to capillary stasis, and the essential change is an increased venous oxygen unsaturation. The oxygen saturation of the arterial blood is normal. Oxygen therapy cannot reduce cyanosis unless capillary stasis results from arterial hypoxia.
1. Peripheral or localized cyanosis
   a. Acrocyanosis of the circumoral region and distal extremities in the first few hours after birth
   b. Local cyanosis owing to constriction of an extremity with a tourniquet
   c. Obstruction of superior or inferior vena cava
   d. Livedo reticularis
   e. Raynaud's disease is characterized by paroxysmal cyanosis or pallor of the fingers and toes. In many instances only the fingers are involved. Characteristically, involvement is bilateral and symmetrical. Symptoms, which occur more frequently in females than in males, may be precipitated by cold or emotional stress.
2. Generalized cyanosis owing in part to increased venous pressure
   a. Cardiac failure
      1. Paroxysmal atrial tachycardia
      2. Coarctation of the aorta of the infantile type. Cardiac failure may develop when the ductus arteriosus closes.
      3. Hypoplastic left heart syndrome
      4. Endocardial fibroelastosis
      5. Anomalous origin of the left coronary artery may be characterized by episodes of cyanosis, especially in relation to feedings, colicky pain, tachycardia, dyspnea and drenching perspiration.
      6. Myocarditis
      7. Rheumatic valvular disease
      8. Patients with left-to-right shunts may demonstrate cyanosis with the onset of congestive heart failure.
   b. Constrictive pericarditis
   c. The cyanosis that occurs during major convulsive seizures may, in part, be attributable to increased venous pressure.
   d. Cyanosis associated with crying
3. Generalized cyanosis owing to poor peripheral perfusion
   a. Capillary stasis owing to polycythemia or hyperviscosity may be an important secondary cause of cyanosis (e.g., in patients with congenital heart disease with hematocrits over 70 per cent).
   b. Localized cyanosis in the newborn (e.g., cord around the neck)
   c. Shock or hypotension may be characterized by cyanosis or an ashen gray color, as well as by pallor. Dehydration is a major cause of shock and capillary stasis

in infants and young children with severe diarrhea, adrenal hemorrhage and hypoadrenalism. Shock may also be caused by acute blood loss. Mottled cyanosis may occur in infants and children with severe, acute infectious diseases such as sepsis, (e.g., Group B beta hemolytic *Streptococcus* in the newborn infant); and, as a result of low cardiac output, hypotension, peripheral vascular collapse and pooling of blood in the skin. Cyanosis associated with profound circulatory collapse may be seen in the Waterhouse-Friderichsen syndrome. The "gray syndrome," characterized by peripheral vascular collapse and a gray pallor, occurs in newborn infants who receive inappropriately large doses of chloramphenicol.

   d. Hypoglycemia in the newborn
   e. Poor perfusion occurs in the hypoplastic left heart syndrome and with primary myocardial disease. Profound congestive heart failure with dyspnea and mild or moderate cyanosis (ashen gray color) occurs in the first hours or days of life in infants with the hypoplastic left heart syndrome.
   f. Cyanosis in the infant with heart failure may be caused, in part, by a low cardiac output. In addition to congenital heart defects, congestive heart failure and cyanosis may be caused by pulmonary disease, sepsis, anemia, myopathy, hypoxia and hypoglycemia.
   g. Peripheral cyanosis owing to chilling of the skin and venostasis. This is often a familial characteristic.
D. Peripheral cyanosis in which the primary factor is an increase in the total hematocrit
   1. Polycythemia and hyperviscosity syndromes in the newborn infant. Polycythemia in the newborn infant is present when the venous hematocrit is above 60 to 65 per cent. Viscosity increases markedly above a hematocrit of 65. Presenting signs and symptoms include peripheral cyanosis, respiratory distress, cardiomegaly, lethargy, and seizures. Several disorders may be associated with neonatal polycythemia, including infants small for gestational age; infants of diabetic mothers; chromosomal abnormalities, (e.g., Down's syndrome); and placental-cord, maternal-fetal and twin-twin transfusion. Since the hyperviscosity syndrome may also occur when the hematocrit is within the upper limits of normal, the blood viscosity should be measured with a microviscometer in infants with suggestive symptoms. Hyperviscosity may also be associated with acidosis and hypothermia.

Black, V. D., and Lubchenco, L. O.: Neonatal polycythemia and hyperviscosity. Pediatr. Clin. North Am. 29:1137, 1982.

   2. Polycythemia secondary to chronic hypoxia. Chronic hypoxia invariably produces polycythemia if the bone marrow is normal. Hypoxia and polycythemia accompany most forms of cyanotic heart disease and are present in patients with a pulmonary arteriovenous fistula. Polycythemia usually accentuates the cyanosis in these cases.
   3. Polycythemia vera

DIAGNOSIS OF CYANOSIS IN THE NEWBORN

The differentiation of pulmonary and cardiac causes of cyanosis in the newborn may be difficult or impossible. Indeed, both etiologies may be simultaneously involved. A few generalizations may be made. The response of cyanosis to crying in the newborn does not permit differentiation between a pulmonary and a cardiac etiology. Severe cyanosis usually implies a congenital heart disorder such as transposition of the great vessels. Similarly, tachypnea accompanied by intense cyanosis without apparent respiratory distress is more characteristic of cyanotic congenital heart disease. Arterial blood gases and pH should be promptly obtained in the infant with cyanosis. The chest x-ray is probably the next most helpful examination, since it may demonstrate the radiologic features of respiratory distress syndrome, the cardiomegaly of cardiac disease or the increased or decreased pulmonary vascular markings associated with specific congenital cardiac disorders. The increase in Pco_2 and the decrease in Pao_2 and pH secondary to severe pulmonary disease may also lead to moderate cardiomegaly.

Whereas both alveolar hypoventilation and a right-to-left shunt may be accompanied by a low Pa_{O_2}, the P_{CO_2} is generally increased in the former but not the latter. In the case of hyaline membrane disease with right-to-left shunting, the low Pa_{O_2} may be accompanied by a normal or decreased P_{CO_2}. The response of the Pa_{O_2} to breathing of 100 per cent oxygen for 10 to 30 minutes is also of differential interest: in alveolar hypoventilation, the Pa_{O_2} will rise, whereas there will be no effect with a right-to-left shunt. A Pa_{O_2} over 50 or 60 while breathing 100 per cent oxygen almost always rules out a cyanotic congenital cardiac defect. Response to oxygen with clinical improvement in color does not, however, always permit differentiation between pulmonary and congenital heart disease. Some babies with right-to-left shunts improve with oxygen; some infants with marked pulmonary disease do not. Infants who remain cyanotic beyond three hours after birth should be evaluated by a pediatric cardiologist.

The diagnostic work-up of a cyanotic infant should generally include the following: arterial blood gases (P_{O_2}, P_{CO_2}), pH, chest x-ray, hematocrit, blood glucose, cultures, possibly an electrocardiogram and response to 100 per cent oxygen (Pa_{O_2} in 100 per cent Fi_{O_2}). An echocardiogram or cardiac catheterization with angiocardiography, or both, may also be indicated.

GENERAL REFERENCES

Emmanouilides, G. C., and Baylen, B. G.: Neonatal cardiopulmonary distress without congenital heart disease. Curr. Probl. Pediatr. 9:4, 1979.

Kitterman, J. A.: Cyanosis in the newborn infant. Pediatr. Rev. 4:13, 1982.

Lees, M. H.: Cyanosis of the newborn infant. J. Pediatr. 77:484, 1970.

Sahn, D. J., and Friedman, W. F.: Difficulties in distinguishing cardiac from pulmonary disease in the neonate. Pediatr. Clin. North Am. 20:293, 1973.

Yabek, S. M.: Neonatal cyanosis. Reappraisal of response to 100% oxygen breathing. Am. J. Dis. Child. 138:880, 1984.

ETIOLOGIC CLASSIFICATION OF CYANOSIS

I. ABNORMAL FORMS OF HEMOGLOBIN, 383
   A. Familial methemoglobinemia, 383
   B. Methemoglobinemia from well-water (nitrate) ingestion, 384
   C. Methemoglobinemia from aniline dyes, wax crayons, benzocaine ointment or suppositories, 384
   D. Low oxygen affinity hemoglobin variants, 384
   E. Carbon monoxide poisoning, 384
II. ABNORMAL AMOUNTS OF REDUCED HEMOGLOBIN, 384
   A. Increased amount of hemoglobin passing in reduced form through aerated portions of the lung, 384
      1. Decreased alveolar ventilation from prematurity, intrauterine hypoxia, intracranial hemorrhage, drug administration or Ondine's curse
      2. Decreased alveolar ventilation from respiratory tract obstruction
      3. Decreased alveolar ventilation from lung structural changes, diffusion impairment, ventilation/perfusion unevenness, shunting
      4. Decreased alveolar ventilation from neuromuscular dysfunction
      5. Breath-holding spells
      6. Decreased alveolar exchange from lowered barometric pressure   ·

      7. Cardiorespiratory syndrome of obesity
   B. Amount of hemoglobin passing in reduced form through unaerated, venoarterial shunts from the heart's right side to the arterial blood in the lungs or through the foramen ovale or ductus arteriosus, 385
      1. Cyanotic congenital heart disease
      2. Pulmonary arteriovenous fistula
      3. Respiratory distress syndrome
      4. Portopulmonary anastomoses or pulmonary arteriovenous fistula in patients with chronic hepatic disease and portal hypertension
   C. Extent of deoxygenation in the capillaries, 387
      1. Peripheral cyanosis
      2. Generalized cyanosis from increased venous pressure
      3. Generalized cyanosis from poor peripheral perfusion
   D. Peripheral cyanosis from an increase in the total hematocrit, 388
      1. Polycythemia and hyperviscosity syndrome in newborn
      2. Polycythemia secondary to chronic hypoxia
      3. Polycythemia vera

ETIOLOGIC CLASSIFICATION OF CHEST PAIN

I. CARDIAC AND MEDIASTINAL. When a cardiac cause for chest pain is suspected, the evaluation should include a posteroanterior and lateral chest x-ray, electrocardiogram, M-mode echocardiogram, 2D echocardiogram, exercise tolerance test, 24-hour Holter monitor, serum cholesterol and, possibly, cardiac catheterization, depending upon the lesion suspected.

A. Pericarditis may be characterized by chest pain, at times sharp and stabbing, usually sudden in onset and localized substernally over the precordium, in the epigastrium, in the interscapular region, referred to the shoulder, or present over the entire thorax. Accentuation of the pain may occur with deep breathing, coughing, swallowing or twisting of the thorax. The child may have grunting respirations or primary pulmonary hypertension.
B. Pulmonary vascular obstructive syndrome may be characterized, in part, by pain on exertion.
C. Rheumatic fever may be accompanied by precordial pain.
D. Ruptured congenital aneurysm of the sinuses of Valsalva. Rupture of an aortic aneurysm is a rare cause of chest pain in the pediatric population.
E. Anginal pain may occur in children with sickle cell anemia, severe aortic stenosis, pulmonic stenosis, aberrant coronary artery, tachyarrhythmia, mitral valve prolapse, idiopathic hypertrophic subaortic stenosis and cardiomyopathy.

Hamilton, W., Rosenthal, A., Berwick, D., and Nadas, A. S.: Angina pectoris in a child with sickle cell anemia. Pediatrics 61:911, 1978.

F. Mitral valve prolapse is an unusual cause for sharp or dull, intermittent, left-side chest pain or precordial discomfort.
G. Takayasu's arteritis may be accompanied by chest pain.
H. Rheumatoid arthritis may cause chest pain owing to pleuritis and/or pericarditis or both.
I. Kawasaki disease with coronary artery involvement may lead to exertional substernal pain.
J. Superior vena cava syndrome
K. Palpitations may be associated with paroxysmal supraventricular tachycardia, hyperventilation syndrome, pheochromocytoma, hypochondriasis and anxiety.
L. Spontaneous mediastinal emphysema is characterized by precordial pain, crunching auscultatory sounds, and subcutaneous air in the neck.

Sturtz, G. S.: Spontaneous mediastinal emphysema. Pediatrics 74:431, 1984.

II. PULMONARY AND DIAPHRAGM. Since the posterior third and the lateral parts of the diaphragm are innervated by the lower six intercostal nerves, pain arising from these areas is referred to the lower part of the thorax or upper part of the abdomen. The central and anterior portions of the diaphragm are innervated by the phrenic nerve with pain referred to the shoulder and trapezius ridge.

A. Pleurisy may occur alone or as a complication of pneumonia. The pain is sharp in intensity, well-localized over the involved area, perceived as superficial and accentuated by deep breathing, coughing and arm movements. The patient attempts to splint the involved side. Localized tenderness may be noted.
B. Epidemic pleurodynia is characterized by sharp or stabbing pain similar to that of pleurisy. Involvement may be unilateral or bilateral. Tenderness and some swelling may be noted over the involved area. The pain may last two or three days and then recur.
C. Familial paroxysmal polyserositis (Mediterranean fever) may be characterized by paroxysmal pleuritis with severe, sharp, stabbing pain. The episodes may occur independently or with peritonitis.
D. Spontaneous pneumothorax may cause acute chest pain.
E. Trichinosis involving the diaphragm is characterized by chest pain as well as systemic manifestations.
F. Pulmonary embolism, which may occur during an elective abortion, is character-

ized by cough, fever, chills, dyspnea and chest pain.

Nudelman, R., and Best, L.: Pulmonary embolism in a 14 year old following an elective abortion. Pediatrics 66:584, 1981.

G. Sickle cell disease may cause episodes of chest pain owing to pulmonary infection, infarction or embolization (acute chest syndrome). Differentiation may be difficult. Findings include fever, dyspnea, pleuritic pain, leukocytosis and pulmonary infiltration. Infarctions of the ribs may cause superficial tenderness. Acute cholecystitis or splenic infarction may cause referred chest pain.
H. Bacterial pneumonia; interstitial pneumonitis; cystic fibrosis
I. Pulmonary sarcoidosis may cause pleuritic pain.
J. Asthma is a frequent cause of chest pain.

III. MUSCULOSKELETAL

A. Muscle strain, spasm and fatigue are probably the most common causes of chest pain in children (chest wall syndrome). The involved muscles may be tender, and the pain is increased by truncal movement. Weight-lifting and other vigorous sports may be etiologic. The pain occurs at rest.
B. Trauma to the chest wall
C. Tumors or other infiltrative processes involving the bony skeleton may give rise to pain.
D. Rib fracture
E. Tietze's syndrome, or costochondritis, is characterized by exquisite point tenderness on pressure over the involved costochondral junction.
F. Tender or painful xiphoid is of unknown etiology.
G. Severe paroxysms of coughing or asthma with bronchospasm may cause chest pain
H. Primary fibromyalgia syndrome, which may occur in school-age children or adolescents, is characterized by chronic, persistent musculoskeletal pain in at least three areas of the body for a minimum of three months, in addition to aching, fatigue and morning stiffness.
I. Slipping rib in which the sudden onset of pain may be caused by the tip of the lower ribs overriding the one above.

Heinz, G., and Zavala, D.: Slipping rib. JAMA 237:794, 1977.

IV. ESOPHAGEAL

A. Achalasia (cardiospasm) with diffuse spasm of the esophagus may cause substernal pain.
B. Hiatus hernia and gastroesophageal reflux

Darling, D. B., Fisher, J. H., and Gellis, S. S.: Hiatal hernia and gastroesophageal reflux in infants and children: Analysis of the incidence in North American children. Pediatrics 54:450, 1974.

C. Esophagitis may cause burning retrosternal pain. Candidiasis may be etiologic in immunosuppressed or deficient patients.

V. PSYCHOGENIC

A. Occasionally, a child seen because of pain over the precordium will be found to have a psychologic basis for the symptom. The interview will frequently disclose that a parent or other relative has angina or some other cardiac disorder. The pain, which the child reasons has been caused by a heart problem, may represent a conversion reaction or somatization associated with depression.
B. Hyperventilation syndrome may present with the complaint of palpitation and left precordial chest pain described as sharp and evanescent.

VI. NEUROLOGIC

A. Radicular pain owing to compression of the spinal cord by tumor, epidural abscess or vertebral collapse.
B. Prodromal phase of herpes zoster

VII. HEARTBURN

A. Gastroesophageal reflux
B. Achalasia

GENERAL REFERENCES

Coleman, W. L.: Recurrent chest pain in children. Pediatr. Clin. North Am. 31:1007, 1984.
Driscoll, D. J., Glicklich, L. B., and Gallen, W. J.: Chest pain in children: A prospective study. Pediatrics 57:648, 1976.
Pantell, R. H., and Goodman, B. W., Jr.: Adolescent chest pain: A prospective study. Pediatrics 71:881, 1983.
Perry, L. W.: Pinpointing the cause of pediatric chest pain. Cont. Pediatr. 2:71, 1985.
Selbst, S. M.: Chest pain in children. Pediatrics 75:1068, 1985.

53 / FREQUENT INFECTIONS

CLINICAL CONSIDERATIONS

In considering the presenting complaint of "frequent infections," the physician must differentiate among parental overestimation of the number and severity of the illnesses; an above average but normal number of infections; allergic airway disease; and the rare occurrence of a true or acquired immunodeficiency.

Dingle's classic study demonstrated that during the second year of life children experience, on the average, eight respiratory infections a year. The frequency of such infections gradually decreases until an average of three to four a year is reached in adolescence. The more than 10 per cent of children who have more than 12 respiratory infections per year are generally those seen for "frequent colds." Other studies suggest that children, on the average, experience 100 infections, most asymptomatic, by the age of 10 years. Environmental factors that predispose to frequent infections include crowding, especially in sleeping areas, the presence of school-age siblings; or attendance in day care centers, nursery school, kindergarten or the primary grades. Reactive airway disease is another common cause for "frequent colds."

Honicky, R. E., Osborne, J. S., III, and Akpom, C. A.: Symptoms of respiratory illness in young children and the use of wood-burning stoves for indoor heating. Pediatrics 75:587, 1985.

The possibility of an immunodeficiency syndrome exists when (1) infections are especially frequent, severe, or persistent, (e.g., two or more serious pyogenic skin infections); (2) persistent or recurrent stomatitis or gingivitis occurs; (3) multiple sites of infection are involved with many etiologic agents, especially organisms not commonly pathogenic; (4) infections to which the child should have acquired immunity recur; or (5) a common disease has an unusually severe and progressive course.

Goodman, R. A., Osterholm, M. T., Granoff, D. M., and Pickering, L. K.: Infectious diseases and child day care. Pediatrics 74:134, 1984.
Loda, F. A.: Day care. Pediatr. Rev. 1:277, 1980.

ETIOLOGIC CLASSIFICATION OF IMMUNODEFICIENCY DISORDERS

I. PHAGOCYTIC DYSFUNCTION

A. Neutropenia. An absolute granulocyte count under 1000/cu mm may be associated with recurrent bacterial infections. With an absolute granulocyte count between 500 to 1000/cu mm, the patient may develop gingivitis, furunculosis or a perianal abscess. Serious infections occur when the granulocyte count is less than 500 polymorphonuclear leukocytes and band forms/cu mm.

1. Cyclic neutropenia is manifested by periodic episodes (approximately every three weeks and each lasting about a week) of fever, mouth ulcers, arthralgia, furunculosis or pneumonia. The diagnosis may be established by obtaining white blood cell and differential counts three times a week for two months, unless the neutropenia is confirmed sooner.

2. Congenital or chronic infantile agranulocytosis (Kostmann's syndrome), an autosomal recessive and usually fatal disease that occurs in the first year of life, is characterized by chronic, recurrent pyogenic infections of the skin and upper respiratory tract or by other serious infections. Although the total white blood count may be normal, the neutrophil count during episodes is usually less than 300 neutrophils per cu mm.

3. Chronic benign granulocytopenia of childhood, which usually becomes symptomatic by the end of the first year and continues for months to years, is characterized by the occurrence of mild infections, mouth ulcers and stomatitis.

4. The Shwachman-Diamond syndrome consists of exocrine pancreatic insufficiency and neutropenia, dwarfism, severe infections and, at times, metaphyseal dysostosis.

5. Drug-induced neutropenia results

from a profound bone marrow suppression involving the myeloid cells.

6. Aplastic anemia
7. Acute leukemia
8. Neutropenia may occur secondary to vitamin B_{12} or folic acid deficiency.
9. Neonatal isoimmune neutropenia
10. Congestive splenomegaly
11. Chronic granulocytopenia of childhood, usually a sclf-limited disorder, is characterized by susceptibility to localized infections such as paronychia, subcutaneous abscesses, impetigo, gingivitis and genital ulcers. The bone marrow responds to infection with the release of immature but functionally adequate white blood cells.
12. Cartilage-hair hypoplasia is characterized by chronic neutropenia and depression of cell mediated immunity.

Lux, S. E., Johnson, R. B., Jr., August, C. S., Say, B., Penchaszadeh, V. B., Rosen, F. S., and McKusick, V. A.: Chronic neutropenia and abnormal cellular immunity in cartilage-hair hypoplasia. N. Engl. J. Med. 282:231, 1970.
Oski, F. A.: Neutropenia in children. Pediatr. Rev. 3:108, 1981.

B. Disorders of neutrophil adherence
1. Absence of a neutrophil membrane glycoprotein may be associated with delayed separation of the umbilical cord and polymicrobial bacterial infections.

Hayward, A. R., Leonard, J., Wood, C. B. C., Harvey, B. A. M., Greenwood, M. C., and Soothill, J. F.: Delayed separation of the umbilical cord, widespread infections and defective neutrophil mobility. Lancet 1:1099, 1979.
Kobayashi, K., Fujita, K., Okino, F., and Kajii, T.: An abnormality of neutrophil adhesion: Autosomal recessive inheritance associated with missing neutrophil glycoproteins. Pediatrics 73:606, 1984.

2. Patients with thalassemia may demonstrate depressed neutrophil adherence.
C. Disorders of phagocyte locomotion
D. Disorders of chemotaxis
1. Lazy leukocyte syndrome is characterized by mild recurrent infections such as rhinitis, gingivitis, stomatitis or otitis media.
2. Ichthyosis is frequently associated with depressed granulocyte chemotactic responsiveness.
3. The Schwachman-Diamond syndrome

4. Hyperimmunoglobinemia E (Job's) syndrome usually becomes manifest within the first three months of life. Recurrent infections include pyoderma, furunculosis, cold abscesses, staphylococcal pneumonia, otitis media, otitis externa, recurrent bronchitis, eczematoid dermatitis and a coarse facies. The serum IgE level may be over 2000 IU/ml. A defect in cell-mediated immunity may also be present.

Buckley, R. H., Wray, B. B., and Belmaker, E. Z.: Extreme hyperimmunoglobulinemia E and undue susceptibility to infection. Pediatrics 49:59, 1972.

E. Defective opsonization
1. Complement deficiencies
2. Antibody deficiencies
F. Defective bactericidal function
1. Chronic granulomatous disease, characterized by defective intracellular killing of phagocytosed or ingested bacteria, occurs in a male to female ratio of 7:1 and is transmitted in an X-linked recessive or, uncommonly, an autosomal recessive form. Suppurative lymphadenopathy and draining cutaneous fistulas usually occur by the end of the first year of life. Other findings include pneumonia; empyema; lung abscess; hepatosplenomegaly; purulent dermatitis around the mouth and ears; chronic pyoderma; hepatic abscesses; persistent diarrhea, perianal abscesses; osteomyelitis, usually of the small bones of the hands and feet; and a special susceptibility to fungal infections. The peripheral blood leukocytes do not reduce nitroblue tetrazolium dye during phagocytosis. The three major immunoglobulins are elevated, and the isohemagglutinin titers are normal.

Hill, H. R., Quie, P. G., Pabst, H. F., Ochs, Clark, R. A., Klebanoff, H. D., and Wedgewood, R. J.: Defect in neutrophic granulocyte chemotaxis in Job's syndrome of recurrent "cold" staphylococcal abscesses. Lancet 2:617, 1974.
Johnson, R. B., Jr., and Baehner, R. L.: Chronic granulomatous disease: Correlation between pathogenesis and clinical findings. Pediatrics 48:730, 1971.
Johnston, R. B., Jr.: Unusual forms of an uncommon disease (chronic granulomatous disease). J. Pediatr. 88:172, 1976.
Johnston, R. B., III, Harbeck, R. J., and Johnston, R. B., Jr.: Recurrent severe infections in a girl with apparently variable expression of mosaicism for chronic granulomatous disease. J. Pediatr. 106:50, 1985.

2. Familial lipochrome histocytosis is characterized by defective phagocytic function similar to that of chronic granulomatous disease.
3. Glutathione synthetase deficiency is accompanied by recurrent infections.
4. Myeloperoxidase deficiency may be associated with recurrent candida infections.
5. Bactericidal activity of Chédiak-Higashi neutrophils is defective.

Blume, R. S., and Wolff, S. M.: The Chédiak-Higashi syndrome: Studies in four patients and a review of the literature. Medicine 51:247, 1972.

6. Tuftsin deficiency, either inherited or acquired secondary to splenectomy, is characterized by increased susceptibility to infection owing to defective granulocyte phagocytosis.

Quie, P. G., and Hetherington, S. V.: Patients with disorders of phagocytic cell function. Pediatr. Infect. Dis. 3:272, 1984.
Winkelstein, J. A., and Drachman, R. H.: Phagocytosis. Pediatr. Clin. North Am. 21:551, 1974.

II. DEFECTS PRIMARILY OF ANTIBODY PRODUCTION are characterized by recurrent, severe pyogenic infections of the skin, bones, joints, lungs, meninges, sinuses and middle ear. Etiologic agents include pneumococci, *Haemophilus influenzae, Staphylococcus aureus,* meningococci and, occasionally, beta-hemolytic streptococci. Giardiasis may cause diarrhea in patients with hypogammaglobulinemia.

A. Transient hypogammaglobulinemia of infancy, attributable to delayed maturation of B-cell function, begins between two and six months of age. The diagnosis may be established by screening the serum of relatives of patients who have a primary immunodeficiency or by the study of infants with a history of recurrent fever, repeated or severe pyogenic infections, chronic mucocutaneous candidiasis or bronchitis. Levels of IgG, IgA and IgM are low. Patients identified on the basis of screening are asymptomatic, whereas those with a history of recurrent infections usually experience no major infectious problems after six months of age. In the former group, the immunoglobulin levels in time become completely normal, whereas the values in the latter improve gradually but may remain subnormal.

Tiller, T. L., Jr., and Buckley, R. H.: Transient hypogammaglobulinemia of infancy: Review of

the literature, clinical and immunologic features of 11 new cases, and long-term follow-up. J. Pediatr. 92:347, 1978.

B. Congenital X-linked agammaglobulinemia (Bruton's type) is characterized by recurrent pyogenic infections in boys after six to nine months of age. Viral and fungal disorders usually elicit a normal response except for those caused by polioviruses (vaccine-associated poliomyelitis), echoviruses (encephalitis), *Giardia lamblia* (diarrhea), *Pneumocystis carinii* (pneumonia) and mycoplasma (arthritis). Because the tonsils and adenoids are absent or underdeveloped, the adenoid shadow is absent on lateral pharyngeal x-rays. Serum IgG is less than 100 mg/dl. About one third of these patients develop a nonbacterial arthritis that closely simulates rheumatoid arthritis.
C. X-linked hypogammaglobulinemia may occur with isolated growth hormone deficiency and micropenis.

Fleisher, T. A., White, R. M., Broder, S., Nissley, S. P., Blaese, A. M., Mulvihill, J. J., Olive, G., and Waldman, T. A.: X-linked hypogammaglobulinemia and isolated growth hormone deficiency. N. Engl. J. Med. 302:1429, 1980.

D. Autosomal recessive agammaglobulinemia in young girls simulates the symptomatology of X-linked agammaglobulinemia in boys.
E. Common variable or late onset hypogammaglobulinemia is characterized by a low serum IgG and variable amounts of IgA and IgM. Clinical manifestations, which begin at a later age than X-linked agammaglobulinemia, include pyoderma, pneumonia, meningitis, tonsillitis, otitis media, sinusitis, diarrhea, giardiasis, bronchiectasis, and, in some cases, an associated autoimmune disorder. The three immunologic findings include intrinsic B-cell defects, immunoregulatory T-cell imbalance or antibodies to T and B cells. B cells may be present.

Hausser, C., Virelizier, J-L., Buriot, D., and Griscelli, C.: Common variable hypogammaglobulinemia in children. Am. J. Dis. Child. 137:833, 1983.
Donabedian, H., and Gallin, J. I.: The hyperglobulin E recurrent-infection (Job's) syndrome. Medicine 62:195, 1983.

F. Partial or selective immunoglobulin deficiencies
1. The clinical significance of selective IgA deficiency (less than 10

mg/dl) is uncertain. Secretory IgA is also deficient in these children, who may be clinically normal or have recurrent respiratory tract infections, intermittent diarrhea, an atopic disorder, autoimmune disease or a collagen-vascular disorder.

Ammann, A. J., and Hong, R.: Selective IgA deficiency: Presentation of 30 cases and a review of the literature. Medicine 50:223, 1971.

2. Partial gamma globulin deficiency, a disorder in which one or more of the four IgG subclasses may be absent, is characterized by recurrent pyogenic infections that are less severe than those secondary to agammaglobulinemia.
3. Selective IgM deficiency, a very rare disorder, may be accompanied by serious or recurrent pyogenic infections, including meningococcemia.
4. Low concentrations of IgG and IgA may be accompanied by an elevated concentration of IgM (and sometimes IgD). Clinical manifestations similar to those in patients with X-linked agammaglobulinemia include pyogenic infections, autoimmune disorders and lymphoproliferative disease. Hematologic findings may include hemolytic anemia, thrombocytopenia or neutropenia.
G. Short-limbed dwarfism may be associated with antibody-mediated immunodeficiency.

Ammann, A. J., Sutliff, W., and Millinchick, E.: Antibody-mediated immunodeficiency in short-limbed dwarfism. J. Pediatr. 84:200, 1974.

III. DEFECTS PRIMARILY OF CELLULAR IMMUNITY

A. Severe, combined immunodeficiency (SCID), a rare disorder in infants, may be inherited in an X-linked recessive manner or an autosomal recessive fashion (with or without adenosine deaminase deficiency). T and B lymphocytes are markedly abnormal in both number and function. Affected infants are markedly susceptible to all types of infections. Clinical characteristics include persistent candidiasis of the buccal mucosa, larynx and skin; marked failure of growth or runting, chronic interstitial pneumonitis owing to *Pneumocystis carinii*; intractable diarrhea; and marked susceptibility to viral infections.

A morbilliform rash may be present in the first few days of life. Later, the dermatitis may resemble that of Letterer-Siwe's disease. Profound lymphopenia is usually present with less than 1000 lymphocytes per cubic millimeter. Serum immunoglobulins are usually low.

Bortin, M. M., and Rimm, A. A.: Severe combined immunodeficiency disease. JAMA 238:591, 1977.

B. Nezelof's syndrome, owing to combined immunodeficiency with predominant T-cell defects, is a poorly defined disorder associated with thymic dysplasia and characterized by failure to thrive, chronic lower respiratory tract infections, otitis media, recurrent pyoderma, chronic candidiasis and diarrhea. Laboratory examinations show lymphopenia, reduction of T-cells and, usually, a normal concentration of serum immunoglobulins.
C. Combined immunodeficiency with enzyme deficiency
   1. Purine nucleoside phosphorylase deficiency, which may be associated with defective T-cell function, is characterized by a marked susceptibility to opportunistic and viral infections. The clinical manifestations resemble those of the acquired immunodeficiency syndrome.

Biggar, W. D., Giblett, E. R., Ozere, R. L., and Grover, B. D.: A new form of nucleoside phosphorylase deficiency in two brothers with defective T-cell function. J. Pediatr. 92:354, 1978.

   2. Adenosine deaminase deficiency
D. Type 1 short-limbed dwarfism may be associated with combined antibody and cell-mediated immunodeficiency.
E. X-linked lymphoproliferative syndrome (Duncan's disease) is characterized by an immunodeficiency with a special susceptibility to the Epstein-Barr virus. Possible sequelae are fatal or chronic infectious mononucleosis; non-Hodgkin lymphoma, including Burkitt lymphoma or nasopharyngeal carcinoma, dysgammaglobulinemia, and acquired hypo- or agammaglobulinemia.

Hamilton, J. K., et al: X-linked lymphoproliferative syndrome registry report. J. Pediatr. 96:669, 1980.
Sullivan, J. L.: Epstein-Barr virus and the X-linked lymphoproliferative syndrome. Adv. Pediatr. 30:365, 1983.

F. Acquired immune deficiency syndrome (AIDS) is characterized by recurrent or persistent opportunistic infections occurring after three to six months of age. Clinical manifestations include failure to thrive, upper respiratory tract infections, otitis media, chronic diarrhea, candidiasis, opportunistic infections, recurrent or persistent pneumonia, hepatosplenomegaly, persistent lymphadenopathy and chronic parotid swelling. Diagnostic evaluation demonstrates lymphopenia, elevated serum immunoglobulins, including IgM in children, selective T-cell deficiency and decreased or absent cutaneous hypersensitivity to antigens.

Rogers, M. F.: AIDS in children: A review of the clinical, epidemiologic and public health aspects. Pediatr. Inf. Dis. 4:230, 1985.

Rubinstein, A.: Acquired immunodeficiency syndrome in infants. Am. J. Dis. Child. 137:825, 1983.

Seligmann, M., et al: AIDS—an immunologic re-evaluation. N. Engl. J. Med. 311:1286, 1984.

Shannon, K. M., and Ammann, A. J.: Acquired immune deficiency syndrome in childhood. J. Pediatr. 106:332, 1985.

G. Short-limbed dwarfism may occur with cell-mediated immunodeficiency. Some of these patients have cartilage-hair hypoplasia.

Virolainen, M., Savilahti, E., Kaitila, I., and Perheentupa, J.: Cellular and humoral immunity in cartilage-hair hypoplasia. Pediat. Res. 12:961, 1978.

IV. COMPLEMENT DISORDERS associated with severe and recurrent infections.

A. C3 or C5 deficiency or absence
B. Dysfunction of C5 is associated with Leiner's syndrome characterized by seborrheic dermatitis, diarrhea, failure to thrive and recurrent gram-negative bacterial and fungal infections.
C. Absence of C6, C7 and C8 and defects in the alternative complement pathway are also associated with serious infections. Infections in patients with sickle cell anemia, or nephrotic syndrome or following-splenectomy may be attributable to the latter defect.

Alper, C. A., Abramson, N., Johnston, R. B., Jr., Jandl, J. H., and Rosen, F. S.: Increased susceptibility to infection associated with abnormalities of complement-mediated functions and of the third component of complement (C3). N. Engl. J. Med. 282:349, 1970.

Jacobs, J. D., and Miller, M. E.: Fatal familial "Leiner's disease": A deficiency of the opsonic activity of serum complement. Pediatrics 49:225, 1972.

McLean, R. H., and Winkelstein, J. A.: Genetically determined variation in the complement system: Relationship to disease. J. Pediatr. 105:179, 1984.

Miller, M. E., and Nilsson, U. R.: A familial deficiency of the phagocytosis-enhancing activity of serum related to a dysfunction of the fifth component of complement (C5) N. Engl. J. Med. 282:354, 1970.

V. IMMUNODEFICIENCY ASSOCIATED WITH OTHER DEFECTS

A. DiGeorge's syndrome (congenital aplasia of thymus and parathyroid glands, pharyngeal pouch syndrome) is manifested by a characteristic facies and recurrent infections. Congenital heart disease is usually the initial presenting problem, with interrupted aortic arch and truncus arteriosus being frequent defects. Neonatal tetany is another early clinical manifestation. Facial and cranial features present in many of these children include micrognathia; anteverted nostrils; low-set, poorly formed ears; a short philtrum; a "fish" mouth; bifid uvula; hypertelorism; clefts in the midline of the nose; and esophageal atresia. Although infection is usually not a problem in the first weeks of life, some infants develop purulent rhinorrhea. Later symptoms include susceptibility to infection, (e.g., *Pneumocystis carinii*), pneumonia, diarrhea, moniliasis and failure to thrive. The severity of the immunodeficiency depends upon the degree of thymic hypoplasia. Serum immunoglobulin concentrations are generally near normal, but IgA may be decreased and IgE elevated. The number of T cells is decreased.

Conley, M. E., Beckwith, J. B., Mancer, J. F. K., and Tenckhoff, L.: The spectrum of the DiGeorge's syndrome. J. Pediatr. 94:883, 1979.

B. Wiskott-Aldrich syndrome, an X-linked recessive disorder manifest in early infancy, is characterized by variable symptomatology including petechiae, severe eczema, skin infections, otitis media and pneumonia. Laboratory findings include marked thrombocytopenia, small platelets, elevated IgA and IgE, decreased IgM and normal IgG levels. T cells demonstrate a steady decline in number and function.

Perry, G. S., III, Spector, B. D., Schuman, L. M., Mandel, J. S., Anderson, V. E., McHugh, R. B., Hanson, M. R., Fahlstrom, S. M., Krivit, W., and Kersey, J. H.: The Wiskott-Aldrich syndrome in the United States and Canada (1892–1979). J. Pediatr. 97:72, 1980.

C. Ataxia telangiectasia, an autosomal recessive disorder, becomes clinically manifest with progressive cerebellar ataxia at the end of the second year. Repeated sinopulmonary infections and bronchiectasis occur after three years of age. Conjunctival and facial telangiectasia often appears between two and eight years of age. IgA is absent in 50 per cent of these patients and very low in an additional 30 per cent. Delayed hypersensitivity may be impaired.

McFarlin, D. E., Strober, W., and Waldmann, T. A.: Ataxia-telangiectasia. Medicine 51:281, 1972.

VI. SECONDARY IMMUNODEFICIENCY DISORDERS

A. Splenectomy may render a child susceptible to overwhelming sepsis, recurrent meningitis and other serious infections. Howell-Jolly bodies may be present on the peripheral blood smear. The functional asplenia that develops in children with sickle cell anemia is associated with serious infections, especially in those under the age of five years.
B. Severe protein-caloric malnutrition is associated with a depression of cell-mediated immunity and an increase in infectious diseases.

Carney, J. M., Warner, M. S., Borut, T., Bryne, W., Ament, M., Cherry, J. D. and Stiehm, R.: Cell-mediated immune defects and infection. Am. J. Dis. Child. 134:824, 1980.
Katz, M., and Stiehm, E. R.: Host defense in malnutrition. Pediatrics 59:490, 1977.

C. Congenital infections such as cytomegalovirus or rubella virus may cause mild, transient immunodeficiency.
D. Long term, high dose corticosteroid treatment; neonatal steroid treatment

Gunn, T., Reece, E. R., Metrakos, K., and Colle, E.: Depressed T cells following neonatal steroid treatment. Pediatrics 67:61, 1981.

E. Malignancies may predispose to frequent infections because of granulocytopenia, quantitative defects in neutrophil function, defects in cell- and humoral-mediated immunity and malnutrition.

Pizzo, P. A.: Infectious complications in the child with cancer. I. Pathophysiology of the compromised host and the initial evaluation and management of the febrile cancer patient. J. Pediatr. 98:341, 1981.

F. Use of immunosuppressive drugs for treatment of neoplasia
G. Immunologic diseases such as lupus erythematosus
H. Transplantation rejection reactions
I. Sickle cell anemia patients have an increased susceptibility to pneumococcal meningitis, bacteremia and pneumonia.
J. Children with the nephrotic syndrome may develop secondary hypogammaglobulinemia owing to urinary protein loss and increased catabolism. Such hypogammaglobulinemia may contribute to increased susceptibility to bacterial infection.
K. Children with intrauterine growth retardation have impaired cellular immunity at birth and for at least the first five years of life. An increased susceptibility to infection and an inadequate response to immunization are characteristically present.

Ferguson, A. C.: Prolonged impairment of cellular immunity in children with intrauterine growth retardation. J. Pediatr. 93:52, 1978.

L. Burns
M. Poorly controlled diabetes mellitus
N. Chronic renal failure

Screening Tests for Presence of Immune Deficiency

I. PHAGOCYTES

A. White blood cell count and differential
B. Nitroblue tetrazolium test
C. Serum IgE concentration

II. CELLULAR IMMUNODEFICIENCY: determination of delayed hypersensitivity to *Candida albicans*, SKSD, DT and *Trichophyton*

III. ANTIBODY

A. Quantitative serum IgA, IgG, IgM
B. Rubella titer
C. Isohemagglutinins

IV. COMPLEMENT

A. Total hemolytic complement activity
B. C3, C4, C5

GENERAL REFERENCES

Ammann, A. S.: T cell and T-B cell immunodeficiency disorders. Pediatr. Clin. North Am. 24:293, 1977.
Hill, H. R.: Laboratory aspects of immune deficiency in children. Pediatr. Clin. North Am. 27:805, 1980.
Johnston, R. B., Jr.: Recurrent bacterial infections in children. N. Engl. J. Med. 310:1237, 1984.
Rosen, F. S., Cooper, M. D., and Wedgewood, R. J. P.: The primary immunodeficiencies. N. Engl. J. Med. 311:235, 300, 1984.
Siegel, R. L.: Clinical disorders associated with T cell subset abnormalities. Adv. Pediatr. 31:447, 1984.

ETIOLOGIC CLASSIFICATION OF IMMUNODEFICIENCY DISORDERS

I. PHAGOCYTIC DYSFUNCTION, 392
   A. Neutropenia, 392
      1. Cyclic neutropenia
      2. Congenital infantile agranulocytosis
      3. Chronic benign granulocytopenia of childhood
      4. Shwachman-Diamond syndrome
      5. Drug-induced neutropenia
      6. Aplastic anemia
      7. Acute leukemia
      8. Vitamin B_{12} or folic acid deficiency
      9. Neonatal isoimmune neutropenia
      10. Congestive splenomegaly
      11. Chronic granulocytopenia
      12. Cartilage-hair hypoplasia
   B. Disorders of neutrophil adherence, 393
      1. Absent membrane glycoprotein
      2. Thalassemia
   C. Disorders of phagocyte locomotion, 393
   D. Disorders of chemotaxis, 393
      1. Lazy leukocyte syndrome
      2. Ichthyosis
      3. Shwachman-Diamond syndrome
      4. Hyper IgE syndrome
   E. Defective opsonization, 393
      1. Complement deficiencies
      2. Antibody deficiencies
   F. Defective bactericidal function, 393
      1. Chronic granulomatous disease
      2. Familial lipochrome histiocytosis
      3. Glutathione synthetase deficiency
      4. Myeloperoxidase deficiency
      5. Chédiak-Higashi syndrome
      6. Tuftsin deficiency
II. DEFECTS PRIMARILY OF ANTIBODY PRODUCTION, 394
   A. Transient hypogammaglobulinemia, 394
   B. X-linked agammaglobulinemia, 394
   C. X-linked hypogammaglobulinemia with growth hormone deficiency, 394
   D. Autosomal agammaglobulinemia, 394
   E. Variable antibody deficiency syndrome, 394
   F. Partial or selective deficiency of major immunoglobulin classes or a subclass of IgG, 394
      1. IgA deficiency

      2. Partial gamma globulin deficiency
      3. IgM deficiency
      4. Low IgG and IgA with normal or high IgM
   G. Short-limbed dwarfism, 395
III. DEFECTS PRIMARILY OF CELLULAR IMMUNITY, 395
   A. Severe combined immune deficiency, 395
   B. Nezelof's syndrome, 395
   C. Combined immunodeficiency with enzyme deficiency, 395
      1. Purine nucleoside phosphorylase deficiency
      2. Adenosine deaminase deficiency
   D. Type l short-limbed dwarfism, 395
   E. X-linked lymphoproliferative syndrome, 395
   F. AIDS (acquired immune deficiency syndrome), 395
   G. Short-limbed dwarfism with cell-mediated immunodeficiency, 396
IV. COMPLEMENT DISORDERS, 396
   A. C3 or C5 deficiency or absence, 396
   B. Dysfunction of C5, 396
   C. Absence of C6, C7, C8 and defects in alternative complement pathway, 396
V. IMMUNODEFICIENCY ASSOCIATED WITH OTHER DEFECTS, 396
   A. DiGeorge's syndrome, 396
   B. Wiskott-Aldrich syndrome, 396
   C. Ataxia-telangiectasia, 397
VI. SECONDARY IMMUNODEFICIENCY DISORDERS, 397
   A. Splenectomy, 397
   B. Severe protein-caloric malnutrition, 397
   C. Congenital infections, 397
   D. Corticosteroid treatment, 397
   E. Malignancies, 397
   F. Immunosuppressive drugs for neoplasia, 397
   G. Lupus erythematosus, 397
   H. Transplantation rejection reactions, 397
   I. Sickle cell anemia, 397
   J. Nephrotic syndrome, 397
   K. Intrauterine growth retardation, 397
   L. Burns, 397
   M. Poorly controlled diabetes mellitus, 397
   N. Chronic renal failure, 397

54 / LYMPHADENOPATHY

Lymph nodes, often small, firm and shotty, are palpable to a variable degree in normal infants and children in the cervical, axillary, inguinal and occipital areas. Lymphadenopathy in the newborn infant is an abnormal finding.

Apart from the enlarged nodes, lymphadenopathy may be accompanied by local pain and tenderness. If suppuration occurs, the overlying skin becomes reddened. Stiffness of the neck and torticollis may accompany cervical adenopathy. Suppuration of retropharyngeal nodes (retropharyngeal abscess) leads to dysphagia and obstructive breathing. Mediastinal adenopathy may cause stridor, cyanosis, dyspnea, dysphagia, cough, pleural effusion, facial edema and venous congestion. Mesenteric and retroperitoneal adenopathy may be characterized by abdominal pain. Iliac adenitis may cause abdominal pain, tenderness, especially above Poupart's ligament, and a limp.

ETIOLOGIC CLASSIFICATION OF LYMPHADENOPATHY

I. INFECTIONS: bacterial, fungal, spirochetal and viral.

A. Acute, unilateral pyogenic adenitis is the most common type of lymphadenopathy. The involved node may be walnut-size, firm and tender with erythema of the overlying skin. Etiologic agents are predominantly group A beta hemolytic *Streptococcus, Staphylococcus* and viruses. Bilateral, acute cervical adenitis is usually caused by viral pharyngitis or infectious mononucleosis. Chronic, localized adenopathy is usually attributable to a persistent regional infection. Submaxillary adenopathy may develop secondary to stomatitis or a periapical dental abscess. Occipital and postauricular adenopathy may accompany infections, seborrheic dermatitis or pediculosis of the scalp. Epitrochlear and axillary lymphadenopathy may result from infections on the arms, whereas inguinal and femoral adenopathy may be secondary to those on the lower extremities. Preauricular adenopathy (Parinaud's syndrome) owing to uniocular granulomatous conjunctivitis may be caused by cat-scratch disease, chlamydial conjunctivitis, listeriosis, tularemia or tuberculosis. Adenovirus type 3 causes pharyngeal-conjunctival fever, a disorder characterized by follicular conjunctivitis with enlarged preauricular and/or posterior cervical nodes. Epidemic keratoconjunctivitis, caused by adenovirus type 8, is also accompanied by preauricular adenopathy. Mediastinal or hilar adenopathy of an infectious etiology may occur in patients with tuberculosis, chronic sinusitis, histoplasmosis, tularemia, infectious mononucleosis, candidiasis, coccidioidomycosis and bronchiectasis.

Hieber, J. P., Davis, A. T.: Staphylococcal cervical lymphadenitis in young infants. Pediatrics 57:424, 1976.

Marcy, S. M.: Cervical adenitis. Pediatr. Inf. Dis. 4:23 (May/June suppl.), 1985.

Margileth, A. M.: Cervical adenitis. Pediatr. Rev. 7:13, 1985.

Shenep, J. L., Kalwinsky, D. K., Feldman, S., and Pearson, T. A.: Mycotic cervical lymphadenitis following oral mucositis in children with leukemia. J. Pediatr. 106:243, 1985.

Zeanah, C. H., and Zusman, J.: Mediastinal and cervical histoplasmosis simulating malignancy. Am. J. Dis. Child. 133:47, 1979.

B. Tularemia. The primary lesion in patients with tularemia may be accompanied by regional adenopathy with local tenderness, pain, suppuration and fever. Generalized lymphadenopathy may also develop.

C. Tuberculosis. Generalized lymphadenopathy in a child with tuberculosis may indicate a hematogenous spread of tubercle bacilli. Localized involvement is most common in the mediastinal, mesenteric or anterior cervical nodes. Early, tuberculosis of the cervical nodes may be confused with lymphadenitis secondary to pharyngitis or with a lymphoma. Tuberculous nodes are initially discrete, firm, mobile and tender. If untreated, they become soft, fluctuant, matted, and adherent to the overlying skin, which may become erythematous. Draining sinuses may develop. Bilateral involvement is the rule, and pulmonary disease is commonly present. A tuberculous etiology is unlikely if the tuberculin test is negative.

D. Atypical mycobacteria also cause cervical or submandibular adenitis clinically similar to tuberculosis except that the involvement is usually unilateral.

Schaad, U. B., Votteler, T. P., McCracken, G. H., Jr., and Nelson, J. D.: Management of atypical mycobacterial lymphadenitis in childhood: A review based on 380 cases. J. Pediatr. 95:356, 1979.

E. Group B streptococcal cellulitis and adenitis, which may occur in infants less than two months of age, is characterized by an abrupt onset of fever, anorexia, irritability and facial or submandibular swelling. The blood culture is usually positive.

Baker, C. J.: Group B streptococcal cellulitis-adenitis in infants. Am. J. Dis. Child. 136:631, 1982.

F. Brucellosis may cause chronic or intermittent lymphadenopathy.

G. *Yersinia enterocolitica* may cause cervical lymphadenitis.

Jaffe, K. M., and Smith, A. L.: *Yesinia enterocolitica* cervical lymphadenitis. J. Pediatr. 97:937, 1980.

H. *Salmonella* infections may be accompanied by generalized lymphadenopathy.

I. Bubonic plague caused by *Yersinia pestis* may cause exquisitely tender lymphadenitis and erythema of the overlying skin in the inguinal, femoral, axillary or cervical regions. The history may disclose that a week prior to the onset of the illness the patient had visited a rural area of the West.

Mann, J. M., Shandler, L., and Cushing, A. H.: Pediatric plague. Pediatrics 69:762, 1982.

J. Cat-scratch disease is a common cause of localized adenopathy. The site of the scratch determines whether axillary, epitrochlear, supraclavicular, femoral, inguinal or submaxillary nodes are affected. Enlarged nodes may also appear in such unusual sites as under the pectoral, trapezius or sternomastoid muscles. Characteristically, the nodes are nontender, discrete, movable and moderately or greatly enlarged. Occasionally, tenderness, redness, warmth and even suppuration may occur. Lymphadenopathy may persist for weeks or months. Other symptoms include malaise, fever and skin lesions that resemble erythema multiforme or erythema nodosum. A red papule, 2 to 5 mm in diameter, at the site of the scratch may precede the appearance of adenopathy by a few days or weeks and persist for one to four weeks.

K. Rubella is characterized by enlargement and tenderness of the posterior auricular, posterior cervical and occipital lymph nodes. Scarlet fever may also be accompanied by cervical adenitis. Generalized superficial lymphadenopathy may occur in patients with measles, chickenpox, mumps or other viral disease.

L. Infectious mononucleosis is accompanied by lymph nodes that are discrete, firm, resilient, usually nontender and 1/2 to 3 inches in diameter. Enlarged anterior and cervical nodes are present, but postauricular and suboccipital lymphadenopathy is also frequent. Generalized lymphadenopathy may also occur. Hepatosplenomegaly is common.

Fernbach, D. J., and Starling, K. A.: Infectious mononucleosis. Pediatr. Clin. North Am. 19:957, 1972.

Ginsburg, C. M., Henle, W., Henle, G., and Horwitz, C. A.: Infectious mononucleosis in children. Evaluation of Epstein-Barr virus-specific serological data. JAMA 237:781, 1977.

Sumaya, C. V., and Ench, Y.: Epstein-Barr virus infectious mononucleosis in children. I. Clinical and general laboratory findings. Pediatrics 75:1003, 1985.

M. Cytomegalovirus infection may cause a mononucleosis-like syndrome with generalized lymphadenopathy, fever, atypical lymphocytes and hepatosplenomegaly.

N. Coxsackie virus may cause a syndrome consisting of cervical or axillary lymphadenopathy, conjunctivitis, painful hepatomegaly and/or splenomegaly, fever, nausea and vomiting.

O. Toxoplasmosis may cause an acquired infection simulating infectious mononucleosis and characterized by cervical, suboccipital, supraclavicular or generalized adenopathy and fever.

Rafaty, M. F.: Cervical adenopathy secondary to toxoplasmosis. Arch. Otolaryngol. 103:547, 1977.

P. Infants with atopic eczema may demonstrate generalized lymphadenopathy. The axillary nodes may become 2 to 3 cm in diameter

Q. Histoplasmosis, with the exception of mediastinal lymphadenopathy, is not a common cause of lymph node enlargement.

R. Rat-bite fever may be characterized by regional lymphadenopathy secondary to the primary lesion. Generalized lymphadenopathy may also occur.

S. Generalized adenopathy may be noted after typhoid immunization. Regional adenitis may follow pertussis vaccine, diphtheria toxoid and tetanus toxoid immunizations.

T. The Gianotti-Crosti syndrome consists of generalized lymphadenopathy, hepatomegaly, nonicteric hepatitis and crops of papular lesions that persist for two to eight weeks. (See page 177).

II. IMMUNOLOGIC OR CONNECTIVE TISSUE DISORDERS

A. Juvenile rheumatoid arthritis is a diagnostic consideration in children with unexplained fever and persistent lymphadenopathy.

B. Serum sickness is often accompanied by generalized, tender lymphadenopathy. The serum sickness type of reaction to penicillin may be characterized by lymphadenopathy, splenomegaly, myalgia and arthritis.

III. Primary Disease of Lymphoid or Reticuloendothelial Tissue; Metastatic Lymphadenopathy. Rapidly enlarging, confluent or fixed nodes and supraclavicular lymphadenopathy may be malignant.

A. Although lymphadenopathy may be an early manifestation of acute leukemia, lymph node enlargement does not become prominent until the disease is advanced. In many children, it never becomes remarkable. Lymphadenopathy is much more prominent, however, with juvenile chronic myelogenous leukemia.

Weisman, S. J., Berkow, R. L., and Baehner, R. L.: Chronic leukemia of childhood. Pediatr. Rev. 6:26, 1984.

B. Lymphosarcoma commonly involves the cervical and mediastinal lymph nodes unilaterally or bilaterally. Initially firm, rubbery, painless and discrete, the nodes soon become matted.
C. Reticulum cell sarcoma
D. Hodgkin's disease is usually characterized by an insidious, painless, unilateral enlargement of regional lymph nodes, most frequently the cervical and less commonly the supraclavicular, mediastinal, axillary, epitrochlear or inguinal nodes. Preauricular nodes may rarely be involved. The right supraclavicular node may enlarge secondary to mediastinal disease, whereas left supraclavicular adenopathy may occur secondary to abdominal involvement. At first the nodes are soft but they later become firm and rubbery. Although discrete, their large size and close proximity cause them to seem adherent and fixed. Pain may ensue with enlargement of the axillary or inguinal nodes. Superimposed infections, such as pharyngitis, may cause further enlargement and pain.

Canellos, G. P.: Hodgkin's disease. Pediatr. Rev. 6:3, 1984.
Gilchrist, G. S., and Evans, R. G.: Contemporary issues in pediatric Hodgkin's disease. Pediatr. Clin. North Am. 32:721, 1985.

E. Non-Hodgkin's lymphoma may present as rapidly enlarging peripheral or mediastinal lymphadenopathy. Tumors of B-lymphocyte origin include Burkitt's and the diffuse large cell lymphoma. The lymphoblastic and the T-immunoblastic lymphomas are of T-lymphocyte derivation. Mediastinal involvement may cause obstruction of the superior vena cava.

Link, M. P.: Non-Hodgkin's lymphoma in children. Pediatr. Clin. North Am. 32:699, 1985.
Murphy, S. B.: Current concepts in cancer: Childhood non-Hodgkin's lymphoma. N. Engl. J. Med. 299:1446, 1978.
Quinn, J.JH.: Non-Hodgkin's lymphoma in children. Curr. Probl. Pediatr. 12:5, 1983.

F. Malignant histiocytosis or histiocytic lymphoma may present with fever, lymphadenopathy, hepatosplenomegaly and weight loss.
G. Non-endemic Burkitt's tumor may present as cervical lymphadenopathy.
H. Rhabdomyosarcoma of the nasopharynx may first be manifest as cervical adenopathy in the upper third of the neck.
I. Neuroblastoma may cause a neck mass that simulates enlarged cervical nodes. In metastatic neuroblastoma, the left supraclavicular (Virchow's) node, involved secondary to extension up the thoracic duct, may be the initial clinical finding.
J. Because of the possibility of thyroid carcinoma, careful palpation of the thyroid is indicated in patients with cervical adenopathy. Enlarged, firm, discrete cervical lymph nodes may be the initial complaint with thyroid carcinoma in the absence of a palpable thyroid nodule. Regional adenopathy may accompany chronic lymphocytic thyroiditis.
K. Histiocytosis X
L. Benign sinus histiocytosis is characterized by painless, bilateral, massive cervical lymphadenopathy that develops insidiously and persists for months or years or recurs. Fever, anorexia, weight loss, anemia, leukocytosis, elevated erythrocyte sedimentation rate and hyperglobulinemia are other findings.

Rosai, J., and Dorfman, R. F.: Sinus histiocytosis with massive lymphadenopathy: A pseudolymphomatous benign disorder. Analysis of 34 cases. Cancer 30:1174, 1972.

M. Angioimmunoblastic or immunoblastic lymphadenopathy is characterized by generalized mild, slightly tender lymphadenopathy, fever, hepatosplenomegaly, pulmonary infiltration, polyarthralgia, skin rash and weight loss.

Lukes, R. J., and Tindle, B. H.: Immunoblastic lymphadenopathy: A hyperimmune entity resembling Hodgkin's disease. N. Engl. J. Med. 292:1, 1975.

N. Chronic pseudolymphomatous lymphadenopathy (chronic benign lymphadenopathy) is characterized by generalized lymphadenopathy, splenomegaly, hypergammaglobulinemia, thrombocytopenia and hemolytic anemia.

IV. IMMUNODEFICIENCY SYNDROMES; PHAGOCYTIC DYSFUNCTION

A. Chronic granulomatous disease of childhood is characterized by chronic suppurative lymphadenitis involving especially the cervical nodes, hepatosplenomegaly, pulmonary infiltration and recurrent infections.
B. Acquired immune deficiency syndrome (AIDS) in infants of high risk parents or hemophilia patients who have received transfusions is characterized by generalized lymphadenopathy, failure to thrive, fever, hepatosplenomegaly, oropharyngeal candidiasis, interstitial pneumonia, chronic diarrhea and hypergammaglobulinemia.
C. Hyper IgE (Job's) syndrome is characterized by recurrent staphylococcal cold skin abscesses and suppurative lymphadenitis.

V. METABOLIC AND STORAGE DISEASES may be accompanied by generalized lymphadenopathy.

A. Gaucher's disease
B. Neimann-Pick disease
C. Histiocytosis X
D. Cystinosis

VI. HEMATOPOIETIC DISEASES may be accompanied by generalized lymphadenopathy.

A. Sickle cell anemia
B. Thalassemia
C. Congenital hemolytic anemia
D. Autoimmune hemolytic anemia may be accompanied by massively enlarged, nontender lymph nodes owing to cytomegalovirus infection.

VII. OTHER DISORDERS CHARACTERIZED BY LYMPHADENOPATHY

A. Kawasaki disease. Cervical lymphadenopathy, the least constant of the principal criteria of Kawasaki disease, is usually unilateral, firm, nontender and over 1.5 cm in diameter. The overlying skin may be erythematous but not warm.

Kawasaki, T., Kosaki, F., Okawa, M. D., Shigematsu, I., and Yanagawa, H.: A new infantile acute febrile mucocutaneous lymph node syndrome (MLNS) prevailing in Japan. Pediatrics 54:271, 1974.

B. Mesantoin may cause enlargement of lymph nodes, most commonly those in the cervical region, fever, eosinophilia, rash and hepatosplenomegaly. Hydantoin may also produce lymphadenopathy as a side effect.

Snead, C., Siegel, N., and Hayslett, J.: Generalized lymphadenopathy and nephrotic syndrome as a manifestation of mephenytoin (mesantoin) toxicity. Pediatrics 57:98, 1976.

C. Sarcoidosis. Almost all patients with sarcoidosis demonstrate either generalized or hilar lymphadenopathy. The bilateral cervical nodes, when enlarged, are firm, rubbery and discrete with little tendency to coalesce. Other symptoms include fatigue, cough, fever, dyspnea and weight loss. Hyperglobulinemia and eosinophilia are common laboratory findings.

Kendig, E. L.: The clinical picture of sarcoidosis in children. Pediatrics 54:289, 1974.

GENERAL REFERENCES

Barton, L. L., and Feigin, R. D.: Childhood cervical lymphadenitis: A reappraisal. J. Pediatr. 84:846, 1974.
Kissane, J. M., and Gephardt, G. N.: Lymphadenopathy in childhood: Long-term follow-up in patients with non-diagnostic lymph node biopsies. Hum. Pathol. 5:431, 1974.
Lake, A. M., and Oski, F. A.: Peripheral lymphadenopathy in childhood. Ten-year experience with excisional biopsy. Am. J. Dis. Child. 132:375, 1978.
Schmitt, B. D.: Cervical adenopathy in children. Postgrad. Med. 60:251, 1976.
Sinclair, S., Beckman, E., and Ellman, L.: Biopsy of enlarged superficial lymph nodes. JAMA 228:602, 1974.
Zuelzer, W. W., and Kaplan, J.: The child with lymphadenopathy. Semin. Hematol. 12:323, 1975.

ETIOLOGIC CLASSIFICATION OF LYMPHADENOPATHY

I. INFECTIONS: BACTERIAL, FUNGAL, SPIROCHETAL AND VIRAL, 399
   A. Pyogenic lymphadenopathy, 399
   B. Tularemia, 399
   C. Tuberculosis, 399
   D. Atypical mycobacteria, 399
   E. Streptococcal cellulitis, 399
   F. Brucellosis, 399
   G. *Yersinia enterocolita*, 399
   H. *Salmonella* infection, 400
   I. Bubonic plague, 400
   J. Cat-scratch disease, 400
   K. Rubella, 400
   L. Infectious mononucleosis, 400
   M. Cytomegalovirus, 400
   N. Coxsackie virus, 400
   O. Eczema, 400
   P. Histoplasmosis, 400
   Q. Rat-bite fever, 400

II. IMMUNOLOGIC OR CONNECTIVE TISSUE DISORDERS, 400
   A. Juvenile rheumatoid arthritis, 400
   B. Serum sickness, 400

III. PRIMARY DISEASE OF LYMPHOID OR RETICULOENDOTHELIAL TISSUE; METASTATIC LYMPHADENOPATHY, 401
   A. Leukemia, 401
   B. Lymphosarcoma, 401
   C. Reticulum cell sarcoma, 401
   D. Hodgkin's disease, 401
   E. Non-Hodgkin's lymphoma, 401
   F. Malignant histiocytosis or histiocytic lymphoma, 401

G. Non-endemic Burkitt's tumor, 401
H. Rhabdomyosarcoma, 401
I. Neuroblastoma, 401
J. Carcinoma of the thyroid, 401
K. Histiocytosis X, 401
L. Benign sinus histiocytosis, 401
M. Angioimmunoblastic lymphadenopathy, 401
N. Chronic pseudolymphomatous lymphadenopathy, 401

IV. IMMUNODEFICIENCY SYNDROMES; PHAGOCYTIC DYSFUNCTION, 402
   A. Chronic granulomatous disease, 402
   B. AIDS (acquired immune deficiency syndrome), 402
   C. Hyper IgE (Job's) syndrome, 402

V. Metabolic and storage diseases, 402
   A. Gaucher's disease, 402
   B. Niemann-Pick disease, 402
   C. Histiocytosis X, 402
   D. Cystinosis, 402

VI. HEMATOPOIETIC DISEASES, 402
   A. Sickle cell anemia, 402
   B. Thalassemia, 402
   C. Congenital hemolytic anemia, 402
   D. Autoimmune hemolytic anemia, 402

VII. OTHER DISORDERS, 402
   A. Kawasaki disease, 402
   B. Mesantoin medication, 402
   C. Sarcoidosis, 402

55 / FATIGUE

Fatigue is a subjective complaint present with or without exertion, whereas weakness is associated with muscular activity. The interview and physical examination, supplemented by appropriate laboratory examinations (mono spot test, SGOT, BUN, serum creatinine, CBC, T_3, T_4, sedimentation rate, and chest x-ray) and, perhaps, a test for pregnancy usually permit a diagnosis to be established readily.

ETIOLOGIC CLASSIFICATION OF FATIGUE

I. EMOTIONAL ETIOLOGIC FACTORS

A. Depression is probably the most common cause of chronic fatigue in children and adolescents. The patient reports awakening tired and has a frequent need to rest during the day. Associated symp-

toms may include headache, insomnia, anorexia, apathy, irritability and dysphoric mood. (See page 445.)
B. Masked school avoidance should be considered in older children and adolescents seen because of chronic fatigue.
C. Grief is characterized by feelings of overwhelming fatigue and lassitude.
D. Hyperventilation syndrome is characterized by fatigue, precordial pain and lightheadedness.
E. Hypochondriasis

II. INFECTIONS

A. Infectious mononucleosis (EBV) is commonly accompanied by easy fatigability. Besides fatigue, lethargy and depressive symptoms may persist for weeks or months after this or other viral illnesses. EBV antibody helps determine the diagnosis.

Jones, J. F., Ray, C. G., Minnich, L. L., Hicks, M. S., Kibler, R., and Lucas, D. O.: Evidence of active Epstein-Barr virus infection in patients with persistent, unexplained illnesses; elevated anti-early antigen antibodies. Ann. Intern. Med. 102:1, 1985.

B. Cytomegalovirus (CMV) mononucleosis may cause persistent malaise and fatigue. Pharyngitis, lymphadenopathy and splenomegaly are usually not present. Lymphocytosis with atypical lymphocytes may be reported. Paired samples for CMV titers may be diagnostically helpful.
C. Subclinical infectious hepatitis may account for fatigue. Determination of SGOT may be indicated.
D. Chronic aggressive hepatitis is characterized by fatigue, anorexia and, at times, splenomegaly and spider angiomata.
E. Tuberculosis
F. Histoplasmosis
G. Chronic infections

III. HEMATOLOGY/ONCOLOGY

A. Anemia
B. Leukemia; lymphoma; chronic myelogenous leukemia

IV. ENDOCRINE

A. Cushing's disease
B. Addison's disease
C. Hypo- and hyperthyroidism. With Graves' disease, insomnia or restless sleep may cause daytime sleepiness and easy fatigability.

D. Primary hyperaldosteronism
E. Pheochromocytoma may cause weakness, exhaustion and fatigue.

V. CONNECTIVE TISSUE DISORDERS

A. Lupus erythematosus. Fatigue is a prominent symptom in patients with this disorder.
B. Dermatomyositis
C. Rheumatoid arthritis
D. Fibromyalgia, a disorder that most frequently occurs in adolescent girls, is manifest by chronic fatigue, stiffness, restless sleep, musculoskeletal aches and pains, and multiple tender points.

VI. ALLERGIC

A. Allergic rhinitis, if severe, causes the child to feel tired.
B. "Tension-fatigue" syndrome, a term applied to a somewhat vague group of symptoms and ascribed to food allergy, is not an established disorder.

VII. SLEEP DISORDERS (See page 317.)

A. Insufficient sleep is a common cause of fatigue in school-age children who stay up late at night.
B. Obstructive sleep apnea is an unusual but important cause of fatigue. Loud snoring and repeated episodes of apnea occur during sleep.
C. Insomnia in the older adolescent patient may cause fatigue. Many middle and late adolescents complain of difficulty sleeping and chronic fatigue although they are not depressed.

VIII. CARDIOVASCULAR

A. Congenital heart disease with hypoxemia
B. Primary pulmonary hypertension
C. Hypertrophic obstructive cardiomyopathy may cause easy fatigability, syncope and dizziness.
D. Takayasu's arteritis may be characterized early by fatigue along with fever, anorexia, arthralgia, asymmetric pulses and hypertension.

IX. OTHER DISORDERS

A. Sarcoidosis presents with fatigue, malaise or lethargy in about one third of patients. Bilateral hilar adenopathy is a frequent finding.
B. Myasthenia gravis

C. Chronic renal disease may be clinically manifest by easy fatigability, pallor, anorexia, poor statural growth and polyuria.
D. Respiratory failure and chronic pulmonary diseases, such as cystic fibrosis, interstitial pneumonitis or hypersensitivity pneumonitis are accompanied by fatigue.

E. Chronic acidosis or ketosis causes a child to be tired and to feel ill.
F. Heat exhaustion, characterized by excessive fatigue, weakness, muscle cramps, headaches and dizziness, is a prodrome to heat stroke.
G. Pregnancy may be characterized by fatigue, nausea and vomiting during the first trimester.

56 / EDEMA; ANGIOEDEMA

Edema represents an abnormal increase in the amount of extravascular, extracellular fluid. The following discussion relates some of the complex and ill-defined mechanisms that are usually concurrently or sequentially involved in edema production to a variety of clinical disorders. See page 163 for a discussion of localized edema.

ETIOLOGIC CLASSIFICATION OF EDEMA

The factors contributing to edema formation and the disease states in which they are operative may be summarized as follows:

I. INCREASED HYDROSTATIC PRESSURE. Increase in the hydrostatic pressure promotes the filtration of fluid from the intravascular to the interstitial spaces. The increased hydrostatic pressure in localized inflammatory states results from capillary dilatation with transmission of a greater than normal head of pressure; however, increased hydrostatic pressure is not always accompanied by edema formation, (e.g., congenital absence of a portion of the inferior vena cava may not lead to edema of the lower extremities). Patients with constrictive pericarditis and chronic elevation of the venous pressure also may or may not demonstrate edema. The role of an elevated venous pressure in patients with congestive cardiac failure is not uniformly clear.

A. Constrictive pericarditis
B. Portal hypertension

C. Congestive heart failure
D. Budd-Chiari syndrome
E. Thrombophlebitis
F. Extrinsic pressure by tumor mass on veins

II. DECREASED ONCOTIC PRESSURE. A low serum albumin permits escape of fluid from the vascular system. As a result, the decreased circulatory volume leads to an increased reabsorption of sodium, perhaps an increased secretion of antidiuretic hormone, and an activation of other compensatory mechanisms. The oncotic pressure, however, may not be the major etiologic factor in edema formation in these disorders. Nutritional edema, for example, may occur without much change in serum protein concentration.

A. Inadequate intake, impaired alimentation, failure of utilization or loss of protein from the gastrointestinal tract, as in protein-losing enteropathy, may be etiologically associated with edema formation. Protein loss into the gastrointestinal tract or protein-losing gastroenteropathy occurs with intestinal lymphangiectasia; Crohn's disease; ulcerative colitis; *Strongyloides stercoralis* infection; constrictive pericarditis; gastrointestinal allergy, including intolerance to cow milk; celiac syndrome; lymphoma; and congenital ileal stenosis. Clinical and laboratory findings include hypoproteinemia, hypogammaglobulinemia, ascites and pleural effusion, as well as edema. Infants with cow's milk intolerance may show iron-deficiency anemia, occult blood in the stools and eosinophilia. Most patients with intestinal lymphangiectasia demonstrate mild diarrhea or steatorrhea. Hypercatabolic hypoproteinemia owing to an increased rate of plasma protein degradation occurs in the nephrotic syndrome. Edema caused by hypoproteinemia is rarely an early manifestation of celiac disease or cystic fibrosis. Kwashiorkor or protein-calorie malnutrition in infants in the United States is usually not associated with poverty but attributable to dietary fads, including vegetarian diets; parents' inadequate nutritional education; mismanagement of food allergies; excessive dilution of infant formula; or the feeding of nondairy creamer to infants.

Chase, H. P., Kumar, V., Caldwell, R. T., and O'Brien, D.: Kwashiorkor in the United States. Pediatrics 66:972, 1980.

Lee, P. A., Roloff, D. W., and Howatt, W. F.: Hypoproteinemia and anemia in infants with cystic fibrosis. A presenting symptom complex often misdiagnosed. JAMA 228:585, 1974.

Sinatra, F. R., and Merritt, R. J.: Iatrogenic kwashiorkor in infants. Am. J. Dis. Child. 135:21, 1981.

B. Impaired production of protein owing to liver disease or in association with chronic constrictive pericarditis
C. Loss of protein in patients with nephrosis or those with ascites, especially associated with inflammatory or malignant disorders. Loss of protein also occurs through the skin, as in Leiner's disease. The cause of edema in the nephrotic syndrome is complex. Increased permeability of the glomerulus permits protein loss into the urine. The resulting hypoproteinemia and decreased plasma colloid osmotic pressure contributes to edema formation by permitting the transudation of fluid into the interstitial spaces. Another etiologic factor is an increase in tubular reabsorption of sodium, possibly secondary to increased renin secretion and aldosterone excretion. Water retention may be an effect of antidiuretic hormone secretion.

Grupe, W. E.: Primary nephrotic syndrome in childhood. Adv. Pediatr 26:163, 1979.

III. INCREASED CAPILLARY PERMEABILITY. The control of capillary permeability is incompletely understood. A possible explanation for the relatively high protein content of ascitic or pleural fluid may be that the capillaries in these serous cavities are relatively more permeable or that lymphatic drainage from these areas is less efficient than elsewhere.

A. Allergic reactions
B. Inflammatory reactions: chemical, thermal, bacterial, rickettsial. Generalized edema may occur as a presenting sign in patients with Rocky Mountain spotted fever owing to generalized vasculitis.

IV. TISSUE TENSION. Before edema can become evident, tissue tension must be relatively low. Low tissue tension may account for the localization of slight edema in the periorbital region, scrotum, vulva and the dorsum of the hands and feet in young infants.

V. SODIUM AND WATER RETENTION. Sodium plays an etiologic role in most instances of edema. Sodium retention is generally accompanied by that of water. Eighty to 90 per cent of the glomerular filtrate of water undergoes obligatory reabsorption in the proximal tubules along with sodium and chloride. The remainder of the water is subject to facultative reabsorption in the distal tubule in response to the action of the antidiuretic hormone. An increased excretion of antidiuretic hormone occurs in some patients with hepatic cirrhosis and ascites, congestive cardiac failure and nephrosis. Peripheral edema and variable hepatomegaly have been reported in a few children with diabetes mellitus during the first three weeks of treatment. The cause of the edema may be related to increased deposition of glycogen accompanied by water retention. Edema of the extremities may occur premenstrually.

A. Congestive cardiac failure. Edema, usually confined to the sacrum and around the eyes, is a much less common manifestation of congestive cardiac failure in infants and children than in adults. The decreased renal plasma flow and diminished glomerular filtration rate associated with cardiac failure result in sodium and water retention. Antidiuretic hormone and aldosterone production may be increased.
B. Hepatic cirrhosis
C. Chronic anemia
D. Acute glomerulonephritis. Glomerular function is relatively more impaired than tubular activity in most patients with acute glomerulonephritis. Normal tubular function in the presence of a decreased glomerular filtration rate facili-

tates increased tubular reabsorption of sodium and water. If the tubular ability to reabsorb sodium is also impaired, abnormal sodium retention may not occur. The congestive cardiac failure present in some of these patients may also contribute to edema formation. Generalized edema may occur with few abnormal findings on urinalysis.

E. Nephrotic syndrome
F. Excessive administration of saline
G. Administration of corticosteroids
H. Diabetes mellitus during early treatment
I. Premenstrual syndrome

VI. IMPAIRMENT OF LYMPHATIC RETURN

VII. IDIOPATHIC CYCLIC EDEMA may occur in adolescent girls with a history of swelling of the face and hands in the morning followed by edema of the abdomen and lower extremities. The swelling is generally worse in hot weather, during menstruation, in the afternoon and evening and with prolonged standing. Bloating and fatigue may be accompanying symptoms. Edema may also be characteristic of the premenstrual syndrome.

ETIOLOGIC CLASSIFICATION OF EDEMA OF THE NEWBORN

I. EDEMA OF PREMATURITY. Transitory edema of the hands, feet, face and genitalia occasionally occurs in premature infants on the second or third day of life. Generalized edema is less frequent. The cause is not established.

II. HYDROPS FETALIS WITH ANASARCA AND ASCITES

A. Fetal
  1. Hematologic
    a. Thalassemia (Bart's hemoglobin)
    b. Twin-to-twin transfusion
    c. Chronic fetomaternal transfusion
    d. Hemolytic disease of the newborn owing to Rh isoimmunization
  2. Cardiovascular
    a. Major congenital cardiac anomaly
    b. Myocarditis
    c. Arteriovenous malformation
    d. Tachyarrhythmias
    e. Bradyarrhythmias; congenital heart block
  3. Pulmonary
    a. Cystic adenomatoid malformation of lung
    b. Pulmonary lymphangiectasia
    c. Hypoplasia of the lung
  4. Renal
    a. Congenital nephrosis
    b. Renal vein thrombosis
  5. Intrauterine infection
  6. Congenital anomalies, including chromosomal disorders and short-rib polydactyly dwarfism of the Saldino-Noonan type.

B. Placental
  1. Umbilical vein thrombosis
  2. Chorioangioma

Sweet, L., Reid, W. D., and Roberton, N. R. C.: Hydrops fetalis in association with chorioangioma of the placenta. J. Pediatr. 82:91, 1973.

C. Maternal
  1. Diabetes mellitus
  2. Toxemia

D. Idiopathic

Etches, P. C., and Lemons, J. A.: Nonimmune hydrops fetalis: Report of 22 cases including three siblings. Pediatrics 64:326, 1979.

III. OTHER CAUSES

A. Edema of the hands and feet may occur in infants with the respiratory distress syndrome.
B. Edema most evident on the lower extremities, feet, labia, and eyelids, along with hemolytic anemia, may occur with vitamin E deficiency in the premature infant.

Oski, F. A.: Anemia in infancy: Iron deficiency and vitamin E deficiency. Pediatr. Rev. 1:247, 1980.

C. Neonatal myotonic dystrophy may be accompanied by edema, especially of the head and extremities, owing perhaps to reduction in the lymphatic return associated with diminished fetal movement.

Pearse, R. G., and Howeler, C. J.: Neonatal form of dystrophia myotonica. Arch. Dis. Child. 54:331, 1979.

D. Zinc deficiency may cause generalized edema and hypoproteinemia in prematurely born infants between five and nine weeks of age.

Kumar, S. P., and Anday, E. K.: Edema, hypoproteinemia, and zinc deficiency in low-birth-weight infants. Pediatrics 73:327, 1984.

ETIOLOGIC CLASSIFICATION OF EDEMA

I. INCREASED HYDROSTATIC PRESSURE, 405
  A. Constrictive pericarditis, 405
  B. Portal hypertension, 405
  C. Congestive heart failure, 405
  D. Budd-Chiari syndrome, 405
  E. Thrombophlebitis, 405
  F. Extrinsic pressure upon veins from tumor mass, 405
II. DECREASED ONCOTIC PRESSURE, 405
  A. Inadequate intake, impaired alimentation, failure of utilization or loss of protein from the gastrointestinal tract, 405
  B. Impaired production of protein owing to liver disease or in association with chronic constrictive pericarditis, 406
  C. Loss of protein in nephrosis or ascites owing to an inflammatory or malignant disorder, 406

III. INCREASED CAPILLARY PERMEABILITY, 406
  A. Allergic reaction, 406
  B. Inflammatory reaction: chemical, thermal, bacterial, rickettsial, 406
IV. DECREASED TISSUE TENSION, 406
V. SODIUM AND WATER RETENTION, 406
  A. Congestive heart failure, 406
  B. Hepatic cirrhosis, 406
  C. Chronic anemia, 406
  D. Acute glomerulonephritis, 406
  E. Nephrotic syndrome, 407
  F. Excessive administration of saline, 407
  G. Administration of corticosteroids, 407
  H. Diabetes mellitus, 407
  I. Premenstrual syndrome, 407
VI. IMPAIRMENT OF LYMPHATIC RETURN, 407
VII. IDIOPATHIC CYCLIC EDEMA, 407

ASCITES

Ascites, the accumulation of serous fluid in the peritoneal cavity, may be caused by a combination of factors including hypoalbuminemia, portal hypertension, overproduction of lymph, increased aldosterone and antidiuretic hormone secretion and enhanced renal reabsorption of sodium and water. The following are some of the clinical disorders associated with ascites.

I. CONGESTIVE CARDIAC FAILURE

II. CHRONIC CONSTRICTIVE PERICARDITIS

Idriss, F. S., Nikaidoh, H., and Muster, A. J.: Constrictive pericarditis simulating liver disease in children. Arch. Surg. 109:223, 1974.
Simcha, A., and Taylor, J. F. N.: Constrictive pericarditis in childhood. Arch. Dis. Child. 46:515, 1971.

III. NEPHROTIC SYNDROME

IV. HEPATIC CIRRHOSIS; CHRONIC AGGRESSIVE HEPATITIS

V. PORTAL HYPERTENSION owing to cirrhosis, Budd-Chiari syndrome or elevated right ventricular pressure. Portal hypertension owing to a prehepatic or presinusoidal obstruction usually does not cause ascites.

VI. BUDD-CHIARI SYNDROME, OBLITERATIVE ENDOPHLEBITIS of the hepatic veins or the hepatic portion of the inferior vena cava

VII. PROTEIN-CALORIE MALNUTRITION

VIII. MALIGNANCY

IX. BILE ASCITES OR BILE PERITONITIS owing to the perforation of the common bile duct may simulate a surgical abdomen with distention, pain and toxicity. Chronic bile ascites is characterized by abdominal distention, acholic stools, fluctuating jaundice, ascites and inguinal hernias. Early, the ascitic fluid may not be bile-stained.

Hansen, R. C., Wasnich, R. D., DeVries, P. A., and Sunshine, P.: Bile ascites in infancy: Diagnosis with ^{131}I-rose bengal. J. Pediatr. 84:719, 1974.

X. PROTEIN-LOSING GASTROENTEROPATHY

XI. Because ASCITES may occur secondary to pancreatitis, serum and ascitic fluid amylase and lipase determinations should be obtained in children with otherwise unexplained ascites.

Kalwinsky, D., Frittelli, G., and Oski, F. A.: Pancreatitis presenting as unexplained ascites. Am. J. Dis. Child. 128:734, 1974.

XII. PRESSURE ON LYMPHATIC OR VENOUS CHANNELS

XIII. INFLAMMATORY PERITONEAL REACTION

XIV. LEUKEMIA, HODGKIN'S DISEASE

XV. CHYLOUS ASCITES, diagnosed by paracentesis and the finding of milky fluid that clears with ether and contains sudan red staining fat particles, may occur secondary to trauma or to an abdominal, retroperitoneal, mediastinal or thoracic neoplasm.

XVI. PERITONITIS, especially the ascitic form of tuberculous peritonitis; tularemia

XVII. CONGENITAL ASCITES may be associated with bilateral hydronephrosis and hydroureters. The cause is not known.

XVIII. ASCITES occurs early in infants with galactosemia.

GENERAL REFERENCE

Wyllie, R., Arasu, T. S., and Fitzgerald, J. F.: Ascites: pathophysiology and management. J. Pediatr. 97:167, 1980.

ETIOLOGIC CLASSIFICATION OF ANGIOEDEMA

Angioedema, which causes pale, well-demarcated, tense, brawny, nonpruritic and nonpitting single or multiple localized swellings, involves the face, tongue, lips, larynx, ear, periorbital tissues, genitalia, extremities and gastrointestinal tract. Lesions, which may be accompanied by urticaria, may persist for only a few hours or up to three days. In over 90 per cent of cases, the cause of angioedema is not known.

I. IgE MEDIATED

A. Episodic angioedema associated with eosinophilia is characterized by attacks of urticaria, angioedema, fever, striking leukocytosis, eosinophilia and a 10 to 18 per cent weight gain.

Gleich, G. J., Schroeter, A. L., Marcoux, J. P., Sacks, M. I., O'Connell, E. J., and Kohler, P. F.: Episodic angioedema associated with eosinophilia. N. Engl. J. Med. 310:1621, 1984.

B. Allergic reactions to food or drugs
C. Physically-induced angioedema
   1. Pressure angioedema of feet, buttocks or hands caused by walking, sitting or manual activities involving the hands. The swelling may follow the activity four to six hours later.
   2. Vibratory angioedema owing to vigorous rubbing
   3. Exercise-induced

II. HYPOCOMPLEMENTEMIC (HEREDITARY) ANGIOEDEMA occurs on an autosomal dominant basis, though a positive family history may not be reported. In the most frequent form, Cl inhibitor is low but functionally normal. Other patients with hereditary angioedema have nonfunctional Cl inhibitor. Recurrent episodes of angioedema, abdominal pain, nausea and vomiting occur either spontaneously or after local trauma, especially of the upper respiratory tract; vigorous exercise; emotional stress; or with menstrual periods.

III. IDIOSYNCRATIC

A. Nonsteroidal anti-inflammatory drugs
B. Other drugs

IV. LUPUS ERYTHEMATOSUS may be a cause of angioedema as well as persistent urticaria.

V. IDIOPATHIC

GENERAL REFERENCES

Buckley, R. H., and Mathews, K. P.: Common "allergic" skin diseases. JAMA 248:2611, 1982.
Kaplan, A. P.: The pathogenic basis of urticaria and angioedema: Recent advances. Am. J. Med. 70:755, 1981.

57 / LIMB AND MUSCULOSKELETAL PAIN

ETIOLOGIC CLASSIFICATION OF LIMB PAINS

I. NONARTICULAR LIMB (GROWING) PAINS that occur principally at night, usually in the thighs, the calves, behind the knees and, at times, in the arms, are common in preschool children but may also occur in older children and adolescents. The pain, which lasts from minutes to hours, varies considerably in frequency and intensity. Though sometimes severe and deep aching, the pain, at other times, may just cause restlessness. Some children awaken crying with pain; others complain less intensely. Usually, massage of the extremities or heat application brings symptomatic relief. Nocturnal limb pains, which may be associated with muscle fatigue, vigorous physical activity or minor orthopedic defects, are almost never attributable to rheumatic fever. Usually the exact cause cannot be determined. Daytime pain may be exacerbated by exercise and interrupt the child's physical activity.

Øster, J., and Nielsen, A.: Growing pains. Acta Paediatr. Scand. 61:329, 1972.

Peterson, H. A.: Leg aches. Pediatr. Clin. North Am. 24:731, 1977.

II. ORTHOPEDIC DISORDERS affecting the lower extremities

A. Pes planus
B. Pronated feet
C. Genu valgum
D. Bowlegs
E. Tight Achilles tendon
F. Contracted or shortened hamstring muscles
G. Hypermobility syndrome. (See page 153.) Children with generalized ligamentous relaxation may complain of leg pains following exercise.

III. JOINT DISORDERS

A. Arthritis. (See page 141.)
B. Hip joint disorders. *A roentgenogram of the hip is indicated in all patients who have unexplained knee pain.*
   1. Osteochondrosis of the femoral capital epiphysis (Legg-Calvé-Perthes disease) is characterized by the insidious appearance of an almost imperceptible limp. Pain, which may be referred along the distribution of the obturator nerve to the medial aspect of the thigh and knee, is usually slight and may simulate that of myalgia or muscle stiffness.
   2. Slipped femoral epiphysis. Pain in the knee or in the medial aspect of the thigh above the knee, referred along the course of the obturator nerve from the hip, is the earliest sign of a slipped epiphysis.
C. Knee
   1. Patellofemoral pain (See page 148.)
   2. Osteochondritis dissecans (See page 149.)

IV. BONE TUMORS. Persistent bone pain may be caused by a bone tumor.

A. Ewing's tumor
B. Osteogenic sarcoma
C. Osteochondroma
D. Osteoid osteoma. Pain, at times described as boring and aching in character, is often present at night and relieved by aspirin. Muscle atrophy develops over time.
E. Metastatic neuroblastoma may cause bone pain, limp and painful joints.
F. Primary lymphosarcoma of the bone may present with bone pain.

V. TRAUMA

A. Sprains
B. Fractures, especially chip and greenstick fractures
C. Traumatic periostitis

VI. OTHER DISEASES AFFECTING BONE

A. Rickets
B. Infantile cortical hyperostosis

410

C. Vitamin A poisoning
D. Hyperparathyroidism
E. Osteomyelitis, including chronic meta-physeal osteomyelitis and chronic mul-tifocal symmetrical osteomyelitis

Meller, Y., Yagupsky, P., Elitsur, Y., Inbar-Ianay, I., and Bar-Ziv, J.: Chronic multifocal symmetrical osteomyelitis. Am. J. Dis. Child. 138:349, 1984.

F. Gaucher's disease may be associated with skeletal pain, either generalized or localized in the large joints and spine.
G. Osseous lesions accompanied by bone pain and soft tissue swelling, polyarthri-tis, fever and tender, erythematous sub-cutaneous nodules may occur with dis-seminated fat necrosis associated with pancreatitis.

Shackelford, P. G.: Osseous lesions and pancrea-titis. Am. J. Dis. Child. 131:731, 1977.

H. Discitis may be accompanied by what may appear to be limb pain when stand-ing or attempting to walk.

VII. Muscle Involvement

A. Muscle pain and cramps occur with McArdle's syndrome, idiopathic rhab-domyolysis, heat cramps, diffuse fasci-itis with eosinophilia and Lyme disease.
B. Infectious myositis is characterized by myalgia and muscle tenderness. (See page 155.)
C. Dermatomyositis; polymyositis
D. Muscle cramps, especially in the gas-trocnemius and soleus muscles and in the feet, may occur at night in older children and adolescents. The cause is unknown.
E. Children with Rocky Mountain spotted fever may cry because of pain if their thigh or calf muscles are squeezed.
F. Epidemic myalgia (Bornholm disease)
G. Trichinosis
H. Poliomyelitis
I. Guillain-Barré syndrome may cause muscle tenderness and weakness.
J. Leptospirosis

VIII. Diseases of the Blood

A. Severe hemolytic anemia may be accom-panied by limb pain.
B. Sickle cell anemia may cause vaso-oc-clusive bone lesions or an acute infarc-tion of long bones that is difficult to differentiate from osteomyelitis. The vaso-occlusive crises may cause limb pain in a single, multiple or migratory sites. Of variable duration and severity, the pain may be severe and can persist for three or four days. Local tenderness, erythema, heat, swelling and low grade fever may be present. Bone scans may not be diagnostically helpful in differ-entiating between osteomyelitis and vaso-occlusive crisis.

Keeley, K., and Buchanan, G. R.: Acute infarction of long bones in children with sickle cell anemia. J. Pediatr. 101:170, 1982.

C. Leukemia may have severe limb pain as an early manifestation.

O'Regan, S., Melhorn, D. K., and Newman, A. J.: Methotrexate-induced bone pain in childhood leukemia. Am. J. Dis. Child. 126:489, 1973.

IX. Other Disorders

A. Although patients with rheumatic fever may have red, hot, painful and swollen joints, these physical signs may be min-imal or absent, especially in young chil-dren. The diagnosis of rheumatic fever cannot be established on the basis of arthralgia or limb pain alone. Limb pains that occur during the night are almost never attributable to rheumatic fever.
B. Connective tissue and hypersensitivity disorders
1. Periarteritis nodosa
2. Serum sickness
3. Dermatomyositis
C. Takayasu's disease may cause claudi-cation in the lower extremities.
D. Infectious diseases are commonly ac-companied by myalgia and limb pains.
E. Reflex neurovascular dystrophy is char-acterized by pain and tenderness, at times exquisite, in an extremity or joint accompanied by distal swelling or vaso-motor changes such as coolness, warmth, pallor, erythema, hyperhi-drosis, limitation of motion or trophic skin changes. Active or passive move-ment is resisted. The pain, which is con-stant, increases on weight bearing or movement. A continuous, burning par-esthesia, accentuated by touch, may be present. As a consequence, the patient does not wish the involved area to be touched, even lightly. In many cases, a history of an antecedent illness or trauma is obtained.

Bernstein, B. H., Singsen, B. H., Kent, J. T., Kornreich, H., King, K., Hicks, R., and Hanson, V.: Reflex neurovascular dystrophy in childhood. J. Pediatr. 93:211, 1978.
Fermaglich, D.: Reflex sympathetic dystrophy in children. Pediatrics 60:881, 1977.

F. Erythromelalgia (See page 176.)

G. Psychogenic factors (psychogenic rheumatism) may account for persistent or recurrent articular and muscular pain in school age children and adolescents in the absence of objective joint findings. Resistance to attending school, chronic fatigue, other somatic complaints and depression may be reported.

H. Primary fibromyalgia syndrome, which may occur in school age children or adolescents, is characterized by chronic, persistent musculoskeletal pain in at least three areas of the body for a minimum of three months. Aching, fatigue and morning stiffness are commonly present. Multiple tender or trigger points are present suboccipitally, in the trapezius muscle, the subscapular bursa, the costochondral junctions, the lateral elbow, the medial knee, the epicondyles of the humerus and the sternomastoid muscle, as well as in other areas. Pressure on these points may produce referred pain. Many of the patients report sleep problems, anxiety, depression, headache and recurrent abdominal pain. No objective evidence of arthritis is present.

Jacobs, J. C., Berdon, W. E., and Johnston, A. D.: HLA-B27–associated spondyloarthritis and enthesopathy in childhood: Clinical, pathologic, and radiographic observations in 58 patients. J. Pediatr. 100:521, 1982.

Yunis, M., and Masi, A.: Juvenile primary fibromyalgia syndrome. Arthritis Rheum. 26(4, Suppl.):544, 1983.

GENERAL REFERENCE

Passo, M. H.: Aches and limb pain. Pediatr. Clin. North Am. 29:209, 1982.

ETIOLOGIC CLASSIFICATION OF LIMB PAINS

58 / TUMORS, SWELLINGS, MASSES

The initial symptom in a child with a malignancy may be an unexplained swelling, lump or mass. Superficial swellings on the forehead, over the eye or elsewhere may at first be thought to be a hematoma secondary to trauma. If the swelling does not regress within a few days, the possibility of malignancy must be seriously considered and roentgenographic studies, excision or biopsy performed. The child with an abdominal or other tumor mass presents an emergency problem. Diagnostic procedures should be completed within 48 hours, followed by surgical removal of the mass or initiation of other therapy. Palpation of the tumor should be limited to those health care professionals immediately concerned in diagnosis and therapy.

Miser, J. S., and Pizzo, P. A.: Soft tissue sarcomas in childhood. Pediatr. Clin. North Am. 32:779, 1985.

59 / SYMPTOMS REFERABLE TO THE URINARY TRACT

Disease of the urinary tract may account for a number of symptoms, including abdominal pain, abdominal tumor, growth retardation, failure to thrive, fever, edema, convulsions and hypertension. Urinalysis is indicated as a routine procedure in each child who is ill. A random normal urinalysis does not eliminate the possibility of renal disease.

I. CHARACTERISTICS OF URINATION

A. *Frequency.* Although over 90 per cent of term and premature infants void during the first day of life, occasionally a newborn infant does not urinate for 36 to 48 hours.

Moore, E. S., and Galvez, M.B.: Delayed micturition in the newborn period. J. Pediatr. 80:867, 1972.

Infants may void between 6 and 30 times a day. During an illness, the number of wet diapers may be a good index of hydration, since dehydrated infants usually do not urinate often. In the second year, many infants are able to remain dry for 2 or more hours. Children between the ages of 3 to 5 years urinate 8 to 14 times a day. The frequency decreases to 6 to 12 times per day in the 5 to 8 year age group and 6 to 8 in children 8 to 14 years of age. The frequency of urination increases during cold weather and with excitement. Children under considerable acute or chronic emotional stress may have frequency (pollakiuria) and urgency in the absence of a urinary tract infection. Such symptoms respond to lessening of the stress. The "sham" or "urge" syndrome consists of a group of symptoms that simulate those of a urinary tract infection, such as frequency, urgency, daytime wetting, cross-leg squeezing or squatting with the heel of one foot pressed into the perineum (curtsy sign) to stop wetting, nocturnal enuresis and dysuria. The wetting, which may be almost continuous, is exaggerated by excitement or other emotional factors.

Disorders that may be characterized by frequency include urinary tract infections, obstruction, megaloureter, foreign bodies and calculi. An inflamed appendix in contact with the right ureter or the bladder may also cause urinary frequency. Polyuria of any cause is accompanied by frequency.

Asnes, R. S., and Mones, R. L.: Pollakiuria. Pediatrics 52:615, 1973.

B. *Oliguria, anuria*
Renal failure
Acute glomerulonephritis
Hyperuricemia secondary to the treatment of leukemia
Hemolytic-uremic syndrome
Severe dehydration
Shock
Acute tubular necrosis
Bilateral renal cortical necrosis
Unilateral or bilateral renal vein thrombosis
Bladder neck obstruction
Transfusion reaction

Dobrin, R. S., Larsen, C. D., and Holliday, M. A.: The critically ill child: Acute renal failure. Pediatrics 48:286, 1971.

C. *Retention of urine* may occur in patients with meningitis, poliomyelitis, jimson weed poisoning, intestinal ascariasis, the Guillain-Barré syndrome, transverse myelitis and in comatose, stuporous and immediately postoperative patients. Phimosis, superficial ulceration of the urethral meatus in infant boys, balanitis, posthitis, hematocolpos or vulvovaginitis may also lead to urinary retention. Rarely, urinary retention may be a manifestation of a conversion reaction. The term "lazy bladder" syndrome has been applied to the occasional child reported to void only once or twice a day and to have had repeated urinary tract infections. The bladder may be palpable, and a vesicoureteral reflux may be present.

D. *Polyuria*
Diabetes mellitus
Diabetes insipidus
Nephrogenic diabetes insipidus
Drinking large quantities of water
Diuresis in edematous patients
Renal tubular acidosis
Fanconi's syndrome
Chronic renal failure
Hypokalemic nephropathy
Primary aldosteronism
Urinary tract infection
Sickle cell disease or trait may be accompanied by a defect in concentration evident by six months of age.

Hypercalcemia
Acute tubular necrosis
Psychogenic water drinking occurs in young children as a result of a disturbed maternal-child relationship. The child asks for liquids almost constantly. Usually, there is no history of dehydration, fever or growth failure. Laboratory examination reveals a normal serum sodium, serum osmolality and urine concentrating ability. Rarely, psychogenic water drinking may accompany diabetes insipidus.

Linshaw, M. A., Hipp, T., and Gruskin, A.: Infantile psychogenic water drinking. J. Pediatr. 85:520, 1974.

Polyuria may follow cessation of supraventricular tachycardia.

Janos, G., Gaum, W., and Kaplan, S.: Polyuria from tachycardia in an infant. N. Engl. J. Med. 302:692, 1980.

E. *Urinary stream.* Inability of a male infant or child to urinate or to produce a forceful, sustained urinary stream warrants urgent urologic investigation. With partial obstruction in the posterior urethra, the urinary stream may be interrupted and without force. A good practice during well-baby visits in early infancy is to routinely ask mothers about the nature of the boy's urinary stream. If a urethral obstruction is suspected, observe the urinary stream for spraying or dribbling. Distention of the urinary bladder may be evident as a lower abdominal mass in infants who have a posterior urethral obstruction.

F. *Incontinence.* Children with chronic bladder distention may dribble constantly or intermittently. Urologic investigation for posterior urethral valves or other partial obstruction is urgently indicated. Overflow incontinence may be the first symptom of a spinal cord tumor. Exstrophy of the bladder is, of course, characterized by incontinence.

Feinberg, T., Lattimer, J. K., Jeter, K., Langford, W., and Beck, L.: Questions that worry children with exstrophy. Pediatrics 53:242, 1974.

Cystitis may cause incontinence owing to bladder irritability and detrusor contraction. Frequency and dysuria may be associated symptoms.

Incontinence may occur during convulsive seizures. The child with nocturnal seizures may be thought to have enuresis.

Severely retarded children may dribble almost constantly.

Combined day and night enuresis in girls may be caused by an ectopic ureter opening near the urethral meatus. Vaginal reflux is a diagnostic consideration when a girl dribbles or wets her underpants when standing up after voiding. Because these patients usually do not abduct their thighs during micturition, the urine refluxes into the vagina.

Giggle incontinence may occur in girls during vigorous laughter. In adolescent girls, daytime wetting may occasionally be caused by bouts of bladder spasm.

A neurogenic bladder with urinary incontinence or retention, or both, may be caused by myelodysplasia or agenesis of the sacrum. A tight filum terminale associated with spina bifida occulta may lead to urinary frequency, urgency and enuresis. In adolescents, bladder dysfunction may occur in achondroplastic dwarfs owing to vertebral deformities or cord compression.

Kaplan, G. W., and Brock, W. A.: Voiding dysfunction in children. Curr. Probl. Pediatr. 10:4, 1980.

Shurtleff, D. B.: Myelodysplasia: Management and treatment. Curr. Probl. Pediatr. 10:7, 1980.

Thompson, I. M., Kirk, R. M., and Dale, M.: Sacral agenesis. Pediatrics 54:236, 1974.

Enuresis is discussed in Chapter 39.

G. *Dysuria.* Suprapubic and urethral pain or burning on voiding accompanied by frequency and urgency may be caused by vaginitis; vulvitis; cystitis; Reiter's disease; non-gonococcal, gonococcal or chlamydial urethritis; viral trigonitis; acute hemorrhagic cystitis; perineal irritation owing to bubble bath or pin worms; crystalluria; prostatitis; or acute epididymitis.

Demetrious, E., Emans, S. J., and Masland, R. P.: Dysuria in adolescent girls: Urinary tract infection or vaginitis. Pediatrics 70:300, 1982.

Ginsburg, C. M., and McCracken, G. H.: Urinary tract infections in young infants. Pediatrics 69:409, 1982.

II. BACTERIURIA/PYURIA

Urine to be examined for bacteriuria or polymorphonuclear leukocytes should be collected with careful avoidance of contamination. In most instances, a cleanly voided specimen will suffice so that catheterization may be avoided. Before the voided specimen is collected in a sterile container, the patient should be as carefully prepared as for catheterization. In uncircumcised boys, the foreskin should be retracted and the area around the meatus cleansed. After the initial few milliliters of urine have been voided, the specimen may be collected. A midstream specimen may be an unrealistic expectation in young girls, but school-age girls can usually obtain a clean midstream specimen once they are given careful instructions. Suprapubic bladder puncture is the only reliable method to obtain urine for culture in infants. Catheterization should be avoided if at all possible, although it may be necessary when the patient is acutely ill and immediate therapy is indicated or when the patient's cooperation cannot be obtained.

In a centrifuged, cleanly voided specimen, the presence of more than 5 to 10 polymorphonuclear leukocytes per high power field is usually considered an abnormal finding.

Urinary tract infection may be defined as the growth of bacteria in the urinary tract. Such infections are commonly asymptomatic, but they may also cause fever, irritability, vomiting, diarrhea, neonatal jaundice, failure to thrive, frequency, burning, urgency and a foul urine odor. Except for the newborn period when the prevalence of urinary tract infection is higher in boys than in girls, the incidence in girls is 30 times that in boys. The prevalence rate in newborn infants is about 1 per cent. In girls between the ages of two and five years, it is also about 1 per cent. The rate increases about 0.5 per cent over each of the next five years. It is estimated that 5 to 10 per cent of girls have a urinary tract infection before 18 years of age.

Escherichia coli is the most common etiologic agent, accounting for 75 to 80 per cent of initial and recurrent infections. *Klebsiella* and *Enterobacter* account for 10 to 15 per cent, *Staphylococcus* and enterococci for 5 to 10 per cent and *Proteus* and *Pseudomonas* for a smaller percentage.

All children thought to have a urinary tract infection must have a urine culture. A number of simple and relatively inexpensive office tests are available for detection of urinary tract infection. Dip-slides (Uricult, Oxoid, Clinicult) have differential bacteriologic media on each side of the slide. Whereas both gram-negative and gram-positive bacteria will grow on one side of the slide, only gram-negative organisms will grow on the other. Although this method is as accurate as standard bacteriologic culture techniques, the latter are needed for identification and antimicrobial sensitivity of the etiologic organism, a desirable procedure once the diagnosis of a urinary tract infection is established. The initial diagnosis of a urinary tract infection is most secure if two cultures showing the same organism are obtained. Microstix is a dipstick that turns pink within a few seconds if nitrite is present in the urine. Because not all gram-negative organisms reduce nitrate, some gram-negative and all gram-positive infections will be missed by this method. Since a large number of organisms are required, optimal results require use of the first morning specimen. Unless the first or second urine cultures are positive, it may be helpful diagnostically if three morning samples are checked. The Microstix strip can also be incubated and used for a colony count. These methods permit the mother to obtain the specimen at home and bring it to the office for processing.

All children with an initial urinary tract infection should have an intravenous pyelogram. A voiding cystourethrogram is indicated in all preschool and older children who demonstrate evidence of upper urinary tract disease. These studies usually need not be repeated if they are normal, if no surgical problem is identified and if the reflux is only minimal or moderate. Cystoscopy is indicated only in the presence of positive x-ray findings of obstructive disease.

Pyuria, insufficient in itself for diagnosis of a urinary tract infection, may be present only intermittently and is frequently absent in the presence of bacteriuria. The diagnosis of a urinary tract infection requires the finding of a significant number of bacteria in the urine. In a specimen obtained by suprapubic aspiration, 1000 or more colonies per milliliter indicate infection.

Differentiation between contamination and a true urinary tract infection can usually be made on the basis of bacterial counts of uncentrifuged "clean catch" urine. Less than 10,000 colonies per milliliter suggests contamination, whereas more than 100,000 colonies per milliliter of a single organism signifies infection. In the asymptomatic child, the diagnosis of significant bacteriuria should be based on two consecutive colony counts of 100,000/ml or more with the same organism. Intermediate counts, since they raise the suspicion of infection, are an indication for repeat examination. Early morning specimens are optimal for culturing. Specimens should be sent to the laboratory on ice and refrigerated at 4° C until cultured.

A drop of clean, uncentrifuged urine that has been dried and gram-stained may also be examined. Organisms are demonstrated on such a preparation in 80 to 95 per cent of cases when colony counts are 100,000 or more per milliliter. No bacteria are seen when the colony count is less than 1000 per milliliter.

Urinary tract infections in infants and children often represent a complication of a congenital anomaly with secondary partial obstruction and stasis. Because significant asymptomatic bacteriuria is present in about 3 per cent of prematures, urine cultures should be obtained at least once during their hospital stay. Hydronephrosis, megaloureters or a ureterocele may also be etiologically responsible for persistent or recurrent pyuria. In boys and in girls under three years of age, both an intravenous pyelogram and a voiding cystourethrogram should be obtained after the first urinary tract infection. Girls between the age of three and ten years should have an intravenous pyelogram. Radiographic studies may be indicated in older girls and adolescents with frequent, symptomatic urinary tract infections.

Sterile pyuria may be caused by mycoplasma, viruses, tuberculosis, urethritis, vaginitis, foreign body, interstitial nephritis, diabetes and glomerulonephritis.

Berger, M., Warren, M. M., and Hayden, C. K.: Urinary tract infection in the infant: The unsuspected diagnosis. Pediatrics 62:610, 1978.

Durbin, W. A., and Peter, G.: Management of urinary tract infections in infants and children. Pediatr. Infect. Dis. 3:564, 1984.

Kunin, C. M.: Urinary tract infections; flow charts (algorithms) for detection and treatment. JAMA 233:458, 1975.

Levitt, S. B.: Medical versus surgical treatment of primary vesicoureteral reflux. Pediatrics 67:392, 1981.

Randolph, M. F., Woods, S. E., Hudson, C. J., and Klauber, G. T.: Home screening for the detection of urinary tract infection in infancy. Am. J. Dis. Child. 133:713, 1979.

Rosenfeld, W. D., and Litman, N.: Urogenital tract infections in male adolescents. Pediatr. Rev. 4:257, 1983.

Screening school children for urologic disease. Statement by the Section on Urology, American Academy of Pediatrics. Pediatrics 60:239, 1977.

III. HEMATURIA

In the presence of massive hematuria, the urine may be bright red or smoky in color. When the urine is grossly red, the bleeding is usually extraglomerular. Clots may be present, but red cell casts should be absent. Brown or reddish brown (tea or cola colored) urine usually denotes glomerular bleeding. Red blood cell casts may be found. No color change occurs with microscopic hematuria. The presence of hematuria may be established by the microscopic examination of freshly voided centrifuged urine sediment or the use of a hemoglobin dip stick. Since hematuria may be transient, the urinalysis should be repeated. A family history of renal disease or recent respiratory infection should be explored.

Causes of Hematuria

Acute post-streptococcal glomerulonephritis. Erythrocytes, white blood cells and proteinuria are noted on urinalysis. Red cell casts may also be present. A positive Streptozyme test and a decrease in the C3 complement level occur in most patients.

Membranous glomerulonephritis accompanied by microhematuria may present with the nephrotic syndrome.

IgA-IgG mesangial nephropathy (Berger disease) begins with sudden gross hematuria one to three days after an upper respiratory infection. With subsidence of the infection, the gross hematuria clears, but intermittent or constant microscopic hematuria and a 1+ level of proteinuria may persist. Gross hematuria may recur with further infections or exercise. The C3 level is normal. The additional presence of proteinuria is an indication for renal biopsy.

Roy, L. P., Fish, A. J., Vernier, R. L., and Michael, A. F.: Recurrent macroscopic hematuria, focal nephritis, and mesangial deposition of immunoglobulin and complement. J. Pediatr. 82:767, 1973.

Nephritis of chronic bacteremia (shunt nephritis) owing to chronic bacteremia is associated with subacute bacterial endocarditis and infected catheters. The serum complement level is depressed.

Membranoproliferative glomerulonephritis (hypocomplementemic persistent glomerulonephritis), more common in adolescents and young adults, is characterized by proteinuria, microscopic and gross hematuria and, occasionally, the nephrotic syndrome. In its silent phase, this disorder may cause only transient hematuria. The serum C3 concentration is often but not invariably depressed. Hypertension may be an early finding. The diagnosis is made by renal biopsy. In some cases the onset may simulate acute glomerulonephritis with azotemia and may demonstrate a rapidly progressive course. Membranoproliferative glomerulonephritis occurs frequently in children with partial lipodystrophy.

Sissons, J. G. P., West, R. J., Fallows, J., Williams, D. G., Boucher, B. J., Amos, N., and Peters, D. K.: The complement abnormalities of lipodystrophy. N. Engl. J. Med. 294:461, 1976.

Membranous glomerulonephritis may cause microscopic hematuria, but its chief clinical manifestation is edema associated with the nephrotic syndrome.

Rapidly progressive glomerulonephritis may be of the post-streptococcal or idiopathic type. Findings include gross hematuria, oliguria, anuria and hypertension. With a low C3, the disorder is likely post-streptococcal in etiology.

Systemic lupus erythematosus nephritis may present with proteinuria and microscopic hematuria. The serum complement level is characteristically low. Since renal changes may occur with systemic lupus erythematosus in the absence of hematuria, a renal biopsy is indicated.

Glomerulonephritis occurs in about half of patients with Henoch-Schönlein purpura. Hematuria and proteinuria may be mild, or the kidney involvement may progress to the nephrotic syndrome or renal insufficiency.

Meadow, S. R., Glasgow, E. F., White, R. H. R., Moncrieff, M. W., Cameron, J. S., and Ogg, C. S.: Schönlein-Henoch nephritis. Q. J. Med. 41:241, 1972.

West, C. D., and McAdams, A. J.: The chronic glomerulonephritides of childhood. J. Pediatr. 93:1, 167, 1978.

Focal segmental glomerulosclerosis

Antiglomerular-basement membrane antibody disease occurs in adolescents and young adults. Goodpasture's syndrome, a form of this disorder, is characterized by hemoptysis, glomerulonephritis, anemia, cough, dyspnea and fever.

Polycystic disease of the kidney is frequently accompanied by hematuria.

Acute urinary tract infection may be accompanied by symptoms and signs of bladder irritation. Gross hematuria may be the initial symptom, but the hematuria is microscopic in character and accompanied by pyuria and bacteriuria. A urine culture should be obtained. Hematuria may be present in such viral diseases as chickenpox, measles and mumps or in parasitic diseases such as schistosomiasis.

Although a relatively rare presentation, gross hematuria may be the initial symptom of Wilms' tumor.

A bladder tumor is usually accompanied by signs of bladder irritation as well as hematuria.

Renal hemangioma may cause severe bleeding, passage of clots and renal colic.

Because of the possibility of preexisting renal anomaly or disease, the urinary tract should be carefully investigated whenever hematuria follows trauma. A previous silent hydronephrosis may be identified in this fashion.

Football hematuria. Both gross and microscopic bleeding may occur transiently after participation in football or other vigorous exercise. Hematuria following strenuous physical activity does not normally persist longer than 24 hours.

Renal calculi may cause generalized abdominal pain or hematuria. Idiopathic hypercalciuria is also a common cause of gross hematuria in the absence of urinary tract infection or proteinuria. A urinary calcium/creatinine ratio is a useful screening examination for hypercalciuria.

Kalia, A., Travis, L. B., and Brouhard, B. H.: The association of idiopathic hypercalciuria and asymptomatic gross hematuria in children. J. Pediatr. 99:716, 1981.

Stapelton, F. B., Roy, S., III, Noe, H. N., and Jerkins, G.: Hypercalciuria in children with hematuria. N. Engl. J. Med. 310:1345, 1984.

Walther, P. C., Lamm, D., and Kaplan, G. W.: Pediatric urolithiases. A ten year review. Pediatrics 65:1068, 1980.

Unilateral or bilateral thrombosis of the renal veins causes hematuria and flank masses. Renal vein thrombosis may occur in the newborn secondary to prematurity, hypoxemia, sepsis, maternal diabetes mellitus or thiazide drug use. In older infants, dehydration or burns may be complicated by renal vein thrombosis.

Oliver, W. J., and Kelsch, R. C.: Renal venous thrombosis in infancy. Pediatr. Rev. 4:61, 1982.

Periarteritis nodosa

Infective endocarditis; other causes of chronic bacteremia

Renal tuberculosis secondary to pulmonary tuberculosis is an unusual cause of hematuria.

Foreign bodies in urethra or bladder

Hemorrhagic disorders: thrombocytopenia, hemophilia

Interstitial nephritis, caused by methicillin, ampicillin and the cephalosporins or associated with Group A beta-hemolytic streptococcal infections, is characterized by fever, rash, abdominal or flank pain, eosinophilia, eosinophiluria, hematuria, proteinuria and, perhaps, renal insufficiency.

Ellis, D., Fried, W. A., Yunis, E. J., and Blau, E. B.: Acute interstitial nephritis in children. A report of 13 cases and review of the literature. Pediatrics 67:862, 1981.

Hydronephrosis

Congestive heart failure

Leptospirosis

Infectious mononucleosis

Gonococcal infection in adolescent males

Transient hematuria may develop during acute febrile illnesses.

Prolapse of the urethra in young girls

Megaloureter

Polycystic kidney disease may be characterized by gross or microscopic hematuria.

Superficial ulceration of the external urethral meatus in circumcised infant boys

Gross hematuria may occur in children with sickle cell trait, sickle cell hemoglobin C disease and, occasionally, sickle cell disease. Infarction of the renal papillae with papillary necrosis may occur.

Renal papillary necrosis may occur in children with juvenile rheumatoid arthritis on high-dose aspirin therapy.

Wortmann, D. W.: Renal papillary necrosis in juvenile rheumatoid arthritis. J. Pediatr. 97:37, 1980.

Hemolytic-uremic syndrome may cause hematuria, proteinuria and pyuria.

Acute hemorrhagic cystitis or viral trigonitis is characterized by a sudden onset of bright red hematuria accompanied by symptoms of bladder irritation, such as marked dysuria and lower abdominal discomfort. Adenovirus (types 11 and 21) is the usual cause in children, especially in boys between 6 and 15 years of age.

Cyclophosphamide may cause hemorrhagic cystitis. Other drugs that may produce hematuria include aspirin, amitriptyline, chlorpromazine and sulfonamides.

Johnson, W. W., and Meadows, D. C.: Urinary-bladder fibrosis and telangiectasia associated with long-term cyclophosphamide therapy. N. Engl. J. Med. 284:290, 1971.

Benign recurrent hematuria, often precipitated by respiratory infections or exercise, is characterized by repeated episodes of microscopic or gross hematuria without proteinuria. Usually no specific cause can be found for the hematuria. Red cell casts may be present. Since the diagnosis is always a tentative one, the child should be reevaluated at intervals with repeated urinalyses for proteinuria.

Benign familial hematuria, inherited as an autosomal dominant, is characterized by constant microscopic hematuria or gross hematuria. Episodes may be associated with infections. Family members should be screened for hematuria. Proteinuria is absent and renal biopsy is not necessary.

Glomerulonephritis of Alport's syndrome (hereditary nephritis) is an uncommon cause of microscopic or gross hematuria. Neurosensory hearing loss, an associated finding, may be overlooked in the absence of audiometric studies. Proteinuria, hypertension and renal failure may also ensue. Nephritis or microscopic hematuria may occur in other family members.

Gubler, M., Levy, M., Broyer, M., Naizot, C., Gonzales, G., Perrin, D. and Habib, R.: Alport's syndrome. Am. J. Med. 70:493, 1981.

The laboratory studies initially indicated in the evaluation of hematuria include urinalysis, urine culture, complete blood count, 24-hour creatinine clearance, 24-hour protein excretion, streptozyme level, C3 complement level and intravenous pyelogram. Additional examinations indicated in some patients include platelet count and other coagulation studies, Coomb's test, sickle cell screen, ANA and voiding cystourethrogram. Renal biopsy may be diagnostically helpful with a history of recurrent episodes of gross hematuria, decreased creatinine clearance, abnormal 24-hour proteinuria and hypertension. Bright red blood in the urine and symptoms of lower urinary tract disease suggest the need for cystoscopy.

Bergstein, J. M.: Hematuria, proteinuria, and urinary tract infection. Pediatr. Clin. North Am. 29:55, 1982.

Emanuel, B., and Aronson, N.: Neonatal hematuria. Am. J. Dis. Child. 128:204, 1974.

Ingelfinger, J. R., Davis, A. E., and Grupe, W. B.: Frequency and etiology of gross hematuria in a general pediatric setting. Pediatrics 59:557, 1977.

Sherman, R. L., Churg, J., and Yudis, M.: Hereditary nephritis with a characteristic renal lesion. Am. J. Med. 56:44, 1974.

IV. PROTEINURIA

Multiple test reagent strips are generally used to test for proteinuria. A false-positive reaction may be obtained if the urine is strongly alkaline. The finding of trace amounts of proteinuria by dipsticks may be checked by the sulfosalicylic acid precipitation method.

The normal upper limit of proteinuria is between 100 and 200 mg/sq m/24 hours. Proteinuria that exceeds 1.5 gm/24 hours usually implies glomerular disease. Persistent proteinuria requires investigation. Transient proteinuria in adolescents and, less frequently, in preschool and school-age children in the absence of other urine abnormalities is usually of no clinical significance. In benign persistent asymptomatic proteinuria, a diagnosis made by exclusion, laboratory findings, intravenous pyelogram and biopsy are normal except for the proteinuria, which ranges from 0.5 to 1.8 gm/24 hours.

Orthostatic proteinuria occasionally occurs in older children and adolescents in whom proteinuria is absent, or nearly so, when recumbent but is regularly or intermittently present up to less than 2 gm/24 hours when standing. Other causes of proteinuria should be ruled out by the history and urinalyses. The child is asked to empty his bladder at bedtime. The first morning specimen obtained either in bed or immediately upon arising and the second sample obtained two hours later, after the child has been normally active, are checked for proteinuria. Specimens should be obtained at home on three separate mornings, identified and frozen until brought to the office. If only the second of the two daily specimens demonstrate proteinuria, the diagnosis of orthostatic proteinuria is established. If both specimens are positive, persistent proteinuria is present.

Investigation of persistent proteinuria includes determination of the 24-hour excretion of protein, urine culture, intravenous pyelogram, CBC and determination of serum electrolytes, serum proteins, BUN, serum creatinine, creatinine clearance, complement and cholesterol. If total protein excretion over 1 gm/day, hypocomplementemia or persistent microscopic hematuria are present, renal biopsy may be indicated. Pseudoproteinuria may result from the reaction between nafcillin or its metabolites and the quantitative reagents used in the sulfosalicylic and trichloroacetic acid methods.

Transient proteinuria may accompany fever over 38.5° C (101.3° F), infectious diseases, vigorous exercise, emotional stress, exposure to extreme cold and seizures.

Other disease processes in which proteinuria may occur include:

Acute and chronic glomerulonephritis. Microscopic hematuria is also often present.

Chronic interstitial nephritis

Membranous and membranoproliferative glomerulonephritis may cause asymptomatic proteinuria. Hematuria is also usually present. The diagnosis is established by renal biopsy.

Nephrotic syndrome is the most likely cause of asymptomatic proteinuria from one to six years of age. Proteinuria with protein loss over 3 gm/day may be present for weeks before edema appears. Serum albumin and IgG levels may be depressed and serum cholesterol elevated. Except in congenital nephrosis, renal biopsy is unnecessary.

Chronic pyelonephritis
Renal hypoplasia or dysplasia
Hydronephrosis
Polycystic disease
Dehydration
Diabetic nephropathy
Congestive cardiac failure
Galactosemia
Fanconi's syndrome

Feld, L. G., Schoeneman, M. J., and Kaskel, F. J.: Evaluation of the child with asymptomatic proteinuria. Pediatr. Rev. 5:248, 1984.

James, J. A.: Proteinuria and hematuria in children: Diagnosis and assessment. Pediatr. Clin. North Am. 23:807, 1976.

V. Reducing Substances

Glycosuria
Diabetes mellitus
Cushing's disease
Excessive glucose ingestion
Fanconi's syndrome
Lead poisoning
Following convulsive seizures
Central nervous system infections, trauma, tumors, hemorrhage
Glycosuria may occasionally occur during acute febrile illnesses.
Advanced tubular damage
Pentosuria may occur after ingestion of fruit or as a manifestation of an inborn error of metabolism. The Benedict's (Clinitest) reaction is positive, but the glucose oxidase dip stick (Clinistix) is negative.
Fructosuria may appear after ingestion of large amounts of fruit or may repesent an inborn error of metabolism. The Benedict's test is positive, but the glucose oxidase dip stick is negative.
Galactosuria occurs in infants with galactosemia. The Benedict's test is positive, but the glucose oxidase dip stick is negative.
Meconium or gas may be present in the urine of the infant with a rectovesical fistula.

VI. Positive Ferric Chloride Test

Phenylketonuria
Histidinemia
Maple syrup urine disease
Oasthouse urine disease

VII. Abnormal Urinary Pigments

Bile produces a golden yellow color in the urine.
The red diaper syndrome, characterized by the appearance of a red color in soiled diapers after 24 to 36 hours, is caused by *Serratia marcescens*.
The blue diaper syndrome may be associated with hypercalcemia and nephrocalcinosis with production of the dye indigotin or with *Pseudomonas aeruginosa* as the predominant organism in the stool.

Libit, S. A., Ulstrom, R. A., and Doeden, D.: Fecal *Pseudomonas aeruginosa* as a cause of the blue diaper syndrome. J. Pediatr. 81:546, 1972.

Hemoglobinuria, usually caused by massive intravascular hemolysis, produces pink, reddish-brown, smoky or black urine. Tests for hemoglobin are positive, but red blood cells are not present on microscopic examination. Spectroscopic examination of the urine confirms the presence of hemoglobin.

Hematuria causes the urine to have a bright red or smoky appearance.
Urates may cause a slight pink or reddish staining of the diaper in newborn and young infants. Orange sand in the diapers may be an early finding in the Lesch-Nyhan syndrome.
Beeturia refers to a pink or deep red pigmentation of the urine that may occur on a genetic basis or in infants with iron deficiency anemia after ingestion of pureed beets.
Porphyria, either congenital or intermittent and acute, causes a burgundy red or dark reddish brown urine color on standing.
Homogentisic acid, excreted in the urine of patients with alcaptonuria, causes the urine to turn dark on standing or after alkalinization. Alkaline urine may be black or dark brown when passed.
Red urine may be caused by drugs such as rifampin, metabolites or dyes, including phenolphthalein.
Myoglobinuria may result from muscle damage and rhabdomyolysis owing to strenuous exercise, infections, trauma, inflammation, poisons, drugs, metabolic disorders and exposure to cold.
Paroxysmal myoglobinuria is characterized by muscle pain, cramps, edema, weakness or paralysis and brown, pink, red or burgundy-colored urine. Myoglobinuria usually is noted 12 to 24 hours after the onset of muscle pain but may appear before or after that time. Both myoglobin and hemoglobin produce a positive test for hemoglobin in the absence of red cells in the urine. Acute porphyria may be excluded by a negative Watson test. The serum is pink or red in patients with hemoglobinuria and normal with myoglobinuria. Myoglobin may be identified spectroscopically.

Robotham, J. L., and Haddow, J. E.: Rhabdomyolysis and myoglobinuria in childhood. Pediatr. Clin. North Am. 23:279, 1976.

VIII. Ketonuria

Diabetic ketoacidosis
Persistent vomiting
Dehydration or starvation. In infants under five months of age, these conditions do not cause ketonuria. Ketonuria in that age period is attributable to a metabolic disorder.
Ketotic hypoglycemia
Fructose l,6-diphosphatase deficiency
Lead poisoning
Acute febrile illnesses in children
Glycogenosis types I and III
Isovaleric acidemia
Propionic acidemia

Pyruvate carboxylase deficiency
Pyruvate dehydrogenase disorders
Methylmalonic aciduria

IX. URINE PH

Determination of the pH of *freshly* passed urine with nitrazine paper may be diagnostically helpful. The finding of an alkaline urine in a patient with systemic acidosis is significant. Patients with renal tubular acidosis, idiopathic hypercalcemia or primary aldosteronism may have a neutral or alkaline urine.

X. OTHER URINARY TRACT FINDINGS

Unusual urine odors may suggest an inborn error of metabolism. (See below.) Meconium or gas may be present in the urine of the infant with a rectovesical fistula.

GENERAL REFERENCE

Edelmann, C. M., Jr. (ed.): Pediatric Kidney Disease. Boston, Little, Brown and Co., 1978.

ETIOLOGIC CLASSIFICATION OF URINARY TRACT SYMPTOMS

60 / UNUSUAL ODORS

I. URINE ODORS

A. Maple syrup or burnt sugar with maple syrup urine disease
B. Musty, mousey with phenylketonuria or tyrosinemia
C. Dried malt, celery or yeast-like with oasthouse urine disease (methionine malabsorption)
D. Boiled cabbage, rancid butter or decaying fish with hypermethioninemia or tyrosinemia
E. Cheesy or sweaty feet with isovalericacidemia
F. Cat urine with beta-methylcrotonoyl-CoA carboxylase deficiency
G. Acetone with diabetic ketoacidosis and other disorders characterized by ketosis

II. HALITOSIS (See page 49.)

III. POOR PERSONAL HYGIENE

IV. ENCOPRESIS

V. URINARY INCONTINENCE

61 / PALLOR; ANEMIA

CLINICAL CONSIDERATIONS

The symptom of pallor is conditioned by the concentration of hemoglobin in the blood, the distribution and state of contraction or dilatation of cutaneous blood vessels, and the presence or absence of edema. Many infants and children appear pale even though they have a normal red blood cell count and hemoglobin concentration. A sallow complexion is often familial. Parents may think their light-complexioned or fair-skinned children are anemic.

Pallor may be noted, even in the absence of anemia, in patients with rheumatic fever, acute glomerulonephritis, urinary tract infection, hypothyroidism, malabsorption syndromes, infantile cortical hyperostosis, chronic ulcerative colitis, other long-term diseases, bacterial endocarditis, Henoch-Schönlein purpura, nephrosis and other diseases characterized by edema. Pallor is a well-known manifestation of shock. It may occur episodically in patients with pheochromocytoma, hypoglycemia, paroxysmal atrial tachycardia and anomalous origin of the left coronary artery. Newborn infants who are deeply sedated or severely hypoxic are also pale.

Anemia is characterized by a diminution in the hemoglobin concentration or oxygen-carrying capacity of the blood. For general purposes, a hemoglobin level below 10 gm/dl of blood or a red blood cell count below 4 million indicates the presence of anemia.

In addition to pallor, a number of other symptoms may occur in anemic patients. The nature of these symptoms depends upon the primary cause of the anemia, its severity, the rapidity with which it developed, and the length of time it has been present. Symptoms may include headache, vertigo, faintness, weakness, easy fatigability, irritability, palpitation, tachycardia, dyspnea, anorexia and edema. Children with hemolytic anemia may demonstrate nausea, vomiting, diarrhea, abdominal pain, arthralgia, limb pain, fever, jaundice, restlessness and, in some instances, hemoglobinuria. Splenomegaly may occur in patients with hemolytic anemia and, occasionally, in those with iron deficiency. Splenomegaly becomes less prominent in patients with sickle cell anemia as the spleen becomes fibrotic. The liver may be enlarged and tender in patients with hemolytic anemia. Hemolytic anemia may be present in the absence of jaundice. Anemia of long duration may cause retardation of physical development. Physiologic adjustments may be surprisingly compensatory, however, as far as physical activity is concerned.

Since the destruction or loss of erythrocytes is normally balanced by production, anemia may be caused by one or more of three mechanisms: (1) decreased production of erythrocytes; (2) increased destruction of erythrocytes; and (3) blood loss.

The presence of anemia may first be established by a determination of the hemoglobin concentration or the hematocrit or by a red blood cell count. Normal hematologic findings are given in Table 61–1. The history and physical examination may assist in classifying the anemia. A history of blood loss, inadequate diet, or anemia in other family members is diagnostically helpful. The physical examination may reveal purpura, jaundice, lymphadenopathy or splenomegaly. Other helpful procedures include examination of a stained blood smear, a white blood cell count and a reticulocyte count. The mean corpuscular volume (MCV) is low with iron deficiency anemia, anemia of chronic disease, thalassemia minor and lead poisoning; normal in the anemia of chronic disease and malignancy as well as in the acute aplastic and hypoplastic anemias; and high with folate or vitamin B_{12} deficiency, chronic hypoplastic anemia and active hemolysis. The urine and stool may be checked for the presence of blood and the urine for bile and urobilinogen. These procedures permit categorization of the anemia according to one of the three basic mechanisms.

ETIOLOGIC CLASSIFICATION OF ANEMIA

I. Decreased Production of Erythrocytes

A. Physiologic anemia of infancy; anemia of prematurity. With the increase in ox-

422

TABLE 61–1. HEMATOLOGIC VALUES DURING INFANCY AND CHILDHOOD

Age	Hemoglobin (gm/dl) Mean	Range	Hematocrit (%) Mean	Range	Reticulocytes (%) Mean	Leukocytes (WBC/cu m) Mean	Range	Neutrophils (%) Mean	Range	Lymphocytes (%) Mean*	Eosinophils (%) Mean	Monocytes (%) Mean	Nucleated Red Cells /100 WBC
Cord blood	16.8	13.7–20.1	55	45–65	5.0	18,000	(9–30,000)	61	(40–80)	31	2	6	7.0 (3–10)
2 wk	16.5	13.0–20.0	50	42–66	1.0	12,000	(5–21,000)	40		48	3	9	0
3 mo	12.0	9.5–14.5	36	31–41	1.0	12,000	(6–18,000)	30		63	2	5	0
6 mo–6 yr	12.0	10.5–14.0	37	33–42	1.0	10,000	(6–15,000)	45		48	2	5	0
7–12 yr	13.0	11.0–16.0	38	34–40	1.0	8000	(4500–13,500)	55		38	2	5	0
Adult													
Female	14	12.0–16.0	42	37–47	1.6	7500	(5–10,000)	55	(35–70)	35	3	7	0
Male	16	14.0–18.0	47	42–52									

*Relatively wide range.

From Behrman, R. E., and Vaughan, V. C., III (eds.): The Nelson Textbook of Pediatrics. Philadelphia, W. B. Saunders Co., 1983, p. 1207.

ygen saturation at birth, a smaller red cell mass is needed. An augmented oxygen unloading capability also develops owing to the change from fetal to adult hemoglobin. Because of physiologic marrow limitations, the rapid increase in blood volume that occurs in early infancy is unaccompanied by a proportionate increase in erythrocyte production. At two months of age, a hemoglobin value of 10.5 gm/dl is normal. At three months of age, the red blood cell count may be about 4 million per cubic millimeter, the hemoglobin concentration about 11 gm/dl, and the hematocrit about 35. Other than the occurrence of pallor in some infants, symptoms attributable to anemia are not present. The erythrocyte count has usually risen again by the seventh month and the hemoglobin by the eighth or ninth month. Until this time the red cells may demonstrate slight hypochromia.

Anemia of prematurity begins shortly after birth and hemoglobin concentrations are lowest between one and three months of age. During this time, a proportionate fall occurs in both the hemoglobin concentration and red blood cell count. The resultant anemia is normochromic. The hemoglobin concentration ranges from 7.0 to 8.0 gm/dl for infants with birth weights between 1000 and 1500 gm. to 9.5 gm/dl for those with birth weights of 2000 to 2500 gm. The fall in hemoglobin concentration is caused by a relatively low amount of erythropoietin along with a slight decrease in the red cell life span.

The intermediate phase, which lasts about two months, is characterized by a steady increase in total circulating hemoglobin mass. Because of the rapid expansion of blood volume that accompanies the rapid growth at this time, the peripheral hemoglobin concentration does not increase.

In the late phase, an iron deficient, hypochromic and microcytic type of anemia develops if the diet has not been supplemented with iron.

Dallman, P. R.: Erythropoietin and the anemia of prematurity. J. Pediatr. 105:756, 1984.
Stockman, J. A., III: The anemia of prematurity and the decision when to transfuse. Adv. Pediatr. 30:191, 1983.

B. Iron deficiency anemia in infants and children is almost always attributable to a long-standing dietary inadequacy, infection or blood loss in the stools. Anemia is a late manifestation of iron deficiency. Irritability is a much earlier complaint. The ingestion of large amounts of milk without other iron-containing foods is usually a reflection of a parenting problem. (See Chapter 64.) With infection, iron is poorly utilized in hemoglobin synthesis, and much of it is stored in the tissues. The anemia accompanying infection may at first be normochromic and normocytic, but with the development of iron deficiency, the erythrocytes become predominantly hypochromic and microcytic. Multiple births or rapid growth in early infancy may predispose to iron deficiency anemia. The adolescent growth spurt and loss of blood during menstruation may contribute to iron deficiency and anemia at that time. Iron deficiency anemia may also occur in patients with chronic diseases such as juvenile rheumatoid arthritis.

The term "relative anemia" describes the hematologic findings in some children with cyanotic congenital heart disease who demonstrate polycythemia in the presence of an average or below-average hemoglobin concentration. The red blood cells in these patients are microcytic and hypochromic. After iron administration, the hemoglobin concentration rises to a level commensurate with the red blood cell count.

In patients with iron deficiency anemia, the erythrocytes have a central pallor. Poikilocytosis and anisocytosis may also be noted. The hematocrit level and the hemoglobin concentration of less than 11.0 gm/dl may reflect the extent of iron deficiency anemia more closely than does the red blood cell count. In iron deficiency, the plasma supernatant in the hematocrit tube is colorless. In some infants, the red cell count may be normal or even elevated in the presence of moderately low hemoglobin and hematocrit levels. The mean corpuscular volume (MCV) will be less than 70 cubic microns in patients under age two. Other findings include a reduced serum ferritin concentration (less than 10 ng/ml), reflecting a decrease in iron stores; elevated free erythrocyte porphyrin (FEP); a decrease in serum transferrin saturation (serum iron/iron binding capacity) of 16 per cent or less; a decreased serum iron level; and an increase in the total iron-binding capacity. The effectiveness of iron therapy may be gauged by the reticulocyte response in 72 hours. Failure of a patient with a hypochromic, microcytic anemia to demonstrate a reticulocyte response after receiving adequate doses of iron in the absence of a large milk intake suggests that the patient has an infectious, chronic inflammatory or neoplastic disease. The hypochromic anemia of thalassemia, which early may be difficult to differentiate from iron deficiency anemia, does not respond to iron therapy. Also, the serum transferrin saturation and the free erythrocyte porphyrin are normal in thalassemia. Patients with juvenile rheumatoid arthritis may have an anemia attributable either to iron deficiency or to inflammation. Cystic fibrosis patients may also demonstrate iron deficiency owing both to impaired iron absorption and to an inadequate erythroid response to hypoxia.

Ater, J. L., Herbst, J. J., Landaw, S. A., and O'Brien, R. T.: Relative anemia and iron deficiency in cystic fibrosis. Pediatrics 71:810, 1983.
Koerper, M. A., Stempel, D. A., and Dallman, P. R.: Anemia in patients with juvenile rheumatoid arthritis. J. Pediatr. 92:930, 1978.

Breast milk, although it has a low iron content, is readily absorbed, so iron supplementation is not essential. Exclusive breast-milk feeding in the term infant for six months is not accompanied by iron deficiency on a nutritional basis. However, for two reasons, cow's milk leads to iron deficiency anemia in infants who ingest a quart or more of homogenized pasteurized whole cow's milk a day. One is that cow's milk is low in iron; the second is that gastrointestinal sensitivity to whole cow's milk may cause occult blood loss. Edema, hypoproteinemia and irritability may occur along with pallor, hypoferremia, hypocupremia and a reduction in iron-binding capacity. The hemoglobin concentration rises following the administration of iron or the substitution of a soy bean or proprietary milk formula.

Shumway, C. N.: Iron deficiency in children. Pediatr. Clin. North Am. 19:855, 1972.
Wilson, J. F., Lahey, M. E., and Heiner, D. C.: Studies on iron metabolism. V. Further observations on cow's milk–induced gastrointestinal bleeding in infants with iron deficiency anemia. J. Pediatr. 84:335, 1974.

C. Copper deficiency may occur in premature infants, in infants on prolonged intravenous alimentation and in those with chronic diarrhea and malnutrition. Presenting signs and symptoms include failure to thrive, apathy, hypotonia, developmental retardation, hypopigmentation of the skin and hair and seborrheic dermatitis. Laboratory examinations reveal hypochromic anemia unresponsive to iron, leukopenia, low serum copper and low ceruloplasmin. X-rays demonstrate osteoporosis with metaphyseal flaring, cupping, spurs and pathologic fractures.

Ashkenazi, A., Levin, S., Djaldetti, M., Fishel, E., and Benvenisti, D.: The syndrome of neonatal copper deficiency. Pediatrics 52:525, 1973.

D. Megaloblastic anemia of infants and children, usually caused by vitamin B_{12} or folic acid deficiency, occurs in some patients who have a history of intestinal resection, recurrent illnesses with dietary disruptions, chronic diarrhea or chronic hemolytic anemia. The red blood cells may be macrocytic, normocytic or, at times, microcytic. Hypersegmentation of polymorphonuclear neutrophils may also occur. Bone marrow examination is diagnostic. Folic acid deficiency may follow feeding with unfortified goat's milk. Megaloblastic anemia and methylmalonic aciduria, perhaps accompanied by ataxia and clonus, may occur in exclusively breast fed infants of mothers who are strict vegetarians.

Higginbottom, M. C., Sweetman, L., and Nyhan, W. L.: A syndrome of methylmalonic aciduria, homocystinuria, megaloblastic anemia and neurologic abnormalities in a vitamin B_{12} deficient breast fed infant of a strict vegetarian. N. Engl. J. Med. 299:319, 1978.

Hereditary orotic aciduria is a rare hereditary disorder of pyrimidine metabolism associated with megaloblastic anemia, leukopenia, retarded growth and the urinary excretion of excessive amounts of orotic acid. Sideroblastic anemias, malignancies of the Di-Guglielmo variety and thiamine dependency are other causes. Megaloblastic anemia may occur during chemotherapy and in patients who are receiving anticonvulsants such as hydantoin, mysoline or phenobarbital. Liver disease may cause a decrease in folic acid stores. Vitamin B_{12} absorption may be impaired in malabsorption disorders, Crohn's disease and intestinal resection.

Transcobalamin II deficiency causes a profound megaloblastic anemia in early infancy, which if untreated leads to agammaglobulinemia.

Juvenile pernicious anemia, an extremely unusual disease in children, may be caused by (1) a congenital lack of intrinsic factor accompanied by gastric achlorhydria. (2) failure of secretion of intrinsic factor with normal gastric acidity, or (3) familial malabsorption of vitamin B_{12}.

Heisel, M. A., et al: Congenital pernicious anemia: Report of seven patients with studies of the extended family. J. Pediatr. 105:564, 1984.

E. Pyridoxine deficiency is a rare cause of a hypochromic microcytic or sideroblastic anemia.
F. Hypoplastic and aplastic anemias
   1. Congenital hypoplastic anemia (Blackfan-Diamond) may have its onset within the first months of life, usually by six months of age. Macrocytosis and an increase in fetal hemoglobin concentration are present. Leukocyte and platelet production are not diminished.

Alter, B. P., and Nathan, D. G.: Red cell aplasia in children. Arch. Dis. Child. 54:263, 1979.

   2. Transient erythroblastopenia of childhood (TEC) is characterized by moderate to severe anemia (3.0 to 9 gm/dl of hemoglobin), reticulocytopenia and decreased erythroid precursors. This generally asymptomatic disorder, which may occur in infancy (usually after six months) or in early childhood, persists from a few weeks to several months, followed by a rapid and complete recovery. The cause is unknown, but the anemia may follow a viral infection. Examination of the bone marrow is necessary for diagnosis. Fetal hemoglobin is absent, and the mean corpuscular volume is normal.

Oski, F. A.: Transient erythroblastopenia. Pediatr. Rev. 4:25, 1982.

   3. Fanconi's anemia consists in pancytopenia; microcephaly; mental retardation; understature; hyperpigmentation; café-au-lait spots; hypogonadism; strabismus; and hypoplastic, absent or supernumerary thumbs. Aplasia of the radii may accompany absent thumbs but otherwise does not occur in this syndrome. The pancytopenia usually does not appear until age four. Examination of the metaphase chromosomes of peripheral blood lymphocytes provides the most specific laboratory examination. The "WT" syndrome, an autosomal dominant disorder, consists of pancytopenia and radioulnar hypoplasia but with normal chromosomes.
   4. Osteopetrosis is characterized by a hypoplastic anemia.
   5. Erythropoiesis may be transiently depressed (aplastic crisis) in patients with sickle cell anemia, thalassemia major, congenital hemolytic anemia, autoimmune hemolytic anemia or repeated blood transfusions.
   6. Aplastic anemias are characterized by normochromic and normocytic erythrocytes, leukopenia and thrombocytopenia. Megakaryocytes, myeloid and erythroid precursors are absent in the marrow. Although the diagnosis of aplastic anemia can

often be postulated from the appearance of the peripheral blood smear, bone marrow biopsy is essential for verification.

   a. Drugs and toxins: chloramphenicol, cancer chemotherapeutic agents, insecticides and benzene compounds.

   b. Radiation

   c. Infection, including viral hepatitis and primary Epstein-Barr virus infection

   d. Malignancy

      1. Neuroblastoma

      2. Leukemia may present with pallor, often accompanied by fever, tiredness, easy bruising, lymphadenopathy and limb pain. Gingival inflammation may occur in myelomonocytic leukemia and with absolute granulocyte counts of less than 1000/cu mm. The anemia is usually normocytic, normochromic, and thrombocytopenia is a frequent finding. The peripheral blood smear in some cases may reveal few or no abnormal cells, or abnormal cells may be found only after a diligent search. Normal or low white blood cell counts are common, but the WBC may also be greater than 50,000/cu mm. Occasionally, the bone marrow examination demonstrates that acute leukemia is the specific cause of agranulocytosis, thrombocytopenic purpura or aplastic anemia.

   e. Familial aplastic anemia

   f. Dyskeratosis congenita is characterized by dystrophic nails; reticulated hyperpigmentation of the face, neck and shoulders; and leukoplakia of mucous membranes.

   g. Idiopathic

Alter, B. P.: Aplastic anemia in children: Diagnosis and management. Pediatr. Rev. 6:46, 1984.

Lipton, J. M., and Nathan, D. G.: Aplastic and hypoplastic anemia. Pediatr. Clin. North Am. 27:217, 1980.

G. Marrow displacement by leukemia, neuroblastoma or granuloma may cause a normocytic, normochromic anemia with teardrop red cells, nucleated red cells, increased platelets and shifts to the left of the white blood cells.

H. Congestive splenomegaly, Gaucher's disease and, at times, other causes of splenomegaly may be accompanied by an anemia.

I. Hypothyroidism may produce an anemia.

J. Lead poisoning causes a hypochromic, microcytic anemia. The transferrin saturation is normal, and the free erythrocyte porphyrin level is increased.

K. Chronic renal disease leads to impaired bone marrow response and decreased production of erythropoietin. Determination of the blood urea nitrogen or serum creatinine is essential in the study of patients with an unexplained anemia.

L. Acute infection or inflammation, if moderately severe, may cause a significant fall in hemoglobin within a week after the onset of the illness.

Abshire, T. C., and Reeves, J. D.: Anemia of acute inflammation in children. J. Pediatr. 103:868, 1983.

M. Chronic diseases, such as juvenile rheumatoid arthritis, cystic fibrosis, Crohn's disease and chronic granulomatous disease of childhood, may lead to anemia owing to sequestration of iron in the reticuloendothelial system. The anemia in these children may be either hypochromic, microcytic or normochromic, normocytic. The serum iron level, transferrin and the iron-binding protein are decreased. The saturation of transferrin is over 30 per cent.

N. Sideroblastic anemias owing to defective iron or heme metabolism are characterized by hypochromic and microcytic erythrocytes in the peripheral blood and sideroblasts in the bone marrow. The serum ferritin level is elevated. Refractory macrocytic sideroblastic anemia may be associated with neutropenia, thrombocytopenia, and exocrine pancreatic dysfunction.

Pearson, H. A., Lobel, J. S., Kocoshis, S. A., Naiman, J. L., Windmiller, J., Lammi, A. T., Hoffman, R., and Marsh, J. C.: A new syndrome of refractory sideroblastic anemia with vacuolization of marrow precursors and exocrine pancreatic dysfunction. J. Pediatr. 95:976, 1979.

O. Congenital atransferrinemia, a rare autosomal recessive disorder, is characterized by a hypochromic microcytic anemia and generalized hemochromatosis.

II. INCREASED DESTRUCTION/SHORTENED LIFE SPAN OF ERYTHROCYTES

The normal life span of the erythrocyte is 100 to 120 days. In the presence of hemolytic disease, the survival time is shortened, at times markedly, owing to an inborn error in the red cell membrane, a hemoglobinopathy, an abnormality of the intracellular enzymes or an acquired extracorpuscular disorder. Increased red cell destruction is accompanied by a fall in free plasma haptoglobin.

Addiego, J. E., Hurst, D., and Lubin, B. H.: Congenital hemolytic anemia. Pediatr. Rev. 6:201, 1985.

Miller, D. R.: The hereditary hemolytic anemias. Membrane and enzyme defects. Pediat. Clin. North Am. 19:865, 1972.

A. Erythrocyte membrane defects. Because of their physical characteristics, red blood cells with membrane defects have a shorter survival time than normal red cells. Their retention by the spleen for a relatively prolonged time accelerates their destruction.

1. Although hereditary spherocytosis may be symptomatic in newborns and during the first year of life, clinical manifestations are usually not present until the latter part of the first decade or later. In the newborn infant, hereditary spherocytosis may have to be differentiated from symptomatic ABO incompatibility. Children seen early as infants or preschool children may have a hemoglobin of 8 to 11 gm/dl. If the hemolytic process is mild and the marrow activity is normal, anemia may not occur. Peripheral blood examination usually reveals spherocytes, but in some patients microspherocytes may be infrequent or the blood smear may be normal. The MCHC is over 36 per cent. Reticulocytosis may be very active. The osmotic fragility of the red cells, commonly increased, may begin at concentrations of about 0.50, instead of the normal 0.45. When the osmotic fragility as determined by the standard procedure is normal, the determination of the fragility of incubated red blood cells may provide useful information. At times, it is difficult to determine whether a patient has an acquired or a congenital hemolytic anemia. The demonstration of spherocytosis in one of the patient's parents makes congenital hemolytic anemia a likely diagnosis; however, in 10 to 20 per cent of patients, a familial incidence cannot be ascertained.

Aplastic crises in patients with hereditary spherocytosis, usually caused by a viral infection, are characterized by depression of erythropoiesis, disappearance of reticulocytosis and increased hemolysis.

2. Hereditary elliptocytosis, a disorder in which the erythrocytes are elliptical or cigar-shaped with possible crenated or spiculated surfaces, is accompanied by a hemolytic anemia in about 10 per cent of patients.

3. Hereditary infantile pyknocytosis, or pyropoikilocytosis, a hemolytic anemia characterized by numerous distorted and contracted erythrocytes or burr cells, may appear in infancy or early childhood. This disorder may cause neonatal hyperbilirubinemia.

4. Hereditary stomatocytosis, an autosomal dominant disorder, is characterized by erythrocytes that have an area of central pallor and resemble a basket, mushroom cap or pinch bottle.

5. Paroxysmal nocturnal hemoglobinuria, caused by an intrinsic erythrocyte defect, is a chronic hemolytic anemia. Hemolysis is increased at night, and hemoglobinuria is present in the morning.

6. Erythropoietic porphyria

7. Abetalipoproteinemia is characterized, in part, by acanthocytosis, reticulocytosis and hemolytic anemia.

B. Hemoglobinopathies. The most frequently encountered hemoglobinopathies in the United States are sickle cell disease, thalassemia and the variants of hemoglobin C disease.

1. Sickle cell disease may occur as sickle cell trait or anemia or as a variant in association with hemoglobins C, D, Punjab, E, G, J, N and O Arab, with beta thalassemia, hereditary spherocytosis and hereditary persistence of F hemoglobin. Patients with the sickle cell trait are asymptomatic. The "trait" cells have a normal span, whereas the sickle cell anemia cells have an abbreviated life span of 15 to 60 days. Both parents of a child with sickle cell anemia demonstrate sickling; however, it occurs in only one parent of a child with the trait. The patient with sickle cell anemia is homozygous for the abnormal sickle cell gene. The "trait" cells contain a mixture of both "A" and "S" types of hemoglobin, whereas the sickle cell anemia cells are composed of "S" and "F" hemoglobin.

Hemoglobin C in combination with sickle cell hemoglobin is responsible for a hemolytic syndrome ("sickle cell-hemoglobin C disease") characterized by mild anemia, sickling and slowly developing hepatosplenomegaly that usually disappears after the age of five years. The hemoglobin concentration in these children ranges between 9 and 10 gm, and the red blood cell count between 3.5 and 4.5 million. The erythrocytes are small and rarely sickle on the routine smear. A striking number (40 to 85 per cent) of target cells are present. One of the parents demonstrates the sickling trait, while the other is an asymptomatic carrier of hemoglobin C. Crises are infrequent and mild. Patients may demonstrate arthralgia, abdominal pain and jaundice. Large numbers of target cells on the peripheral smear of a patient thought to have mild sickle cell anemia raises the possibility of sickle cell–hemoglobin C disease. Patients with the hemoglobin C trait (hemoglobin C plus normal hemoglobin) have many target cells. Rarely, homozygous hemoglobin C disease occurs as a compensated hemolytic anemia with a large number of target cells on the peripheral smear.

Transient "aplastic" crises, which may persist for about ten days, follow acute infectious diseases in children with sickle cell anemia. During these periods, almost no red blood cells are released from the marrow. The child becomes weak and pale and demonstrates high output failure. Splenic sequestration crises are characterized by a sudden massive enlargement of the spleen and a rapid drop in the hemoglobin level.

Sickle cell anemia is normochromic and normocytic. In addition to sickling, the peripheral blood smear may show polychromasia, nucleated red blood cells, spherocytes, siderocytes, Howell-Jolly bodies and target cells. The reticulocyte count is increased. The hemoglobin ranges from 5.5 to 9.5 gm/dl. Because of failure of rouleau formation, the sedimentation rate is not increased. Although sickling usually cannot be regularly demonstrated in infants under three or four months of age, a few sickled cells may be seen. Hemoglobin electrophoresis· is the recommended screening test. A positive Sickledex test, based on the precipitation of hemoglobins

in alkali, confirms the presence of hemoglobin S.

In infants, painful swelling of the hands and feet (hand-foot syndrome) or dactylitis may occur. Hemolytic crises may be manifest by fever, pain, jaundice, increased anemia and dark urine. Arthralgia, muscle pains, cardiac dilatation and murmurs may simulate acute rheumatic fever. Severe abdominal pain and rigidity (abdominal crises) may be difficult or impossible to differentiate from an acute surgical abdomen. Severe pain in an extremity may be caused by a vaso-occlusive complication or salmonella osteomyelitis. Neurologic manifestations include hemiparesis and seizures. Children with sickle cell anemia, especially those under five years of age, are very susceptible to pneumococcal bacteremia. Because the child may not initially appear ill, the clinician must be alert to this possibility. Dyspnea, high fever, leukocytosis and pain on breathing are usually associated with pneumonia, with *Diplococcus pneumoniae* as the etiologic organism. Pulmonary infarction may also occur.

Davis, J. R., Vichinsky, E. P., and Lubin, B. H.: Current treatment of sickle cell disease. Curr. Probl. Pediatr. 10:5, 1980.

Powars, D. R.: Natural history of sickle cell disease—the first ten years. Semin. Hematol. 12:267, 1975.

2. The thalassemia syndromes, a heterogenous group of hereditary anemias caused by impaired synthesis of adult hemoglobin, occur chiefly in persons of Mediterranean extraction. Classification is based on the specific globin chain that is diminished or absent: beta globin is decreased or absent in beta thalassemia; alpha globin in alpha thalassemia. Hereditary persistence of fetal hemoglobin is another variant. The thalassemias have both ineffective erythropoiesis and a hemolytic component.

Beta thalassemia, the most frequent type, occurs in either a heterozygous or a homozygous form. The heterozygous form, termed thalassemia trait or minor, is asymptomatic except for slight splenomegaly. The red blood cells are microcytic and hypochromic. Poikilocytosis, target cells, basophilic stippling and ovalocytosis are present. HbA_2 is increased, and HbF is normal or slightly increased. The MCV and MCH are very low, 60 and 22 respectively. Serum ferritin and transferrin saturation are normal.

Homozygous beta thalassemia (thalassemia major or Cooley's anemia) becomes evident in infancy with a hemoglobin concentration frequently under 5 gm, marked poikilocytosis, anisocytosis, hypochromasia, polychromatophilia, basophilic stippling, target cells, oval cells, macrocytes and microcytes. Hepatosplenomegaly appears early. Osseous changes are apparent on roentgenographic examination. Usually HbF is increased to 30-60 per cent with a range from 3 to 100 per cent. The iron binding capacity is fully saturated.

Thalassemia intermedia, a milder form of homozygous beta thalassemia, is characterized by slight splenomegaly and hemoglobin over 6.5 gm and does not require blood transfusions.

Alpha-thalassemia, which has a higher prevalence in the Chinese, occurs, in order of increasing severity, in (1) an asymptomatic carrier state with normal erythrocyte morphology; (2) alpha thalassemia trait characterized by either hypochromic microcytosis or normal morphology without anemia; and (3) HbH disease or fatal hydrops fetalis in which only HbBarts and HbH are present. Sickle cell–thalassemia disease (microdrepanocytic anemia) results when the gene for thalassemia is inherited from one parent and that for sickle cell from the other. The peripheral blood smear simulates that of Cooley's anemia. Only a few sickle cells may be noted on the fixed smear, but up to 100 per cent sickling is observed on special preparations.

Bank, A.: The thalassemia syndromes. Blood 51:369, 1978.
Orkin, S. H., and Nathan, D. G.: The thalassemias. N. Engl. J. Med. 295:710, 1976.
Poncz, M., Cohen, A., and Schwartz, E.: Thalassemia. Adv. Pediatr. 31:43, 1984.

3. Hemoglobin variants (hemoglobin Zurich, Koln), some 60 in number and known as "unstable" hemoglobins, may be associated with a chronic severe or compensated hemolytic state referred to as congenital Heinz body hemolytic anemia. See also page 432.

4. Hereditary persistence of fetal hemoglobin causes mild polycythemia in the homozygote.

C. Hereditary enzymatic defects of the erythrocytes leads to nondeformable cells that become entrapped in the reticuloendothelial system. The hereditary enzymatic defects may be classified into three groups.

1. Defects of the Embden-Meyerhof or anaerobic pathway
   a. Pyruvate kinase deficiency, transmitted in an autosomal recessive fashion, is the most common enzymatic defect in this group. The severity of the hemolytic process is variable. Hemolytic anemia and jaundice in newborn infants are common. Splenomegaly may be present.
   b. Diphosphoglyceromutase deficiency
   c. Glucose phosphate isomerase deficiency
   d. Hexokinase deficiency
   e. Phosphofructokinase deficiency
   f. Phosphoglycerate kinase deficiency
   g. Triose phosphate isomerase deficiency

2. Defects of the hexose monophosphate shunt
   a. Glucose-6-phosphate dehydrogenase (G6PD) deficiency, likely the most common inborn error of metabolism, linked in its transmission to the X chromosome and described in over 100 variants, occurs most frequently in blacks (10 to 15 per cent of black Americans), Chinese, Italians, Greeks and Sephardic Jews. When present, the hemolysis may be acute or chronic, spontaneous, or precipitated by exposure to oxidant drugs such as acetophenetin, acetylsalicylic acid, sulfonamides, nitrofurans, naphthalene, fava beans, vitamin K and antimalarials. Acute hemolysis appears two to four days after drug exposure, leading to a drop in hemoglobin concentration, hemoglobinuria, jaundice, reticulocytosis, decreased or absent haptoglobin and a peripheral smear that is characterized by fragmented erythrocytes, crenated forms, Heinz bodies and occasional spherocytes.

Hemolytic reactions may also be precipitated by infections. G6PD deficiency is a cause of neonatal hyperbilirubinemia.

  b. 6-phosphogluconic dehydrogenase deficiency.
3. Defects in glutathione synthesis. GSH synthetase deficiency.
4. Abnormalities of erythrocyte nucleotide metabolism
   a. Pyrimidine 5′-nucleotidase deficiency
   b. Increased adenosine deaminase

Sullivan, D. W., and Glader, B. E.: Erythrocyte enzyme disorders in children. Pediatr. Clin. North Amer. 27:449, 1980.

D. Extracorpuscular mechanisms. In this group of hemolytic anemias, extrinsic factors cause intrinsically normal erythrocytes to be destroyed or their susceptibility to destruction to be increased. Transfused red blood cells are also rapidly destroyed. Occasionally, acquired extracorpuscular mechanisms complicate the course of anemia associated with an intrinsic erythrocyte abnormality, perhaps as a result of repeated blood transfusions.
1. Immune hemolytic anemias
   a. Isoimmune
      1. Mismatched blood transfusion
      2. Rh or ABO sensitization (hemolytic disease of the newborn)
   b. Autoimmune
      Autoimmune hemolytic anemias may be transient or chronic. IgM-induced hemolytic anemia is associated with cold hemagglutinin as in *Mycoplasma pneumoniae* infection, infectious mononucleosis, cytomegalovirus infection, mumps, non-Hodgkin's lymphoma or systemic lupus erythematosus. Most autoimmune hemolytic anemias involve IgG antibodies. The onset is usually acute or hyperacute, and the degree of anemia usually mandates transfusions, at least initially. Hemoglobinuria may also occur. The direct Coombs' test is positive.
      1. Viral infection: (infectious mononucleosis, influenza, Coxsackie B, measles, mumps, varicella, cytomegalovirus)
      2. Bacterial infection (*Escherichia coli*, streptococcal sepsis, tuberculosis, typhoid fever)
      3. *Mycoplasma pneumoniae* infection

4. Malaria
5. Drugs (phenacetin, cephalosporin, penicillin)
6. Connective tissue disorders (lupus erythematosus, periarteritis nodosa, scleroderma, dermatomyositis, rheumatoid arthritis)
7. Oncologic disorders (leukemia, lymphoma)
8. Paroxysmal cold hemoglobinuria
9. Idiopathic thrombocytopenic purpura may be accompanied by acute hemocytic anemia (Evans syndrome) in connective tissue disorders such as systemic lupus erythematosus or with chronic lymphocytic thyroiditis.
10. Chronic inflammatory disorders such as ulcerative colitis

Habibi, B., Homberg, J-C., Schaison, G., and Salmon, C.: Autoimmune hemolytic anemia in children. A review of 80 cases. Am. J. Med. 56:61, 1974.
Pui, C-H., Williams, J., and Wang, W.: Evans syndrome in childhood. J. Pediatr. 97:754, 1980.

2. Nonimmune hemolytic anemia
   a. Idiopathic
   b. Secondary
      1. Infections (as above, plus malaria, histoplasmosis)
      2. Drugs (vitamin K, benzene, phenacetin). The hemolytic action of drugs may be related to an enzymatic red cell deficiency, a hemoglobinopathy or antibodies to the drug.
      3. Hematologic disorders (leukemia, megaloblastic anemia, congestive splenomegaly, histiocytosis)
      4. Burns
      5. The venom of certain reptiles and arachnids may act as hemolysins. The bite of the brown recluse spider (*Loxosceles reclusa*) causes both a local necrotic lesion and a severe systemic reaction characterized by fever, nausea, hemolytic anemia, hemoglobinuria and thrombocytopenia.
      6. Porphyria
      7. Microangiopathic hemolytic anemia
         a. The hemolytic uremic syndrome in infants and young children commonly begins with vomiting, diarrhea,

mild fever and an upper respiratory infection followed by a severe hemolytic anemia, thrombocytopenia, hemoglobinuria, bleeding, acute renal failure, hypertension, irritability, seizures, stupor and coma. The red blood cells may be distorted, fragmented, contracted and deeply stained. Burr and helmet cells may be noted.

Drummond, K. N.: Hemolytic uremic syndrome—then and now. N. Engl. J. Med. 312:116, 1985.

    b. Disseminated intravascular coagulation
    c. Hemolytic anemia may rarely occur after surgical repair of an endocardial cushion defect or of tetralogy of Fallot.

Maurer, H. M.: Hematologic effects of cardiac disease. Pediatr. Clin. North Am. 19:1083, 1972.

    d. Marked neonatal microangiopathic hemolytic anemia, thrombocytopenia and persistent hemolysis may occur in association with a large placental chorioangioma.

Bauer, C. R., Fojaco, R. M., Bancalari, E., and Fernandez-Rocha, L.: Microangiopathic hemolytic anemia and thrombocytopenia in a neonate associated with a large placental chorioangioma. Pediatrics 62:574, 1978.

    e. Spur cell anemia with bizarre, thorny red cell projections may occur in association with progressive intrahepatic cholestasis.
    f. Severe hypertension
  8. Vitamin E deficiency may cause a hemolytic anemia in infants by four to six weeks of age. The disorder has a predilection for premature infants who weigh less than 1500 gm. The hemoglobin in these patients is 7 to 9 gm/dl, and the reticulocyte count ranges between 4 and 20 per cent. The peripheral blood smear shows spherocytes, red cell fragments and spiculated red blood cells. The platelet count is markedly elevated. Peripheral edema may be present. Owing to formula supplementation, vitamin E–dependent anemia is now rare.

Oski, F. A., and Barness, L. A.: Vitamin E deficiency: A previously unrecognized cause of hemolytic anemia in the premature infant. J. Pediatr. 70:211, 1967.

  9. Wilson's disease in adolescence may cause acute hepatic failure with hemolysis.

III. BLOOD LOSS. Acute hemorrhage causes a normochromic, normocytic anemia, leukocytosis and an increase in the percentage of polymorphonuclear leukocytes. Reticulocytosis develops within a day or two. Chronic hemorrhage in disorders such as Crohn's disease causes a hypochromic, microcytic anemia with moderate reticulocytosis. Further discussion of blood loss is included in Chapter 62 on Hemorrhage. A stool guaiac test should be routine in patients with an unexplained anemia. The platelets may be increased in the presence of gastrointestinal blood loss.

Idiopathic pulmonary hemosiderosis may be characterized by iron deficiency anemia and episodes of fatigue, dyspnea, cyanosis, fever and cough, progressive pulmonary changes and reticulocytosis.

The possibility of intrauterine fetal-fetal or fetal-maternal hemorrhage is an important consideration in infants with pallor or shock at birth or in the first few hours of life. Neonatal blood loss may also occur secondary to placenta previa, placenta abruptio, velamentous insertion of the cord, tears in the placental vessels during delivery, surgical incision into the placenta during cesarean section or rupture of the umbilical cord. The newborn infant may also experience an internal hemorrhage.

Gill, F. M., and Schwartz, E.: Anemia in early infancy. Pediatr. Clin. North Am. 19:841, 1972.
Pearson, H. A.: Posthemorrhagic anemia in the newborn. Pediatr. Rev. 4:40, 1982.

LABORATORY EXAMINATIONS

Special examinations that may be indicated in patients thought to have increased blood destruction include the following:
  1. Blood smear. Examination of the peripheral blood smear may demonstrate polychromasia, nucleated red cells, immature myeloid cells and an increase in the percentage of polymorphonuclear leukocytes. The

morphologic characteristics of the red cells may be diagnostic or very suggestive in patients with red cell membrane defects or hemoglobinopathies. Spherocytes may occur in hereditary spherocytosis, autoimmune hemolytic anemias, ABO incompatibility, congestive splenomegaly and microangiopathic hemolytic anemias. In the presence of an active hemolytic process, spherocytes are usually readily evident on the stained smear. Target cells are frequently present in patients with an abnormal type of hemoglobin (e.g., sickle cell anemia and thalassemia), in liver disease and after splenectomy. Twenty to 95 per cent of the erythrocytes may appear as target cells in patients with hemoglobin C or sickle cell hemoglobin C disease. Basophilic stippling of red cells may be noted in patients with lead poisoning. Stippling, which becomes even more evident when the smear is stained with brilliant cresyl blue, is not specific for lead poisoning but may occur in other hematologic disorders. Heinz bodies, aggregates of denatured cell-membrane proteins and visible on slides stained with brilliant cresyl blue, occur in anemias caused by enzymatic defects. Malaria may also be diagnosed by examination of a peripheral blood smear. Hypochromic, microcytic red blood cells may be seen with iron deficiency, chronic disease, lead poisoning, copper deficiency, congenital transferrin deficiency and chronic blood loss. An increased number of platelets may be noted on the smear in patients with gastrointestinal blood loss.

2. Reticulocyte count. The presence of anemia and reticulocytosis should suggest a hemolytic process even in the absence of jaundice. Reticulocytosis disappears during aplastic crises in the hemolytic anemias. With iron deficiency anemia, a reticulocyte response to iron therapy should be observed in 5 to 10 days.
3. Osmotic fragility
4. Serologic studies
   a. Test for blood group incompatibility if a transfusion reaction occurs.
   b. Rh antibodies; ABO incompatibility in hemolytic disease of the newborn
   c. Coombs' test. A positive direct Coombs' test indicates the presence of an immunohemolytic anemia. The Coombs' test is often positive in extracorpuscular anemias and almost always negative in those caused by intracorpuscular anomalies. Although the direct Coombs' test is almost always positive in hemolytic disease of the newborn with Rh incompatibility, it is usually negative with ABO incompatiblity.
   d. Autohemagglutinins: cold agglutinins, warm agglutinins
   e. Procedures utilizing trypsin-treated red blood cells and acidification of the patient's serum have been used to help demonstrate circulating antibodies in patients with acquired hemolytic anemia.
5. Antinuclear and anti-DNA antibodies
6. Screening examinations for the presence of infection, including blood cultures and chest roentgenogram.
7. The serum bilirubin level may be increased in patients with hemolytic anemia. In the presence of good hepatic function, however, elevation of the serum bilirubin may be minimal or absent.
8. Hemoglobinuria is an indication of intravascular hemolysis.
9. Bilirubin may appear in the urine in some patients with hemolytic anemia owing to the development of regurgitation jaundice.
10. Hemoglobin electrophoresis is required when a hemoglobinopathy is suspected.
11. Screening test for G6PD deficiency
12. Free erythrocyte porphyrin is increased in iron deficiency, lead poisoning and protoporphyria.

GENERAL REFERENCES

Dickerman, J. D.: Anemia in the newborn infant. Pediatr. Rev. 6:131, 1984.

Nathan, D. G., and Oski, F. A. (eds.): Hematology of Infancy and Childhood. Philadelphia. W. B. Saunders Co., 1974.

Oski, F. A., and Naiman, J. L.: Hematologic Problems in the Newborn, 3rd. ed. Philadelphia, W. B. Saunders Co., 1982.

ETIOLOGIC CLASSIFICATION OF ANEMIA

62 / HEMORRHAGE, PURPURA

Hemorrhage requires prompt diagnosis and management. Bleeding may be caused by local causes, such as a Meckel's diverticulum, or by systemic disorders, such as thrombocytopenic purpura. In most instances, the cause can readily be identified by the history, the physical examination and a few laboratory procedures. The two chief pathophysiologic processes involved in the pathogenesis of hemorrhagic disorders are an increase in capillary fragility (vascular factors) and a defect in the blood-clotting mechanism (intravascular factors). Systemic hemorrhagic disorders may range in severity from spontaneous hemorrhage or bleeding after insignificant trauma, to a mild tendency to bleed only after dental extraction or tonsillectomy, to recurrent epistaxis or easy bruising. Because extensive bruising raises the possibility of physical abuse, a skeletal survey may be indicated.

Epistaxis is discussed on page 46.
Hematemesis is discussed on page 216.
Hemoptysis is discussed on page 381.
Melena is discussed on page 258.
Hematuria is discussed on page 416.
Dysfunctional uterine bleeding is discussed on page 289.

ETIOLOGIC CLASSIFICATION OF HEMORRHAGE AND PURPURA

I. VASCULAR FACTORS

The factors that control or influence capillary fragility and the vascular factors in hemostasis are not well understood. The Rumpel-Leede test permits only a crude evaluation of capillary fragility. Diseases in which hemorrhage or purpura may be attributed to vascular factors are listed below. Vascular factors may be responsible for the presence or absence of bleeding in patients with thrombocytopenia.

A. Trauma or other physical cause for sudden rupture of a vessel
B. Infectious diseases may be accompanied by hemorrhagic manifestations as a result of bacterial emboli or endothelial damage. Hemorrhagic manifestations may accompany the acute exanthems, typhoid fever, infectious mononucleosis, infective endocarditis, the rickettsial diseases, congenital toxoplasmosis, septicemia and other disease processes. Meningococcemia must always be a diagnostic consideration in patients with acute, unexplained petechiae and purpura.
C. Drugs, chemicals, toxins
D. Scurvy
E. Allergic or anaphylactoid purpura (Henoch-Schönlein) may be characterized by distinctive rash with purpura (see page 165); severe, cramping abdominal pain; painful, hot, swollen joints; localized edema; and, possibly, melena, epistaxis, hematemesis or hematuria, convulsions, encephalopathy, facial palsy and bleeding into the scrotum. Recurrences of the rash may continue for months, and there may be chronic renal sequelae. Allergic purpura may follow an acute infectious disease, such as streptococcal pharyngitis, rheumatic fever, acute glomerulonephritis or periarteritis nodosa.
F. Irradiation
G. Metabolic diseases
   1. Histiocytosis X in infants may be characterized by petechial skin lesions.
   2. Cushing's syndrome
H. Hereditary telangiectasia usually does not appear in young children but may be a rare cause of epistaxis in adolescents.
 I. Ehlers-Danlos syndrome may be characterized by capillary hemorrhage, large hematomas and fragile skin that breaks with slight trauma. Cutis hyperelastica and subcutaneous lipomas may also be present.

II. INTRAVASCULAR FACTORS: defects in the blood-clotting mechanism

When the wall of a vessel is ruptured, reflex vasoconstriction and retraction temporarily prevent further blood loss. The platelets in contact with the subendothelial collagen release ADP (adenosine diphosphate), which causes a loose platelet plug owing to platelet aggregation and adhesion. Simultaneously, the collagen fibers activate the intrinsic clotting mechanism beginning with the conversion of proenzyme factor XII (Hageman) to the active enzyme XIIa. The cascade of enzymatic reactions continues with XIIa acting on factor XI (PTA) as its substrate to produce XIa, which acts on factor IX (PTC or Christmas factor) to produce IXa, which converts factor X (Stuart) to Xa. This reaction is catalyzed when IXa forms a complex with factor VIII, phospholipid contributed from platelets, and calcium. Factor X is also activated to Xa by tissue juice or thromboplastin, forming a complex with factor VII (stable factor) and calcium via the extrinsic pathway.

A complex of Xa, factor V (labile factor), phospholipid and calcium then converts prothrombin (factor II) to thrombin, which (1) converts fibrinogen (factor I) to fibrin and (2) activates fibrin-stabilizing factor XIII. Screening tests that permit identification of deficiencies in this hemostatic cascade include the PTT (partial thromboplastin time), PT (prothrombin time) and fibrinogen levels.

With circulating anticoagulants and fibrinolysins, whole blood clotting time is usually prolonged.

The clinical states associated with intravascular deficiencies include the following.

A. Hemorrhagic diseases characterized by thrombocytopenia or qualitative platelet disorders.

Gilchrist, G. S.: Platelet disorders. Pediatr. Clin. North Am. 19:1047, 1972.

   1. Thrombocytopenia
      a. Idiopathic (immune) thrombocytopenic purpura is a diagnosis made by the exclusion of other specific etiologies. Idiopathic thrombocytopenic purpura may follow within one to six weeks an upper respiratory tract infection, measles, measles vaccination, rubella, mumps, chickenpox, infectious mononucleosis, hepatitis or cytomegalovirus infection. Occasionally, ITP occurs before or concomitantly with an autoimmune disorder such as acute hemolytic anemia (Evans syndrome). In other instances, an obvious preceding infection cannot be identified.

In children, idiopathic thrombocytopenic purpura is usually a self-limited disorder; however, intracranial hemorrhage may be a rare complication. Whereas congenital thrombocytopenic purpura is often associated with maternal thrombocytopenia or purpura, and maternal platelet antibody is postulated to cross the placenta, the mother's platelet status may be normal.

In addition to the contribution that thrombocytopenia makes to hemorrhage, vascular changes are probably an even more important determinant of whether or not bleeding occurs. Bleeding or bruising tendencies in idiopathic thrombocytopenic purpura may diminish even without an increase in the platelet count.

McClure, P. D.: Idiopathic thrombocytopenic purpura in children. Pediatrics 55:68, 1975.
Ozsoylu, S., Kanra, G., and Savas, G.: Thrombocytopenic purpura related to rubella infection. Pediatrics 62:567, 1978.

b. Secondary thrombocytopenic purpura
1. Infections
   a. Systemic or local bacterial or viral infections are frequent causes of thrombocytopenic purpura. Infectious mononucleosis may rarely be complicated by thrombocytopenic purpura.

Overall, J. C., Jr., and Glassgow, L. A.: Virus infections of the fetus and newborn. J. Pediatr. 77:315, 1970.

   b. Disseminated intravascular coagulation
2. Drugs: sulfonamides, chloramphenicol, iodides, arsenicals, phenolphthalein, valproic acid
3. Poisons and toxins
4. Irradiation
5. Neoplasms, especially leukemia and neuroblastoma
6. Congestive splenomegaly
7. Systemic lupus erythematosus
8. Giant hemangiomas
9. Storage diseases: histiocytosis X, Gaucher's disease, Niemann-Pick disease
10. Exchange transfusion
11. Isoimmunologic hemolytic disease of the newborn
12. Idiopathic hyperglycinuria
13. Inborn metabolic errors
14. Aplastic anemia. Hemorrhage owing to thrombocytopenia may be the first manifestation of aplastic anemia.
15. Megaloblastic anemia with ineffective thrombopoiesis
16. Hemolytic-uremic syndrome
17. Acquired immune deficiency
c. Wiskott-Aldrich syndrome, a sex-linked, recessive disorder characterized by thrombocytopenia, small platelets, petechiae, bloody diarrhea, eczema, chronically draining ears, recurrent infections and selective abnormalities of B- and T-cell function. Gross melena may be the initial manifestation in the newborn infant.

Perry, G. S., III, Spector, B. D., Schuman, L. M., Mandel, J. S., Anderson, V. E., McHugh, R. B., Hanson, M. R., Fahlstrom, S. M., Krivit, W., and Kersey, J. H.: The Wiskott-Aldrich syndrome in the United States and Canada (1892–1979). J. Pediatr. 97:72, 1980.

d. Familial hemophagocytic reticulosis is a fatal familial disease characterized by fever, hepatosplenomegaly, abnormal liver functions, lymphadenopathy, pancytopenia, thrombocytopenia, hypofibrinogenemia and bone marrow histiocytic hyperplasia with erythrophagocytosis. The virus-associated hemophagocytic syndrome (VAHS) may be caused by the cytomegalovirus, herpes simplex virus, Epstein-Barr virus, adenovirus and other viruses.

McClure, P. D., Strachan, P., and Saunders, E. F.: Hypofibrinogenemia and thrombocytopenia in familial hemophagocytic reticulosis. J. Pediatr. 85:67, 1974.
Risdall, R. J., et al.: Virus-associated hemophagocytic syndrome: A benign histiocytic proliferation distinct from malignant histiocytosis. Cancer 44:993, 1979.

e. Thrombotic thrombocytopenic purpura is characterized by hemorrhage, hemolytic anemia, fever, neurologic symptoms and azotemia.
f. Bernard-Soulier syndrome, an autosomal recessive disorder, is characterized by giant platelets and shortened platelet survival.

g. Osteopetrosis

h. May-Hegglin syndrome, an autosomal dominant disorder, is characterized by unusually large platelets, blue cytoplasmic inclusions in the neutrophils and thrombocytopenia.

i. Fanconi's pancytopenia

j. Thrombocytopenia with absent radii (TAR) syndrome is characterized by neonatal thrombocytopenia and absent radii but with both thumbs present.

2. Qualitative and functional platelet disorders are characterized by easy bruising, epistaxis, oozing after dental extraction, spontaneous petechiae and bleeding as a complication of surgery.

Hathaway, W. E.: Bleeding disorders due to platelet dysfunction. Am. J. Dis. Child. 121:127, 1971.

a. Glanzmann's thrombasthenia, a hemorrhagic disease transmitted as an autosomal recessive trait and usually symptomatic in infancy, is manifested by epistaxis, prolonged oozing, ecchymoses and petechiae that occur spontaneously in response to slight trauma or following surgery. Although normal in number, the platelets are physically or functionally abnormal. The bleeding time is prolonged, clot retraction is defective and platelet aggregation and adhesion are decreased or absent.

b. von Willebrand's disease, a group of hemorrhagic syndromes usually transmitted as an autosomal dominant disorder, is associated most frequently with severe epistaxis. Menorrhagia may be another presenting symptom, along with easy bruising and hemorrhage after trauma and surgery. In its severe form, both functional components of the factor VIII system (e.g., antihemophilic factor and von Willebrand factor) are decreased. The best screening test depends upon the ability of the patient's plasma to support ristocetin-induced aggregation of normal platelets. The bleeding time is prolonged, the partial thromboplastin time abnormal and platelet adherence to glass beads decreased.

Gralnick, H. R., Sultan, Y., and Collier, B. S.: Von Willebrand's disease. Combined qualitative and quantitative abnormalities. N. Engl. J. Med. 296:1024, 1977.
Green, D., and Chediak, J. R.: Von Willebrand's disease: Current concepts. Am. J. Med. 62:315, 1977.

c. ADP release defect (thrombopathia, Portsmouth's disease). The platelet count and clot retraction are normal. Platelet adhesion and aggregation are decreased.

d. PF3 release defect (thrombocytopathy). The platelet count, clot retraction, platelet adhesion and aggregation are normal, but PF3 release is decreased.

e. Platelet "storage pool" disease with defective endogenous stores of adenosine diphosphate.

f. Aspirin, antihistamines, phenothiazides, glycerol and guaiacolate interfere with the release of endogenous adenosine diphosphate and, therefore, prevent platelet aggregation and plug formation.

Schwartz, A. D., and Pearson, H. A.: Aspirin, platelets and bleeding. J. Pediatr. 78:558, 1971.

g. Platelet dysfunction occurs in connective tissue disorders, glycogen storage disease, Type I, uremia and cirrhosis.

h. Wiskott-Aldrich syndrome is accompanied by platelet dysfunction and shortened survival.

B. Inherited deficiencies of coagulation factors

1. Deficiency of antihemophilic globulin (AGH, factor VIII) is the most frequent cause of hemophilia (hemophilia A). About one half of severely affected patients report no family history of hemophilia. Whereas bleeding may occur after circumcision, hemophilia often is not symptomatic until the toddler age when the child bruises easily in response to slight trauma or bleeds from his mouth or frenulum of the tongue after a fall. The disorder is regarded as severe if the factor VIII level is less than 1 per cent, and mild if the factor VIII level is over 1 to 5 per cent. Hemarthroses, which develop after the age of two or three years, always suggest hemophilia as the cause.

The correlation between the whole blood coagulation time and hemorrhage is not a constant one. Although it is usually greatly prolonged, the clotting time may be normal in very mild disease. Although the bleeding time is normal, hemorrhage may persist if too large a skin puncture is made. The partial thromboplastin time is increased, the thromboplastic generation test abnormal and the factor VIII level decreased. Factor VIII antihemophilic factor may be reduced in von Willebrand's disease.

Abildgaard, C. F.: Progress and problems in hemophilia and von Willebrand's disease. Adv. Pediatr. 31:137, 1984.
Buchanan, G. R.: Hemophilia. Pediatr. Clin. North Am. 27:309, 1980.

2. Deficiency of factor IX or plasma thromboplastin component (hemophilia B, or Christmas disease), transmitted as a sex-linked recessive disorder and clinically indistinguishable from hemophilia A, is present in about 15 per cent of patients with hemophilia. Laboratory findings are similar to those of hemophilia A except that the factor IX assay is decreased.
3. Factor XI deficiency (hemophilia C)
4. Hereditary deficiency of the other coagulation factors is much rarer than those of VIII and IX.

Strauss, H. S.: Diagnosis and treatment of inherited bleeding disorders. Pediatr. Clin. North Amer. 19:1009, 1972.

C. Acquired clotting factor deficiencies
   1. Disseminated intravascular coagulation (DIC) is characterized by the intravascular consumption of factors I, II, V, VIII and platelets; deposition of fibrin thrombi within the vascular system; and a generalized hemorrhagic state. Clinical manifestations include hemorrhage (purpura, oozing from venipuncture sites or other bleeding); thrombotic and embolic phenomena (hematuria, renal failure and thrombotic skin lesions); central nervous system symptoms such as convulsions or coma; gastrointestinal manifestations such as ileus, vomiting and diarrhea; pallor; jaundice; and shock. In addition to evidence of consumption of the clotting factors as noted above, laboratory findings include the presence of fibrin split products and microangiopathic hemolytic anemia.
      Disseminated intravascular coagulation is a complication of bacterial sepsis, viral and rickettsial infections, burns, trauma, neonatal respiratory distress, malignancies, snake bite, purpura fulminans, cyanotic congenital heart disease, the hemolytic uremic syndrome, head injury and the virus-associated hemophagocytic syndrome, among other disorders.

Corrigan, J. J.: Disseminated intravascular coagulopathy. Pediatr. Rev. 1:37, 1979.
Hathaway, W. E.: Care of the critically ill child: the problem of disseminated intravascular coagulation. Pediatrics 46:767, 1970.
Miner, M. E., Kaufman, H. H., Graham, S. H., Haar, F. H., and Gildenberg, P. L.: Disseminated intravascular coagulation fibrinolytic syndrome following head injury in children. Frequency and prognostic implications. J. Pediatr. 100:687, 1982.

   2. Vitamin K deficiency causes decreased levels of prothrombin and factors VII, IX and X. The PT and PTT are greatly prolonged. The normal, physiologic deficiency of prothrombin between the second and tenth days of life may be prevented by vitamin K administration; otherwise, hemorrhagic disease of the newborn may occur. Acquired deficiency of vitamin K may be a complication of chronic diarrhea, cystic fibrosis, malabsorption syndromes and coumarin administration. A bleeding disorder may be the presenting problem in infants with cystic fibrosis. Hemorrhage usually does not occur unless the prothrombin time is less than 20 per cent of normal.

Lane, P. A., and Hathaway, W. E.: Vitamin K in infancy. J. Pediatr. 106:351, 1985.

   3. Liver disease, such as hepatitis, Reye's syndrome or Wilson's disease may cause a fall in factors I, II and V.
   4. Uremia may be accompanied by thrombocytopenia and an increase in PT and fibrin split products.
   5. Acyanotic and cyanotic congenital heart disease may be accompanied by a clotting disorder characterized by a tendency to bruise or to bleed excessively after trauma or surgery. A number of hemostatic abnormalities may occur.

Montgomery, R. R., and Hathaway, W. E.: Acute bleeding emergencies. Pediatr. Clin. North Am. 27:327, 1980.
Naiman, J. L.: Clotting and bleeding in cyanotic congenital heart disease. J. Pediatr. 76:333, 1970.

III. Psychogenic Hemorrhage

A. Erythrocyte sensitization (psychogenic purpura, Gardner-Diamond syndrome) is characterized by spontaneous ecchymoses, preceded, at times, by painful stinging or burning sensations, warmth, erythema or puffiness at the site. The bruises, which may range from one to several centimeters in diameter, undergo color change and gradually disappear over a one- to two-week period. The face and hands are the most frequent sites. Some patients report bleeding through the skin. Other somatic symptoms include severe headaches, syncope and abdominal pain.

Ratnoff, O. D.: The psychogenic purpuras: A review of autoerythrocyte sensitization, autosensitization to DNA, "hysterical" and factitial bleeding, and the religious stigmata. Semin. Hematol. 17:192, 1980.

B. Factitious hemorrhage owing to Munchausen's syndrome by proxy implies that the history of hemorrhage in an infant or young child (e.g., melena or hematuria) has been fabricated by a parent.

Kurlandsky, L., Lukoff, J. Y., Zinkham, W. H., Brody, J. P, and Kessler, R. W.: Munchausen syndrome by proxy: Definition of factitious bleeding in an infant by ^{51}Cr labeling of erythrocytes. Pediatrics 63:228, 1979.

ETIOLOGIC CLASSIFICATION OF HEMORRHAGE OR PURPURA IN THE NEWBORN

I. Hemorrhagic Disease of the Newborn occurs on the second or third days of life owing to transient deficiencies of vitamin K–dependent clotting factors (II, VII, IX and X). Clinical manifestations include bleeding from the umbilical cord, nose, gastrointestinal tract or circumcision site. In infants whose mothers received drugs, (e.g., phenytoin or phenobarbital), severe prenatal vitamin K deficiency may cause bleeding in the first 24 hours of life.

II. Hemorrhagic Manifestations at this time may also be caused by congenital deficiency of coagulation factors such as V, VII, X, XI and XII.

III. Hemophilia

IV. Severe Liver Disease

V. Neonatal Thrombocytopenic Purpura or platelet dysfunction may cause generalized showers of petechiae.

Pearson, H. A., and McIntosh, S.: Neonatal thrombocytopenia. Clin. Haematol. 7:111, 1978.

A. Passive immune neonatal thrombocytopenia associated with fetal-maternal platelet antigen incompatibility, maternal idiopathic thrombocytopenia purpura or systemic lupus erythematosus

Kelton, J. G., Blanchette, V. S., Wilson, W. E., Bowers, P., Pai, K. R. M., Effer, S. B., and Barr, R. D.: Neonatal thrombocytopenia due to passive immunization. N. Engl. J. Med. 302:1401, 1980.

B. Intrauterine infections: rubella, cytomegalovirus, toxoplasmosis and syphilis

Hanshaw, J. B., Dudgeon, J. A., and Marshall, W. C.: Viral Diseases of the Fetus and Newborn. 2nd ed. Philadelphia. W. B. Saunders Co., 1985.

C. Sepsis
D. Enterovirus infection

Lake, A. M., Lauer, B. A., Clark, J. C., Wesenberg, R. L., and McIntosh, K.: Enterovirus infection in neonates. J. Pediatr. 89:787, 1976.

E. Disseminated intravascular coagulation in sick infants may be initiated by acidosis, hypoxia, infection, endothelial damage, tissue necrosis and shock.

Woods, W. G., Luban, N. L. C., Hilgartner, M. W., and Miller, D. R.: Disseminated intravascular coagulation in the newborn. Am. J. Dis. Child. 133:44, 1979.

F. Increased consumption of platelets may be associated with renal vein thrombosis, giant hemangioma, necrotizing enterocolitis and infection.
G. Megakaryocytic hypoplasia
H. Wiskott-Aldrich syndrome may cause bloody diarrhea in the newborn male owing to thrombocytopenia.
I. Thrombocytopenia with absent radii (TAR) syndrome may cause neonatal bleeding.
J. Hemolytic disease of the newborn; exchange transfusion
K. Congenital leukemia
L. Suppression of platelet production by prenatal medications (e.g., sulfonamides, tolbutamide, quinine, benzothiadiazines)
M. Congenital deficiency of thrombopoietin
N. In most instances of neonatal thrombocytopenia, the etiology is unknown but may be related to neonatal complications.

Mehta, P., Vasa, R., Neumann, L., and Karpatkin, M.: Thrombocytopenia in the high-risk infant. J. Pediatr. 97:791, 1980.

VI. QUALITATIVE AND FUNCTIONAL PLATELET DEFECTS

VII. PETECHIAE may transiently occur around the head, neck or other presenting part in normal infants in the absence of thrombocytopenia.

Glader, B. E., and Buchanan, G. R.: The bleeding neonate. Pediatrics 58:548, 1976.

Hathaway, W. E.: The bleeding newborn. Semin. Hematol. 12:175, 1975.

Hathaway, W. E., and Bonnar, J.: Perinatal Coagulation. New York. Grune and Stratton. 1978.

McIntosh, S., O'Brien, R. T., Schwartz, A. D., and Pearson, H. A.: Neonatal isoimmune purpura: Response to platelet infusion. J. Pediatr. 82:1020, 1973.

Merenstein, G. B., O'Loughlin, E. P., and Plunket, D. C.: Effects of maternal thiazides on platelet counts of newborn infants. J. Pediatr. 76:766, 1970.

PROCEDURES USEFUL IN THE DIAGNOSIS OF HEMORRHAGIC STATES

1. A careful history of an abnormal bleeding tendency in the child or the family (e.g., easy bruising or unusual bleeding after dental extraction or tonsillectomy) is a valuable screening tool. In the presence of a positive history, complete coagulation studies are indicated.
2. Laboratory test selection depends upon the findings in the history, physical examination and screening tests.
   a. The Lee-White clotting time is as suitable as any other test for determination of the clotting time, which is normally between 6 and 15 minutes.
   b. The bleeding time, normally between one and 5 minutes, depends upon the status of capillary contractility and platelet function, as well as extravascular factors. The Ivy method, which uses the forearm with blood pressure cuff inflated to 40 mm of mercury, is preferred. The bleeding time may be prolonged with thrombocytopenic purpura, von Willebrand's disease or hypoprothrombinemia.
   c. Clot retraction, which requires the presence of platelets, correlates well with the platelet count. Retraction is impaired or absent if the platelet count is less than 70,000 and poor in patients with thrombasthenia.
   d. Red blood cell count; hemoglobin; hematocrit; white blood cell count
   e. Platelet count
   f. The peripheral smear may be helpful in the diagnosis of infectious mononucleosis and leukemia. The presence of platelets in clumps tends to rule out thrombocytopenia.
   g. When meningococcemia is suspected, a petechial smear may be performed by nicking a petechial lesion moderately deeply with a Bard-Parker blade, making and staining a smear and examining it for gram-negative intracellular diplococci.
   h. Examination of the bone marrow may be indicated to determine the status of the megakaryocytes and to rule out aplasia or leukemia. The presence of at least one megakaryocyte per low-power field in a cellular bone marrow is normal.
   i. Prothrombin time, partial thromboplastin time and a fibrinogen level. Deficiencies in the intrinsic pathway (XII, XIII, IX, X, XI) show an abnormal thromboplastin time while prothrombin and fibrinogen levels are normal. Deficiencies in the extrinsic pathway (II, V, VIII and X) show an abnormal thromboplastin time and prothrombin time, but normal fibrinogen level. With congenital absence of fibrinogen, clotting does not occur.
   j. Liver function tests
   k. A positive tourniquet test raises the possibility of a vascular defect; a negative result does not exclude this possibility.

LABORATORY FINDINGS IN THROMBOCYTOPENIC PURPURA

1. Deficient clot retraction or absence of retraction
2. Lowered platelet count, usually under 75,000. The number of platelets and the patient's tendency to bleed may be poorly correlated.
3. Diminution or absence of platelets on the peripheral blood smear. In ITP

the young platelets are increased in size.

4. Bleeding time may be normal or increased. If the platelet count is under 60,000, the bleeding time is usually prolonged.
5. Coagulation time of whole blood is normal.
6. The capillary fragility may be increased. Since a good correlation exists between capillary fragility and the patient's tendency to bruise and

bleed, the tourniquet test may offer a better guide than the platelet count.

7. The bone marrow should be examined for blast cells, neuroblastoma, other foreign cells and aplasia. In idiopathic thrombocytopenic purpura, the megakaryocytes are normal or increased in number; in secondary thrombocytopenic purpura, the megakaryocytes are normal, increased or absent.

ETIOLOGIC CLASSIFICATION OF HEMORRHAGE AND PURPURA

ETIOLOGIC CLASSIFICATION OF HEMORRHAGE, PURPURA OR PETECHIAE IN THE NEWBORN

63 / PSYCHOSOCIAL SYMPTOMS: GENERAL

Psychologic or biosocial symptoms may be approached by understanding the significance of the developmental and psychologic challenges that a child is attempting to master at a given age. Certain psychosocial symptoms are more commonly seen in one age period than another. Table 63–1 illustrates this developmental spectrum of problems from infancy to adolescence. Reference is made to the page on which further discussion of the problem may be found in this volume.

Green, M. (ed.): The Psychosocial Aspects of the Family: The New Pediatrics. Lexington, MA, Lexington Books, 1985.

TABLE 63–1. DEVELOPMENTAL SPECTRUM OF PSYCHOSOCIAL PROBLEMS FROM INFANCY TO ADOLESCENCE

Developmental delay (See page 442.)
Failure to thrive (See page 272.)
Feeding problems (See page 273.)
Anorexia (See page 255.)
Rumination (See page 215.)
Breath-holding spells (See page 327.)
Excessive rocking and head banging (See page 13.)
Resistance to sleep; sleep awakening (See page 319.)
Unmanageable behavior (See page 449.)
Biting, scratching or hitting the mother (See page 445.)
Temper tantrums (See page 449.)
Pica (See page 256.)
Autism (See page 312.)
Resistance to separation from the mother (See page 448.)
Problems in toilet training (See page 236.)
Constipation with withholding of stools (See page 238.)
Delayed speech (See page 57.)
Phobias (See page 450.)
Destructiveness (See page 449.)
Hyperactivity (See page 315.)
Munchausen's syndrome by proxy (See page 438.)
Night terrors and fears (See page 318.)
Nightmares (See page 318.)
Excessive shyness; elective mutism (See page 57.)
Withdrawn behavior (See page 447.)
Cruelty to animals (See page 451.)
Fire setting (See page 451.)
Nervousness (See page 315.)

Resistance to attending school; school phobia (See page 448.)
Failure to do well in school (See page 302.)
Encopresis (See page 239.)
Enuresis (See page 320.)
Excessive or public masturbation (See page 450.)
Effeminate behavior in boys (See page 297.)
Lying (See page 451.)
Stealing (See page 451.)
Excessive fighting (See page 451.)
Prolonged grief reaction (See page 443.)
Poor peer relations; lack of friends (See page 451.)
Hyperventilation syndrome (See page 362.)
Psychogenic pain disorders (abdominal pain; headaches; chest pain) (See page 250.)
Conversion symptoms (See page 451.)
Psychogenic purpura (See page 438.)
Pseudoseizures (See page 329.)
Depression (See page 445.)
Low self-esteem (See page 447.)
School underachievement (See page 302.)
Truancy (See page 449.)
Conduct disorder (See page 451.)
Running away (See page 451.)
Alcohol and drug abuse (See page 451.)
Anorexia nervosa (See page 256.)
Suicide gestures and attempts (See page 447.)
Homicide (See page 451.)
Facitious fever (See page 210.)

64 / PSYCHOSOCIAL SYMPTOMS IN INFANCY

This chapter is concerned with infants in the first year of life and with their parents, who are usually in their late adolescence or early adulthood, though often younger. The psychosocial signs, symptoms or observations listed below often are secondary to an impairment in the parent-infant interaction.

1. Failure to thrive. Whether attributable to inadequate caloric intake or to anorexia, a disturbance in the parent-infant relationship is a frequent cause of failure to thrive. Indeed, periodic determination of an infant's weight and length offers a simple screening method that can alert the physician to such difficulties.
2. Feeding problems such as anorexia and refusal of solid or unfamiliar foods (See Chapter 26.)
3. Developmental delay, especially in vocalization and gross motor development. The baby may show other evidence of environmental deprivation such as "hot cube" behavior, a reluctance to accept from the examiner one of the one-inch cubes used in infant testing.
4. Recurrent vomiting or rumination
5. Recurrent diarrhea
6. Irritability, fretful and unconsolable crying, marked reactivity
7. Listlessness, decreased motor activity, withdrawal, lethargy or apathy; sad, apprehensive expression, minimal smiling
8. Sleep disturbances
9. Unusual watchfulness, increased visual alertness with "radar-like" behavior
10. Withdrawal from or disinterest in people. Crying when approached
11. Lack of cuddling behavior
12. Poor physical care
13. Evidence of physical abuse
14. Passive behavior or rapid shifts in behavior
15. Stereotypic behavior or tonic immobility. The elbows are held in 90-degree flexion, the upper arms are abducted and the hands held near or behind the head. The lower extremities may be flexed and abducted with the legs and feet held an inch or two above the mattress for periods of time.
16. Breath-holding
17. Iron deficiency anemia
18. Mother is unable to report what has been going on
19. Infant is held stiffly and facing away from the mother
20. Separation problems (e.g., the infant clings and insists on being held all the time)
21. Excessive maternal worry about illness in the infant
22. Temper tantrums

Krieger, I., and Sargent, D. A.: A postural sign in the sensory deprivation syndrome in infants. J. Pediatr. 70:332, 1967.

Powell, G. F., and Low, S.: Behavior in nonorganic failure to thrive. J. Dev. Behav. Pediatr. 4:26, 1983.

Parenting problems often represent the current sequelae of many historically predisposing factors. These past life experiences do not always lead to problems, but they increase the odds against successful parenting. The list below includes those life events that are commonly reported by women who experience difficulties in their mothering roles.

HISTORICALLY PREDISPOSING FACTORS

1. A history of a poor relationship between the mother and her own mother or between the father and his father is a frequent antecedent to a parenting problem. Being subjected as a child to emotional deprivation, rejection, derogation, lack of affection and constant criticism appears to be a major handicap to successful mothering. The parents of physically abused children seem almost always to have had highly unsatisfactory rearing experiences themselves.

Steele, B. F., and Pollock, C. B.: A psychiatric study of parents who abuse infants and small children. In Kempe, C. H., and Helfer, R. E. (eds.): The Battered Child. Chicago, University of Chicago Press, 1974, pp. 103-147.

2. Lack of social supports from spouse, boyfriend, other relatives, friends, and neighbors and an inability to turn to others for help.
3. Long-term emotional disturbance or maladaptation, such as alcoholism, drug abuse, intellectual limitation, immaturity, psychosis or personality disorder.
4. Unresolved maternal grief, perhaps over the previous loss of an infant owing to the sudden death syndrome or the recent death of her husband or one of her parents. More unusually, the mother may be handicapped in her mothering ability because the new baby comes to represent for her an important person in her past (e.g., her own mother who died prematurely). The mother is secretly convinced that the new baby will also die prematurely.
5. Marital discord, separation or desertion during pregnancy
6. Maternal prenatal illness, especially one that may possibly be injurious to the baby or mother
7. Many pregnancies at short intervals
8. A very much unwanted pregnancy
9. Family illness, especially when the expectant mother has to provide care for the sick relative
10. A disruptive move late in pregnancy
11. A threatened miscarriage
12. A serious complication of pregnancy, including being informed of the possibility of fetal death
13. Financial worries
14. Unemployment

The current life situation of a pregnant woman or new mother greatly affects her child-rearing behavior. Such women may be vulnerable to a breakdown in their mothering capacities when overwhelmed by unexpected perinatal contingencies. The pediatrician should be especially diagnostically alert in the following contemporary situations in which mothering may be vulnerable.

PERINATAL CONTINGENCIES

1. Prematurity. The potentially deleterious effects that the birth of a premature baby may have on mother-ing arise from such considerations as a guarded prognosis, the anticipatory mourning that may occur, the sense of failure that the woman may endure, and the separation from and infrequent contact with the baby that may be experienced in some settings. Such babies also appear to be at higher risk of being physically abused than those who are full-term.
2. The birth of an infant with a congenital anomaly or birth injury. The birth of a handicapped infant may lead to parental feelings of inadequacy, distortion of child-rearing practices, lack of communication within the family, increased physical demands on the parents and social isolation. If a baby is severely retarded, the feedback and positive reinforcement that optimal parenting requires are seriously constrained. With the birth of a malformed baby, the parents' previously formed notion of what their baby would be like—the infant's anticipated identity—is either modified strikingly or lost almost completely, depending upon the character of the malformation.

Green, M.: Care of infants and children with long-term handicaps. Bull. N.Y. Acad. Med. 55:832, 1979.

3. An early critical illness or a long-term life-threatening illness is psychologically, as well as physically, dangerous. Unexpected recovery from an illness in which the mother thought the baby would die may be followed by the "vulnerable child syndrome," a constellation of symptoms that includes difficulty in separation, sleep problems, delay in the acquisition of self-help skills, the mother's inability to set limits, and maternal overconcern about the child's health. Because she is unable to tell whether the baby is well or ill, the mother may call the physician frequently about symptoms that appear to the doctor to be trivial or about signs (e.g., rapid respiration) that the physician is unable to confirm.
4. Maternal depression in the first year of life (See page 445.)
5. A difficult delivery in which a complication threatened the life of the mother or baby
6. Multiple births

7. Psychologic or physical absence of the father
8. Marital discord
9. Isolation, lack of a supportive social network and inability to mobilize social supports. Many young mothers and fathers are isolated from the support that might come from friends, neighbors, or older relatives experienced in parentcraft. Parents who abuse their children have great difficulty in turning to others for help in a crisis. They are often alienated from their parents or from community agencies.
10. Failure of the infant to meet parental expectations. The infant or young child's temperament, sex, activity, and style of responsiveness obviously have major influences on parenting. Thomas, Chess and Birch have pointed out that the infants who have the greatest susceptibility to behavioral disturbances show the following characteristics: extreme irregularity in biological functions, such as sleeping and feeding; withdrawal from new stimuli; negative mood; excessive and loud crying; and intense reactions and nonadaptability to changes in foods, routines, places and activities. Some parents who abuse their children seem to expect the child, in a kind of role reversal, to reassure and comfort the parent.
11. Financial insecurity, sudden loss of a job, unexpected expenses, and other financial crises obviously have an important impact on parenting.
12. Parents who find parenthood unrewarding may have little interest in infant and child care.
13. Illness of the mother or of a relative for whom the mother must provide care
14. Guilt about returning to work or not working
15. Mother with an external locus of control views her immediate future as unpredictable and life's contingencies as uncontrollable.

Prevention of developmental problems manifested in the first year necessitates that the clinician identify those high-risk parents who are vulnerable to the development of a parenting disability. This requires that parents be screened for these possibilities just as they are evaluated for other biologic vulnerabilities or problems. These data could facilitate diagnostic alertness on the part of the physician.

Greenspan has published a helpful screening outline of clinical landmarks for adaptive and disordered infant development for the periods from birth to three months (homeostasis); two to seven months (attachment); three to ten months (somatic-psychological differentiation); and nine to 24 months (behavioral organization, initiative, and internalization). Table 64–1, adapted from this screening outline, describes disordered maternal behaviors that suggest maladaptive patterns.

Successful intervention and secondary prevention require that the physician and other health professionals be alert to early evidence of disturbance in the infant. Such signs and symptoms in the baby may provide the only diagnostic clue since a mother will not likely spontaneously volunteer that she is depressed or that she is enduring other stressors that limit her functioning. It is not difficult to recognize parenting disturbances when one knows that the child has lived in an institution, but it may be a diagnostic challenge to be aware of the same problems when the infant lives with his own family.

Whenever possible, the father should be seen along with the mother to facilitate communication within the family. Mothers who are experiencing difficulties need to sense the physician's empathy for what they are feeling and experiencing. Expressions such as "How are *you* feeling?" or "You sound kind of tired," or "You seem a little blue" may open a channel for communication and support. Clarification and identification of the problem linked to the offer of an accepting relationship impressively facilitate successful parenting. The right word or phrase at the appropriate time may be extremely effective in early intervention.

TABLE 64–1. Maternal Behavior Associated with Mothering Disability

1. Inability to comfort infant
2. Inability to provide developmentally appropriate environmental stimuli
3. Overstimulation of baby
4. Maternal responses not contingent upon or reciprocal with infant's needs or states; misreading or missing of infant's signals
5. Care given mechanically and impersonally without positive interaction
6. Failure to look or smile at, talk to, reach out for, hug or caress infant; withdrawn or aloof maternal demeanor
7. Overly anxious or overprotective maternal behaviors
8. Mother's response limited to one modality (feeding, swinging), regardless of infant's immediate need

Once full-blown symptoms such as failure to thrive or severe sleep or discipline problems are present in the baby, one may anticipate secondary reactions in the parent such as extreme sensitivity to any implication of blame owing to feelings of inadequacy, extreme frustration, guilt, anxiety and anger. These nonverbalized feelings may masquerade as overt hostility or apparent disinterest shown by failure to visit the baby in the hospital. Such defenses need to be understood. The parents benefit not from criticism but from acceptance and support.

GENERAL REFERENCES

Green, M. (ed.): Guidelines for Health Supervision. Elk Grove Village, American Academy of Pediatrics, 1985.

Greenspan, S. J.: Psychopathology and Adaptation in Infancy and Early Childhood. Principles of Clinical Diagnosis and Preventive Intervention. New York, International Universities Press, Inc., 1981.

Greenspan, S. J.: Developmental morbidity in infants in multi–risk-factor families. Clinical perspectives. Public Health Rep. 97:16, 1982.

Greenspan, S. I., and Greenspan, N. T.: First Feelings: Milestones in the Emotional Development of the Infant and Young Child. New York, Viking Press, 1985.

65 / DEPRESSION

Depression, a common symptom, syndrome or disorder in pediatric patients and their parents, causes a variety of symptoms and signs, significant morbidity and occasional mortality. Depressive symptoms in the parent may secondarily affect the child; they may appear only in an infant, child or adolescent; or both parent and child may be depressed. When depression represents a symptom, the dysphoric mood, often related to a recent precipitating event, is usually relatively transient. Anxiety may be an accompanying affect. The depressive syndrome is more chronic and persistent. Depressive symptoms may also accompany such chronic illnesses as malignancies, inflammatory bowel disease, asthma and diabetes.

MATERNAL DEPRESSION

Depression in the mother may be suspected from symptoms and signs in the infant or child. A depressed mother generally does not initially report that she is depressed, nor does she spontaneously relate the symptoms in her child to her own affective state. ("You mean my baby knows how I feel?") That the mother's depression has only rarely been perceived by others may reflect the pioneer heritage that expects a mother to keep going as a matter of course, regardless of her condition. Unable herself to understand the reason for her incapacitating symptoms, she customarily expects or receives little understanding or help from other adults. Rather, the mother is commonly viewed as just being highly "emotional," irritable and nagging. Because of her depression, she appears to lose her *mothering presence*, that nonverbal projection of an effective mother that is somewhat analogous to *command presence*. As a result, she is unable to provide the guidance and sense of security that young children require. She may not appear to be depressed enough to require psychiatric hospitalization, but she is too ill to function effectively as a mother.

Maternal depression may begin in the postpartum period, follow the death of a significant person, accompany the mother's chronic or life-threatening illness or be reactive to marital difficulties. Since the mother tends to conceal her depression outside the house and recovers well with adults, there is no substitute for the physician's observation of the baby, as well as the mother. The infant's or young child's behavior may provide the only clue to maternal depression.

Wolkind, S.: Depression in mothers of young children. Arch. Dis. Child. 56:1, 1981.

Symptoms and signs in the child that may alert the physician to the possibility of maternal depression include

I. IN THE INFANT AND TODDLER

A. Marked lack of discipline. The child seems to dominate the household, ignores the mother's disciplinary efforts and may strike back at her. Although victimized, the mother appears powerless and afraid to deal appropriately with the child's behavior.

B. Severe temper tantrums, which occur with great frequency, often end with both the mother and child in tears.

C. Oppositional behavior is marked

D. Abusive behavior toward the mother, (e.g., scratching, slapping, pinching and kicking) is often observed or reported on specific inquiry.

E. Hyperactivity is a frequent presenting complaint.

F. Crying and harassing irritability, most marked in the presence of the mother and worse on days when the mother is most depressed, is common.

G. Difficulty in separation so that the mother is rarely, if ever, away from the child.

H. Overprotection

I. Sleep problems, especially resistance to going to sleep, are often the precipitating cause for visiting the doctor.

J. The infant demonstrates a delayed achievement of self-help skills such as feeding.

K. Rumination may occur secondary to unsatisfying maternal-infant interactions.

L. Developmental delay may be manifest by slow gross motor development.

M. Maternal overconcern about the child's health is manifest by frequent calls to the doctor or visits to the office or emergency room because of complaints that cannot be verified or that are judged to be inconsequential and to present no threat to the infant's health.

II. IN THE SCHOOL-AGED CHILD AND ADOLESCENT

A. School avoidance or resistance to going to school may be associated with maternal depression.

B. Chronic depression in an adolescent may be accompanied by chronic or recurrent depression in one of the parents.

C. Hyperactivity may be secondary to depression in the mother.

DEPRESSION IN INFANTS, CHILDREN AND ADOLESCENTS

A child or adolescent generally does not think of his or her problem as representing depression or spontaneously report a depressed mood. Similarly, parents usually do not associate the presenting complaint with childhood depression. Consequently, the doctor must suspect this possibility largely on the basis of the patient's appearance, affect, symptoms and the history. Parents often find it difficult to accept that depression causes fatigue, hyperactivity and headache. ("How can you tell since you haven't done any tests?") In eliciting the history from the child or adolescent, a thoughtful, gently stated observation by the physician such as, "I would guess that things aren't going so well for you," will often evoke an acknowledging glance or other nonverbal affirmation. The physician can then say, "Tell me about it." Other questions that may be posed are: "What kind of things make you sad?" "What do you worry about?" "How do you feel about yourself?" "Do you tend to blame yourself . . . feel guilty?" "What do you do for fun?" If the child denies depression, the doctor, with a nod to convey his awareness of the child's hesitancy to talk about such upsetting feelings, may simply say, "Well, O.K. . . . I just thought that maybe you were kind of down. We can talk about it some other time." This statement conveys the doctor's understanding and his availability to help when the child is ready to discuss his or her unhappiness more openly.

The patient's facial expression, especially if he or she is unaware of being observed, may be highly suggestive. Other clues include somber dress, flat affect, slow speech, gaze avoidance, and a mendicant posture. While the child may sit erect at the onset of the interview, as time goes on, he slowly leans forward with his head down. The patient may become tearful if the physician touches upon a significant subject, situation or person.

Experiences and contingencies that may make children vulnerable to an acute depressive reaction are listed below. Generally, the depressive reaction in these instances is transient but, in some cases, it may be persistent.

I. SEPARATION EXPERIENCES, especially clusters of losses

A. Death of a loved relative, friend or pet

B. Serious illness in a relative

C. Recent move of the family or of an especially close friend

D. Onset in the child of a chronic illness or handicap with loss of normal health and change in the child's self-image

E. Rejection (e.g., a unilateral termination

of a close boy-girl relationship or failure to achieve admission to a desired college or career track)

F. Parental separation, desertion or divorce

II. STRESSORS, especially clusters of stressors

A. Entrance to a new school (e.g., a large, consolidated middle or junior high school)
B. The first year in college, especially when the adolescent is a long distance from home and without close friends
C. School learning problems
D. Mothers and fathers with whom the child has relatively little physical contact or close relationship because of the parents' work or social schedules
E. Lack of friends
F. A generally unhappy life with few or no experiences of joy or success
G. Inability of a child to maintain a high level of achievement or accomplishment
H. Severe acne
I. Obesity
J. Infectious mononucleosis and other viral syndromes may be followed by continuing depressive symptoms.
K. Post-traumatic syndrome following a head injury may be accompanied by depressive symptoms.
L. Remarriage of a parent to a spouse whom the child does not like or with whom the child is uncomfortable
M. Birth of a sibling with a handicap or the onset of a chronic or life-threatening illness in a sibling
N. Unwanted pregnancy
O. Sexual abuse

III. DEPRESSION IN A PARENT

Although children and adolescents who are acutely depressed usually have a history of previous emotional health, some have a long record of poor adjustment. Persistent symptoms raise the possibility of a depressive syndrome or a bipolar affective disorder. Often one of the parents is also chronically or recurrently depressed.

The symptoms of a depressive reaction are developmentally determined. In infants, symptoms may include apathy, withdrawn behavior, irritability, lethargy, decreased responsiveness, regression, developmental delay or rumination and failure to thrive. The preschool depressed child may demonstrate marked separation anxiety, hyperactivity, oppositional behavior, withdrawal, irritability, crying, temper tantrums and regression in developmental achievements such as speech and toilet training.

In the school-age child and adolescent, the symptoms include a dysphoric mood of sadness or ill-being, anhedonia or inability to have fun, social withdrawal with loss of interest or pleasure in usual activities, loneliness, loss of energy, apathy, indifference, chronic fatigue, increased or decreased appetite and weight, insomnia or hypersomnia, self-deprecatory feelings of worthlessness, self-reproach, excessive or inappropriate guilt, diminished ability to concentrate, self-recrimination, pessimism, impairment of school or work performance, suicidal thoughts, recurrent thoughts of dying, a feeling of abandonment, episodes of crying, irritability, hyperactivity, excessive anger, somatic complaints (e.g., persistent headache, chest pain, chronic fatigue), conduct disorder, truancy, resistance to attending school, running away, promiscuity and substance abuse.

SUICIDE RISKS AND ATTEMPTS

In the presence of depression, the physician needs to determine whether the child is at risk of suicide. High risk situations are those in which the child feels helpless, hopeless and trapped in an intolerable situation from which he sees no way of extrication; has thought out in detail how he would commit suicide; seems extremely guilty; and has not considered the devastating impact of the suicide on his family. The management of children at risk of suicide or those who make actual suicide attempts is optimally a joint pediatric–child psychiatric endeavor.

Early recognition and intervention in the case of a child at risk of suicide are enhanced if the physician has seen the child or adolescent regularly and has established the kind of relationship that permits the doctor to be psychologically accessible to the patient. The physician needs also to be alert to the adolescent who is at special risk of suicide. Such vulnerability is associated with loss of a parent or close friend, alcohol or drug abuse, presence of a major psychiatric illness, loss of family or other close relationships, recent onset of depressive behaviors, family history of suicide, previous suicide attempts, unwanted pregnancy, school failure, arrest and incarceration.

GENERAL REFERENCES

Cytryn, L., and McKnew, D. H.: Proposed classification of childhood depression. Am. J. Orthopsychiatry 129:149, 1972.

Eisenberg, L.: Adolescent suicide: On taking arms against a sea of troubles. Pediatrics 60:315, 1980.

Friedman, S. B., and Sarles, R. M.: "Out of control" behavior in adolescents. Pediatr. Clin. North Am. 27:97, 1980.

Malmquist, C. P.: Depression in childhood and adolescence. N. Engl. J. Med. 284:887, 155, 1971.

Marks, A.: Management of the suicidal adolescent on a nonpsychiatric adolescent unit. J. Pediatr. 95:305, 1979.

Poznanski, E. O., Cook, S. C., and Carroll, B. J. A.: Depression rating scale for children. Pediatrics 64:442, 1979.

Schowalter, J. E.: Depression in children and adolescents. Pediatr. Rev. 3:51, 1981.

66 / SCHOOL REFUSAL (AVOIDANCE)

School refusal, at times inappropriately referred to as school phobia, requires prompt intervention. In this disorder, the child refuses to attend school or to go outside during school hours. Although a child or adolescent may be brought to the doctor with the chief complaint of refusal to attend school, more commonly a somatic symptom is given as the reason for the visit.

School avoidance may be accompanied by vomiting, abdominal pain or pallor that quickly abates once the child is told he will not have to attend school. When persistent or recurrent symptoms such as fever, sore throat, fatigue, abdominal pain or dizziness constitute the chief complaint, school absence is usually not mentioned by the parents as a problem. In such instances, it is diagnostically helpful for the physician to ask how much school the illness has caused the child to miss.

Separation anxiety is the most common cause of school refusal. Many five- and six-year-old children show a transient reluctance to separate from their mothers to attend school during the first few months of the first school year. These children rarely have physical symptoms and are relatively easy to manage with parental firmness and the understanding support of their teachers. However, other children with persistent school refusal have a developmentally inappropriate level of dependency. They worry that something devastating will happen to their mother or that she will leave home while they are at school. The mother herself may find it difficult to tolerate separation

from her child. Fully illuminating these irrational fears in the interview can be helpful. For example, "Tell me what you are afraid will happen? What else? And . . . ?" The child may quietly report that he is afraid of a teacher who seems irritable and has scolded other children or of classmates who push other children around. Generally, however, such school-based fears do not account for school refusal. This is not to deny that a frightening experience going to and from school or while at school may have been the precipitating cause of the problem.

School avoidance may also be a late manifestation of the vulnerable child syndrome in which the child and the mother share an unspoken agreement that the child is safe only in the presence of the mother. Reluctance to attend school may also occur in children with chronic illness owing to feelings of anxiety or vulnerability, concern about their appearance (alopecia, cushingoid facies, understature), and inability to keep up with the academic pace because of frequent absences owing to recurrent hospitalization or visits to the doctor.

Environmental stressors that may contribute to school refusal include the birth of a sibling, physical or mental illness of a parent or sibling, death of a significant person, separation or divorce, parental alcoholism, a move that requires transfer to a new school, entrance to a middle or junior high school, harassment on the way to school and the lack of privacy when undressing or showering for physical education classes. In addition, depressed mothers, especially if they have thought of suicide, may feel safer when someone is with them at home.

An occasional older child who has missed school because of an acute illness may find it difficult to resume a previous pattern of overachievement. Depression and incipient psychosis are other diagnostic considerations in the older child or adolescent with school refusal. Truancy differs from school refusal in a number of ways. The parents are usually unaware of or indifferent to the child's school absence. Although the child ostensibly leaves for school, he neither arrives there nor returns home during school hours. Truants have usually been poor students with a history of disciplinary and learning problems at school. Many are in-

volved in antisocial and delinquent behavior symptomatic of a rebellion against authority. Some may be chronically depressed. Others come from multi-problem families. In contrast, children with school refusal generally are excellent students who enjoy school but are afraid to leave home.

GENERAL REFERENCES

Nader, P. R., Bullock, D., and Caldwell, B.: School phobia. Pediatr. Clin. North Am. 22:605, 1975.

Schmitt, B. D.: School phobia—the great imitator: A pediatrician's viewpoint. Pediatrics 48:433, 1971.

Weitzman, M., Klerman, L. V., Lamb, G., Menary, J., and Alpert, J. J.: School absence: A problem for the pediatrician. Pediatrics 69:739, 1982.

67 / OUT-OF-CONTROL TODDLER BEHAVIOR

The physician is occasionally consulted about a toddler who is described by his parents as "out-of-control" (e.g., disobedient, stubborn, intrusive, resistant or hyperactive). In addition to temper tantrums, the child is reported to cry, scream, fight, swear, bite, hit, disturb and destroy. Sleeping, eating and bowel training problems may be prominent.

ETIOLOGIC CONSIDERATIONS

Inexperienced parents unfamiliar with young children may misinterpret and poorly tolerate normal oppositional or autonomous behavior. Those who are insecure in their parental roles may be ambivalent about or reluctant to set limits because of an uneasy apprehension that firmness may harm their child emotionally. If the parent had been harshly reared as a child, she may try to compensate by being overly permissive and overindulgent. Parents of children who are chronically ill or handicapped often find it difficult to set limits. Mothers who are depressed, grieving, have low self-esteem or worry about their child dying (vulnerable

child syndrome) have inadequate parenting *presence* or authority. A grandmother living in the household may dilute a mother's leadership. Working mothers, especially single parents, may be too exhausted at the end of the day to be effective. Disagreement between parents may result in inconsistent expectations. Divorce, illness or other family crisis may lead to a moratorium for parenting. Some children evoke negative parental feelings and expectations because they consciously or unconsciously remind their parents of themselves or some other relative. Other toddlers may be used as scapegoats for family problems.

Neurologic impairment or the attention deficit syndrome with hyperactivity may also account for "out-of-control" behavior. Some toddlers have been unsupervised, unsocialized, emotionally deprived and insecure owing to family discord, placement in a succession of foster homes or frequent moves. Some children are temperamentally more difficult to rear than others, especially those who are extremely irregular in sleeping and feeding, withdraw from new stimuli, cry frantically and respond highly negatively to changes in foods, routines, places and activities. Unrecognized giftedness in a young child may so tax the parents' patience that they regard him as "out-of-control."

The toddler's environment may be disorganized, chaotic, crowded, overstimulating or depriving, with frequent exposure to parental fights, alcoholism, violence, sexual activity, hunger and cold. Children who live in mobile homes or small apartments often have little opportunity for appropriate motor activity, especially in cold or rainy weather.

The management of the toddler with "out-of-control" behavior depends upon the number and duration of complaints, the cause, and whether the problem is pervasive or limited to interactions with only one parent. The physician's skill and time, the severity of the symptoms, the number of other problems in the family, the marriage's status, the parents' level of understanding and their ability to follow advice determine whether the problem is to be managed by the physician alone, by collaboration with other professionals or by referral.

The first step is to define the problem, clarify the etiology, observe the child and family interactions and perform a physical and developmental assessment. Problems primarily caused by a misunderstanding of stage-related behavior may respond readily to advice, explanation, reeducation, and support. Behavior that is reactive to specific environmental circumstances, places, persons, objects, or activities may be prevented by minimizing exposure to such provocative stimuli. Schedules and routines for sleeping and eating may help structure the child's environment. Proximal physical presence may be advised so that the parent is immediately available to distract the child or interrupt the process.

GENERAL REFERENCES

Chamberlin, R. W.: Management of preschool behavior problems. Pediatr. Clin. North Am. 21:33, 1974.
Drabman, R. S., and Jarvie, G.: Counseling parents of children with behavior problems: The use of extinction and time out techniques. Pediatrics 59:78, 1977.
Smith, E. E., and VanTassel, E.: Problems of discipline in early childhood. Pediatr. Clin. North Am. 29:167, 1982.

68 / OTHER BEHAVIORAL COMPLAINTS

CHANGES IN PERSONALITY

Changes in personality or behavior may be reported in children in the presence of a brain tumor; degenerative, post-traumatic or postinfectious central nervous disease; Sydenham's chorea; Wilson's disease; depression; hyperthyroidism; substance abuse; sexual abuse; an overwhelming psychologic stressor; or schizophrenia.

PANIC ATTACKS

Panic attacks are characterized by apprehension, fear, hyperventilation, feelings of unreality, hot and cold flashes, trembling and fear of dying or "going crazy." A familial predisposition may be present.

VanWinter, J. T., and Stickler, G. B.: Panic attack syndrome. J. Pediatr. 105:661, 1984.

PHOBIAS

Simple phobias in children are not infrequent. They occur as a persistent, involuntary and irrational fear and attempt to avoid a specific object, activity or situation. A phobia of animals, especially dogs; the dark, thunder; elevators; or school may be transiently present in young children. Persistent phobias are rare in the pediatric population.

DuPont, R. L.: Phobias in children. J. Pediatr. 102:999, 1983.

PUBLIC OR COMPULSIVE MASTURBATION

Excessive, public or compulsive masturbation may be caused by a number of etiologic factors, including anxiety; the birth of a sibling; a disturbed mother-child relationship with lack of parental affection; sexual molestation and abuse; exposure to adult sexual behavior; depression; lack of interaction with peers; retardation; prolonged absence of a parent; or parental loss by divorce or death.

McCray, G. M.: Excessive masturbation of childhood: A symptom of tactile deprivation. Pediatrics 62:277, 1978.

LYING AND STEALING

Although these symptoms may occasionally occur as transient problems in normal children, a careful psychosocial assessment is indicated when they have become sufficiently troublesome or persistent to concern the parents or others. The seriousness of the behavior depends upon the child's age, whether the child knows the difference between right and wrong, whether the behavior is evident only at home or elsewhere as well, whether the child can control this behavior, and the presence of additional behavioral complaints or characteristics of a conduct disorder.

CONDUCT DISORDERS

Children or adolescents with conduct disorders may demonstrate a number of behavioral characteristics such as manipulativeness, lack of concern for others, poor peer relations, absence of guilt or remorse, physical violence, theft, stealing, homicide, truancy, substance abuse, running away, lying, vandalism, fire setting, cruelty to animals, precocious sexual activity and chronic violation of rules at home or school. Comprehensive psychologic evaluation is required in these instances.

PSYCHOTIC BEHAVIOR

Signs and symptoms of psychotic behavior, which may occur in pervasive developmental or schizophrenic disorders, include bizarre and unpredictable social behavior, inappropriate mood and affect, decreased impulse control, withdrawal, delusions, hallucinations, disturbed forms of thinking, inappropriate or flat affect, loose associations and strange mannerisms.

69 / CONVERSION SYMPTOMS

Conversion symptoms include paralysis or weakness of an extremity, blindness, blurring of vision, deafness, aphonia, whispering, anesthesia or paresthesia, abnormal gait, tics, pain (abdominal, chest or musculoskeletal), headache, urinary retention, fatigue, hyperventilation, anorexia, dysphagia, convulsions, syncope, vertigo, nausea and vomiting. The symptom chosen may be unconsciously modeled after that in a relative or other significant person, current or in the past; or it may be one that the child has previously experienced. Often a precipitating emotional stress (e.g., sexual abuse, a family crisis, marital discord, critical school examinations, an illness, physical trauma, surgery or other major life change) can be identified in the history. The onset may be either acute or insidious and the symptoms persistent, intermittent or shifting.

DIAGNOSIS

Diagnosis requires the simultaneous exclusion of an organic etiology and the identification of those psychologic findings consistent with a conversion reaction. In many instances, the symptom is clearly inconsistent with an organic disorder, and the criteria for a conversion reaction are readily evident; in other cases, the differentiation may be very difficult, especially as the symptomatology of either etiology may be almost identical. Organic and psychologic disease may co-exist, and the early manifestations of some serious organic disorders (e.g., dystonia musculorum deformans, degenerative central nervous system disease, brain tumor or osteoid osteoma) may be misinterpreted.

Conversion reactions most commonly occur in school aged children and adolescents and are unlikely in children under five years of age. The psychologic attitude of *la belle indifference*, or a seeming lack of concern, is not a reliable diagnostic feature.

The prognosis is best when the onset is acute; when an identified precipitating stressful experience can be clearly identified; when the child has been previously emotionally healthy; and when the family is developmentally or psychologically minded so as to be able to accept a psychologic etiology. The diagnosis and treatment of conversion symptoms is best done on an ambulatory basis, since hospitalization tends to fix the symptom. In the interview, an effort should be made to identify possible precipitating emotional stresses. Unnecessary diagnostic procedures are to be avoided. Since the conversion mechanism is an unconscious one, the parents and child usually do not spontaneously associate the emotional stressor with the symptom. Indeed, the occurrence of such a stressor may be denied.

Mass or epidemic hysteria is characterized by the contagious appearance in a group, most commonly of school-age or adolescent girls, of symptoms such as syncope, nausea, abdominal pain, hyperventilation, dizziness, headache, weakness and tingling sensations.

Moffatt, M. E. K.: Epidemic hysteria in a Montreal train station. Pediatrics 70:308, 1982.

GENERAL REFERENCE

Lazare, A.: Conversion symptoms. N. Engl. J. Med. 305:745, 1981.

Appendix

CHARTS OF GROWTH STATISTICS ON BOYS AND GIRLS FROM BIRTH TO 18 YEARS*

*Courtesy of the National Center for Health Statistics, U.S. Government Department of Health, Education and Welfare, 1978.

BOYS FROM BIRTH TO 36 MONTHS

WEIGHT FOR AGE

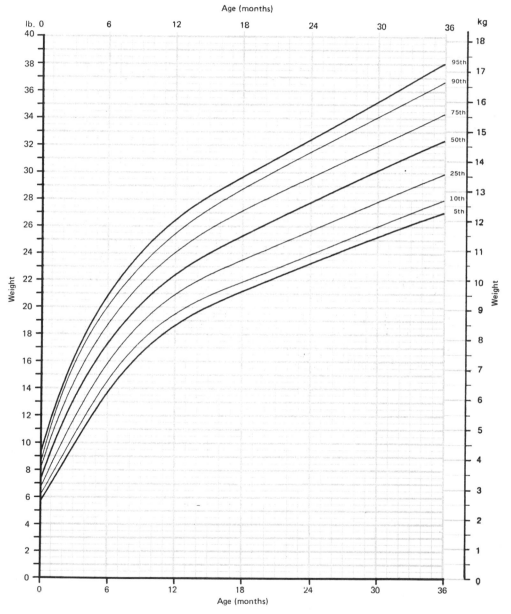

BOYS FROM BIRTH TO 36 MONTHS

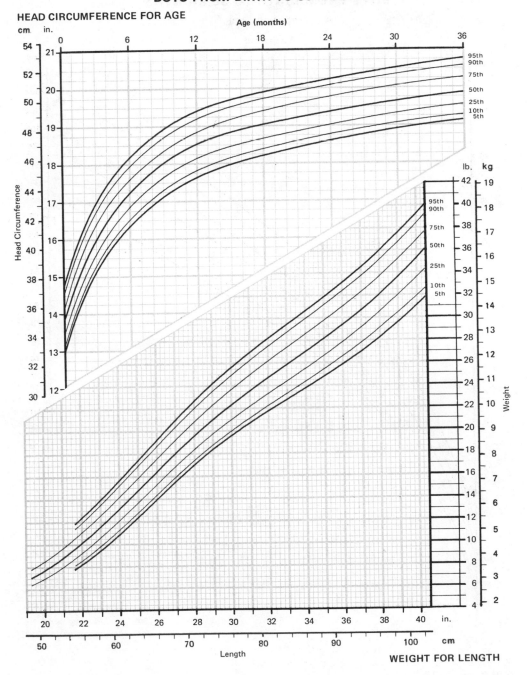

HEAD CIRCUMFERENCE FOR AGE

WEIGHT FOR LENGTH

BOYS FROM BIRTH TO 36 MONTHS

LENGTH FOR AGE

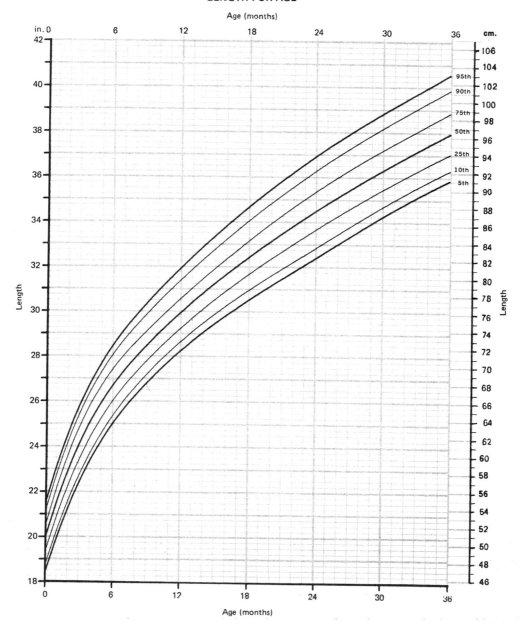

BOYS FROM 2 TO 18 YEARS

WEIGHT FOR AGE

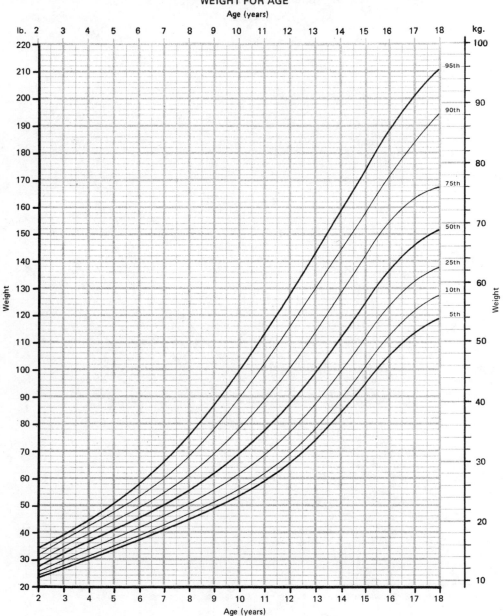

PRE-PUBERTAL BOYS FROM 2 TO 11½ YEARS

WEIGHT FOR STATURE

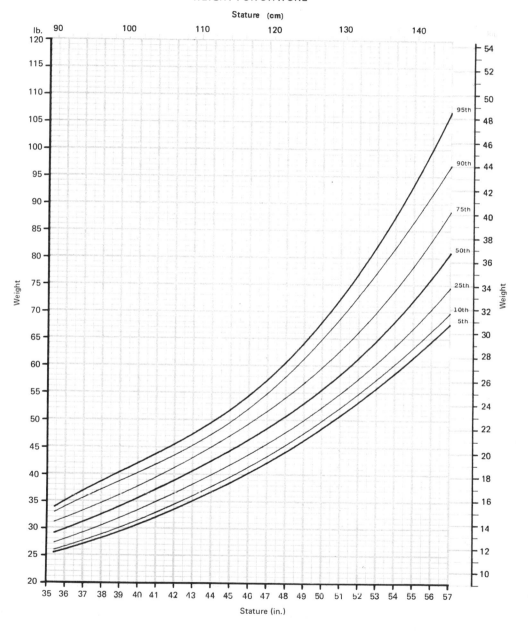

BOYS FROM 2 TO 18 YEARS

STATURE FOR AGE

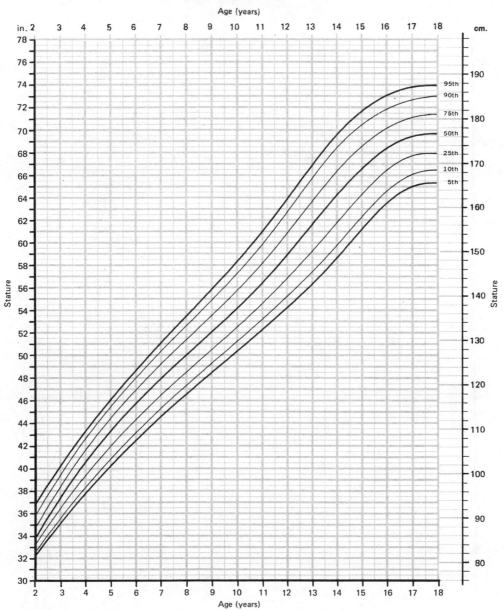

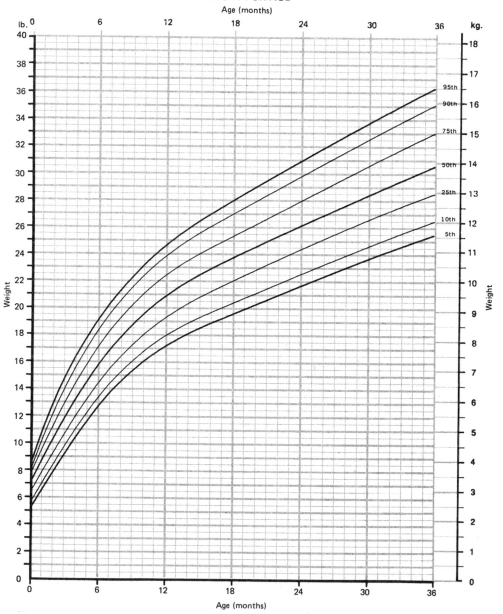

GIRLS FROM BIRTH TO 36 MONTHS

WEIGHT FOR AGE

GIRLS FROM BIRTH TO 36 MONTHS

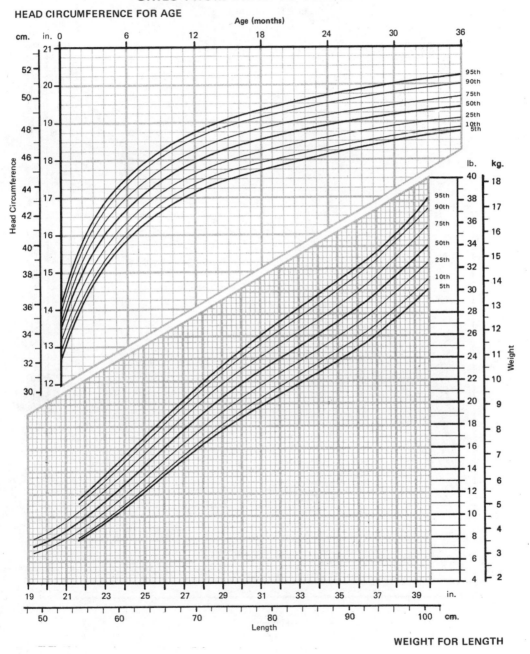

HEAD CIRCUMFERENCE FOR AGE

WEIGHT FOR LENGTH

GIRLS FROM BIRTH TO 36 MONTHS

LENGTH FOR AGE

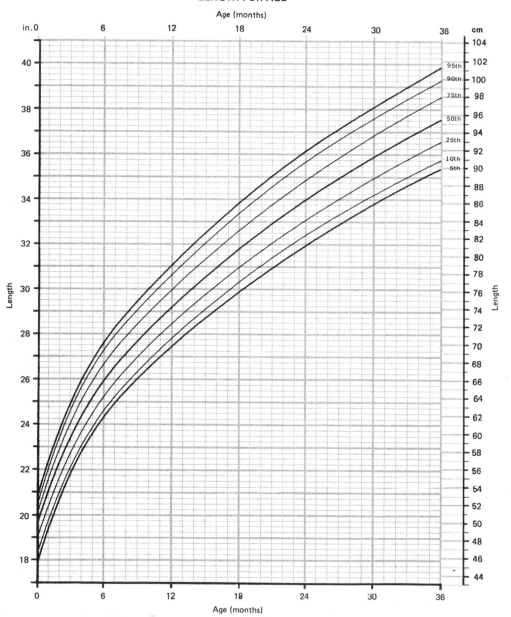

GIRLS FROM 2 TO 18 YEARS
WEIGHT FOR AGE

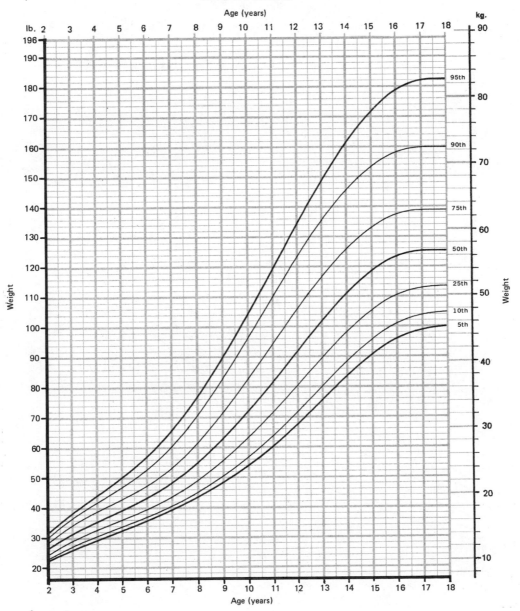

PRE-PUBERTAL GIRLS FROM 2 TO 10 YEARS

WEIGHT FOR STATURE

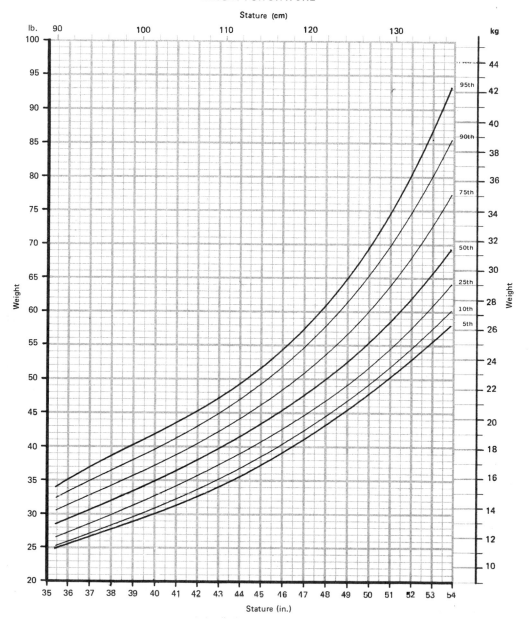

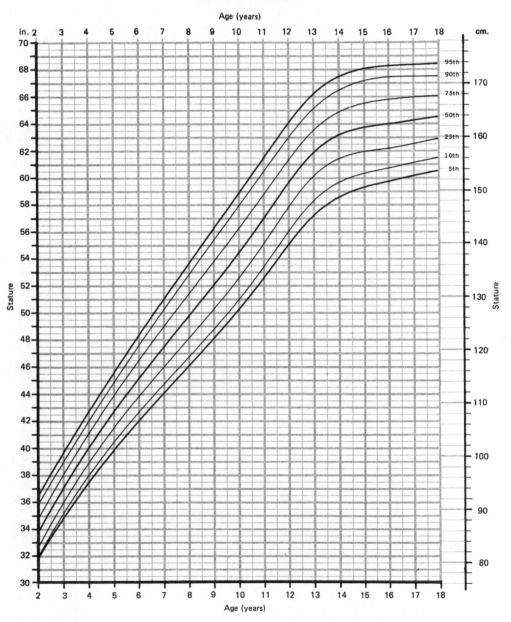

GIRLS FROM 2 TO 18 YEARS
STATURE FOR AGE

INDEX

Italic numbers refer to illustrations; (t) indicates tables.

Burns, 187
electrical, of mouth, 187
encephalopathy in, delirium due to, 335
in child abuse, 187
Byler's disease, 268-269

Café au lait spots, 161
Caffey's syndrome, 132
Calcification, subcutaneous, 159
Calluses, 138
Campodactyly, 134
Canal of Nuck, hydrocele of, 88
Canavan's disease, 9, 312
Candida, in vaginitis, 100
Candida albicans, as cause of thrush, 50
Candidiasis, cutaneous, congenital, 159
Canicola fever, jaundice due to, 265-266
Canker sores, 50
Capillaries, fragility of, in hemorrhage, 433-434
increased permeability of, in edema, 406
pulsation of, 173
Caput succedaneum, 14
Carbohydrate malabsorption, diarrhea due to, 229
Carbon monoxide poisoning, cyanosis due to, 384
lips in, 49
Carcinoma, nevoid basal cell, 180
Cardiac disease. See also Heart, disease of.
failure to thrive due to, 274
gallop rhythm in, 76
Cardiac failure. See Heart failure.
Cardiac murmurs. See under Murmur(s).
Cardiac tamponade, pulsus paradoxus with, 74
Cardiomegaly, 74
apex beat in, 72
Cardiospasm, 242
Cardiovascular hypertension, 82
Carditis, 74
rheumatic, 78
Caries, nursing bottle, 55
Carnosinemia, 310
Caroli disease, 268
Carotenemia, 161
Carotenoderma, 161
Carotid artery, unusual pulsation of, 64
Carotid bruit, 78
Carpenter's syndrome, 12
Carpopedal spasm, 118
Cartilage, discoid lateral, 148
Cartilage-hair hypoplasia, neutropenia due to, 393
syndrome, 15
Cartilaginous tags, of neck, 62
Cataplexy, 317
Cataracts, 28
congenital, 28
Catheterization, cardiac, fever due to, 210
"Cat's eye" pupillary reflex, 27
"Cat's eye" syndrome, 29, 104
Cat-scratch disease, adenopathy due to, 400
conjunctiva in, 25
Cat-scratch fever, 207
Cattel scale, for mental retardation, 305
Caudal regression syndrome, 129, 152
Cebocephaly, 23
Celiac syndrome, diarrhea due to, 227-228
failure to thrive due to, 273-274
understature due to, 282
vomiting due to, 219

Cellular immunity, impaired, frequent infections due to, 395-396
Cellulitis, facial, 159
mandibular, 159
orbital, 21
perianal, 105
Central nervous system, degenerative disorders of, irritability in, 351
disturbances of, coma due to, 335
fever due to, 205
obesity due to, 300
infection of, coma due to, 337
fever due to, 205
seizures due to, 326
lesions of, male isosexual precocity due to, 290
sexual precocity due to, 292
leukemia, headache due to, 348
spongy degeneration of, 9
Cephalohematoma, 14
Cerebellar ataxia, 120
Cerebellum. See also Brain.
tumors of, of hemispheres, 126
of posterior midline, 126
Cerebral dysgenesis, 9-10
Cerebral gigantism, 286-287
Cerebral hypertension, 82
Cerebral palsy, 111
atonic, 112
hemiparetic, hands in, 133-134
mental retardation due to, 311
poor head control in, 6
tremor in, 117
Cerebro-costo-mandibular syndrome, 59, 68
respiratory distress due to, 356
Cerebrohepatorenal syndrome, 312
Cerebrospinal fluid, decreased absorption of, 8
increased production of, 8
Cerebrum. See also Brain.
concussion, coma due to, 336
edema in, vomiting due to, 221
hemorrhage in, coma due to, 336
thrombosis of, coma due to, 337
vascular occlusion in, coma due to, 337
Ceroid lipofuscinosis, 309
Cerumen, cough due to, 381
removal of, 41
Cervical adenopathy, 61
Cervical aortic arch, 64
Cervical masses, 61-62
Chaddock's sign, 116
Charcot-Marie-Tooth disease, 124
Chédiak-Higashi syndrome, 36
Cheilitis, 49
Cherry red spot, 31
Cherry red spot myoclonus syndrome, 308-309
Cherubism, 60
Chest, 65-72
pain in, 390-391
due to heart disorders, 390
due to rib fracture, 391
etiologic classification of, 390-391
psychogenic, 391
structural anomalies of, 67
"Chest syndrome," respiratory distress due to, 360
Chewing, 255
Chiari's syndrome, abdominal pain due to, 247
Chickenpox, 185-186
and mouth, 51
Children. See also Infant(s) and Newborn.